Clinical Trials in Neurology

Design, Conduct, Analysis

Clinical Trials in Neurology

Design, Conduct, Analysis

Edited by

Bernard Ravina, MD, MS
Medical Director, Translational Neurology, Biogen Idec, Cambridge, MA, USA

Jeffrey Cummings, MD
Director, Cleveland Clinic Lou Ruvo Center for Brain Health in Nevada, Ohio, and Florida, USA

Michael P. McDermott, PhD
Professor of Biostatistics, and Professor of Neurology,
University of Rochester School of Medicine, Rochester, NY, USA

R. Michael Poole, MD, FACP
Head, CNS and Pain Innovative Medicine Unit, AstraZeneca PLC, Waltham, MA, USA

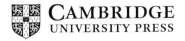

CAMBRIDGE
UNIVERSITY PRESS

CAMBRIDGE UNIVERSITY PRESS
Cambridge, New York, Melbourne, Madrid, Cape Town,
Singapore, São Paulo, Delhi, Mexico City

Cambridge University Press
The Edinburgh Building, Cambridge CB2 8RU, UK

Published in the United States of America by Cambridge University Press, New York

www.cambridge.org
Information on this title: www.cambridge.org/9780521762595

First published 2012

Printed in the United Kingdom at the University Press, Cambridge

A catalogue record for this publication is available from the British Library

Library of Congress Cataloguing in Publication data
Clinical trials in neurology : design, conduct, analysis / edited by Bernard Ravina ... [et al.].
    p.   cm.
  Includes bibliographical references and index.
  ISBN 978-0-521-76259-5 (hardback)
  1. Neurology – Research – Methodology.   2. Clinical trials.   I. Ravina, Bernard.
  RC337.C62   2012
  616.80072′4–dc23   2012000303

ISBN 978-0-521-76259-5 Hardback

To J, Gers, Double Reh, and Bewds

Contents

List of contributors   ix
Preface   xiii
Acknowledgements   xv

Section 1. The role of clinical trials in therapy development

1 **The impact of clinical trials in neurology**   1
E. Ray Dorsey and S. Claiborne Johnston

2 **The sequence of clinical development**   8
R. Michael Poole

3 **Unique challenges in the development of therapies for neurological disorders**   19
Gilmore N. O'Neill

Section 2. Concepts in biostatistics and clinical measurement

4 **Fundamentals of biostatistics**   28
Judith Bebchuk and Janet Wittes

5 **Bias and random error**   42
Susan S. Ellenberg and Jacqueline A. French

6 **Approaches to data analysis**   52
William R. Clarke

7 **Selecting outcome measures**   69
Robert G. Holloway and Andrew D. Siderowf

Section 3. Special study designs and methods for data monitoring

8 **Selection and futility designs**   78
Bruce Levin

9 **Adaptive design across stages of therapeutic development**   91
Christopher S. Coffey

10 **Crossover designs**   101
Mary E. Putt

11 **Two-period designs for evaluation of disease-modifying treatments**   113
Michael P. McDermott

12 **Enrichment designs**   127
Kathryn M. Kellogg and John Markman

13 **Non-inferiority trials**   135
Rick Chappell

14 **Monitoring of clinical trials: Interim monitoring, data monitoring committees, and group sequential methods**   147
Rickey E. Carter and Robert F. Woolson

15 **Clinical approaches to post-marketing drug safety assessment**   160
Gerald J. Dal Pan

Section 4. Ethical issues

16 **Ethics in clinical trials involving the central nervous system: Risk, benefit, justice, and integrity**   173
Jonathan Kimmelman

17 **The informed consent process: Compliance and beyond**   187
Scott Y. H. Kim

Section 5. Regulatory perspectives

18 **Evidentiary standards for neurological drugs and biologics approval**   197
Russell Katz

19 **Premarket review of neurological devices**   206
Eric A. Mann and Peter G. Como

Section 6. Clinical trials in common neurological disorders

20 **Parkinson's disease**   215
Karl Kieburtz and Jordan Elm

21 **Alzheimer's disease**   227
Joshua D. Grill and Jeffrey Cummings

22 **Acute ischemic stroke** 242
Devin L. Brown, Karen C. Johnston, and
Yuko Y. Palesch

23 **Multiple sclerosis** 257
Richard A. Rudick, Elizabeth Fisher, and
Gary R. Cutter

24 **Amyotrophic lateral sclerosis** 273
Nazem Atassi, David Schoenfeld, and
Merit Cudkowicz

25 **Epilepsy** 284
John R. Pollard, Susan S. Ellenberg, and
Jacqueline A. French

26 **Insomnia** 295
Michael E. Yurcheshen, Changyong Feng, and
J. Todd Arnedt

Section 7. Clinical trial planning and implementation

27 **Clinical trial planning: An academic and industry perspective** 309
Cornelia L. Kamp and Jean-Michel Germain

28 **Clinical trial implementation, analysis, and reporting: An academic and industry perspective** 338
Cornelia L. Kamp and Jean-Michel Germain

29 **Academic-industry collaborations and compliance issues** 352
D. Troy Morgan

Index 362

Contributors

J. Todd Arnedt, PhD
Assistant Professor, Departments of Psychiatry and Neurology; Director, Behavioral Sleep Medicine Program, University of Michigan Health System, Ann Arbor, MI, USA

Nazem Atassi, MD, MMSc
Instructor in Neurology, Harvard Medical School and Massachusetts General Hospital, Boston, MA, USA

Judith Bebchuk, ScD
Statistical Scientist, Statistics Collaborative Inc., Washington, DC, USA

Devin L. Brown, MD, MS
Associate Professor, Department of Neurology, University of Michigan Health System, Ann Arbor, MI, USA

Rickey E. Carter, PhD
Associate Professor of Biostatistics, Department of Health Sciences Research, Mayo Clinic, Rochester, MN, USA

Rick Chappell, PhD
Professor, Department of Biostatistics and Medical Informatics, University of Wisconsin School of Medicine and Public Health, Madison, WI, USA

William R. Clarke, PhD
Professor of Biostatistics, The University of Iowa, Iowa City, IA, USA

Christopher S. Coffey, PhD
Professor, Department of Biostatistics; Director, Clinical Trials Statistical and Data Management Center, The University of Iowa, Iowa City, IA, USA

Peter G. Como, PhD
Lead Reviewer /Neuropsychologist, Center for Devices and Radiological Health, Division of Opthalmic Neurological and ENT Devices, US Food and Drug Administration, Silver Spring, MD, USA

Merit Cudkowicz, MD, MMSc
Professor of Neurology, Harvard Medical School and Massachusetts General Hospital, Boston, MA, USA

Jeffrey Cummings, MD
Director, Cleveland Clinic Lou Ruvo Center for Brain Health in Nevada, Ohio and Florida, USA.

Gary R. Cutter, PhD
Department of Biostatistics, University of Alabama at Birmingham, Birmingham, AL, USA

Gerald J. Dal Pan, MD, MHS
Director, Office of Surveillance and Epidemiology, Center for Drug Evaluation and Research, US Food and Drug Administration, Silver Spring, MD, USA

E. Ray Dorsey, MD, MBA
Associate Professor of Neurology, Johns Hopkins University School of Medicine, Baltimore, MD, USA

Susan S. Ellenberg, PhD
Professor of Biostatistics, Center for Clinical Epidemiology and Biostatistics, Perelman School of Medicine at the University of Pennsylvania, Philadelphia, PA, USA

Jordan Elm, PhD
Research Assistant Professor, Department of Biostatistics, Medical University of South Carolina, Charleston, SC, USA

Changyong Feng, PhD
Assistant Professor of Biostatistics, Department of Biostatistics and Computational Biology, University of Rochester School of Medicine, Rochester, NY, USA

Elizabeth Fisher, PhD
Department of Biomedical Engineering, Lerner Research Institute, Cleveland Clinic, Cleveland, OH, USA

Jacqueline A. French, MD
Director, Epilepsy Study Consortium, Department of Neurology, NYU Langone Medical Center, New York, NY, USA

Jean-Michel Germain, PhD
Global Trial Director, Wyeth Pharmaceuticals France, a Division of Pfizer Inc., Collegeville, PA, USA

Joshua D. Grill, PhD
Mary S. Easton Center for Alzheimer's Disease Research; Katherine and Benjamin Kagan Alzheimer's Disease Treatment Development Program, Department of Neurology, David Geffen School of Medicine, University of California Los Angeles, Los Angeles, CA, USA

Robert G. Holloway, MD, MPH
Professor of Neurology and Community and Preventive Medicine, University of Rochester Medical Center, Rochester, NY, USA

Karen C. Johnston, MD, MSc
Harrison Distinguished Professor and Chair, Department of Neurology, University of Virginia, Charlottesville, VA, USA

S. Claiborne Johnston, MD, PhD
Professor of Neurology and Epidemiology, University of California San Francisco, San Francisco, CA, USA

Cornelia L. Kamp, MBA
Department of Neurology, University of Rochester Medical Center, Rochester, NY, USA

Russell Katz, MD
Director, Division of Neurology Products, US Food and Drug Administration, Silver Spring, MD, USA

Kathryn M. Kellogg, MPH, BA
Research Fellow, Department of Emergency Medicine, University of Rochester School of Medicine, Rochester, NY, USA

Karl Kieburtz, MD, MPH
Robert J. Joynt Professor Neurology; Director, Center for Human Experimental Therapeutics; Professor, Community & Preventive Medicine and Environmental Medicine; University of Rochester Medical Center, Rochester, NY, USA

Scott Y. H. Kim, MD, PhD
Associate Professor of Psychiatry and Co-Director, Center for Bioethics and Social Sciences in Medicine, and Department of Psychiatry, University of Michigan Medical School, Ann Arbor, MI, USA

Jonathan Kimmelman, PhD
Clinical Trials Research Group, Biomedical Ethics Unit, Department of Social Studies of Medicine, Faculty of Medicine, McGill University, Montreal, QC, Canada

Bruce Levin, PhD
Professor, Department of Biostatistics, Mailman School of Public Health, Columbia University, New York, NY, USA

Michael P. McDermott, PhD
Professor, Department of Biostatistics and Computational Biology and Department of Neurology, University of Rochester Medical Center, Rochester, NY, USA

Eric A. Mann, MD, PhD
Clinical Deputy Director, Division of Ophthalmic, Neurological, and ENT Devices, Center for Devices and Radiological Health, US Food and Drug Administration, Silver Springs, MD, USA

John Markman, MD
Director , Translational Pain Research, Department of Neurosurgery, University of Rochester School of Medicine, Rochester, NY, USA

D. Troy Morgan Esq.
Director of Corporate Compliance, Biogen Idec, Cambridge, MA, USA

Gilmore N. O'Neill, MB, MMedSc
Vice President, Multiple Sclerosis – Clinical Development, Biogen Idec, Cambridge, MA, USA

Yuko Y. Palesch, PhD
Professor of Biostatistics and Director of the Division of Biostatistics and Epidemiology, Medical University of South Carolina, Charleston, SC, USA

John R. Pollard, MD
Penn Epilepsy Center, University of Pennsylvania, Philadelphia, PA, USA

R. Michael Poole, MD, FACP
Head, CNS and Pain Innovative Medicine Unit,
AstraZeneca PLC, Waltham, MA, USA

Mary E. Putt, PhD, ScD
Associate Professor of Biostatistics and Epidemiology,
Center for Clinical Epidemiology and Biostatistics,
Department of Biostatistics and Epidemiology,
University of Pennsylvania School of Medicine,
Philadelphia, PA, USA

Bemard Ravina, MD, MS
Medical Director, Translational Neurology, Biogen
Idec, Cambridge, MA, USA

Richard A. Rudick, MD
Director, Mellen Center for Multiple Sclerosis Treatment
and Research, Department of Neurology, Neurological
Institute, Cleveland Clinic, Cleveland, OH, USA

David Schoenfeld, PhD
Professor of Medicine, Harvard Medical School and
Massachusetts General Hospital, Boston, MA, USA

Andrew D. Siderowf, MD, MSCE
Associate Professor of Neurology at the Pennsylvania
Hospital, University of Pennsylvania, Philadelphia,
PA, USA

Janet Wittes, PhD
President, Statistics Collaborative Inc., Washington,
DC, USA

Robert F. Woolson, PhD
Professor Emeritus, College of Medicine, Medical
University of South Carolina, Charleston, SC;
Center for Health Services Research in Primary
Care, Durham VAMC, Durham; Department of
Biostatistics and Bioinformatics, Duke University
Medical Center, Durham, NC, USA

Michael E. Yurcheshen, MD
Assistant Professor, Departments of Neurology
and Internal Medicine; Director, Sleep Medicine
Fellowship, University of Rochester School of
Medicine, Rochester, NY, USA

Preface

The aging population is increasing the global burden of neurological diseases and the need for safe and effective therapeutics for these disorders. While therapeutic targets for neurological disorders are increasingly tractable, neurology also has one of the highest failure rates in late stage clinical trials. There is an increasing need for proficiency in the design, conduct, analysis, and interpretation of clinical trials in neurology. This is especially true in the early and middle stages of therapeutic development, which determine if and how comparative efficacy studies should be conducted.

The goal of this book is to describe how the principles of clinical trials can be applied to the challenges that arise in developing therapies for neurological disorders. The fundamentals of clinical trials are explored in several existing texts and are the same across different fields of medicine. Here we describe the application of those principles to the specific clinical questions that arise with the study of neurological diseases.

There is no one trial design that meets all objectives for a particular phase of development. Rather there are parameters that need to be optimized for each intervention, question, and study. A clinical trial can be defined as an experiment in humans that is designed to test a medical, surgical, behavioral, or other type of intervention. This definition does not presuppose a particular design, type of control group, or analysis plan. When designing a trial and consulting this text for guidance, the reader should carefully consider the clinical question they are facing and how that question fits in the overall program of research for the intervention. The next step is to select a design that can practically and efficiently answer the question and guide decision-making about the intervention and the steps to further develop it.

The underlying motivation for this text is the notion that better clinical trial design and conduct will improve the efficiency of the development process by eliminating interventions with a low likelihood of success and focusing resources on those with more promise. This does not mean that all trials will be positive. By carefully selecting the appropriate dose, design, population, measure, and analytical approach we can best test the intervention's mechanism and its relevance for treating patients with neurological disorders. Rather than a high volume of clinical trials, we seek high quality trials that have the potential to lead to improvements in patient care and quality of life.

Audience

This text is intended for those who conduct clinical trials in academia, the pharmaceutical and biotechnology industries, and government and is written by experts from each of these areas. The intended audience is meant to include the broad spectrum of medical researchers, statisticians, data managers, trial managers, regulators, and program officials. Clinical trials are by nature multidisciplinary, social undertakings that are accomplished by teams. Those teams work most effectively when the members have a common understanding of goals and principles that unite their different areas of expertise.

Organization and terminology

The text is written to emphasize key concepts, with examples from neurology and other fields and references that can provide additional detail. It should be regarded as a starting point for learning about clinical trials and a companion to formal coursework and practical experience.

The text begins with a description of the growing need for progress in the treatment of neurological disorders, the sequence of clinical development, and a discussion of the unique challenges of neurology research, such as measuring drug disposition in the central nervous system. While this is not a book specifically about drug development, any clinical trial must be nested within an overall development plan to determine how to optimize the intervention (learning) and then to actually test it (confirming) for its hypothesized benefit. Subsequent sections focus on core principles of clinical trials: control of bias and random error, basic aspects of statistical inference, notable clinical trial designs in the neurology literature, clinical measurement and assessment of outcomes, interim monitoring, ethics, and the regulatory framework for drugs and devices using the US as an example. We then consider how these principles manifest in clinical trials for several common neurological disorders.

We have devoted two chapters to clinical operations, which is unusual in a clinical trials text. It is not sufficient to merely design an elegant experiment. The experiment must be conducted in a manner that ensures the integrity of the intervention and the study data. The steps involved in planning and implementing studies are often neglected in texts and courses and many trials fail on aspects of execution, timeline, and budget. This is especially true for many neurological disorders, where clinical trials are relatively new and researchers are often working in uncharted or unfamiliar territory. Our objective is to provide direction from what has been learned through experience to help researchers avoid costly mistakes. The final chapter of the text focuses on issues of financial relationships and compliance in industry-academic collaborations. This issue is of growing importance and transparency is necessary to facilitate these essential collaborations and ensure trust in the clinical research enterprise.

Disclaimer

Any views or opinions presented in this book are solely those of the authors, and not necessarily those of the US Food and Drug Administration or the authors' employers or institutions.

Acknowledgements

This is a multi-author text and this diverse group in many ways reflects the multidisciplinary teams needed to conduct clinical trials and develop new therapies. Many of the authors and my co-editors have been mentors and colleagues through my positions at the National Institute of Health (NIH), academic medicine, and now the biotechnology industry. I am grateful to them not only for contributing to this text but for facilitating my own interest in and understanding of clinical trials. The NIH/NINDS Neurology Clinical Trials Methods Course brought many of us together. The focused discussions and debates with faculty and trainees alike have helped to shape my approach to clinical trials. I would like to thank Janine Fitzpatrick and Briana Bouchard for their administrative and technical support and Nancy Richert for the MRI cover image. The otherwise un-named contributor to this text is my wife Joanna. Her unwavering support and critical thinking skills have been essential for this text and for the many studies, large and small, that fill a career in clinical research.

Bernard M. Ravina
Cambridge, MA

Chapter

1

The impact of clinical trials in neurology

E. Ray Dorsey and S. Claiborne Johnston

Overview

Fueled by the aging global population and economic growth of developing countries, the demand for new, safe, and effective therapeutics for neurological conditions in the US and globally will increase dramatically over the next generation. Scientific discovery and clinical investigation are critical for developing and evaluating new treatments and can have substantial public health benefits. However, several challenges confront the development of new therapies. Some of these are generic (e.g., rising costs of drug development, misaligned incentives, recruitment of research participants) and some are specific to neurological conditions (e.g., slow course of neurodegenerative conditions, limited availability of biomarkers). Along with these challenges are potential advances that could accelerate development, including scientific progress in the platforms that support discovery and development (e.g., in genetics and biotechnology) and in the more active participation of patients and advocacy groups that can help fuel the development of new treatments, even for the rarest of disorders. Beyond drugs for neurological conditions, clinical trials will examine other promising therapeutic interventions, including devices and procedures. Meeting the great need for effective therapeutics will not only require continued scientific discovery but also modifications in commercial incentives, improvements in the conduct of clinical trials, and advocacy and participation by the growing number of individuals affected by neurological conditions.

The burden of neurological disease is growing globally

The increase in life expectancy that occurred in the twentieth century has led to substantial increases in the number of individuals with neurological conditions, a trend that is expected to accelerate during this century.

In China, for example, the number of individuals over 65 will more than double from 110 million in 2010 to nearly 240 million by 2030 (Figure 1.1) [1]. This change in population structure – occurring in many countries – will increase the burden of neurological disease globally [2]. Cerebrovascular disease currently accounts for the majority of global disability for neurological disorders as measured in disability-adjusted life years and will account for 4% of total disability-adjusted life years globally by 2030 [2]. Other conditions, such as Alzheimer's disease and Parkinson's disease, will see the number of individuals affected increase, and that increase will be greatest in developing countries [3], [4]. The number of individuals with Parkinson's disease in the world's most populous nations is projected to more than double from approximately 4 million in 2005 to over 8 million in 2030 (Figure 1.2) [4].

The growth in the burden of neurological disease coupled with the economic growth of developing economies, especially in Asia, will increase the global demand for neurotherapeutics. As the income of countries increases (as measured by per capita gross domestic product), countries tend to devote a greater proportion of their gross domestic product to health care [5]. Access to care for individuals with neurological conditions is severely limited in many parts of the world; however, with increasing income, a larger proportion of individuals in developing economies will have the resources necessary to benefit from current and future treatments for their conditions.

Clinical investigations can have a substantial public health impact

The development of new drugs and treatments is costly. The current estimate for the successful development of a drug, including opportunity costs, is $800 million,

Clinical Trials in Neurology, ed. Bernard Ravina, Jeffrey Cummings, Michael P. McDermott, and R. Michael Poole. Published by Cambridge University Press. © Cambridge University Press 2012.

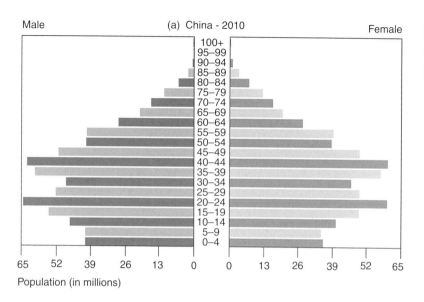

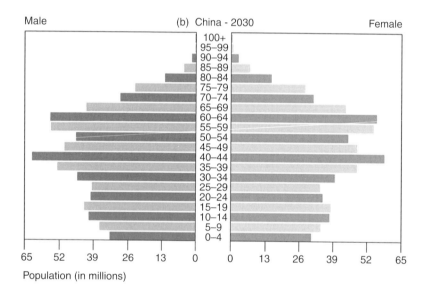

Figure 1.1. Population pyramids for China, 2010 (a) and 2030 (b). Source: US Census Bureau, International Data Base available at http://www.census.gov/ipc/www/idb/

[6] and the estimate for the successful development of a new neurological drug exceeds $1 billion [7]. While the resources required to develop a new therapy are substantial, the societal return on this investment in improved health can be even larger.

One economic study suggests that the societal return from improved health on a handful of proven interventions would justify total US health care expenditures, including the research to produce the new therapies [8]. A detailed analysis of clinical trials funded by the National Institute of Neurological Disorders and Stroke found that the public return on investment in

clinical trials has been substantial [9]. In that study, the investigators examined the costs associated with 28 clinical trials and resulting health care expenditures from adoption of interventions with benefit and compared those costs to resulting improvements in health over 10 years following completion of the trial. The study found that the total cost of the clinical trials was $335 million and that over ten years the total cost associated with the clinical trials and adoption of the beneficial intervention was $3.6 billion. However, the estimated net health benefit was $18.1 billion, which was calculated as the incremental health benefit from

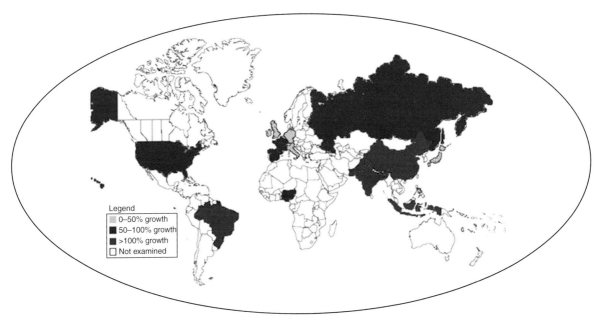

Figure 1.2. Change in number of people with Parkinson's disease in the world's most populous nations from 2005 to 2030*.
*Among individuals over 50 in the world's ten most and Western Europe's five most populous nations.
Reproduced with permission from ref [4].

the intervention (measured in quality-adjusted life years and then multiplied by the per-person annual gross domestic product) projected over ten years. The net societal benefit was, therefore, $15.5 billion ($18.1 billion less $3.6 billion), a 40-fold return on the research investment.

The results of the study highlight two additional important findings (Table 1.1). First, only a small minority (6 of the 28 or 21%) of the clinical trials were associated with any incremental societal benefit. And, second, most (80%) of the societal benefit came from two clinical trials. These points highlight the substantial risk of drug development for neurological conditions and the need to reduce and spread that risk effectively.

Developing new and novel drugs is increasingly difficult

In addition to the inherent risks involved in clinical trials, the challenges of translating scientific advances into new therapeutic advances are increasing. From 1994 to 2003, funding for US biomedical research from industry and government doubled [10]. Funding grew at a slower rate from 2003 to 2008 and now exceeds $100 billion annually [11]. However, despite this increase

in financial support, the number of novel treatments approved by the US FDA has remained relatively stagnant [10, 11], even when allowing for time lags between when the investments were made and when new products might be expected [12]. Thus, the return on the research investment over at least the last 10 years – measured as new therapies – is decreasing.

Coupled with the lack of increase in the number of new drugs is the rising cost of drug development [13]. In 1979, the estimated cost for the clinical development of a new drug was $54 million. By 2003, that number had increased nine-fold to $467 million [6]. Larger scale and longer duration trials may account for some of the increase in costs.

Another large cost and barrier to the development of new therapies is the recruitment of research participants [14]. Public participation may be the most critical challenge. Despite bearing the burden of disease and expressing a strong desire to participate in clinical trials, the public is not always encouraged to participate in research [15]. Only 7% of Americans report their physician ever suggested that they participate in a research study [15], and when they do participate, participants often are not informed of the research results [16, 17]. Dedicated efforts to informing individuals of research opportunities, reducing the travel burden of

Table 1.1 Estimated use, health benefits, treatment costs, and net societal benefits from eight clinical trials funded by the National Institute of Neurological Disorders and Stroke[a]

	Quality-adjusted life years per use	Societal cost per use ($)	Total net uses	Quality-adjusted life years	10-year projections Treatment costs ($)	Incremental net benefits ($)
Randomized Indomethacin Germinal Matrix/Intraventricular Hemorrhage Prevention Trial	1.00	–632	146 837	146 837	–92 857 340	6 003 009 978
Diazepam for acute repetitive seizures	NA	849	1 050 776		–891 839 458	890 276 155
Recombinant beta interferon as treatment for multiple sclerosis	0.014	3213	297 256	4038	955 140 007	–800 131 189
Asymptomatic Carotid Artery Stenosis Collaborative Study	0.25	11552	371 282	92 820	4 288 862 203	–590 564 802
Stroke prevention in atrial fibrillation I	0.24	984	147 736	35 457	145 402 116	1 267 774 453
North American Symptomatic Carotid Endarterectomy Trial	0.35	1819	163 669	57 120	297 716 385	1 940 786 211
Tissue plasminogen activator in ischemic stroke	0.75	–6074	178 517	134 066	–1 084 314 904	6 469 781 905
Extracrania/Intracranial Arterial Anastomosis Study	NA	30 998	–10 500	..	–325 476 690	296 277 864
Total	..	..	..	470 339	3 292 632 319	15 477 210 576

NA: not available. Incremental net benefits include trial treatment costs, and quality-adjusted life years valued at 2004 per capita gross domestic product $40 310. Products of per use and net use data vary slightly from 10-year projections because of rounding.

[a] The clinical trials are from a set of 28 phase 3 clinical trials whose funding was completed before January 1, 2000 and for which data on use, health benefits, and costs were available. Reproduced with permission from ref [9].

studies [18], and communicating research results [19] can facilitate participation in clinical trials.

The public is increasingly looking for roles beyond passive participation as research 'subjects' in clinical trials. Some, especially those affected by rare conditions, are creating their own research networks [20], funding their own studies [21], and even forming their own virtual biotechnology firms. Active participation by the public can lead to creative solutions to many of the challenges industry currently faces and may ultimately reduce the costs of development and increase the impact of proven therapies.

Developing neurotherapeutics has its own set of challenges

Many of the challenges of drug development are particularly acute for treatments of neurological conditions. Like biomedical research as a whole, increases in funding for neuroscience research have not translated into an increase in the number of novel treatments [22]. Particular challenges include a paucity of validated biomarkers [23] – with the notable exception of imaging for multiple sclerosis – that can assess efficacy (or lack thereof) of experimental therapeutics, longer duration of clinical trials [7], and higher failures rates due to lack of efficacy [24].

The scope of investigations for neurological treatments is growing

The scope of clinical trials for neurological conditions is rapidly expanding to address orphan indications, biologics, medical devices, surgeries, and comparative effectiveness studies. Interest in orphan drugs is increasing, due in part to advances in the understanding of rare neurological disorders and the high profile commercial success of some drugs for orphan indications. For example, the drug imiglucerase (Cerezyme) for Gaucher's disease generated nearly $800 million of revenue in 2009 [25].

The design of the pivotal studies that have led to the approval of drugs for orphan indications within neurology differs from that for non-orphan indications, and this may reduce the costs of clinical development. For example, 68% of drugs with orphan indications did not have at least two pivotal studies that were randomized, double-blind, or placebo-controlled even though the standard regulatory requirements are the same for products with an orphan drug designation [26].

By contrast, 100% of pivotal studies for non-orphan indications included at least two randomized, double-blind, placebo-controlled studies.

Scientific advances have also led to the development of new biological therapies for neurological conditions. Some of these have addressed conditions with previously very limited treatment options (e.g., botulinum toxin for focal dystonia) and others have demonstrated substantial efficacy (e.g., natalizumab for multiple sclerosis). However, along with these benefits have come risks, including manufacturing and safety. The emergence of significant safety concerns (e.g., progressive multifocal leukoencephalopathy) with natalizumab [27] has led to restrictions on its use and has increased the need and interest for long-term safety monitoring of drugs [28].

In addition to drugs, clinical trials frequently evaluate devices for neurological conditions. The number of devices approved by the FDA is actually more than ten-fold greater than the number of drugs [29]. Part of this difference is due to the lower US regulatory threshold for the approval of devices compared to drugs [29, 30]. The FDA classifies devices into three levels. As described in more detail in the chapter on device regulation, Class I devices are generally low-risk devices and Class II devices represent an intermediate risk. Both are generally exempt from premarket review by the FDA unless the manufacturer desires to market the device for a new indication. Class II devices are evaluated by a Premarket Notification, or 510(k), process that only requires that the new device is as safe and effective ('substantially equivalent') to another marketed Class II device. Most 510(k) submissions, which the FDA has 90 days to review, do not require clinical data to demonstrate substantial equivalence. Class III devices, which comprise only 5% of products, are more complex and high-risk, and must demonstrate a 'reasonable assurance of the safety and effectiveness' for their desired indication [30]. Some class III devices, such as deep-brain stimulators, have undergone rigorous assessments in clinical trials [31, 32].

The scope of clinical trials for neurological interventions also includes surgeries. High quality data on surgical interventions, such as temporal lobe resections for epilepsy [33], are critical to understanding their relative risks and benefits in the target populations. The challenge, like that for drugs and devices, is that once benefit has been established for a given target population in a rigorous study, the intervention quickly spreads to populations for which the benefit is lower or not established. For example, while carotid endarterectomy offers significant benefit for symptomatic carotid disease [34, 35], the vast majority are done for individuals with asymptomatic disease for whom the benefits are much smaller and less clear. Similar to outcomes of device trials, surgical outcomes in clinical trials is a function of the investigators – often the most experienced surgeons operating in the most experienced centers – which raises questions about the generalizability of results to the broader population.

A final frontier for clinical investigations in neurology is comparative effectiveness studies. Comparative effectiveness research 'is the generation and synthesis of evidence that compares the benefits and harms of alternative methods to prevent, diagnose, treat, and monitor a clinical condition or to improve the delivery of care [36].' While comparative effectiveness has gained more attention recently due to the $1.1 billion dollars in funding for these studies as part of the American Recovery and Reinvestment Act of 2009 [37], comparative effectiveness studies in neurology are not new. For example, about half of the 31 trials the National Institute of Neurological Disorders and Stroke funded prior to 2000 could qualify as comparative effectiveness research [38]. Among these trials were the comparison of low-dose warfarin plus aspirin vs. standard warfarin for stroke prevention for those with atrial fibrillation and a comparison of valproate vs. phenytoin for seizure prophylaxis after brain trauma. Trials like these, including trials comparing ways health care is delivered, will likely become more common in the future, especially because many of the top priorities for comparative effectiveness research identified by the Institute of Medicine involve neurological conditions [37].

Conclusions

The need and impact of clinical trials for neurology will increase in the future. Demographic and economic factors will fuel this demand and increase the geographic reach of clinical trials, which will raise its own challenges [39]. Continued scientific advances will allow better characterization of clinical conditions, new biomarkers will provide for more efficient and informative investigations, and increased public participation will lead to more creative funding and organization of clinical trials. The scope of clinical trials for neurology is rapidly expanding and has moved past drugs to devices, surgeries, and comparative effectiveness research. The ultimate success of these expanded investigations will require continued attention to rigorous methodology, measures to reduce the burden of participation, and expanded collaboration among industry, other sponsors, and investigators.

Acknowledgement

We thank Mr. Nick Scoglio for his assistance in the preparation of this chapter.

References

1. U.S. Census Bureau, International Data Base. 2010. http://www.census.gov/ipc/www/idb/ (Accessed March 8, 2010.)

2. World Health Organization. Global burden of neurological disorders estimates and projections. 2006. http://www.who.int/mental_health/neurology/chapter_2_neuro_disorders_public_h_challenges.pdf. (Accessed February 5, 2010).

3. Ferri CP, Prince M, Brayne C, et al. Global prevalence of dementia: a Delphi consensus study. Lancet 2005; 366: 2112–7.

4. Dorsey ER, Constantinescu R, Thompson JP, et al. Projected number of people with Parkinson disease in the most populous nations, 2005 through 2030. Neurology 2007; 68: 384–6.

5. Reinhardt UE, Hussey PS, and Anderson GF. U.S. health care spending in an international context. Health Aff 2004; 23: 10–25.

6. DiMasi JA, Hansen RW, and Grabowski HG. The price of innovation: new estimates of drug development costs. J Health Econ 2003; 22: 151–185.

7. Adams CP and Bratner W. Estimating the cost of new drug development: is it really 802 million dollars? Health Aff 2006; 25: 420–8.

8. Cutler DM and McClellan M. Is technological change in medicine worth it? Health Aff 2001; 20: 11–29.

9. Johnston SC, Rootendberg JD, Katrak S, et al. Effect of a US National Institutes of Health programme of clinical trials on public health and costs. Lancet 2006; 367:2057–8.

10. Moses H, Dorsey ER, Matheson DH, et al. Financial anatomy of biomedical research. JAMA 2005; 294:1333–42.

11. Dorsey ER, de Roulet J, Thompson JP, et al. Funding of US biomedical research, 2003–2008. JAMA 2010; 303: 137–43.

12. Dorsey ER, Thompson JP, Carrasco M, et al. Financing of U.S. biomedical research and new drug approvals across therapeutic areas. PLoS One 2009; 4: e7015.

13. Booth B and Zemmel R. Prospects for productivity. *Nat Rev Drug Discov* 2004; **3**: 451–6.

14. Sung NS, Crowley WF, Genel M, *et al.* Central challenges facing the national clinical research enterprise. *JAMA* 2003; **289**: 1278–87.

15. Research! America: An Alliance For Discoveries in Health: 2008 Poll Data. http://www.researchamerica. org/advocacy_awards (Accessed February 20, 2010).

16. Meier, B. Participants left uninformed in some halted medical trials. *New York Times*, October 30, 2007. (Accessed February 23, 2010).

17. Berenson A. After a trial, silence. *New York Times* November 21, 2007. (Accessed February 23, 2010).

18. Karlawish J, Cary MS, Rubright J, *et al.* How redesigning AD clinical trials might increase study partners' willingness to participate. *Neurology* 2008; **71**: 1883–8.

19. Dorsey ER, Beck CA, Adams M, *et al.* Communicating clinical trial results to research participants. *Arch Neurol* 2008; **65**: 1590–5.

20. Frydman GJ. Patient-driven research: rich opportunities and real risks. *J Particip Med* 2009; **1**: e12.

21. Merz, J. Finding a cure: paying to keep your drug trial alive. Wall Street Journal, April 10, 2007 (Accessed February 20, 2010).

22. Dorsey ER, Vitticore P, and de Roulet J. Financial anatomy of neuroscience research. *Ann Neurol* 2006; **60**: 652–9.

23. Dunckley T, Coon KD, and Stephan DA. Discovery and development of biomarkers of neurological disease. *Drug Disc Today* 2005; **10**: 326–334.

24. Gordian MA, Singh N, and Zemmel RW. Why drugs fall short in late-stage trials? *McKinsey Q* November 2006. (Accessed February 20, 2010).

25. Morrison T. Big biotechs preview earnings as JPM conference continues. BioWorld.com. January 13, 2010 (Accessed February 5, 2010).

26. Mitsumoto J, Dorsey ER, Beck CA, *et al.* Pivotal studies of orphan drugs approved for neurological disease. *Ann Neurol* 2009; **66**: 184–90.

27. Kleinschmidt-DeMasters BK, and Tyler KL. Progressive multifocal leukoencephalopathy complicating treatment with natalizumab and interferon beta-1a for multiple sclerosis. *N Engl J Med* 2005; **353**: 369–74.

28. The Pink Sheet, November 3, 2008, p. 27–28.

29. Johnston SC and Hauser SL. Neurology and medical devices. *Ann Neurol* 2006; **60**: 11A–12A.

30. Yustein A. The FDA's process of regulatory premarket review for new medical devices. http://www.gastro.org/ user-assets/Documents/08_Publications/06_GIHep_ Annual_Review/Articles/Yustein.pdf. (Accessed February 20, 2010).

31. Deuschl G, Schade-Brittinger C, Krack P, *et al.* A randomized trial of deep-brain stimulation for Parkinson's disease. *N Engl J Med* 2006; **355**: 896–908.

32. Weaver FM, Follet K, and Stern M. Bilateral deep brain stimulation vs best medical therapy for patients with advanced Parkinson disease: a randomized controlled trial. *JAMA* 2009; **301**: 63–73.

33. Wiebe S, Blume WT, Girvin JP, *et al.* A randomized, controlled trial of surgery for temporal-lobe epilepsy. *N Engl J Med* 2001; **345**: 311–8.

34. North American Symptomatic Carotid Endarterectomy Trial Collaborators. Beneficial effect of carotid endarterectomy in symptomatic patients with high-grade carotid stenosis. *N Engl J Med* 1991; **325**: 445–53.

35. Burton TM and Kamp, J. Study boosts stents in stroke prevention. *Wall Street Journal*, February 27, 2010. (Accessed March 5, 2010).

36. Chaturvedi S, Bruno A, Feasby T, *et al.* Carotid endarterectomy – an evidence-based review: report of the Therapeutics and Technology Assessment Subcommittee of the American Academy of Neurology. *Neurology* 2005; **65**: 794–801.

37. Institute of Medicine. Initial Priorities for Comparative Effectiveness Research. 2009. http:// www.iom.edu/~/media/Files/Report%20Files/2009/ ComparativeEffectivenessResearchPriorities/CER%20 report%20brief%2008–13–09.ashx (Accessed February 8, 2010).

38. Johnston, SC and Hauser SL. Comparative effectiveness research in the neurosciences. *Ann Neurol* 2009; **65**: A6–A8.

39. Glickman SW, McHutchison JG, Peterson ED, *et al.* Ethical and scientific implications of the globalization of clinical research. *N Engl J Med* 2009; **360**: 816–23.

Chapter

2

The sequence of clinical development

R. Michael Poole

Introduction

Clinical development can be described as a process of asking and answering specific scientific and operational questions at specific times to learn about the risks and benefits of drugs or devices that may be useful for human health. Good clinical development requires the involvement of skilled scientists from many different disciplines working together under the guidance of a thoughtful plan that describes the program of research that will provide the data to answer these questions. Because the human, monetary, and time resources required to initiate and complete a clinical development program are significant, every such plan involves careful articulation and sequencing of the questions to be answered.

It is especially important at the outset to state clearly the ultimate objective for a clinical program and how the approach being undertaken may improve on what is currently known or practiced. Is the purpose of the trial to improve prognostication, or provide a better understanding of disease or biomarkers? Is the objective to demonstrate efficacy, safety, or economic advantages of a drug or device over current standards of care? Is there an expectation that the approach will offer improved survival or long-term outcome? Each of these objectives requires a very different clinical plan and sequence of experiments.

Typically, clinical programs are described as involving several specific phases (phases I–IV). By convention, this scheme provides some understanding of the kinds of trials employed and the subjects being studied, but the specific phase does not provide a good basis for understanding exactly what kinds of questions are being asked. Trials typically thought of as being performed during a specific phase (such as a human volunteer study, phase 1) can be performed at multiple times during a development program. It is preferable when creating a clinical development plan to organize one's thinking into stages of information gathering that will accomplish specific objectives.

Table 2.1 provides an illustration of this concept and shows that, in the simplest way of thinking, clinical programs can be divided into early, middle and late stages. Although there is some overlap, each development stage has unique objectives that are required to progress further into development. The information collected at each stage builds upon what has already been learned and influences how decisions are made with respect to study design, population, indication, and program size.

What follows is a brief description of the questions that are typically asked and answered at each stage of clinical development and the kinds of clinical trials that are utilized in the effort. This chapter focuses specifically on the activities and questions that are involved in the generation of data to support the registration and approval of a drug candidate. The ultimate objective in this case is to demonstrate the use of a drug for management of symptoms or signs of an illness or to cure or slow progression of a disease. However, a similar framework and discipline can be used when ordering the sequence of questions for medical devices or for more academic clinical programs aimed at improving diagnosis, gaining better understanding of a disease state, or prevention of illness. Lastly, some important sources of information apart from the general scientific and medical literature are provided.

Clinical Trials in Neurology, ed. Bernard Ravina, Jeffrey Cummings, Michael P. McDermott, and R. Michael Poole. Published by Cambridge University Press. © Cambridge University Press 2012.

Table 2.1 Early, middle, and late development: objectives and examples of studies performed

Objectives	Development stage		
	Early	Middle	Late
Human pharmacology and biomarker exploration	'First in human', single and multiple ascending dose trials ('phase 1')	Targeted special safety studies in patients and volunteers	Special formulation pharmacology; drug-drug interaction studies; drug metabolism in renal and liver impairment
Exploratory efficacy and safety studies	Early, 'first in patient' studies	Dose-ranging efficacy and safety studies in patients ('phase 2')	Dose-ranging studies in new indications
Confirmatory efficacy trials		Seamless exploratory dose ranging and confirmatory efficacy	Pivotal confirmatory trials in primary indication; comparative efficacy trials ('phase 3')
Therapeutic use studies, new indications expansion		Comparative efficacy trials	New indications, expanded population studies, combination trials ('phase 4')

Early stage clinical development

Early stage clinical research involves the design and conduct of studies aimed at understanding the basic human pharmacology of a drug. The program of early research is built upon knowledge gained from preclinical *in vitro* and *in vivo* experiments that define and justify an initial assessment of potential benefit and risk to human subjects. Clinical studies are then designed and performed to produce data that will enable initial determinations of safety and tolerability, pharmacokinetics, pharmacodynamics, and aspects of drug action and CNS penetration for the drug.

Every early stage clinical development program requires information derived from basic laboratory and animal experiments that define the fundamental pharmacologic properties of a drug. Basic information about the biological target, cellular pathways and the biochemical mechanism of action should be known. Information about the potency and selectivity of the compound for its target and the nature of concentration vs. response relationships is critical to the design of an early clinical program. Typically, data is available from more than one *in vivo* efficacy model that provides justification for exploration in humans. This data should include information about the time course of onset and duration of effect, dose vs. response characteristics, and the no-pharmacologic effect dose. Any information on biomarkers from *in vivo* models is also enormously useful at this stage.

In addition, safety and toxicology data from both *in vitro* and animal testing is needed to justify exposure in humans. Data from acute and chronic studies in animals as well as safety pharmacology studies help to define the dose range that can be used safely in humans and can highlight specific toxicity issues that may need to be monitored. In certain settings, special studies examining the potential for reproductive toxicity and carcinogenicity are required. Additional information on drug metabolizing enzymes, drug metabolites, the potential for drug interaction, and initial estimates of preclinical pharmacokinetics help to define parameters for early studies. When they are available, data from animals on pharmaceutical properties such as absorption and bioavailability are also useful in helping to design an early clinical program.

The main goals of early clinical studies are to provide initial assessments of safety, tolerability and pharmacokinetics and to estimate the dose range that will be deployed in later trials. This is usually accomplished through a combination of single ascending dose and multiple ascending dose trials that help to determine the maximum tolerated dose and regimen that provides adequate drug exposure for the proposed indications.

The key objectives of single ascending dose studies are to define safety, tolerability, pharmacokinetics and pharmacodynamics of a drug. The dose range deployed usually covers approximately two logs and is framed by a starting dose that is a fraction of the preclinical pharmacologic no-pharmacologic effect dose (NOPED) in the most appropriate or sensitive species and limited to a top dose that is guided by the preclinical exposure (drug concentration in plasma) at the no-adverse effect level (NOAEL). Although designs are highly variable, as many as 6–8 dose levels are used with dose increments typically >2-fold at the lowest doses and <2-fold at the highest doses. Commonly, about eight subjects are exposed in each dose cohort at a placebo-to-drug ratio of one to three. Close assessments of vital signs, hematology and blood chemistry, electrocardiography, and adverse events are collected in each cohort and advancement to the next dose level is allowed only after thorough review of these data. Intensive plasma sampling for pharmacokinetics is also performed in each cohort although typically these data are not available before advancement to the next dose level. At study end, an assessment is made of the overall tolerability and safety across the examined dose range along with any defined dose-limiting toxicity whether defined by adverse event or laboratory evidence. Detailed analysis of pharmacokinetic samples adds to the profile of the medication. This information is then used to help define design parameters for multiple ascending dose studies.

Multiple ascending dose studies extend observations on human pharmacology to longer periods of dosing. Again, the key objectives are to provide data on safety, tolerability and pharmacokinetics with prolonged dosing. In most studies, the duration of dosing ranges from 7 to 14 days with dosing frequency determined by the pharmacokinetic parameters defined in single-dose studies. Typically, 4–5 dose levels are examined in the single ascending dose study, with the dose range covering a little over 1 log.

Single and multiple ascending dose human pharmacology studies are usually conducted in healthy volunteers whose age may reflect the target population for the intended indication for the drug. Healthy volunteers are often preferred at this stage since the assessments of the tolerability and pharmacokinetic profile of the drug are less likely to be contaminated by disease-related adverse events and concomitant medications. However, there are several situations where early assessments of human pharmacology should be supplemented by data from the target patient population.

For some medications the tolerability profile in patients differs markedly from that in healthy volunteers. For example, patients with chronic epilepsy and schizophrenia who are chronically exposed to anticonvulsant or antipsychotic medications respectively, typically report fewer central nervous system adverse events than normal volunteers exposed to the same doses of a new medication. To ensure an accurate determination of the tolerable dose range, during early development both single-dose and multiple-dose studies are conducted in parallel in patients and normal volunteers. The combined data set provides the best overall initial picture of safety, tolerability and pharmacokinetics: studies in normal volunteers provide an assessment of normal human pharmacokinetics and determine which adverse events can reasonably be attributed to drug exposure; studies in patients provide a more accurate assessment of the tolerable dose range. Other studies specifically designed to characterize drug–drug interactions and effects on pharmacokinetic parameters can be performed to provide information about effects of concomitant medications used in patient populations.

Some initial studies in humans can only be conducted in patients. Medications with substantial potential toxicity risks such as cytotoxic or genotoxic drugs cannot be administered to normal volunteers and for this reason, early studies are conducted in patients. The most common setting where this occurs is in oncology drug development where initial single- and multiple-dose studies are virtually always conducted in cancer patients. Examples from neurological therapeutics include the use of specific B-cell depleting therapies for multiple sclerosis and immunotherapeutic vaccines for Alzheimer's disease [1, 2].

Data generated from the kinds of experiments described thus far provide an initial picture of the human pharmacology of a drug. Ideally, early research efforts should also provide evidence of drug exposure at the target site of action over a period of time that is consistent with what is believed to be needed for efficacy in the human disease state. Further confidence is gained by demonstrating that the drug binds to the target at the site of action and that binding to the target results in a measurable pharmacologic effect. In these respects, wherever possible both single- and multiple-dose studies should include measures of central nervous system penetration and pharmacodynamic properties of drugs that are related to both primary and secondary mechanisms of action. Conducting these kinds of early assessments in patients rather than healthy volunteers may be easier to justify ethically and may generate data that is more relevant for decision-making.

Estimates of exposure in the brain can be determined by direct assessment of drug concentration in the cerebrospinal fluid or indirectly by effects on physiological or imaging measures. Both efficacy and safety pharmacologic dose–response relationships can be assessed by the addition of targeted clinical measurements to the standard data collection. A simple example comes from the early development of serotonin-norepinephrine reuptake inhibitors where investigators made assessments of pupillometry and pulse/blood pressure measures in each cohort to estimate the dose relationship for adrenergic effects. More complex assessments of serotoninergic effects can be provided by quantitative polysomnography [3]. These examples show that substantial insights on dose–response pharmacology can be provided with relatively small sample sizes.

Neuroimaging can provide important evidence of distribution of drug in areas of the CNS with known target expression. For example, the cerebral distribution of C-11 labeled donepezil in the brains of Alzheimer's patients has been demonstrated using PET imaging [4]. In addition, imaging studies can provide important evidence of specific drug effects in the brain. Another PET ligand, Pittsburgh Imaging agent B (PIB), a C-11 labeled thioflavin ligand that binds to fibrillar beta-amyloid, was used to confirm the clinical diagnosis and demonstrated the ability of a monoclonal antibody to lower cerebral beta-amyloid in patients with Alzheimer's disease [5]. Important information on brain function that may be modulated with drug therapy may eventually come from other measures like functional MRI [6, 7]. The evolving importance of brain imaging studies in drug development was borne out in a recent review of new drug applications in the Neuropharmacology Division at the US FDA. This review showed that a substantial number of those projects utilized neuroimaging during early stage development [8].

The data generated in early stage studies provide confidence for deciding whether to advance a drug into more complicated and expensive trials in specific patient populations. Further, they provide evidence for the selection of safe doses to be used in those studies and insights into specific safety or tolerability issues that may need further clarification. Increasingly, pharmaceutical companies are utilizing pharmacokinetic and pharmacodynamic modeling to build confidence in their assessments of the dose-response relationship for drugs in early development. Lalonde and colleagues provided a useful review of the role that model-based

development can play in determining dose-response relationships [9]. They make a strong case for the more routine use of quantitatively defined, model-based decision criteria in early development and point to several organizational challenges for broader implementation of model-based development. These include the need for early development scientists to be more specific about the assumptions made in creating the models and for team members with less training in quantitative scientific disciplines to become comfortable with the process of defining and applying quantitative decision rules.

Middle stage clinical development

The middle stage of clinical development typically involves more significant exploration of therapeutic efficacy in patients. The issues that need to be addressed at this stage include defining the specific patient population to be studied, the determination of the dose range and regimen, and the selection and evaluation of endpoints for use in later confirmatory studies. Trials conducted in this stage of clinical research carry a special burden within an overall development program because the data generated in them have a significant impact on future trial size, expense, and risk. It is especially important that the limitations of trial design and data interpretation at this stage are clearly understood and communicated to investigators, patients, and other stakeholders.

During middle stage development it is critical to begin to characterize the dose-response relationship for efficacy and safety endpoints in the selected population. Determination of the likely effective and safe dose range is a critical objective of middle stage development that affects not only the design of later stage trials but other aspects of non-clinical development as well. An important study from the FDA showed that a substantial percentage of new drugs approved were relabeled to correct dose ranges, and the majority of these changes were for safety reductions [10]. Of all therapeutic areas examined, drugs for nervous system indications had the highest percentage of dosing changes. Establishment of the optimal dose range requires that substantial attention be paid to selection of the appropriate patient population, efficacy endpoints, and safety evaluations.

Patient selection during middle stage evaluation of efficacy typically is more restrictive than in later stages of development because there is a desire to provide control over aspects of the disease state that might influence the therapeutic response to a drug. The specific restrictions that are employed depend on the clinical setting. For example, in the evaluation of a new analgesic medication a protocol may exclude patients whose pain is refractory to multiple medications on the premise that those patients would be unlikely to respond to any new medication. Similarly, initial proof-of-efficacy trials for new anticonvulsants typically require that patients have recurrent seizures despite treatment with more than one medication. Here, the drug to be tested needs to demonstrate anticonvulsant efficacy above background therapy in order to advance to further studies in less severely affected patients. In certain clinical trial settings where placebo response rates are known to be high (major depressive disorder, painful diabetic neuropathy, generalized anxiety disorder), protocols may require that patient selection be based upon responses to evaluation instruments prior to randomization or after a period of placebo run-in. In each of these settings the external validity of a positive efficacy signal is limited by the bias introduced by the restricted patient selection.

Endpoint selection in early efficacy trials depends on the nature of the drug effect expected, previous experience with measurement scales used in the disease state, and the kind of decision problem faced by the study team. The specific endpoints selected should balance the need to measure the effect of the drug on the disease state, provide some initial reassurance that the drug effect is clinically meaningful, and have adequate operating characteristics for studies that typically are of somewhat smaller sample size. If the ultimate goal of the development program is the approval of a new medication, the endpoints selected for pivotal trials must be acceptable to regulatory authorities wherever the drug will be registered. When a new instrument is used, substantial evidence of its measurement properties and appropriateness for efficacy assessment will be needed.

This is particularly true for patient-reported outcomes (PRO), which are used commonly in CNS development. A PRO is a report of a patient's health status or condition that comes directly from the patient, without interpretation of the patient's response by another person. A simple example is the Numeric Pain Rating Scale, a measurement tool used to evaluate the efficacy of analgesic medications. On this scale, patients rate their pain using a number from 1 to 10, where the extreme ends of the scale are anchored with the descriptions 'no pain' or 'worst imaginable pain'. More complicated examples of PRO include various quality of life rating instruments. Regulatory agencies review and evaluate the suitability of PRO assessments based upon several characteristics including the medical condition and population for intended use, concepts being measured, number of items, conceptual framework, data collection method, scale administration, response options, scoring and weighting of items or domains, and availability of translations or cultural adaptations.

Because the properties of a measurement instrument like a PRO need to be well understood prior to collecting definitive efficacy data in pivotal confirmatory trials, this important groundwork must be initiated and is often largely completed during middle stage development. The FDA has published a useful guidance document that is aimed at ensuring that the process for evaluating new instruments is adequately understood by clinical researchers [11].

Although general safety data collection at this stage is important, the strategy for learning about specific safety issues needs special attention. The development plan should take into account what has already been learned in the initial experience with healthy volunteers and what is known or believed to be an issue in the patient population of interest. For example, some anticonvulsants are known to have adverse effects on cognitive function in epilepsy patients and specific scales aimed at quantifying the dose-response relationship for these effects may be needed. Similarly, in the evaluation of certain psychoactive agents, rather than relying on spontaneous reporting to detect withdrawal effects, specific instruments such as the Physicians Withdrawal Checklist are often deployed at this stage to gain insight into the dose-response relationship [12]. Separate study visits specific to this objective may be necessary and special care is taken when determining the appropriate schedule for study drug dosing relative to the evaluation of withdrawal effects. Another example comes from the evaluation of drugs for neuroprotection in the setting of acute stroke where often there is a need to be certain that the drug is compatible with concomitant use of recombinant tissue plasminogen activator (rtPA). These agents can have both pharmacokinetic and pharmacodynamic interactions with rtPA that may require specific plasma sampling, blood tests, or imaging to understand fully.

Another specific safety issue particularly important to CNS drug development is the assessment of abuse liability. Although some components of this assessment are undertaken at middle stages of development, efforts may begin earlier with preclinical assessments in animals and extend well into late stage development and post-marketing. The drug's primary and secondary pharmacology, absorption and metabolism, intended patient population, and final formulation all affect the timing and extent of the overall assessment [13]. Initial abuse liability studies in humans may be undertaken at middle stage; however, these studies should only be considered and designed in the context of an overall strategy for abuse assessment. Careful planning and decision-making are essential since the data generated during assessment of abuse liability can have profound impacts on the overall value and availability of a new treatment.

Another critical objective of middle stage development is the assessment, understanding and mitigation of patient access, and study feasibility issues that may arise during later studies. Every experienced clinical researcher has dealt with the gap between expectations and reality that comes from incorrectly projecting large numbers of suitable patients for a specific trial. This common problem was described by the clinical pharmacologist Louis Lasagna, who stated that the number of patients actually available for a clinical trial is between 10% and 33% of original estimates [14]. The gap is usually a result of the particular requirements and design of the clinical experiment. For example, narrow inclusion and exclusion criteria or restrictions on concomitant medications may eliminate many patients from participation. Similarly, the period of study participation may be too long or the study procedures too onerous for some patients. These issues require objective evaluation and an honest assessment of the scientific and pragmatic trade-offs that need to be made in order for later trials to be successful. Much of this assessment can and should be done during clinical trials conducted in middle stage development. Failure to do so can have significant, negative effects on later trials.

The specific clinical trial designs deployed in the middle development stage typically utilize a broad dose range derived from the early experience in volunteers and patients. Ideally, the program of research will provide an early determination of the doses that provide no effect, maximum effect, and the best overall balance of efficacy and adverse effects. This can be accomplished by conducting multiple dose-ranging, parallel-group studies with overlapping dose ranges

or, under the right circumstances, by utilizing adaptive randomization schemes and assessments [15].

Adaptive trials can be designed to assist with specific decision problems related to efficacy or safety endpoints and can be used effectively in assessments of performance relative to comparator agents. Because of the promise they hold for efficient clinical decision-making, particularly around identification of the optimal dose range, trials utilizing adaptive designs are becoming more commonplace in industry settings. An in depth review of this topic is provided in Chapter 9 of this text.

Active controls are frequently employed in middle stage development, particularly in areas where placebo response rates can be high and failed trials are common (neuropathic pain, Alzheimer's disease, depression and generalized anxiety disorder). In this setting the positive control mainly functions to demonstrate that the experiment has adequate assay sensitivity to detect treatment effects with the new agent. In some circumstances the positive control also serves as a comparator to evaluate efficacy or safety advantages of a new treatment. Although the study may not be powered to test the question of superiority of the new treatment over the comparator, sufficient insight may be gained to help with decision-making about whether to proceed to definitive efficacy trials. This assessment, the ensuing discussions and decision-making are aided by careful articulation, in advance of seeing data, of the specific efficacy or safety criteria advantage that must be demonstrated by the new treatment. This is one of the most important activities undertaken during middle stage development.

Late stage clinical development

Clinical trials conducted during late stage development are aimed at extending efficacy and safety observations in larger populations. The two key objectives of late stage development are confirmation of efficacy and firmer establishment of the general safety profile with enhanced understanding of special safety issues. These data provide an adequate basis for assessing the benefit/risk relationship of a new treatment. Typically, additional efforts are made to confirm the optimal dose–response relationship and to provide evidence of quality of life benefits. In large pharmaceutical companies, significant resources are also expended in late stage development on comparative efficacy trials that are sometimes necessary for initial regulatory approval and for making cost-benefit arguments with third party payers in the US and government pricing authorities in other parts of the world.

Late stage confirmatory clinical trials often utilize a broader study population than was studied during early development. This is done to ensure that the studies performed provide evidence of efficacy and safety that is relevant for the majority of patients with a particular disease. This often necessitates loosening the entry criteria that were used in middle stage trials, which can involve significant risks since a less highly selected population may respond less predictably to a drug. More and more however, late stage trials are focusing on specific subsets of patients determined either by genetic makeup or specific biomarkers to be particularly suited for a new treatment. The best examples of this approach are currently being pursued in oncology, a simple example of which is the use of estrogen antagonists in estrogen-positive breast cancer. In neurology, the previously mentioned use of imaging methods to determine the presence of fibrillar amyloid in the brains of patients with Alzheimer's disease might ultimately be used to define the appropriate patient population for anti-amyloid drugs.

Regardless of whether it is narrowly or broadly defined, careful description of the patient population is essential to the interpretation of study results. For example, study protocols should describe the method for determining that study subjects have the correct diagnosis and that the stage or severity of their disease has been determined adequately. This is particularly important in late stage trials where the study population may be less strictly defined by exclusion or inclusion criteria. The methods used for patient selection in late stage studies that are used to support regulatory approval and product labeling are evaluated and interpreted carefully during regulatory review.

Late stage studies are usually powered at higher levels than in earlier development, with sample size estimation typically employing smaller type-2 error rates. Partly this is done to ensure the robustness of any positive efficacy signal. The additional power provided by the larger sample size may be necessary for validation of novel endpoints, and can help to add confidence to the interpretation of secondary efficacy measures and supplementary analyses of the primary endpoint.

In addition, larger sample sizes provide a more substantial basis for interpreting safety and tolerability results from a single study or from a program of clinical research. Confidence in the accuracy of the safety and tolerability profile is derived from the number of patients exposed and their duration of treatment with a medication. For chronically administered drugs for non-life threatening conditions, the International Committee on Harmonisation (ICH) Guidelines recommend an overall exposure of 1500 patients with 300–600 patients exposed for 6 months and 100 patients exposed for one year [16]. These exposures must occur at the dose or dose range believed to be efficacious. There are circumstances where these guidelines can be relaxed (for example, when the number of patients affected is small), but occasionally the required number can be even larger (for example, when there is a need to quantify the frequency of rare but serious adverse events known to occur in a particular drug class). Most often, development teams plan carefully to ensure that the basic exposure requirements set forth by ICH will be met by the time that applications for regulatory approval are submitted and reviewed. These requirements underscore the need to understand the effective dose range as early as possible during development; failure to do so can lead to significant delays while additional patient exposures are accrued.

The plan for broadening the understanding of specific safety issues needs to be articulated at the beginning of late stage clinical trials. For example, certain CNS drugs are believed to increase the risk for suicidal behaviors. If the risk is known or believed to be particularly high for a given drug class, specific data collection instruments may be needed for the program and investigators should be specifically instructed in the handling of adverse events related to suicidality. When a particular safety or tolerability issue is uncovered in middle stage development, a specific plan for the data collection needed to fully describe and understand the issue should be created for all late stage trials. For example, initial efficacy trials in middle stage may uncover that peripheral edema complicates the use of a medication in a significant percentage of patients. For any patient presenting with a complaint of edema, specific additional medical history is recorded, limb measures are taken and additional blood, urine or other testing is performed to more fully understand the nature of the edema in specific cases. At the end of the late stage program, these data are summarized and described in aggregate and can provide significant insight into a particular safety or tolerability issue. Having a plan for uniform data collection across studies for important safety issues makes this effort much easier and the resulting interpretation more robust.

It is very common for healthy human volunteer studies to be performed during late stage development. These trials often have as their specific objectives the generation of data on drug-drug interactions, drug metabolism and pharmacokinetics. Alternate dosing formulations are also frequently studied during late stage, such as liquid formulations that may be appropriate for pediatric populations. These formulations may be required in order to conduct pediatric studies, which are typically not initiated until there is some assurance that a drug will be successful in adult populations. Sometimes specific tolerability and safety issues are more robust when studied in trials utilizing healthy volunteers. For example, a placebo-controlled clinical trial to assess the effect of the drug pregabalin on sperm motility was conducted in 30 healthy male subjects [17]. This study would have been difficult to complete with a high level of data quality in the diabetic, psychiatric, and epileptic patient populations for which the drug was ultimately approved.

Clinical trial designs deployed in late stage development typically involve large and relatively simple parallel group assignment to drug, placebo and sometimes, active comparators. In late stage experiments, active controls are usually employed to provide direct evidence of comparative efficacy for the purpose of demonstrating advantages of the new drug over existing agents. Here, the data generated with the comparator is mainly used to support superior efficacy claims, to justify the additional investment needed to market a new product, and to meet the requirements of regulatory agencies around the world for pricing decisions.

Since earlier studies conducted during middle stage can almost never detect small differences in efficacy and do not provide a complete safety profile, it is appropriate to continue to explore dose-response in late stage development. For antihypertensives, antidepressants, anti-migraines, and anti-psychotics most or all pivotal trials include some degree of dose-ranging. Robert Temple, Deputy Director for Clinical Science in the Center for Drug Evaluation & Research at FDA has stated publicly his opinion that dose-ranging designs should be utilized more commonly in pivotal trials performed during late stage development [18].

In certain special circumstances, novel designs may be used in late stage development that accomplish a seamless transition from the typical dose-ranging trial used in middle stage to a parallel group, pivotal proof-of-efficacy study normally used in late stage [19]. These 'seamless phase 2–3' studies should be deployed very selectively based upon several factors. When the eligible population of patients is small and there is an urgent need for a new treatment, these designs may help to save time required for development and may make the most efficient use of eligible patients. This 'adaptive' approach is not appropriate for programs in which efficacy measurements or surrogates need validation or are poorly understood in the patient population. In any circumstance, close discussion with regulatory agencies is essential before embarking on a study with this design.

Another trial adaptation that can be useful in late stage development is sample size re-estimation. At the beginning of a clinical trial, the assumptions that underlie sample size calculations may not be well understood. In particular, the variability in the primary efficacy parameter may be over- or underestimated and can significantly affect the likelihood of observing a statistically significant result at study end. This may be a particular problem when entry criteria change from middle stage to late stage trials. Sample size re-estimation involves examining blinded efficacy data at a predetermined point in study enrollment and calculating the variability in the primary parameter. If the variability observed is significantly larger than the estimate that was used for original sample size calculations, the sample size is adjusted upward to reflect the observed value for variability in the primary parameter. No statistical penalty needs to be paid for this adjustment, but the procedure must be carefully documented in the statistical analysis plan.

Open-label safety extension studies are also frequently used during late stage development. Typically, these studies follow directly after pivotal, double-blind, proof-of-efficacy studies and have as a primary objective the collection of long-term safety data for a drug used for a chronic condition. In these studies, participants enter a transition period from receiving blinded study medication in the preceding controlled trial, following which they immediately enroll and receive active study drug in the open-label extension. The duration of patient participation in an open-label extension study is typically planned for at least one year. In addition to collecting safety data, open-label trials sometimes include efficacy data collection for the purpose of observing longer-term responses to a medication. Because an open-label study is uncontrolled, the interpretation of both efficacy and safety data is limited. The interpretation of both can be enhanced somewhat by ensuring a blinded transition from the double-blind to the open-label phase; that is, neither the patients nor the investigators are informed of the preceding double-blind treatment assignment at the time of transition to open-label. Patients may benefit from participating in open-label studies by being allowed access to a potentially effective medication that would otherwise be unavailable. Access to active medication in a follow-on open-label study also provides incentive for some patients to enroll in the preceding double-blind trials where they may receive placebo. Sponsors benefit by the generation of long-term safety data that would otherwise not be collected easily in prolonged double-blind studies.

Important sources of information

Besides the general scientific and medical literature, there are several important sources of information that can help with the strategy for clinical development programs and the design of specific trials and their questions. Some of these resources are free and available on government-sponsored internet sites while others are proprietary collections of information that require subscription fees for access.

The FDA provides access to guidance documents that outline regulatory requirements related to the development of drugs and devices [20]. There are general guidance documents related to both preclinical and clinical requirements for development in any therapeutic area, as well as specific guidance for some, but not all CNS indications. Clinical guidance documents describe design requirements, endpoints, and analytic approaches to consider when conducting trials aimed at registration and marketing approval. Regulators work diligently to keep up with the latest science related to clinical trials; in this respect, guidance documents may be somewhat outdated and not completely reflect the current thinking of regulatory scientists. These documents can therefore provide a starting point for strategic thinking, but fulsome and contemporaneous discussion with reviewing scientists at regulatory agencies is essential before making significant commitments to program or trial designs.

Another important resource provided by FDA are documents describing their review of data submitted in New Drug Applications (NDA) for drugs approved for marketing in the US [21]. This database, indexed alphabetically by drug name, provides access to PDF files of reviews conducted by regulatory scientists from clinical pharmacology, statistics and medical disciplines,

correspondence between the sponsor and FDA, and approved labels and labeling changes. The reviews cover assessments of pharmacokinetics, efficacy and safety, and detail the concerns raised by FDA scientists in their assessment of the drug's risk and benefit. These reviews provide an important and detailed source of information on design elements, entry criteria, and performance of endpoints in clinical trials. Importantly, data is available from trials that were submitted in support of the drug application but sometimes not submitted for publication in peer-reviewed journals. In this respect, a more complete view of the data that supports a drug's efficacy and safety profile is available and can help to frame the challenges that may be expected in a clinical program aimed at the same indication. The database does not contain information for all drugs approved in the US but there are significant additions to the document database every year.

European regulators also provide access to documents that describe requirements for drug evaluation and registration. Similar to the FDA, the European Medicines Agency (EMEA) web site contains links to development guidance documents, reviews of approved products and administrative requirements [22]. Since the labels created for the EU differ depending on the country where the drug is marketed, there is not the same access to product labeling that is available on the FDA web site. Agency scientists working in different countries can have different opinions of the data that is necessary to support usage of a drug for a particular indication, and therefore it is necessary to compare requirements in the US and EU when considering the strategy for a clinical trial program aimed at registration in both regions. Sometimes, regulatory conclusions on risk and benefit differ substantially from region to region. A careful comparative review of information from EMEA and FDA web resources can provide essential insights for the clinical development plan when global registration is a primary objective.

The FDA also provides public access to meeting materials and transcripts from public advisory committee meetings [23]. These meetings are organized by the FDA in order to obtain independent expert advice on scientific, technical, and policy matters. The meetings are open to the public and are a good source of information on drugs that are under review for regulatory approval, scientific matters such as safety issues related to particular drug classes, and public discussion prior to the promulgation of guidelines. Although the best insight is gained by attending advisory committee meetings in person, transcripts, briefing documents, and presentation materials are enormously useful by themselves.

The US National Institutes of Health (NIH), through the National Library of Medicine, provides access to information on clinical trials currently underway at sites in the US and around the world. The web site, ClinicalTrials.gov is a registry of federally and privately supported clinical trials conducted in the US and around the world. The registry is a searchable, online database that provides information on study objectives, requirements for participation, locations of investigative sites, and contact information. As of this writing, ClinicalTrials.gov contained information on 94 215 trials conducted in the US and 173 countries, including those sponsored by US federal government agencies (such as NIH) and private industry [24].

Pharmaceutical companies provide data on trials that are underway and results for trials that have completed. For example, Novartis posts information on clinical trials that are currently recruiting subjects as well as results from completed trials in searchable, online databases [25, 26]. Most large pharmaceutical companies provide similar internet access to information on their projects in development. Although the information posted in these documents is sometimes not highly detailed, considerable insight can be gained into design considerations and performance of endpoints used in studies.

Proprietary databases also exist which gather publically available information into a searchable format. One example of this kind of database, TrialTrove, is marketed by Citeline Intelligence Solutions [27]. TrialTrove provides surveillance of planned, ongoing, and completed clinical trials from numerous public domain sources. The information is reviewed by a scientific analyst staff and sorted into topic and discipline areas. The database can be searched by drug name, indication or disease state, and specific pharmacologic approaches. The information is similar to that available from government and company databases but in general is more detailed and provides information reported from sources such as press releases that are not typically cited by companies or government sites. Access to databases of this kind requires subscription payments.

Conclusions

Clinical development is an expensive and time consuming effort that must be carefully planned in order to provide essential information to characterize the risks and benefits of a drug or device. In planning a clinical research program, it is useful to consider the sequence of questions that must be posed and answered in order to proceed through each stage of data gathering, keeping the ultimate objective in mind. As the plan for development unfolds, the specific tactics used to answer questions may change as results become available. Although studies typically become progressively larger and operationally more complicated as development proceeds into late stage, the specific questions posed are usually more focused as the specific characteristics of a drug are revealed. There are numerous information resources apart from scientific literature that should be used when creating a clinical development plan.

References

1. Gilman S, Koller M, Black RS, *et al.* Clinical effects of Abeta immunization (AN1792) in patients with AD in an interrupted trial. *Neurology* 2005; **64**: 1553–62.

2. Mehta LR, Schwid SR, Arnold DL, *et al.* Proof of concept studies for tissue-protective agents in multiple sclerosis. *Mult Scler* 2009; **15**: 542–6.

3. Chalon S, Pereira A, Lainey E, *et al.* Comparative effects of duloxetine and desipramine on sleep EEG in healthy subjects. *Psychopharmacology (Berl)* 2005; **177**: 357–65.

4. Okamura N, Funaki Y, Tashiro M, *et al.* In vivo visualization of donepezil binding in the brain of patients with Alzheimer's disease. *Br J Clin Pharmacol* 2008 **65**: 472–9.

5. Rinne JO, Brooks DJ, Rossor MN, *et al.* 11C-PiB PET assessment of change in fibrillar amyloid-beta load in patients with Alzheimer's disease treated with bapineuzumab: a phase 2, double-blind, placebo-controlled, ascending-dose study. *Lancet Neurol* 2010; **9**: 363–72.

6. Wong DF, Tauscher J, and Gründer G. The role of imaging in proof of concept for CNS drug discovery and development. *Neuropsychopharmacology* 2009; **34**: 187–203.

7. Pihlajamäki M and Sperling RA. Functional MRI assessment of task-induced deactivation of the default mode network in Alzheimer's disease and at-risk older individuals. *Behav Neurol* 2009; **21**: 77–91.

8. Uppoor RS, Mummaneni P, Cooper E, *et al.* The use of imaging in the early development of neuropharmacological drugs: a survey of approved NDAs. *Clin Pharmacol Ther* 2008; **84**: 69–74.

9. RL Lalonde, KG Kowalski, MM Hutmacher, *et al.* Model-based drug development. *Clin Pharm Therap* 2007; **82**: 21–32.

10. Cross J, Lee H, Westelinck A, *et al*. Postmarketing drug dosage changes of 499 FDA-approved new molecular entities, 1980–1999. *Pharmacoepidem Drug Safety* 2002; **11**: 439–46.

11. Guidance for Industry: Patient-Reported Outcome Measures: Use in Medical Product Development to Support Labeling. 2009. www.fda.gov/downloads/Drugs/…/Guidances/UCM193282.pdf.

12. Rickels K, Garcia-Espana F, Mandos LA, *et al*. Physician withdrawal checklist (PWC-20). *J Clin Psychopharmacol* 2008; **28**: 447–51.

13. Mansbach RS, Feltner DE, Gold LH and Schnoll SH. Incorporating the assessment of abuse liability into the drug discovery and development process. *Drug Alcohol Depend* 2003; **70**: S73–85.

14. van der Wouden JC, Blankenstein AH, Huibers MJ, *et al*. Survey among 78 studies showed that Lasagna's law holds in Dutch primary care research. *J Clin Epidemiol* 2007; **60**: 819–24.

15. Quinlan J, Gaydos B, Maca J, *et al*. Barriers and opportunities for implementation of adaptive designs in pharmaceutical product development. *Clin Trials* 2010; **7**: 167–73.

16. International Conference on Harmonisation of Technical Requirements for Registration of Pharmaceuticals for Human Use. ICH Harmonised Tripartite Guideline: The extent of population exposure to assess clinical safety for drugs intended for long-term treatment of non-life-threatening conditions, E1. http://www.ich.org/MediaServer.jser?@_ID=435&@_MODE=GLB (Accessed August 2010.)

17. Lyrica package insert. http://www.pfizer.com/pfizer/download/uspi_lyrica.pdf (Accessed August 2010.)

18. Temple R, Comments made at presentation at Drug Information Association meeting, June 14, 2004. Washington, DC.

19. Maca J, Bhattacharya S, Dragalin V, *et al*. Adaptive Seamless Phase II/III Designs—Background, Operational Aspects, and Examples. *Drug Inf J* 2006; **40**: 463–73.

20. US Food and Drug Administration, Guidances (Drugs). http://www.fda.gov/drugs/guidancecomplianceregulatoryinformation/guidances/default.htm (Accessed August 2010.)

21. US Food and Drug Administration, Drugs@FDA. http://www.accessdata.fda.gov/scripts/cder/drugsatfda/index.cfm (Accessed August 2010.)

22. European Medicines Agency. http://www.ema.europa.eu/ema/index.jsp?curl=pages/home/Home_Page.jsp&murl=&mid=&jsenabled=true (Accessed August 2010.)

23. US Food and Drug Administration, Advisory Committees. http://www.fda.gov/AdvisoryCommittees/default.htm (Accessed August 2010.)

24. ClinicalTrials.gov. http://clinicaltrials.gov/ (Accessed August 2010.)

25. Novartis Research and Development, Clinical Trials. http://www.novartis.com/research/clinical-trial.shtml (Accessed August 2010.)

26. Novartis Clinical Trial Results Database, Neuroscience. http://www.novctrd.com/ctrdWebApp/clinicaltrialrepository/public/products.jsp?divisionId=2&diseaseAreaID=3 (Accessed August 2010.)

27. Citeline Products and Services: Citeline TrialTrove. http://www.citeline.com/trialtrove (Accessed August 2010.)

Unique challenges in the development of therapies for neurological disorders

Gilmore N. O'Neill

Introduction

The ultimate goal of clinical science is to identify novel therapeutics to relieve human suffering. Therapies for neurological diseases, including amyotrophic lateral sclerosis (ALS), Parkinson's disease (PD), Alzheimer's disease (AD), schizophrenia and neuropathic pain aim to arrest or slow the progression of disease, the worsening of disability and/or relieve symptoms.

The challenge of any therapeutic development plan is to deliver, with confidence, the appropriate concentration of an intervention to the intended target on the intended cell type(s), in the intended tissue type for the intended duration of time. To do this, it is necessary to confirm that the target of interest is expressed in humans, and most particularly, in human disease of interest and then to confirm one's ability to hit the target and drive the expected downstream effects (Figure 3.1). In this chapter we will discuss the unique challenges to answering these questions when developing CNS therapies. Difficulties arise because of the elusive nature of the targets, the challenges of delivering therapies across the blood brain barrier (BBB) (delivery and efflux equilibrium), the intricacies of models of CNS biologies and the handicaps to measuring drug concentrations and pharmacodynamic markers in the CNS. In addition, clinical trials suffer from the insidious course followed by many neurological diseases, from the limitations of functional outcome measures, which have been often developed as descriptors or classifiers of disease rather than clinical trial endpoint, e.g., Expanded Disability Status Scale (EDSS), and from the challenges posed by diseases that may only clinically manifest after the accumulation of significant pathologic burdens. It is these difficulties that are largely responsible for the greater than average attrition rates in late CNS drug development. Therefore, every effort

should be made to develop the techniques, early in a drug's development, that are necessary to answer these questions as soon as possible after entry into human studies. Indeed, serious consideration should be made not to advance a drug or therapeutic program in the absence of these techniques to avoid exposing patients to risks not balanced by a reasonable probability of efficacy and to avoid squandering critical resources.

Notwithstanding this thesis in support of rational drug development, if empirically compelling human trial data appear then an opportunistic approach is reasonable.

In the previous chapter (Chapter 2), you will have read about the general principles of drug development and will have seen how specific questions are posed and answered at different stages of a drug's development. In Chapter 1, you will read about the enormous and ever increasing human and economic burden of neurological and psychiatric disease on this planet. This chapter will focus on the key early phase questions that must be answered prior to starting pivotal or registrations trials. Prior to initiating phase 3 studies, which use considerable resources and expose a large number of patients to risks associated with a novel therapeutic, the early studies should have:

- identified the optimal population(s) in which to develop the new therapeutic
- preliminarily defined the dosing paradigm for the novel therapeutic so that investigators can be confident that the biology under investigation is being impacted by the investigational therapeutic.

Rational drug development identifies biological targets that may be important to a disease's pathophysiological process and then creates interventions that impact these targets. The key challenge to drug development is the translation of these discoveries from the laboratory

Clinical Trials in Neurology, ed. Bernard Ravina, Jeffrey Cummings, Michael P. McDermott, and R. Michael Poole. Published by Cambridge University Press. © Cambridge University Press 2012.

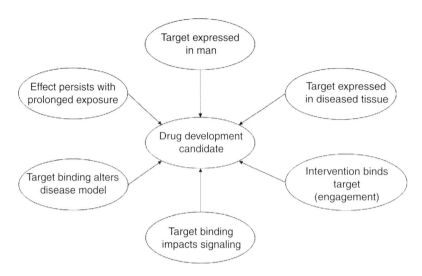

Figure 3.1. Examples of factors that determine the ability to translate from a potential target to a clinical development candidate.

bench into the human patient. It is in this endeavor that clinical biomarkers can be used.

In considering clinical biomarkers it is important to distinguish between pharmacodynamic markers that measure the biological effect of a therapeutic intervention and other biomarkers that reflect the pathophysiological processes of the targeted clinical disease. A pharmacodynamic biomarker allows the investigator to ascertain if the study drug is interacting with and affecting its desired target and helps to identify the dosage range and exposures required to affect this target. A pharmacodynamic marker will not necessarily predict a therapeutically meaningful effect in the studied disease and population, but it will allow the investigator to confirm that the biological hypothesis has been tested in clinical trials leading to a definitive 'positive' or 'negative' outcome. Such a clear binary outcome is eminently more desirable than a 'failed' study where the clinical outcome in the disease population is negative but it is not known if the targeted biology was altered by the study drug.

Examples of pharmacodynamic markers include assays of dystrophin in studies of therapeutic ribosomal read-through of premature termination codons in Duchenne muscular dystrophy and Aβ clearance from the brain in AD. Biomarkers that reflect the pathophysiological process of the target neurodegenerative disease are used to identify the optimal test population for a new therapeutic, to monitor disease progression, and to measure slowing of disease progression. Examples of biomarkers of disease pathophysiology include MRI brain lesion number and volume in

multiple sclerosis (MS) and Pittsburgh Compound B PET scanning to confirm the presence of Aβ plaque in the brains of AD disease (AD) patients. In some instances, changes in these biomarkers (MS MRI) are also highly predictive of a clinical effect [1].

Development of pharmacodynamic (Pd) biomarkers for CNS drug development should be a high priority. For timely delivery of such biomarkers, their development should occur in parallel with transition of a molecule from non-clinical to clinical development.

Why are CNS diseases difficult to treat?

It is well recognized that few drugs (~11%) entering clinical trials will be approved for human use [2]. Indeed, the rate of successful development is poorer for CNS drugs than other therapeutic areas, averaging only 8% [3] with half of these failures occurring late in development (see Chapter 2).

Unfortunately, many of these failed development programs have been associated with persisting uncertainty about the relevance of their biological targets to human diseases. The story of neurotrophic factor development in ALS and PD is a great example, where clinical trials were conducted without any certainty that the interventions actually entered the CNS in adequate concentrations or impacted their cognate receptors [4–6].

In addition, difficulties arise because of the complexity of the CNS and the challenges of developing clinical endpoints to capture therapeutic effects on multiple functional domains controlled by complex brain circuits. Some of these problems have arisen because we have historically used clinical scales that were developed to describe subgroups of domains affected by CNS diseases. One example is the EDSS in MS which is largely influenced by lower extremity walking function, but less so by cognition or upper extremity function. Furthermore, it has been extremely difficult to determine and agree on what degree of change represents a clinically meaningful outcome. All of these factors have contributed to a high degree of failure in late stages of development (see Chapter 2).

This chapter will focus on the challenges presented by therapeutic targets in the CNS, the manner in which animal models have and can be used to support the translation of therapeutic biologies to the human CNS, the BBB, and the uncertainties of CNS drug exposures. This chapter will also attempt to address how these challenges can be met and the associated risks of CNS therapeutic development mitigated.

Targets

CNS targets traditionally tend to be proteins that are critical to neural signaling, trophic signaling, or guidance of neural projections. Neural signaling proteins include neurotransmitter receptors, ion channels, and neurotransmitter transporters. Other proteins include members of the glial cell line-derived factor (GDNF), neurotrophin and other trophic factor receptor families. Finally, a complex network of repulsion and attraction guidance factors includes the Nogo receptor, Lingo receptor, and semaphorin families.

Target selection is always difficult in the drug development process. It is particularly challenging for neurological indications owing to the relative complexity of the human CNS, the paucity of validated targets (most neurological targets, while tantalizing, are poorly validated and thus very risky) and the 'orphan' nature of many neurological diseases.

CNS targets that have been clinically validated in human CNS disease include the dopamine D2, serotonin 5HT1b, gamma amino butyric acid-A (GABA-A), N-methyl-D-aspartate (NMDA) receptors, norepinephrine and 5HT transporters and monoamine oxidase and catechol-O-methyl transferase (COMT). Additionally MS, which is the most successful field of neurotherapeutics when one considers disease modification, has several robustly validated targets that include the VLA-4 integrin and type 1 interferon receptors.

Non-validated targets are numerous and have and will be identified through the understanding

and modeling of putative disease related pathways. Analyses of human neuropathology and disease genetics have identified targets such as $A\beta$ amyloid and tau in Alzheimer's disease, and NGF, TRPV1 and voltage-gated sodium channels in pain.

When considering such high risk targets, it is necessary to develop as much information as possible around the target's expression in human disease and to predict the behavior of the target's specific pharmaceutical effects, including affinities, metabolism and CNS concentrations, and biological effects prior to making decisions to advance through clinical trials.

Animal models of CNS biology and 'human disease'

Animal CNS disease models are unique tools that have led to a significant increase in the number of potential new therapeutic targets and an improved understanding of the biologies underlying disease processes. They have, however, proven disappointing in predicting therapeutic efficacy in humans in many areas including neuropathic pain, ALS, PD, stroke, spinal cord injury and MS [7–9]. This has led to considerable debate about the use of animal models in drug discovery. Nevertheless, models have clear utility and have largely suffered from the use of incorrect assumptions, inappropriate endpoints, and a failure to understand their limitations. Models attempt to extend human pathology to other species or to in vitro systems. Few models succeed in perfect replication of human disease. The modeling of human nervous system biologies to lower species such as rodents is particularly difficult. Some reasons for this include the enormous relative complexity of the human cerebral cortex required to support language, self-awareness, and comprehension, in addition to the deep nuclear development required for upright walking. This significantly impacts human drug development. In pain, for example, the main burden of pain is spontaneous while animal models can only be interrogated using evoked pain outcomes such as thermal hyperalgesia. Similar issues can be expected in cognitive research and drug development for spinal cord injury and psychiatric disease. The reasons for the translational disconnect between rodents and humans have been recently summarized [8].

Many targets lack homology across species and thus have quite different affinities for drug molecules. In addition, animal models are quite susceptible to changes in genetic background and transgenic animal models

21

in humans [39]. Non-clinical radio-pathological correlation experiments have confirmed the feasibility of imaging Aβ clearance [40] from the CNS. In addition, a reduction in Pittsburgh B signaling in human brain PET scan following passive immunotherapy has been demonstrated [41], further supporting the validity of this methodology for deriving biological proof of principle in human CNS trials. There are no human data that these interventions or CNS Aβ clearance mitigate AD dementia, but the biologically relevant doses have been defined allowing the necessary Phase 3 confirmatory studies that use clinical dementia outcome measures to confidently test the hypothesis that Aβ deposition in the brain is a key pathophysiological event that drives AD dementia.

Similar non-clinical and phase 0 clinical preparatory non- and clinical studies are warranted for the development of Pd biomarkers for proof of biological principle studies. Such tools can markedly reduce the risk of moving forward in CNS drug development by providing robust proof of biology and by identifying a biologically relevant dose range for further clinical studies.

Conclusions

All clinical trials, as any scientific experiment, must give a clear answer that supports a clear decision. This goal is particularly challenging for CNS therapeutics development and has resulted in a high historical rate of attrition. Nevertheless new imaging and biochemical and electrophysiological methods offer opportunities to mitigate the risks of failure. To do this, a CNS drug development plan must define clear parameters to test a biological hypothesis through the direct or indirect confirmation of target engagement and alteration within the CNS (through CNS imaging, electrophysiological, or biochemical assays) followed by correlation of that biology to a clinical outcome that is clinically meaningful. In other words, the goal of early Phase 1 and 2 development is to confirm biological effect prior to embarking on phase 3 comparative efficacy clinical protocol.

References

1. Sormani MP, Bonzano L, Roccatagliata L, *et al.* Magnetic resonance imaging as a potential surrogate for relapses in multiple sclerosis: a meta-analytic approach. *Ann Neurol* 2009; **65**: 268–75.

2. Kola I, Landis J. Can the pharmaceutical industry reduce attrition rates? *Nature Rev* 2004; **3**: 711–5.

3. Miller G. Is pharma running out of brainy ideas? *Science* 2010; **329**: 502–4.

4. Gill SS, Patel NK, Hotton GR, *et al.* Direct brain infusion of glial cell line-derived neurotrophic factor in Parkinson disease. *Nature Med* 2003; **9**: 589–95.

5. A controlled trial of recombinant methionyl human BDNF in ALS: The BDNF Study Group (Phase III). *Neurology* 1999; **52**: 1427–33.

6. Ochs G, Penn RD, York M, *et al.* A phase I/II trial of recombinant methionyl human brain derived neurotrophic factor administered by intrathecal infusion to patients with amyotrophic lateral sclerosis. *Amyotroph Lateral Scler Other Motor Neuron Disord* 2000; **1**(3): 201–6.

7. Rothstein JD. Current hypotheses for the underlying biology of amyotrophic lateral sclerosis. *Ann Neurol* 2009; **65**(Suppl 1): S3–9.

8. Geerts H. Of mice and men: bridging the translational disconnect in CNS drug discovery. *CNS Drugs* 2009; **23**: 915–26.

9. Akhtar AZ, Pippin JJ, Sandusky CB. Animal models in spinal cord injury: a review. *Rev Neurosci* 2008; **19**: 47–60.

10. Ludolph AC, Bendotti C, Blaugrund E, *et al.* Guidelines for preclinical animal research in ALS/MND: A consensus meeting. *Amyotroph Lateral Scler* 2010; **11**: 38–45.

11. Gold R, Linington C, and Lassmann H. Understanding pathogenesis and therapy of multiple sclerosis via animal models: 70 years of merits and culprits in experimental autoimmune encephalomyelitis research. *Brain* 2006; **129**: 1953–71.

12. Wilcock DM, Rojiani A, Rosenthal A, *et al.* Passive amyloid immunotherapy clears amyloid and transiently activates microglia in a transgenic mouse model of amyloid deposition. *J Neurosci* 2004; **24**: 6144–51.

13. Ghersi-Egea JF, Leininger-Muller B, Cecchelli R, and Fenstermacher JD. Blood-brain interfaces: relevance to cerebral drug metabolism. *Toxicol Lett* 1995; **82–83**: 645–53.

14. Terasaki T and Ohtsuki S. Brain-to-blood transporters for endogenous substrates and xenobiotics at the blood-brain barrier: an overview of biology and methodology. *NeuroRx* 2005; **2**: 63–72.

15. Loscher W and Potschka H. Blood-brain barrier active efflux transporters: ATP-binding cassette gene family. *NeuroRx* 2005; **2**: 86–98.

16. Patel MM, Goyal BR, Bhadada SV, *et al.* Getting into the brain: approaches to enhance brain drug delivery. *CNS Drugs* 2009; **23**: 35–58.

17. Neuwelt E, Abbott NJ, Abrey L, *et al.* Strategies to advance translational research into brain barriers. *Lancet Neurol* 2008; **7**: 84–96.

18. Rambeck B, Jurgens UH, May TW, *et al.* Comparison of brain extracellular fluid, brain tissue, cerebrospinal fluid, and serum concentrations of antiepileptic drugs measured intraoperatively in patients with intractable epilepsy. *Epilepsia* 2006; **47**: 681–94.

19. Norinder U and Haeberlein M. Computational approaches to the prediction of the blood-brain distribution. *Adv Drug Deliv Rev* 2002; **54**: 291–313.

20. Lohmann C, Huwel S, and Galla HJ. Predicting blood-brain barrier permeability of drugs: evaluation of different in vitro assays. *J Drug Target* 2002; **10**: 263–76.

21. Rubenstein JL, Combs D, Rosenberg J, *et al.* Rituximab therapy for CNS lymphomas: targeting the leptomeningeal compartment. *Blood* 2003; **101**: 466–8.

22. Pardridge WM. Drug delivery to the brain. *J Cereb Blood Flow Metab* 1997; **17**: 713–31.

23. Kroll RA and Neuwelt EA. Outwitting the blood-brain barrier for therapeutic purposes: osmotic opening and other means. *Neurosurgery* 1998; **42**: 1083–99; Discussion 99–100.

24. Salvatore MF, Ai Y, Fischer B, *et al.* Point source concentration of GDNF may explain failure of phase II clinical trial. *Exper Neurol* 2006; **202**: 497–505.

25. Lonser RR, Schiffman R, Robison RA, *et al.* Image-guided, direct convective delivery of glucocerebrosidase for neuronopathic Gaucher disease. *Neurology* 2007; **68**: 254–61.

26. Krewson CE, Klarman ML, and Saltzman WM. Distribution of nerve growth factor following direct delivery to brain interstitium. *Brain Res* 1995; **680**: 196–206.

27. Blasberg RG, Patlak C, and Fenstermacher JD. Intrathecal chemotherapy: brain tissue profiles after ventriculocisternal perfusion. *J Pharmacol Exper Ther* 1975; **195**: 73–83.

28. Frank R and Hargreaves R. Clinical biomarkers in drug discovery and development. *Nature Rev* 2003; **2**: 566–80.

29. Biomarkers Definitions Working Group Biomarkers and surrogate endpoints: preferred definitions and conceptual framework. *Clin Pharmacol Therap* 2001; **69**: 89–95.

30. Helmy A, Carpenter KL, and Hutchinson PJ. Microdialysis in the human brain and its potential role in the development and clinical assessment of drugs. *Curr Med Chem* 2007; **14**: 1525–37.

31. Lin JH. CSF as a surrogate for assessing CNS exposure: an industrial perspective. *Curr Drug Metab* 2008; **9**: 46–59.

32. Weinmann O, Schnell L, Ghosh A, *et al.* Intrathecally infused antibodies against Nogo-A penetrate the CNS and downregulate the endogenous neurite growth inhibitor Nogo-A. *Mol Cell Neurosci* 2006; **32**: 161–73.

33. Brooks DJ, Papapetropoulos S, Vandenhende F, *et al.* An open-label, positron emission tomography study to assess adenosine A2A brain receptor occupancy of vipadenant (BIIB014) at steady-state levels in healthy male volunteers. *Clin Neuropharmacol* 2010; **33**: 55–60.

34. Finkel RS. Read-through strategies for suppression of nonsense mutations in Duchenne/ Becker muscular dystrophy: aminoglycosides and ataluren (PTC124). *J Child Neurol* 2010; **25**: 1158–64.

35. Welch EM, Barton ER, Zhuo J, *et al.* PTC124 targets genetic disorders caused by nonsense mutations. *Nature* 2007; **447**: 87–91.

36. Siemers ER, Friedrich S, Dean RA, *et al.* Safety and changes in plasma and cerebrospinal fluid amyloid beta after a single administration of an amyloid beta monoclonal antibody in subjects with Alzheimer disease. *Clin Neuropharmacol* 2010; **33**: 67–73.

37. DeMattos RB, Bales KR, Cummins DJ, *et al.* Peripheral anti-A beta antibody alters CNS and plasma A beta clearance and decreases brain A beta burden in a mouse model of Alzheimer's disease. *Proc Natl Acad Sci USA* 2001; **98**: 8850–5.

38. Blennow K, Zetterberg H, Minthon L, *et al.* Longitudinal stability of CSF biomarkers in Alzheimer's disease. *Neurosc Lett* 2007; **419**: 18–22.

39. Bacskai BJ, Frosch MP, Freeman SH, *et al.* Molecular imaging with Pittsburgh Compound B confirmed at autopsy: a case report. *Arch Neurol* 2007; **64**: 431–4.

40. Maeda J, Ji B, Irie T, *et al.* Longitudinal, quantitative assessment of amyloid, neuroinflammation, and anti-amyloid treatment in a living mouse model of Alzheimer's disease enabled by positron emission tomography. *J Neurosci* 2007; **27**: 10957–68.

41. Rinne JO, Brooks DJ, Rossor MN, *et al.* 11C-PiB PET assessment of change in fibrillar amyloid-beta load in patients with Alzheimer's disease treated with bapineuzumab: a phase 2, double-blind, placebo-controlled, ascending-dose study. *Lancet Neurol* 2010; **9**: 363–72.

Fundamentals of biostatistics

Judith Bebchuk and Janet Wittes

Statistical formulation of clinical questions

While in vitro and animal experimentation can yield valuable information about the action of a new drug or other intervention, only clinical trials on human beings can determine a drug's safety profile and clinical efficacy in humans. The necessity for using people as subjects in potentially risky experiments makes clinical trials difficult to perform well, since they must be conducted in accordance not only with scientific rigor but also observing ethical guidelines, regulatory codes, and legal statutes. Furthermore, the investigators designing and carrying out a clinical trial must be fully aware of the serious consequences of their findings and must maintain high standards of scientific probity. The large number of competing therapies, the high cost of conducting a clinical trial, the ethical considerations that mandate against further testing of therapies shown to have an unfavorable profile of risks and benefits, and the desire for the timely introduction of new and effective therapies into general application all sharply limit the redundancy of clinical research and increase the importance of the integrity of individual studies. For example, if a clinical trial wrongly declares a beneficial therapy to be ineffective, the potential gains from use of the therapy will most likely be lost indefinitely because the therapy will probably not be tested again. Conversely, the falseness of a finding that an unsafe drug is safe or that a worthless therapy is beneficial may not be detected until large amounts of resources are wasted or until many people are hurt.

This chapter highlights some important aspects of the design and analysis of clinical trials and sketches a number of relevant statistical concepts [1–3]. The remainder of this book presents more complete discussions of various topics addressed in this chapter. The chapter begins with some general ideas about the design of controlled clinical trials. It then sketches in basic statistical principles with an introduction to calculating the necessary sample size for trials. A basic formula is presented for sample size that can be adapted to continuous, binary, and time-to-failure variables. Because of the importance in neurology of trials studying time to failure, analyses relevant to this type of outcome are then introduced. Issues related to the effect of multiplicity on sample size are addressed and issues that affect sample size are mentioned. Finally, Bayesian analysis is briefly introduced. Throughout, we illustrate the methods using an example from a hypothetical trial that tests the cognitive subscale of the Alzheimer's Disease Assessment Scale (ADAS-Cog).

General principles of the design of controlled clinical trials

A controlled clinical trial of a medical intervention should have at least one primary hypothesis that drives its design. Typically, the hypothesis is expressed in terms of the effect of the intervention on one or more outcomes of primary interest. For example, investigators studying a new drug that potentially decreases the rate of loss of cognitive functioning may hypothesize that the drug will lead to a lower decline of score on a cognitive assessment test than the control treatment. In general, the more explicit the stated primary purpose, the more likely one can design a feasible study to answer the question of interest.

Well-designed and well-executed trials include an unambiguous protocol approved by the Institutional

Clinical Trials in Neurology, ed. Bernard Ravina, Jeffrey Cummings, Michael P. McDermott, and R. Michael Poole. Published by Cambridge University Press. © Cambridge University Press 2012.

Review Boards (IRBs) or Ethics Committees of the participating clinics, laboratories, and data centers. The comprehensiveness of both the protocol and its supporting manuals of operation should reflect the size and complexity of the investigation and the length of the follow-up, as well as the number of clinical centers, laboratories, and other organizations involved. During a trial, unexpected events may occur that necessitate changes in the protocol. The protocol should include explicit, well-documented procedures for making amendments after the study has begun in order to protect the scientific integrity of the trial.

Primary outcome

A clinical trial should include at least one explicit, unambiguously defined primary outcome that forms the basis for calculating the sample size of the trial. For example, in a study of the effect of a new anti-dementia drug on progression of Alzheimer's disease, the protocol should state the outcome in terms of the measure that will be used. For example, the endpoint may be 'cognitive function' or 'functional ability' as assessed by a specific instrument but not a vague reference to 'measures of disease progression.'

Most neurological clinical trials have one of three types of primary outcome: a continuous or ordinal variable, a binary variable, or a time-to-failure variable. These three types of outcomes lead to different types of studies.

A continuous variable is a quantity like a score that is measured on a continuous, or nearly continuous, scale. (In the specific example of ADAS-Cog, the score ranges from 0 to 70.) An ordinal variable has several ordered classes. For example, the Clinical Global Impression is a 7-point scale that measures the global functional status of a patient. A binary variable has two possible values, for example, a score above or below 40 on the ADAS-Cog or, for trials studying the effect of an intervention on mortality, dead or alive.

A time-to-failure variable measures the time from randomization to the occurrence of an event. (Some trials use time from initiation of treatment, but using any time different from randomization compromises the expected equivalence of the study groups assured by the process of randomization.) Time to death and time to loss of 20 points on the ADAS-Cog are examples of time-to-failure variables. See Chapter 7 for a fuller discussion on issues related to measurement.

Secondary and exploratory outcomes

Most clinical trials in neurology study more than the primary outcome. Secondary outcomes are measures that are of clinical interest but are less important to the aims of the trial than the primary outcome.

The protocols of many clinical trials list a host of secondary outcomes with little consideration of their relative importance in terms of the inferences to be made from the trial. A helpful rule of thumb is to consider as secondary outcomes only those for which the investigators have formal hypotheses. Using that guideline, the investigators should include in the protocol of a clinical trial a list of the secondary outcomes with the planned methods of measurement and analysis as well as the magnitude of treatment effect the study is likely to detect. When secondary outcomes are specified, investigators should in general use the same degree of care in collecting relevant data for these outcomes as for the primary outcomes.

In addition to formal secondary outcomes, the protocol may list many variables to be measured as exploratory outcomes. Often, the sample size of the trial is too small to expect precise assessments of the effect of the experimental intervention on these outcomes. In other cases, too little information is available to calculate power for these explanatory outcomes. Moreover, the degree of care in collecting and validating these outcomes may be less intense than the care exerted for the primary and secondary outcomes.

Study population

A clinical trial must achieve a balance between the advantages of homogeneity and the advantages of heterogeneity. Ideally, the study cohort is sufficiently homogeneous to yield a high probability of learning whether a therapy is safe and effective while sufficiently heterogeneous to provide assurance that the observed results are applicable to a wide range of people with the condition under study. No rule provides reliable guidance for planning the composition of the study cohort for a single study or for structuring a series of studies to investigate a therapy in different populations. Failure to anticipate fully the consequences of overly rigid inclusion and exclusion criteria for a clinical trial may lead to great difficulty in recruiting patients [4].

Designers of clinical trials should not overestimate the ability of investigators to recruit participants into the trial. We recommend as simple a set of entry and exclusion criteria as possible:

1. The criteria should mimic as closely as possible the patient population to which the results are intended to refer.

2. The criteria may exclude people who are unlikely to comply with the requirements of the protocol. For example, the study may exclude people who have severe underlying illnesses not under study, who are substance abusers, or who are likely to move to another geographic area during the study. Many trials exclude people who, because of cognitive problems, are not able to comply with the study regimen. In trials of neurological disorders, the patient population of interest may be cognitively impaired; in that case, the entry criteria should allow them to participate in the trial, but the protocol should be written in such a way as to facilitate compliance and the statistical analysis plan should deal explicitly with how to handle missing data arising from non-compliance. Similar considerations are relevant to trials of psychiatric conditions where the nature of the disease may lead to considerable non-compliance with the study regimen.

3. The criteria may exclude people taking medications that are not appropriate for use with the intervention being tested.

4. Exclusions on the basis of demographic criteria alone (e.g., sex, age, and race) are not often scientifically justifiable and may make recruitment unnecessarily difficult. In trials of new drugs, however, the standards of local IRBs and general ethical considerations may exclude women of childbearing potential. Furthermore, in trials of primary prevention of disease, a trial may reasonably exclude demographic subgroups with very low incidence rates to limit the sample size of the study and to focus the question of prevention on subgroups at high risk.

5. If possible, before the protocol is written, the entry and exclusion criteria should be applied to a database of people potentially eligible for the study in order to estimate the likely rate of recruitment.

Reference population

In planning a clinical trial, investigators often specify in the protocol the population to which the treatment is expected to apply. In particular, if a trial excludes a specific subgroup of people but investigators intend to generalize to a population more heterogeneous than that represented in the study cohort, the protocol should address both the justification for excluding the subgroup and the rationale for generalization to the reference population. Furthermore, the publications describing the results of the trial should include a description of the population to which the results are to be applied.

Projected timeline

Plans for a clinical trial should describe explicitly the timeline for an individual participant in the study. In studies in which the outcome is measured very soon after the participants are recruited, the timeline is uniform for each participant and follows calendar time, while in trials with long-term follow-up the timeline may differ for each participant [5]. In many long-term studies, patient enrollment takes place throughout the course of the trial, and follow-up for each participant continues until the trial ends. Some trials end on a pre-specified date; some end at a fixed number of months after the last participant has entered; and some end after a fixed number of primary outcome events have occurred. Because the rate of recruitment often differs from expected, the average follow-up time may be considerably longer or shorter than planned so that the probability of finding an effect of treatment may be higher, or lower, than expected. In particular, when recruitment is slower than anticipated, average follow-up time is likely to be longer than expected; conversely, rapid recruitment may lead to shorter follow-up time than planned.

Control group

Comparing observations from an experimental group to observations from a control group is central to science. In a few very unusual medical settings, the control group need not be explicit, for the new observation is so surprising that it defies all previous experience. Penicillin provides the classic example of a new drug that had an immediately obvious benefit and needed no control group to show efficacy. Almost always, however, the medical condition being studied varies in its presentation, and the treatment being studied elicits variable response. Therefore, rigorous, unbiased inference about the effect of a drug or other intervention requires comparison to a concurrent, randomized control. In very early phases of drug development a control group may not be necessary, but for clinical trials that aim to evaluate both safety and efficacy, a control group is important. Since adverse events in a treatment group may be either a result of the medical condition being treated or a reaction to the new drug, the safety of a drug can only be accurately assessed by comparison with a control group. Similarly, the beneficial effect of a treatment can be measured only in relation to a control. The control group may be a group treated with a number of interventions, including placebo, 'usual care', 'standard of care', 'other therapy' plus a placebo [5], a non-drug intervention (e.g., surgery or a behavioral intervention), or a competing drug. A control group should be as comparable as possible to the experimental group so that differences in the endpoint being studied are attributable solely to the difference in therapy. Randomization assures that the experimental and control groups have identical expected distributions of measured and unmeasured baseline variables. The larger the sample size, the more likely the two groups will be very similar to each other with regard to baseline characteristics. In small samples, while randomization ensures identical expected distributions, the actual distributions may differ sizably from each other by chance.

Basic statistics for randomized clinical trials

This section briefly describes the basic frequentist statistical testing paradigm used by the typical randomized clinical trial with particular reference to ideas necessary in selecting sample size. We do not address estimation because that topic is covered in Chapter 6. We introduce hypothesis testing and confidence intervals insofar as they are relevant to sample size calculation. Chapter 6 includes more detail.

Null and alternative hypotheses

The study question in a typical clinical trial is formulated in terms of two opposing hypotheses: the 'null' hypothesis and an 'alternative' hypothesis. The study is designed to provide evidence that will disprove the null and therefore 'accept' the alternative. For example, consider a trial of a drug whose purpose is to slow the rate of decline of the score on the ADAS-Cog. If the study has two arms, drug and placebo, the null hypothesis might be, 'Mean change in score from baseline in patients treated with drug is the same as among those treated with placebo.' A 'one-sided' alternative hypothesis would be, 'Mean decrease in score from baseline

is less among patients treated with drug than among those treated with placebo.' The use of a one-sided alternative implies that the investigators do not entertain the possibility that the drug might lead to a greater decrease in mean change in score from baseline compared to placebo. A 'two-sided' alternative hypothesis would state, 'Mean change in score from baseline is different among patients treated with drug than among those treated with placebo.' Adoption of a two-sided alternative allows the data to provide evidence of either favorable or unfavorable effect of drug on cognitive function. For most comparative efficacy studies in neurology, two-sided alternative hypotheses are considered appropriate.

The type I error, or 'α-level'

Having specified the null and alternative hypotheses, the investigators select an α-level, the probability of erroneously concluding that the null hypothesis is false if the null hypothesis is indeed true. Although the choice of α-level is arbitrary, many clinical trials use $\alpha = 0.05$ or $\alpha = 0.01$. To continue our example, suppose the new drug had no effect on the mean change in ADAS-Cog score from baseline and the investigators selected a two-sided α-level of 5%. Then, the probability would be 0.05 that the clinical trial would 'reject' the null hypothesis and falsely find that the mean change in score from baseline differs (either better or worse) in the treatment and control groups.

Many investigators view an experiment that produces a p-value less than 0.05 two-sided, or less than 0.025 one-sided, as strong evidence, even 'proof', that the treatment under study was effective. We caution that 0.05 is not a very stringent criterion – the probability that a single toss of a pair of dice yields two sixes is $1/36 = 0.028$. If you were playing a game of backgammon and your opponent rolled a pair of sixes on the first toss, you would think the opponent was lucky; you would not think the dice were loaded.

The type II error, or 'β-level'

To calculate sample size, the investigators must predict the degree of effect Δ_A of the therapy under study (the subscript A denotes 'alternative'). In our example, they might specify that drug treatment might lead to a decline in ADAS-Cog subscale that is less than 10 points lower than the decline in the control group. The β-level, or type II error rate, is the probability of failing to reject the null hypothesis if the true effect of the drug is Δ_A. The choice of β-level, like the choice of α-level, is arbitrary. Typical values used in many clinical trials are 5, 10, or 20%. The smaller the α- and β-levels, the less likely the clinical trial is to make an incorrect conclusion. In our example, β = 0.20 would imply, for example, that if the true effect of treatment were to halt average decline in the ADAS-Cog over the period of the study by a mean of 10 points more than the decline in the control group, the probability of failing to reject the null hypothesis would be 0.20, in which case we would not learn that the treatment was truly efficacious.

Statistical tests of significance

A test of significance is a procedure that calculates whether the observed data provide sufficient evidence to reject the null hypothesis. The choice of test depends on the nature of the outcome under study. Standard textbooks on statistics provide many tests tailored to different settings [6–8].

Sample size

Selection of the α- and β-levels and hypothesizing the effect Δ_A of drug, allow calculation of sample size. The required sample size increases with any of the following:

1. decreasing α-level
2. decreasing β-level
3. increasing variability of the outcome
4. decreasing Δ_A

Thus, although ideally the α- and β-levels would both be very small, practical and economic constraints limit the sample size and preclude arbitrarily low error rates.

Power

The power γ of a statistical test is 1 − β: the probability of rejecting the null hypothesis when the true effect of treatment is Δ_A. Power is often expressed in terms of percentages. In our example, the β-level is 0.20 so the power γ is 0.80, or, as usually expressed, 80%, when Δ_A = 10 points. Therefore, if the true effect of drug is to decrease the decline by 10 points relative to control, the power is 1 − 0.2 or 80%.

The power decreases with any of the following:

1. decreasing α-level
2. decreasing Δ_A

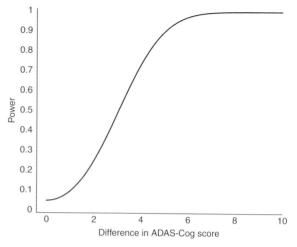

Figure 4.1. Power of a test of the difference in ADAS-Cog score between anti-dementia treatment and placebo. The standard deviation of ADAS-Cog score in each group is assumed to be 10.

3. decreasing sample size
4. increasing variability of the outcome

Note that while we speak of power at the alternative Δ_A, in fact power is a function of the class of possible alternatives. Rather than speak simply of power as a single number, a more useful construct is to consider power as a function γ(Δ) where the power is calculated over a range of values of effect sizes Δ (see Figure 4.1).

Figure 4.1 shows the power as a function of difference in ADAS-Cog scores for a test of a new anti-dementia drug compared with placebo. The study, which has been designed to have a two-sided α-level of 5%, has 84 participants each in the active and standard of care arms. The standard deviation of the ADAS-Cog score is assumed to be 10 points. Note that if the true difference in treatment effect between the anti-dementia drug and placebo is 5 points, the power to detect the difference is roughly 90%. If, however, the true difference is 2 points the power is only about 25%.

For fixed power, sample size increases proportionately to the variance (which is the square of the standard deviation) and inversely proportionately to the square of the difference to be detected. Thus, if for a given α-level and power, 100 people per group are needed to detect a difference of four points, then 400 are needed to detect a difference of two points.

The p-value

When all data from a study have been gathered, the primary hypothesis is tested. The p-value is the probability of observing an apparent effect of treatment at least as large as shown by the data if the null hypothesis is in fact true. The smaller the *p*-value, the more confidence in the conclusion that the null hypothesis is not true.

Confidence intervals

Closely related to statistical tests are confidence intervals. A statistical test asks whether one can reject the null hypothesis. A confidence interval is the set of null hypotheses that the data could have rejected had the statistical test been performed at the stated α-level. Suppose, for example, that the clinical trial of ADAS-Cog reports that the 95% confidence interval for the difference between the change from baseline in ADAD-Cog for the new drug and placebo is (4, 8). We can interpret the interval in one of two ways. One correct interpretation is that if we did an infinite number of identical clinical trials, 95% of the confidence intervals calculated would cover the true difference between the changes. Another interpretation is that the data from this trial would reject any null hypothesis less than 4 and greater than 8. In particular, it rejects the null hypothesis that the true difference is zero. Note the confidence interval does not mean that the probability is 95% that the true difference is between 4 and 8. Chapter 6 describes confidence intervals in more detail.

Sample size for controlled clinical trials

A basic formula for sample size

The statistical literature contains formulas for determining sample size in many specialized situations. This part describes a simple generic formula that provides a first approximation of sample size and that forms the basis of variations appropriate to specialized situations. To understand these principles, consider a trial that aims to compare two treatments with respect to a parameter of interest, again, say ADAS-Cog. For simplicity, suppose that half of the participants will be randomized to a new drug and the other half to a control group. The trial investigators may be aiming to compare mean values, proportions, odds ratios, hazard ratios, or some other statistic. Suppose that with proper mathematical transformation, the difference between the parameters in the treatment and control groups has an approximately normal distribution. These conditions allow construction of a generic formula for the required sample size. Typically, in comparing means or proportions, the difference between the sample statistics has an approximately normal distribution. In comparing odds ratios or hazard ratios, the logarithm of the ratio, or, equivalently, the difference in the logarithms, has this property.

Consider three different trials using a new drug called 'COG-Plus' to improve relative cognitive function score relative to control in a study group of people with Alzheimer's disease and a baseline cognitive functioning score of 20 or more.

The first hypothetical study, to be called the Slower COG Decline Trial, tests whether COG-Plus in fact lowers the rate of decline of cognitive functioning scores relative to placebo. The trial, which randomizes patients to receipt of COG-Plus or placebo, measures the cognitive functioning score at the end of the sixth month of therapy. The outcome is the continuous variable 'score on the ADAS-Cog.'

The second study, to be called the Low COG Prevention Trial, compares the proportions of people in the treated and control groups with cognitive functioning scores above 25 points at the end of 1 year of treatment with COG-Plus or placebo.

The third study, called the Time to COG-loss, follows patients for at least 5 years and compares times to loss of 10 points in the two groups. This type of outcome is a time-to-failure variable.

The formulas for determining sample size use several statistical concepts. Throughout this chapter, Greek letters denote a true or hypothesized value, while italic Roman letters denote observations.

Under the above conditions, a generic formula for the total number of persons needed in each group to achieve the stated type I (α) and type II (β) error rates is:

$$n = 2\sigma^2 \left\{ \left[\xi_{1-\alpha/2} + \xi_{1-\beta} \right] / \Delta_A \right\}^2$$

where σ^2 is the variance of the outcome measure and its square root σ is its standard deviation.

The formula assumes one treatment group and one control group of equal size and two-tailed hypothesis testing. The quantity ξ_x is the value that corresponds to the xth percentile of the standard normal distribution (e.g., $\xi_{0.975} = 1.96$ and $\xi_{0.8} = 0.84$). Typical controlled trials in neurology set the statistical significance level at 0.05 or 0.01 and the power at 80 or 90%. Table 4.1 shows the sample sizes required for

Table 4.1 Relative sample sizes as a function of statistical power and α level

			Power		
α	50%	70%	80%	90%	95%
0.05	0.5	0.8	**1.0**[a]	1.3	1.7
0.01	0.9	1.2	1.5	1.9	2.3
0.001	1.5	1.8	2.2	2.7	3.1

[a] Reference group.
To read the table, choose a power and an α level. Suppose one is interested in a trial with 90 percent power and an α level of 0.01. The entry of 1.9 in the table means that such a trial would require 1.9 times the sample size required for a trial with 80 percent power and an α level of 0.05.

various levels of α and β relative to the sample size needed for a study with a two-sided α equal to 0.05 and 80% power ($\beta = 0.20$).

Some people in using sample size formulae mistakenly interpret the '2' as meaning two groups and hence incorrectly use half the sample size necessary.

For tests at significance level 0.05, the sample size needed to achieve high power is considerably larger than the sample size needed to observe a p-value of 0.05. Thus, many people get confused by what appears to be a very large sample size needed to show statistical significance. They point to studies where a much smaller sample size demonstrated a statistically significant effect. In fact, that observation is correct: if a trial is designed with a two-sided α-level test of 0.05 and power of 80%, the expected p-value under the alternative is 0.005. Similarly, if the same trial had 90% power, the expected p-value would be 0.001 (see p. 43 of Proschan, *et al.* [3] for a proof). One way to understand this apparent contradiction is to consider the sample size required for 50% power. In that case, the sample size formula reduces to $N = 2\sigma^2 [\xi_{1-\alpha/2}/\Delta_A]^2$ because $\xi_{1-0.5} = \xi_{0.5} = 0$. In other words, the 'just barely significant' cut-off occurs at 50% power. The reason to design studies with larger sample sizes (e.g., studies with 80% or 90% power) is to ensure a high probability of actually showing statistical significance.

Continuous variables: testing the difference between mean responses

To calculate the sample size needed to test the difference between two mean values, one makes several assumptions.

1. The responses of participants are independent of each other. The formula does not apply to studies that randomize in groups, for example, trials that assign the same treatment to all students in a classroom, or all people in a village, or all visitors to a clinic, or to studies that match patients or parts of the body and randomize pairwise. For this type of randomization in groups (i.e., cluster randomization), see, for example, Donner and Klar [9]. Analysis of studies with pairwise randomization focuses on the difference between the results in the two members of the pair.
2. The variance of the response is the same in both the treated and control groups.
3. The sample size is large enough that the observed difference in means is approximately normally distributed. In practice, for reasonably symmetric distributions, a sample size of about 30 in each treatment arm is sufficient to apply normal theory. The central limit theorem legitimizes the use of the standard normal distribution. For a discussion of its appropriateness in a specific application, consult any standard textbook on statistics.
4. In practice, the variance is unknown. Therefore, the test statistic under the null hypothesis replaces σ with s, the sample standard deviation. The resulting statistic has a t distribution with $2(n-1)$ degrees of freedom (df). Under the alternative hypothesis, the statistic has a non-central t-distribution with non-centrality parameter $\sqrt{2n} \, \Delta_A$ and, again, $2(n-1)$ df. Standard software packages for sample size calculations employ the t and non-central t-distributions [10–12]. Except for small sample sizes, the difference between the normal distribution and the t-distribution is quite small, so the normal approximation yields adequately close sample sizes in most situations. Table 4.2 presents the necessary sample size for a two-arm study using the normal approximation under the assumption of no non-compliance with protocol.

Binary variables: testing the difference between two proportions

Calculation of the sample size needed to test the difference between two proportions requires several assumptions.

1. The responses of participants are independent.

Table 4.2 Approximate total sample size for a controlled clinical trial that compares two groups when the primary outcome is a continuous variable

	Power = 90%	Power = 80%
Δ/σ	(n)	(n)
0.1	4200	3100
0.2	1100	790
0.3	470	350
0.4	270	200
0.5	170	130
0.6	120	88
0.7	88	66
0.8	68	50
0.9	54	40
1.0	44	34
1.5	20	16
2.0	12	10

$\alpha = 0.05$; Δ is the difference to be detected and σ is the population standard deviation. The sample size per group is half the value in the table.

Table 4.3 Approximate total sample size for a controlled clinical trial that compares two groups when the primary endpoint is a binary variable

Proportion with the event in group 2	Proportion with the event in group 1					
	0.05	0.1	0.2	0.3	0.4	0.5
0.1	1242					
0.2	228	572				
0.3	102	178	824			
0.4	62	94	238	992		
0.5	42	58	116	268	1076	
0.6	32	40	66	122	280	1076
0.7	24	32	46	74	122	268
0.8	18	22	21	46	66	116
0.9	14	16	22	21	40	58

α – 0.05; power = 90%; table assumes no loss to follow up, no non-compliance, no multiple looks at the data, and uses the Fisher's exact test. The sample size per group is half the value in the table.

2. The probability of an event is π_c and π_t for each person in the control group and the treated group, respectively. Because the sample sizes in the two groups are equal, the average event rate is $\bar{\pi} = \dfrac{\pi_c + \pi_t}{2}$. This assumption of constancy of proportions within each group is rarely strictly valid. If the proportions vary considerably in recognized ways, one may refine the sample size calculations to reflect that heterogeneity. Often, however, one hypothesizes average values of π_c and π_t and calculates sample size as if those proportions applied to each individual in the study.

Under these assumptions, the binary outcome variable has a binomial distribution, and the following simple formula provides the sample size for each of the two groups:

$$n = 2\bar{\pi}\,(1-\bar{\pi})\,\frac{\left(\xi_{1-\alpha/2} + \xi_{1-\beta}\right)^2}{\left(\pi_c - \pi_t\right)^2}$$

The simple formula uses the same variance under both the null hypothesis and the alternative hypothesis. A more accurate approach would acknowledge that the variance under the null is proportional to $2\bar{\pi}(1-\bar{\pi})$ while under the alternative it is proportional to $\pi_c(1-\pi_c) + \pi_t(1-\pi_t)$.

The formula, which uses the normal approximation, becomes inaccurate as $n\pi_c$ and $n\pi_t$ become very small (e.g., less than 5). If one employs a correction for continuity in the final analysis, or if one will be using Fisher's exact test, one should replace n with the formula given by Fleiss [13]:

$$n' = \frac{n}{4}\left(1 + \sqrt{1 + \frac{4}{n|\pi_c - \pi_t|}}\right)^2$$

Table 4.3 presents the necessary sample size for a two-arm study using the test for proportions under the assumption of no non-compliance with protocol.

Failure time studies

Many neurological clinical trials compare therapies with respect to time to occurrence of the primary outcome. This time is often called *failure time* or *time to failure*. More optimistically, the time may be measured not as the time to failure but as the length of time the participant has not failed, or the *survival time*. Here we introduce several important concepts related to failure time distributions [14]. Specifically, we mention censoring, hazard, survival curves, the Kaplan-Meier representation of the estimated survival curves, the log-rank test, and the Cox proportional hazard model.

Censoring

Trials that compare time to failure usually end before all the participants experience the primary outcome under study. These participants are said to be 'censored' at the time of their last observation. In the usual methods of time-to-failure analysis, censoring is assumed to be 'non-informative;' that is, the mechanism causing the censoring favors neither those who are more likely to fail nor those who are less likely to fail [15]. Several mechanisms lead to censoring in clinical trials. The simplest type of censoring is so-called administrative censoring: the study ends before all persons experience the primary outcome. For example, in a 10-year study of survival among a low risk group, only a small proportion of the study group is expected to die by the time the study ends. At the end of the study, no one knows when an administratively censored person will die.

In some clinical trials, each participant has a fixed follow-up time. More typically, the trial ends on a 'common closeout date.' Since participants are recruited over a period of months or years, the length of the follow-up time is specific for each person. This 'staggered entry' leads to unequal time of administrative censoring. Because the degree of administrative censoring is independent of treatment, such censoring is non-informative. Standard life-table methods are appropriate for handling the resulting unequal follow-up times (see, for example, Collett [16]).

A second type of censoring is caused by loss to follow-up. In this case, the endpoint cannot be measured because the participant or the participant's medical records become unavailable to the study. A person is then censored at the time of loss. Vigorous efforts by the investigator can often minimize loss to follow-up. Some participants who have moved residences are willing to be measured at a clinic near their new home. Sometimes routinely collected data like the National Death Index can be used to ascertain vital status at the common closeout date even if the participant is not following study protocol. Loss to follow-up is conceptually more difficult to deal with than administrative censoring because such losses may be informative. The life-table methods appropriate to administrative censoring are strictly valid when some participants are lost to

follow-up only if the mechanism that leads to loss favors neither those who would have experienced the outcome nor those who would not have. In an effort to show that losses did not occur differentially by treatment group, many investigators use baseline parameters to compare those lost to follow-up to those who were not lost or compare the patients lost to follow-up from the treatment and the control groups. The fact that such a comparison shows no difference is not sufficient to preclude informative censoring. Imagine, for example, a study of memory agents that compares two groups of people with identical baseline parameters. During the course of the study, a number of people in the placebo group who have experienced a decrease in memory drop out of the study because they perceive that they are not receiving any benefit from the study agent and wish to switch to an efficacious treatment. Since functioning is associated both with memory loss and dropping out of the study, this censoring is informative in spite of the fact that all people in the study had identical baseline characteristics. Although standard life-table methods are very often used when patients are lost to follow-up, investigators should be aware of potential bias arising from loss to follow-up. Similar problems occur when participants withdraw from the trial. Such withdrawals are often not at random so that censoring them as if the withdrawal were non-informative can introduce bias into the analysis.

Another important type of censoring is that caused by competing risks. For example, in a long-term survival study of patients with Alzheimer's disease, many people die of causes other than those due to progression of their Alzheimer's disease during the course of the study. Such non-Alzheimer's death is a competing event that precludes the occurrence of the study outcome. This type of censoring is often informative. Censoring occurs only when the outcome cannot be measured. The standard methods of statistical analysis (e.g. life tables, Kaplan-Meier survival curves, the log-rank test, and Cox models) can deal with censoring computationally. All, however, make the assumption that the censoring is non-informative.

In summary, at any given time during the study only a subset of the study cohort is at risk for experiencing the primary outcome. This subset decreases each time a primary outcome occurs and each time a person leaves the study by loss to follow-up or by competing risk. Losses due to administrative censoring do not lead to bias in the inference about the estimated effect of treatment (except when the statistical methods confound loss and effect), but losses due to non-independent

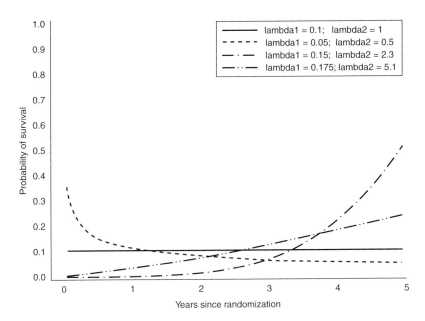

Figure 4.2. *Four hazard functions. The four hazard curves correspond to different clinical settings. A flat curve represents constant risk, the curve with lambda1 = 0.05 and lambda2 = 0.5 represents high immediate risk but diminishing risk as time proceeds. The two increasing curves show functions that describe deteriorating conditions.*

competing risks may lead to bias in the estimated size of the treatment effect.

Hazard rate

Consider a study that assigns time 0 to the date a patient was randomized. For any small interval of time Δt about a specific time t, the probability that a person will experience the event under study is represented by $h(t)\Delta t$. The function $h(t)$ is called the hazard function. Figure 4.2 plots four hazard curves that correspond to very different clinical settings. The flat line represents constant hazard; that is, the risk of mortality, or more generally, the risk of the event under study, is constant over time. The curve with $\lambda_1 = 0.05$ and $\lambda_2 = 0.5$ represents typical hazards after surgery: high immediate post-surgical mortality, but diminishing mortality risk as time proceeds. The two increasing curves show functions that describe deteriorating conditions. The curve with $\lambda_1 = 0.15$ and $\lambda_2 = 2.3$ represents a cohort of initially healthy people whose risk of death increases fairly steadily during the first 5 years after randomization. The curve with $\lambda_1 = 0.175$ and $\lambda_2 = 5.1$ depicts a cohort of people at low risk for death during the first 2 years, but rapidly increasing risk thereafter.

Survival curve

The function that describes the proportion of participants alive at time t is the survival curve $S(t)$. Figure 4.3 shows the four survival curves associated with the

hazard curves of Figure 4.2. In all cases, since $S(5) = 0.6$, 60% of the people live beyond 5 years. The hazard curve $h(t)$ is related mathematically to $S(t)$:

$$h(t) = \frac{-d\{\log[S(t)]\}}{dt}.$$

Kaplan-Meier curve

Perhaps the most common representation of the survival curve in clinical trials is the Kaplan-Meier curve, which interprets the survival curve as a product of probabilities. For example, in a 7-year trial of mortality following diagnosis of Alzheimer's disease the two-year survival rate can be written as:

$$S(2) = S(1)S(2|1)$$

where $S(2|1)$ is the probability of surviving at least 2 years for a participant who has survived for 1 year. Similarly, the 3-year survival rate is:

$$S(3) = S(1)S(2|1)S(3|2)$$

where $S(3|2)$ is the probability that a person who has survived for 2 years will survive for at least 3 years. Finally, the 7-year survival rate is:

$$S(7) = S(1)S(2|1)S(3|2)S(4|3)S(5|4)S(6|5)S(7|6)$$

To construct the Kaplan-Meier curve, we estimate each component probability from the set of

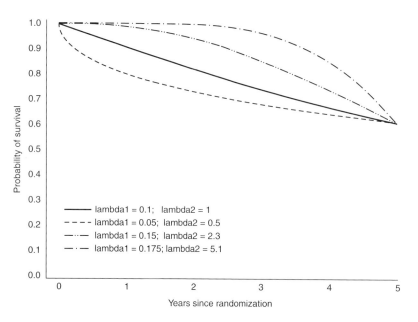

observations. In the typical Kaplan-Meier curve, each time a person dies the curve steps down; the height of the step represents the probability of death within the preceding horizontal time interval. The height of the graph from zero at each time t represents the overall probability of survival to time t. Figure 4.4 shows a typical Kaplan-Meier curve. Here, failure time is death. The curve starts at the point $(t,S(t)) = (0,1)$ because the entire patient cohort is alive at randomization. In most neurological clinical trials, $S(t)$ does not drop to zero because the study ends while some participants are still alive. To determine the median survival time, draw a horizontal line at 0.5 on the y-axis and when this line hits the survival curve draw a vertical line down to the x-axis. In this simple case, the median survival time is 38 months $[S(38)=0.5]$ and the dotted lines are shown on Figure 4.4. Many standard statistical software packages have subroutines that plot Kaplan-Meier curves. Note that the Kaplan-Meier estimator of the survival curve does not make any assumptions about the shape of either the survival curve or the hazard function. As previously mentioned, it does assume that censoring occurs non-informatively.

Log-rank test

The log-rank test is a widely used method for comparing survival curves in randomized clinical trials.

The test, which requires no assumptions regarding the shapes of the survival curves, compares treatment and control groups each time a person experiences the primary study outcome. Suppose, for example, at the time of the dth study outcome n_1 patients remain in the control and n_2 in the treated group. If treatment has no effect on the outcome, the death would have occurred in the control group with probability $n_1/(n_1 + n_2)$. The log-rank test compares the expected number of events in the control group during the study with the actual number observed. Standard texts on survival analysis present formulas for performing the calculation [16]. Because the calculation requires meticulous accounting for each person's time of event or censoring, we recommend using a standard computer program.

Sample size formulae

Consider a trial that compares time to some specified event – for example, loss of 10 points from baseline on the ADAS-Cog scale in a study of Alzheimer's disease. Let π_c and π_t be the probability that a person in the control group and a person in the treated group, respectively, experience an event during the trial. The relative risk is π_t/π_c. Define $\theta = \ln(1 - \pi_c)/\ln(1 - \pi_t)$.

Assume that the event rate is such that within each of the two groups every participant in a given treatment group has approximately the same probability of experiencing an event. Assume that no participant

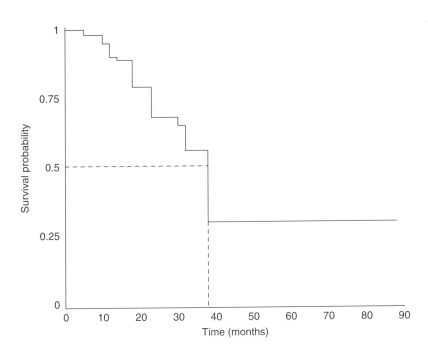

Figure 4.4. Example of a Kaplan-Meier curve for a small study.

withdraws from the study. In a study in which half of the participants will receive experimental treatment and half will be controls, Freedman [17] presents the following simple formulas.

Total number of events in both treatment groups:

$$\left(\frac{\theta+1}{\theta-1}\right)^2\left(\xi_{1-\frac{\alpha}{2}}+\xi_{1-\beta}\right)^2$$

Sample size in each group:

$$\frac{1}{\pi_c+\pi_t}\left(\frac{\theta+1}{\theta-1}\right)^2\left(\xi_{1-\alpha/2}+\xi_{1-\beta}\right)^2$$

An even simpler formula is due to Schoenfeld [18] who derived it for the log-rank test without assuming an exponential model. Under their models, the *total* number of events required in the two treatment groups is:

$$4\frac{\left(\xi_{1-\frac{\alpha}{2}}+\xi_{1-\beta}\right)^2}{[\ln(\theta)]^2}$$

Then the total sample size required in *each* treatment group is:

$$\frac{4}{\pi_c+\pi_t}\frac{\left(\xi_{1-\alpha/2}+\xi_{1-\beta}\right)^2}{[\ln(\theta)]^2}$$

If the ratio of allocation to treatment and control is m:1 rather than 1:1, the '4' in the above formula becomes $(m+1)^2/m$. Neither of the above formulae explicitly incorporates time. In fact, time appears only in the calculation of the probabilities π_c and π_t of events.

Table 4.4 presents the necessary sample size for a two-arm study using the log-rank test under the assumption of no non-compliance with protocol.

General problems of multiplicity as it relates to sample size

Most clinical trials study more than one outcome of interest. A trial of treatment after diagnosis of Alzheimer's may compare 5-year mortality, 10-year mortality, and time to a score of <20 on the ADAS-Cog. A trial to study the effect of treatment on cognitive function might compare memory loss and ability to perform activities of daily living. The probability of type I error increases with the number of endpoints considered (as discussed earlier in this chapter, type I error, or α-error, is the error incurred by falsely finding two treatments to be different when they truly have equivalent effects). The standard approach to statistical testing in clinical trials presupposes a single outcome; if there is more than one outcome of interest, the statistical test procedure must be adjusted if the experiment is to preserve the stated type I error rate. Many

Table 4.4 Approximate total sample size for a controlled clinical trial that compares time to event in a treatment and control group

Proportion with the event in group 2	Proportion with the event in group 1					
	0.05	0.1	0.2	0.3	0.4	0.5
0.1	758					
0.2	120	356				
0.3	53	107	554			
0.4	31	53	153	694		
0.5	21	33	73	182	773	
0.6	15	22	43	83	195	785
0.7	12	16	28	47	86	190
0.8	9	13	20	30	46	79
0.9	8	10	14	20	27	39

$\alpha = 0.05$; power = 90%; table assumes no loss to follow-up, no non-compliance, no multiple looks at the data and uses the Lakatos method. The sample size per group is half the value in the table.

approaches are available to adjust for multiplicity; different people support approaches that range from no adjustment to extreme adjustment [19] with follow-up time twice recruitment time [20]. The simplest approach, the so-called Bonferroni method, counts the number of statistical tests k to be performed and then divides the α-level by k. The resulting α-level is used to declare significance. This conservative approach will lead to large sample sizes if there are many tests. For example, consider a study with an α-level of 5%. If the sample size were 100 per group in an experiment with a single primary outcome, under a Bonferroni adjustment the size would need to be 118 if there were two primary outcomes, 136 for four, and 159 for 10. Similarly, in a trial that compares more than two drugs, the α-level should adjust the sample size to account for the multiple comparisons possible among treatments.

How should investigators address the issue of multiple outcomes? When feasible, they can severely limit the number of outcomes to be formally tested. If having a limit of one or two outcomes is scientifically or medically unacceptable, the investigators should decide to whom they are addressing the results of the study and use a method of adjustment acceptable to their intended audience. If the results of the experiment will support a submission to the US FDA, the investigators should discuss the appropriate methods of adjustment with the FDA.

Many statisticians, the two authors of this chapter included, recommend statistical adjustments to maintain the type I error rate at the stated level. If, however, the results are to be reported in a professional journal that does not require such adjustment, then the investigators may decide to adopt the methods standard for the work previously published in the journal.

If the experiment is to be used as a pilot for the design of a larger study, then the degree of adjustment may not need to be very rigorous.

One rigorous approach to multiplicity is to declare a single primary outcome variable and assign to it the entire type I error rate. Then list a set – preferably a small set – of important secondary outcomes. Apply a rule to adjust for multiplicity of these secondary outcomes. See, for example, Dmitrienko, *et al.* [21] for a discussion of various approaches for adjusting for multiplicity. In their α-preserving paradigm, if the primary outcome is not statistically significant, then one cannot declare significance for any of the secondary outcomes. Problems of multiplicity also arise in sequential analysis of clinical trials. See Chapter 14 for details on this type of multiplicity.

Other considerations in calculating sample size

The sample size discussion in this chapter introduces the basic concepts and alludes to such complicating factors as multiplicity and loss to follow-up. Actual sample size calculations must account for a host of deviations from ideal in addition to the two already mentioned. Participants may stop taking study medication; they may cross over to the active medication either by the design of the protocol or, if the medication or a similar one is already available, they may do so in violation of the protocol. They may be only partially compliant, taking their medication sometimes but not always, or taking more than prescribed. The population itself may be too heterogeneous to assume that all participants share the same underlying parameters of interest. The centers involved in the study may recruit patients of very different severities of disease and the centers may use quite different standards of care.

In general, the more variability in the population studied and the more variability in the investigators' patterns of treating patients, the larger the sample size must be to maintain adequate power. In designing a randomized clinical trial, the prudent investigator will seriously consider the ways in which the assumptions underlying the planned statistical methods are likely to fail and the potential for deviations from the protocol to occur. The investigators, including the statisticians, should deal carefully with the consequences of the likely failure of assumptions and violations of protocol. In certain types of studies in neurology, for example, in prevention of stroke in high risk populations, these types of problems are no more severe than in many other fields of medicine. In other areas, however, for example, Alzheimer's disease, severe epilepsy, and ALS, the nature of the population under study is such that many participants fail to complete the protocol as planned. To the extent feasible, the design of such trials should incorporate features that either allow large enough sample sizes to overcome the resultant increases in variability or that redefine outcome variables in such a way as to avoid violations of protocol.

Bayesian statistics

Our discussion thus far has assumed that the clinical trial will be conducted in the classical, or frequentist, framework. Philosophically, a frequentist considers that the parameter of interest is fixed; that is, if the sample size were large enough, the estimated value of the parameter would converge to the true value. In, Bayesian statistics, on the other hand, the parameter itself is viewed as having a distribution. One starts with a 'prior' distribution for that parameter and one uses the data from the clinical trial to modify one's prior. In the past, few clinical trials were performed in the Bayesian framework, but Bayesian methods have become more widely used recently. See Berry [22] for a basic description of the approach.

References

1. Meinert CL. *Clinical Trials*. Oxford: Oxford University Press, 1986.

2. Friedman LM, Furberg C, and DeMets DL. *Fundamentals of Clinical Trials*, 4th ed. New York: Springer, 2010.

3. Proschan M, Lan KKG, and Wittes JT. *Statistical Monitoring of Clinical Trials: A Unified Approach*. New York: Springer, 2006.

4. Yusuf S, Held P, and Teo KK. Selection of patients for randomized controlled trials: Implications of wide or narrow eligibility criteria. *Stat Med* 1990; **9**: 73–86.

5. Lan K and DeMets D. Group sequential procedures: calendar versus information time. *Stat Med* 1989; **8**: 1191–8.

6. Moore D and McCabe, GP. *Introduction to the Practice of Statistics*, 3rd edition. New York: W.H. Freeman and Company, 1999.

7. Altman DG. *Practical Statistics for Medical Research*. London: Chapman & Hall, 1991.

8. Pagano M and Gauvreau K. *Principles of Biostatistics* 2nd ed. Duxbury, MA: Duxbury Press, 2000.

9. Donner A and Klar N. *Design and Analysis of Cluster Randomized Trials in Health Research*. London: Arnold, 2000.

10. Borenstein M, Rothstein H, Cohen J, *et al. Power and Precision*. Englewood, NJ: Biostat, Inc., 2001.

11. Elashoff J. *nQuery Advisor Version 4.0 User's Guide*. Los Angeles, CA: Statistical Solutions, 2000.

12. Hintze J. *PASS 2008*. NCSS LLC, Kaysville, UT, 2008.

13. Fleiss J, Tytun A, and Ury H. A simple approximation for calculating sample sizes for comparing independent proportions. *Biometrics* 1980; **36**: 343–6.

14. Cox DR and Oakes D. *Analysis of Survival Data*. New York: Chapman and Hall, 1984.

15. Lagakos SW. General right censoring and its impact on survival data. *Biometrics* 1979; **35**: 139–156.

16. Collett D. *Modelling Survival Data in Medical Research*. 2nd ed. Boca Raton, FL: Chapman and Hall/CRC, 2003.

17. Freedman L. Tables of the number of patients required in clinical trials using the logrank test. *Stat Med* 1982; **1**: 121–9.

18. Schoenfeld D. The asymptotic properties of nonparametric tests for comparing survival distributions. *Biometrika* 1981; **68**: 316–9.

19. Lakatos E. Sample sizes based on the log-rank statistic in complex clinical trials. *Biometrics* 1988; **44**: 229–241.

20. Miller JRG. *Survival Analysis*. New York: John Wiley & Sons, Inc., 1981.

21. Dmitrienko A, Tamhane AC, Wang X, *et al.* Stepwise gatekeeping procedures in clinical trial applications. *Biometr J* 2006; **48**; 984–91.

22. Berry D. Bayesian clinical trials. *Nature Rev Drug Discov* 2006; **5**: 27–36.

Bias and random error

Susan S. Ellenberg and Jacqueline A. French

Introduction

The goal of a controlled clinical trial, as it is for any controlled experiment, is to compare the effects of interventions on outcomes of interest. In order to draw valid and reliable conclusions from a trial, one must believe that any observed difference between groups treated differently is due to the difference in interventions and not to any inherent differences between the groups, or simply to the play of chance.

Bias is the existence of systematic differences between groups that will lead to differences in outcomes regardless of any difference in treatment effect. A major focus of clinical trial methodology, in regard to design, conduct, and analysis, relates to the control of bias, as bias can arise in any of these areas. For example, a trial designed with a historical control group consisting of previously treated individuals identified from medical records might be biased since there are many reasons why individuals treated in the past might be different, and have different prognoses for the outcome of interest, from those treated currently. A trial conducted so that those evaluating outcomes are aware of the treatment assignments might be biased if the evaluators believe that one treatment is likely superior. A trial analysis that excludes individuals who did not comply with the assigned treatment might be biased if non-compliance is associated with prognosis for outcome.

Random error refers to differences that occur by chance. If we flip a fair coin 20 times we are not likely to observe exactly 10 head and exactly 10 tails, although that is the expected outcome. In coin flips, the random error may result from the force going into the flip, air currents in the room, or other conditions extraneous to the fairness of the coin. Similarly, in a clinical trial, if two treatments were in fact equivalent, and if we treated 50 subjects with each treatment, we would not expect to observe precisely identical outcomes. In a clinical trial, we need to plan our trial so that, if there is a true difference in outcomes, we will expect to observe a large enough difference to be able to distinguish it from a difference attributable to chance. As with bias, the control of random error is important to consider throughout the process of a clinical trial.

In this chapter, we consider methods to limit bias and random error at each stage of a clinical trial – design, conduct, analysis and interpretation of results.

Study design

Bias

Many aspects of study design relate to control of bias. The one of greatest importance is the method of assignment to treatment. Since the middle of the twentieth century it has been widely accepted that the best way to minimize bias related to subject characteristics is to assign treatment at random. This means using a truly random mechanism to determine the treatment assignment for each successive subject. Alternative approaches all have the potential for creating treatment groups that are systematically different, thereby confounding any attempt to estimate treatment effect by comparing outcomes in the treatment groups. Some types of non-randomized control groups, and the problems they raise, are as follows:

- Historical controls: may have received differing concomitant therapies; may have been treated by different physicians, using different protocols to manage therapy; may not have met all inclusion criteria for current study; may have differing distributions of prognostic factors [1]
- Concurrent subjects choosing not to receive investigational treatment: choice of treatment may be associated with prognosis

Clinical Trials in Neurology, ed. Bernard Ravina, Jeffrey Cummings, Michael P. McDermott, and R. Michael Poole. Published by Cambridge University Press. © Cambridge University Press 2012.

- Concurrent subjects at other sites: similar to problems with historical controls
- Systematic assignment according to birthdate, first letter of last name, etc.: assignment of each patient will be known to recruiting investigator, may influence decision to approach patient for study
- Alternating treatment assignments: Similar to systematic assignment above.

When a true randomized design is used, there can be no reason other than chance (whose influence can be controlled by sample size, as we will discuss later) for outcomes to differ between arms other than the different treatment assigned to each arm.

Probably the tool of next greatest importance in the control of bias is blinding (or masking; these terms are used interchangeably). Ideally one would wish to use a double-blind design, in which neither the subject nor treating physician knows to which treatment the subject is assigned. In this way, neither the subject's perception of his/her health status, nor the physician's decisions about patient management can be influenced by the knowledge of the treatment assignment.

Studies of new drugs in which subjects on the control arm can be untreated are typically designed with placebo controls, which maintain the double-blind. The placebo must match the active drug in route and schedule of administration, appearance, smell and taste. When two active drugs are being compared, double-blinding can be more complicated. It is usually not feasible to prepare different active drugs so that they look, smell and taste the same. The approach commonly used is a 'double-dummy' design in which a placebo for each drug is prepared and subjects receive one active drug and one placebo but of course do not know which is which. In this way, drugs with different routes and schedules can still be compared in a double-blind fashion. An excellent example is the Heparin in Acute Embolic Stroke Trial (HAEST) in which subcutaneous heparin (dalteparin 100 IU/kg) twice a day was compared to aspirin tablets 160 mg once a day [2]. To maintain study blind, patients received either aspirin tablets and subcutaneous injection of a saline placebo, or subcutaneous heparin and an aspirin placebo.

Double-blind designs are not always feasible due to ethical or logistical considerations. In a trial of surgery versus medication, for example, the treating physician cannot be blinded, but if a sham surgical procedure can be done ethically, it may still be done as a single-blind study with all subjects undergoing either the real or sham procedure, and taking either an active or placebo medication. Many single-blind studies involving transplantation of experimental tissue and therefore requiring a sham surgical procedure in the control group have been performed in Parkinson's disease [3,4]; the known high rate of placebo response in single-arm trials have led researchers to insist on double-blind designs and these studies have largely been accepted by institutional review boards and research participants.

In many cases, however, an unblinded design will be necessary, and other approaches to control bias will have to be implemented. Sham surgeries, while largely accepted in Parkinson's disease, arthroscopic knee surgery, and a few other areas, are always controversial and are complicated to conduct. Even in trials comparing medication strategies a blinded design is not always possible or ethical. Some medications have distinctive side effects that make it difficult to blind. Further, some drugs with narrow therapeutic indices or potentially serious toxicities may be difficult to manage in a fully blinded way, or clinicians may not feel comfortable managing a serious medical condition without fully understanding which therapies have been employed. Such was the case when a blinded active control comparison trial involving the currently best available therapies for status epilepticus, a life-threatening condition, was suggested. The clinical investigators were initially hesitant about managing the intravenous administration of four different treatments (diazepam (0.15 mg per kilogram of body weight) followed by phenytoin (18 mg per kilogram), lorazepam (0.1 mg per kilogram), phenobarbital (15 mg per kilogram), or phenytoin (18 mg per kilogram)) in a blinded way. Ultimately, however, the trial was successfully performed [5].

Random error

Sample size

Suppose we randomize twenty subjects between two therapies, ten to each. Suppose then that six subjects have a good outcome with drug A but only four with drug B. Can we conclude then that drug A is superior? Certainly not with any high confidence; even though drug A's success rate is 50% higher, this degree of variation from the expected finding under the assumption that they have the same effect (five successes on each arm) is entirely consistent with chance. Just as we would not be surprised to flip a fair coin twenty times and get six heads in the first ten flips and then four heads in the next ten, the comparison of six versus four is not at all inconsistent with the two drugs having identical effects. If however, we treated not 10 but 100 subjects with each drug, and observed 60 successes with drug A and 40 with drug B, we would have a much stronger case for concluding that drug A is superior—the probability that we would observe this much of a difference if the drugs really had the same effect is less than 1%.

Thus, the key to controlling random error in designing a trial is to ensure that the sample size is large enough to permit an observed difference of a specified size to be considered documentation of a true difference in effect. The method of determining the required sample size depends on the type of variable being assessed. If the variable is binomial (e.g., success vs. failure), the comparison will be of the proportion of successes; if the variable is a continuous (or approximately continuous) measure (e.g. weight, blood pressure, IQ score), the comparison will be of the means or medians; if the variable is the time until the event of interest occurs, the comparison will be of these times, accounting for the length of time the subject has been under study and whether or not the subject has had the event.

The goal in calculating sample size is to limit two kinds of random errors: 1) the error of falsely concluding that the two treatments being compared produce different effects when in fact there is no difference; and 2) the error of falsely concluding that the treatments being compared produce similar effects when in fact one is better than the other. The first is referred to as type I error (or 'alpha error' as in sample size formulae this error is designated by the Greek letter α); the second is referred to as type II error (or 'beta error', designated β). Other commonly used terms relating to these errors are 'significance level,' which is equivalent to type I error and 'power,' which is the complement of type II error and therefore represents the probability that we will correctly identify a treatment effect as large as or larger than the difference the study was intended to identify.

The key factors in determining sample size are the difference between the experimental and control group that is deemed important to identify; the variability of the outcome measure in the study population; and the magnitude of type I and type II error we are willing to accept. The smaller the difference we wish to identify, the larger the variability of the outcome measure, and the smaller the risk of type I and type II errors we can accept, the larger the sample size will be.

Details of sample size calculations in different scenarios are given in Chapter 4.

Inclusion criteria

Another way to reduce random error is by selecting eligibility criteria that exclude individuals who have little chance of showing a treatment effect, either because of their underlying health status or because of environmental factors that might affect their adherence to the study protocol. Making the study sample more homogeneous with respect to prognosis for showing a treatment effect will reduce variability. (On the other hand, a highly homogeneous study population will yield study results that may be less clearly generalizable to the target population for the intervention.)

Study conduct

Bias

Experimentation with human beings is an imperfect science; it is impossible to exercise the extent of control over the study implementation as it would be for a laboratory or animal experiment. Many aspects of study conduct have the potential to bias study results.

Allocation concealment

Some of the benefits of randomization may be lost if study personnel involved in recruiting and entering subjects are aware of the treatment assignment for the next subject to be entered. This is primarily an issue in unblinded (sometimes called 'open label') studies, for which a computer-generated assignment list will provide this information. In a multi-center study with a central or web-based randomization process, the upcoming assignment would remain hidden from site investigators, but for single-site studies it can be a concern. If an investigator knows that the next subject to be entered will be assigned a specific treatment, he/she will be able to make a subjective judgment about whether to try to recruit a particular subject. This could lead to systematic differences between arms despite the randomization [6]. The use of sealed envelopes to be opened when the subject agrees to be randomized has been shown to be particularly problematic; investigators may be tempted to open the envelope to learn the assignment and only then decide whether to try to recruit the subject. Implementation of randomization should always consider how to ensure that the allocation schedule remains concealed from investigators.

Blinded outcome evaluation

The evaluation of subject outcomes, the primary focus of the trial, should be done without knowledge of the subject's treatment assignment whenever possible in order to avoid influencing the evaluator who may have a prior belief about the relative efficacy of the treatments being compared. When outcomes are assessed by means of imaging, laboratory measures or subject questionnaires, blinding the evaluators is generally straightforward, even when the trial is not conducted in a single- or double-blind fashion. When the primary outcome results from a clinical evaluation, however, it may be more difficult to arrange for a blinded evaluation, especially when there are subjective aspects to the evaluation, or when one treatment involves surgery. For example, in a study comparing bilateral deep brain stimulation to best medical therapy in patients with advanced Parkinson's disease, patients were required to wear caps to blind the raters to the presence or absence of surgical scars [7].

Non-compliance and dropout

In nearly all clinical trials, it is inevitable that some subjects will not receive the study treatment according to protocol. They may forget to take drugs, stop taking them (or take them inconsistently) because of side effects; they may fail to return for study visits at which treatment is administered or provided; they may refuse to undergo testing. In unblinded studies, they may refuse the assigned treatment if they had hoped to be assigned to the other treatment group. It is generally not possible to know on an individual basis whether a non-compliant subject is more or less likely to have a favorable outcome than a compliant subject, but studies have suggested that there can be a strong systematic difference in prognosis between those who are and are not compliant with the study protocol [8–10]. Thus, it is important to try to maintain information on non-compliant subjects and to obtain the data necessary to include them in the primary analysis. Even subjects who refused assigned treatment, for whatever reason, should be kept in the study if at all possible and encouraged to undergo evaluation for outcome. This issue is elaborated further in the account of analysis.

Random error

Random error in the conduct of a study is commonly referred to as 'noise.' Such errors increase the variability of study outcomes and hence reduce the precision of estimation and the power of the study to detect differences between treatment strategies. Errors in data entry, missing data due to lost lab slips or other records, randomization of a subject who does not meet eligibility criteria, and faulty measures of study outcomes all contribute to increased variability and thereby reduce the chance that the study will be able to document a true difference in treatment effects.

Operations manual and training

There are many ways to minimize random error in the conduct of clinical studies. First and foremost is the development of a detailed manual of procedures and the training of study personnel in these procedures. Training may need to occur more than once during a study, especially if important new procedures are introduced. A manual of procedures should ideally be available electronically with a search function that facilitates accessing the information of interest.

In developing the manual of procedures, it is important to consider how best to reduce variability of certain measurements. Standardizing the time of day may be important for some measures, or timing of the measure with respect to last food intake. Symptoms of some neurological disorders such as Parkinson's disease can vary substantially on a diurnal basis. Serum concentrations will be much less variable if they are taken at a predetermined interval from the time of dosing. If the measure requires subject input, it will be important to provide instructions to the site that will be relayed to the subject on how to complete the measure.

Data entry and audit

Quality control of the data entry process can also reduce error. Missing values, out-of-range data or data inconsistent with other entered data can be identified, either at time of data entry (for web-based data entry systems) or by regular batch edits of the entire database. Resolving such errors is not always possible but in many cases the database can be updated with the correct information. The sooner errors are identified and referred back to the clinical sites for their attention, the more likely such errors can be corrected, so quality control systems should give high priority to timely feedback to clinical sites.

Centralization of operations

Centralization of some study functions can help minimize variability associated with differences among participating clinical sites in a multi-center study. Having laboratory samples run by a central laboratory, rather than at each site, will eliminate variability due to use of different equipment and different protocols. If laboratory results are not needed for patient management, running all study samples in a single batch at the end of the study will reduce variability even further.

Study assessments that incorporate some element of subjectivity can also be centralized. Many trials rely on a central adjudication group to make outcome assessments for all subjects in a study. Such groups may be employed to read scans, assess pathology samples, or review medical charts, and come to consensus on individual subject outcomes. For example, in a recent highly successful randomized blinded trial that assessed the effects of three different antiepileptic drugs (valproic acid, ethosuximide, and lamotrigine) in children with absence seizures, all EEGs were read by a centralized group. This group determined patient eligibility in the trial, and also determined response to treatment. In the eligibility review, the central readers disagreed with the local reader in only three cases; these cases were then excluded [11]. In some trials, however, differences between local and central readers can be substantial.

Case report forms

The design of study forms can influence the quality of data. The items on each form must be crystal clear with regard to what information is being asked for, and possible answers offered must be mutually exclusive and exhaustive. A common error in study form design is omission of an 'other' option when the respondent is asked to select one of several responses; it is difficult for the person entering data to know what to enter when none of the options offered appears appropriate, and this may lead to selection of an available but inaccurate response. When there are many possible options investigators may be tempted to simply have the response entered as free text. While in some cases there may be good reasons for collecting data as free text, this should be avoided when possible as it allows for substantially more errors in transcription and creates major difficulties in data analysis.

Conducting an initial pilot test of data forms prior to initiating data collection on study subjects is highly recommended. Review of the forms by investigators is insufficient as many unclear questions or questions with inadequate response options will not be identified until someone actually tries to complete the forms for specific individuals.

On-site monitoring

Electronic data editing is a form of quality control monitoring, but for many studies electronic editing is supplemented by on-site monitoring conducted by someone otherwise independent of the study who reviews study records on a regular basis to identify errors or other problems in study conduct, and to verify at least some portion of the computerized data by checking them against original source records such as hospital charts, lab slips, etc. Checking of every data item is almost always unnecessary. An approach used in some studies is to verify all data pertaining to the primary outcome and to eligibility, and then some fraction (e.g., 10%) of the remaining data, with expansion of the review if problems arise in the data that are initially checked. Many studies incorporate even more limited on-site checking; studies sponsored by pharmaceutical companies generally perform substantial on-site checking, in many cases involving 100% of data elements, but the slight improvement one might have in accuracy is unlikely to warrant the extensive resources required to verify every data element in most cases.

Analysis of study data

Bias

Even in a study that is designed and conducted with a meticulous eye to avoiding bias, results may still be severely biased if inappropriate methods of data analysis are adopted. Methods that can bias results are those that involve removing subjects from analysis for a systematic reason, thereby undermining the assumption that the treatment groups generated by randomization are prognostically equivalent.

Intention-to-treat

The cornerstone of an unbiased analysis is the intention-to-treat principle. An intention-to-treat (ITT) analysis is one in which everyone who was randomized into the study is included in the analysis – no one is dropped out because they switched treatments, stopped taking treatment, or otherwise failed to comply with the protocol. This often seems counterintuitive to investigators – why count the outcome for someone assigned to arm A who did not get the arm A treatment (or only a minimal amount of it)? The reason this is important is easiest to see for a trial comparing an active treatment with a placebo. The conventional approach to such a trial is to try to show a treatment effect by 'disproving' the assumption that there is no difference between the treatment and placebo. Under that assumption, called the 'null hypothesis,' it wouldn't matter if someone didn't get treatment, since they would be receiving either an ineffective treatment or a placebo. If one

Table 5.1 Five-year mortality in patients given clofibrate or placebo, according to cumulative adherence to protocol prescription

	Treatment group			
	Clofibrate		Placebo	
Adherence[a]	No. of patients	% mortality[b]	No. of patients	% mortality[b]
< 80%	357	24.6 ± 2.3 (22.5)	882	28.2 ± 1.5 (25.8)
> 80%	708	15.0 ± 1.3 (15.7)	1813	15.1 ± 0.8 (16.4)
Total study group	1065	18.2 ± 1.2 (18.0)	2695	19.4 ± 0.8 (19.5)

[a] A patient's cumulative adherence was computed as the estimated number of capsules actually taken as a percentage of the number that should have been taken according to the protocol during the first five years of follow-up or until death (if death occurred during the first five years).

[b] The figures in parentheses are adjusted for 40 base-line characteristics. The figures given as percentages ± 1 SE are unadjusted figures whose SEs are correct to within 0.1 unit for the adjusted figures.

Reproduced with permission from Massachusetts Medical Society and the *New England Journal of Medicine*.

drops out subjects who refused or stopped taking their assigned treatment, however, those dropped out might be sicker on average than others, and that could lead to an apparent difference in outcomes by arm, even if the treatment being studied had no effect at all.

A dramatic example of this potential bias was seen in an NIH trial conducted in the 1970s, the Coronary Drug Project (CDP) [12]. In this trial, several drugs were tested against a placebo control to assess whether any of them improved survival rates in men at high risk for cardiovascular mortality. Treatments were taken as pills, and subjects were asked to bring their supplies to the clinic at each return visit. Compliance was a problem in the trial; analysis of pill counts revealed that a substantial proportion of study subjects failed to take 20% or more of their required medication. A naïve approach to this situation might have been to perform an analysis that compared those in the treatment groups who took 80% or more of their medication with those who took less than 80%. The results of such analyses, as shown in Table 5.1 were quite surprising. Those who took less than 80% of their medicine had about a 60% higher mortality rate than those who were more adherent. The results for the placebo group, however, were even more extreme. Since taking more or less placebo could not influence mortality, it was clear that men with worse prognosis were more likely to be non-adherent to medication [8]. The CDP investigators tried to account for the result in the placebo group by adjusting for all known prognostic factors but were able to explain only a small proportion of the difference between better and worse adherers by such adjustment. The clear lesson of this example is that people who take medication as prescribed may be substantially

prognostically different from those who do not, for reasons that we cannot explain by factors that we can measure. Hence, eliminating non-compliers from analyses raises the real danger of introducing a major bias into the analysis. In the case of the CDP, eliminating the poor compliers from both arms would have produced the same close-to-zero estimate of treatment effect as doing the standard intention-to-treat analysis, with all randomized subjects included; in general, however, one cannot be certain that those who comply with one of the study treatments will be prognostically similar to those who comply with the other.

Intention to treat is an important tool in preventing bias, but a true ITT analysis requires that data on all randomized subjects are available for analysis. When subjects drop out and are not evaluated for the primary outcome, the approach to handling these dropouts can introduce bias. In a study that compared donepezil to rivastigmine as treatments for mild to moderate Alzheimer's disease, there were many more dropouts due to side effects in the rivastigmine arm. These dropouts were included in the analysis with the outcome at their last assessment prior to dropout substituting for the outcome at study completion. Subjects in the rivastigmine arm tended to drop out earlier and thus to have the cognitive assessment earlier in their disease, favoring the less-well-tolerated treatment [13]. In epilepsy studies, treatments which cause very early dropout due, for example, to rapid titration, can cause individuals to drop out before they have had a seizure after randomization. Some studies, attempting to include all randomized subjects, define these patients as seizure-free, driving up the seizure-free percentages in the treated arm, as compared to placebo [11].

The analytical approach that uses the last measure prior to dropout as the primary outcome for subjects who do not complete the study is generally referred to as 'last observation carried forward (LOCF).' As noted above, this approach can lead to biased estimates of treatment effect. A variety of other methods have been proposed for handling missing data; these are discussed in more detail in Chapter 6. No method can guarantee absence of bias in the presence of missing data, however; exploratory analyses should always be conducted to assess the possible extent of bias caused by lack of primary outcome data on some subjects. Such analyses, referred to as sensitivity analyses, can use a variety of approaches to impute the missing data; for example, a 'worst case scenario' analysis might assume that all subjects with missing outcome data were treatment successes if on the control arm and treatment failures if on the investigational arm. If the treatment still showed significant benefit in an analysis with such extreme assumptions one could be certain that the missing data were not hiding information that could change the conclusions. Other types of sensitivity analyses making less extreme assumptions should also be performed; if multiple methods lead to the same conclusions one can feel reasonably confident that the missing data are not leading to errors in interpretation of the data.

Eligibility assessment

It might seem logical that eliminating subjects who are found upon review to have not fully met the inclusion criteria should not lead to any bias – after all, these subjects should not have been entered in the first place. But if the eligibility review is performed by individuals with knowledge of treatment assignment and study outcome, bias could enter in as reviewers made judgments when adjudication of baseline eligibility criteria was not straightforward [15]. Eligibility reviews should always be performed by individuals blinded both to treatment and to study status.

Random error

Random error can be reduced by performing analyses that account for prognostic factors.

Stratification factors

Randomization is often stratified by factors that are expected to be related to prognosis for the primary study outcome. These factors often include study site, demographic factors such as age and gender, and baseline measures of clinical relevance. Study analyses should always account for stratification factors, calculating the treatment comparison within strata and then aggregating across all strata. Since the data within strata will be more homogeneous than the data overall, stratifying the analysis reduces variability [16–18] (also see Chapter 6).

Adjustment for covariates

In most studies, the sample size is too small to permit stratification by more than two or three factors. There may be additional factors that are known to be prognostic for study outcome. When analyses are performed that account for the influence of these factors, the variability with which the treatment comparison is assessed will be reduced, thereby increasing power to detect differences [19–21].

Interpretation of study results

Bias

The multiple comparisons problem

In most studies, the treatments are compared with regard to multiple outcomes. The more comparisons are made, the more likely it is to observe a spurious 'significant' finding. Ideally, one outcome is selected by investigators as the primary outcome, so that analysis of that outcome is readily interpretable without concern about inflation of the false positive rate. That still leaves the problem of interpreting analyses of other outcomes of interest and importance.

It can be difficult to quantify this problem, and thereby correct for it, since the degree to which the false positive rate is increased depends on how closely correlated the outcomes are. For example, there are multiple stroke scales, and they are very similar. If one performed a study of treatment for stroke and compared the treatment groups on each scale, it is highly unlikely that one would give a statistically significant result if the others were not at least strongly suggestive of an effect. For example, in the placebo-controlled NINDS study of R-tpa the investigators looked at the Barthel Index, modified Rankin score, Glasgow Outcome Score, and the NIHSS and all scales demonstrated that the drug was beneficial [22]. On the other hand, in a study of antiepileptic drug therapy, if one outcome was number of seizures occurring during a defined interval and the other outcome was results of a quality of life assessment at the end of that interval, the results would likely have only a modest correlation and it is not unimaginable that a significant effect might be shown for one with little or no effect suggested for the other. If one did not clearly specify which outcome was primary, the investigators would have two opportunities to declare the study positive, thereby doubling the possibility of a false positive finding if the drug were truly inactive.

Subsets

One of the most common ways to introduce the problem of multiple comparisons is to evaluate results in subgroups of the study populations. It can be readily calculated that if 14 independent tests are performed at the 0.05 level of significance, the chance is better than 50% that at least one comparison will produce a p-value less than 0.05 even when there are no true differences. Such findings can arise from a study in which there is no overall treatment difference but when subgroups are examined, a subgroup is found that appears to benefit [23, 24]. It is often difficult for investigators to take a realistic view of the likelihood that the subgroup effect is a 'false positive.'

Of comparable importance is the situation where there is a true difference but when subgroups of the study population are examined separately. In that case it may well happen that by chance, the data from one subgroup show no treatment effect, or a trend in the wrong direction. To illustrate this problem, investigators conducting a large cardiovascular study analyzed their outcome data by signs of the zodiac and showed that study subjects born under the signs of Gemini and Libra appeared to do worse with the tested treatment, while subjects born under the other signs showed a strong benefit that was highly statistically significant [25]. The investigators appreciated that readers of their paper would not believe that signs of the zodiac could influence the likelihood of treatment success, and included this analysis in their publication to demonstrate that great skepticism is needed when examining results in the other subgroups they considered.

Interim analyses

Another multiple comparisons issue arises when the accumulating data are analyzed multiple times during the course of a study with the idea that the study can be stopped, or at least reported, as soon as the primary outcome shows a significant difference between treatment arms. Allowing multiple opportunities to answer the same question raises the same concerns as addressing multiple different questions. It has been shown

that testing for a difference at the nominal 0.05 level ten times during the course of a study raises the type I error, or false positive rate, to 19% [26]. Methods for study monitoring and interim analyses are described in Chapter 14.

Methods to account for multiple comparisons

What can be done about the multiple comparisons problem? The answer surely cannot be to perform only a single significance test when many questions will be of legitimate importance. A variety of statistical methods to allow definitive conclusions to be made when multiple tests are to be performed have been developed. All require either testing at reduced significance levels (Bonferroni and related procedures [27–29]) or setting up nested testing systems whereby secondary hypotheses can be tested only when there is a significant effect on the primary outcome (gatekeeping procedures [30–32]). In the case of multiple tests of a single hypothesis over time, as in the monitoring of accruing clinical trial results, the available methods, such as the commonly used O'Brien-Fleming procedure [33], mostly require testing at reduced significance levels at interim analyses so as to ensure that the probability of a false positive result overall remains less than 0.05 (or whatever significance level has been selected). For multiple testing of different outcomes, the gatekeeping strategies have become more popular. What is most important, however, is the interpretation of the results. Whatever methods are used to account for multiple testing, or even (especially) when no such methods are used at all, authors must describe their approach to multiple testing and how their results should be interpreted given the expected increase in risk of false positives.

Pre-specification of analytical plan

Even when the study objectives are clearly stated and there is a single primary outcome, the details of the primary analyses may not be as clearly defined. For example, the primary objective in a study of an anti-epileptic drug might be to reduce the risk of seizures; this could be quantified in several ways, however. We might compare the simple frequency of seizures over the interval of observation; we might do a seizure-free day assessment; or we might determine how many subjects have had a 50% reduction in seizures. If the intended primary analysis is not specified clearly, multiple analyses could be conducted and the one producing the lowest p-value could be selected. Thus, even if the data remain unbiased, the interpretation of the analysis might be biased.

Random error

Random error is frequently misinterpreted in discussion sections of clinical trials reports. Our significance tests are intended to quantify random error; they tell us the probability we would see a difference as large as or larger than what we have observed if there were truly no difference between groups. Thus, a very low p-value indicates that the observed results are highly inconsistent with an assumption that the two treatment approaches have the same effect. A large p-value indicates that the data provide inconclusive evidence about the existence of a treatment effect but may suggest that if there is an effect it is probably not large.

One ubiquitous error is stating that 'no difference was found between treatments X and Y' whenever the p-value for testing the difference did not cross the 0.05 threshold. The convention that permits us to claim a definitive difference if the significance level dips below 0.05 does not imply that one can definitively conclude that there is no difference when the significance level is above 0.05. A comparison of treatment outcomes resulting in a p-value of 0.07 sends quite a different message from a comparison yielding a p-value of 0.67. The first indicates that a difference this large or larger might be expected 7% of the time when there was truly no treatment difference; the second indicates that a difference this large or larger might be expected 67% of the time when there was truly no treatment difference. These results should not lead to identical statements of 'there was no difference.'

Another common problem is attributing an insignificant p-value to an insufficient number of subjects, resulting in power too low to have detected a true difference. Low power is, of course, a possible reason for failing to document a difference at the conventional 0.05 level of significance, but the competing reason is, of course, the lack of a true treatment difference. Just as it is misleading to interpret any p-value above 0.05 as evidence of no difference, it is equally misleading to interpret such a p-value as the result of low power, implying that there truly is a difference. In fact, a p-value above the conventional significance level (0.05) means only that a difference attributable to treatment cannot be confirmed with high confidence.

Summary

Control of bias and random error underlies virtually all considerations for the design, conduct and analysis of clinical trials. From sample size considerations to central pathology review, from eligibility reviews to interim monitoring plans, all methodological considerations relate in one way or other to minimizing the potential for bias and reducing random error. The more successful researchers can be in these efforts, the more reliable and informative their clinical trial results will be.

References

1. Byar DP, Simon RM, Friedewald WT, *et al.* Randomized clinical trials—perspectives on some recent ideas. *N Engl J Med* 1976; **295**: 74–80.

2. Berge E, Abdelnoor M, Nakstad PH, *et al.* Low molecular-weight heparin versus aspirin in patients with acute ischaemic stroke and atrial fibrillation: a double-blind randomised study. *Lancet* 2000; **355**: 1205–10

3. Freed CR, Greene PE, Breeze RE, *et al.* Transplantation of embryonic dopamine neurons for severe Parkinson's disease. *N Engl J Med* 2001; **344**: 710–19.

4. Olanow CW, Goetz CG, Korower JH, *et al.* A double-blind controlled trial of bilateral fetal nigral transplantation in Parkinson's disease. *Ann Neurol* 2003; **54**: 403–14.

5. Treiman DM, Meyers PD, Walton NY, *et al.* A comparison of four treatments for generalized convulsive status epilepticus. Veterans Affairs Status Epilepticus Cooperative Study Group. *N Engl J Med* 1998; **339**: 792–8.

6. Schulz KA, Grimes D. Allocation concealment in randomised trials: defending against deciphering. *Lancet* 2002; **359**: 614–18.

7. Weaver FM, Follett K, Stern M, *et al.* Bilateral deep brain stimulation vs. best medical therapy for patients with advanced Parkinson disease: a randomized controlled trial. *JAMA* 2009; **301**: 63–73.

8. [no authors listed]. Influence of adherence to treatment and response of cholesterol on mortality in the coronary drug project. *N Engl J Med* 1980; **303**: 1038–41.

9. Lee YJ, Ellenberg JH, Hirtz DG, *et al.* Analysis of clinical trials by treatment actually received: is it really an option? *Statistics in Medicine* 1991; **10**: 1595–1605.

10. Oakes D, Moss AJ, Fleiss JL, *et al.* Use of adherence measures in an analysis of the effect of diltiazem on mortality and reinfarction after myocardial infarction. *J Am Stat Assoc* 1993; **88**: 44–49.

11. Glauser TA, Cnaan A, Shinnar S, *et al.* Ethosuximide, valproic acid, and lamotrigine in childhood absence epilepsy. *N Engl J Med* 2010; **362**: 790–9.

12. Coronary Drug Project Research Group. The Coronary Drug Project. Design, methods and baseline results. *Circulation* 1973; **47** (Suppl 1): I1–I79.

13. Wilkinson DG, Passmore AP, Bullock R, *et al*. A multinational, randomised, 12-week, comparative study of donepezil and rivastigmine in patients with mild to moderate Alzheimer's disease. *Int J Clin Pract* 2002; **56**: 441–6.

14. Gazzola DM, Balcer LJ, and French JA. Seizure-free outcome in randomized add-on trials of the new antiepileptic drugs. *Epilepsia* 2007; **48**: 1303–7.

15. Schulz KF and Grimes DA. Sample size slippages in randomized trials: exclusions and the lost and wayward. *Lancet* 2002; **359**: 781–5.

16. Green SB and Byar DP. The effect of stratified randomization on size and power of statistical tests in clinical trials. *J Chron Dis* 1978; **31**: 445–54.

17. Lipchik GL, Nicholson RA, and Penzien DB. Allocation of patients to conditions in headache clinical trials: randomization, stratification and treatment matching. *Headache* 2005; **45**: 419–28.

18. Friedman LM, Furberg CD, and DeMets DL. *Fundamentals of Clinical Trials*, 3rd ed. New York: Springer-Verlag, 1998.

19. Hernandez AV, Steyerberg EW, and Habbema JD. Covariate adjustment in randomized controlled trials with dichotomous outcomes increases statistical power and reduces sample size requirements. *J Clin Epidemiol* 2004; **57**: 454–60.

20. Pocock SJ, Assman SE, Enos LE, *et al*. Subgroup analysis, covariate adjustment and baseline comparisons in clinical trial reporting: current practice and problems. *Statistics in Medicine* 2002; **21**: 2917–30.

21. Hauck WW, Anderson S, and Marcus SM. Should we adjust for covariates in nonlinear regression analyses of randomized trials? *Control Clin Trials* 1998; **19**: 249–56.

22. The National Institute of Neurological Disorders and Stroke r-TPA Stroke Study Group. Tissue plasminogen activator for acute ischemic stroke. *N Engl J Med* 1995; **333**: 1581–7.

23. Yusuf S, Wittes J, Probstfield J, *et al*. Analysis and interpretation of treatment effects in subgroups of patients in randomized clinical trials. *JAMA* 1991; **266**: 93–8.

24. Assman SF, Pocock SJ, Enos LE, *et al*. Subgroup analysis and other (mis)uses of baseline data in clinical trials. *Lancet* 2000; **355**: 1064–9.

25. ISIS-2 Collaborative Group. Randomised trial of intravenous streptokinase, oral aspirin, both or neither among 17187 cases of suspected acute myocardial infarction: ISIS-2. *Lancet* 1988; **2**(8607): 349–60.

26. McPherson K. Statistics: the problem of examining accumulating data more than once. *N Eng J Med* 1974; **290**: 501–2.

27. Simes RJ. An improved Bonferroni procedure for multiple tests of significance. *Biometrika* 1976; **73**: 751–4.

28. Hochberg Y. A sharper Bonferroni procedure for multiple tests of significance. *Biometrika* 1988; **75**: 800–2.

29. Holm S. A simple sequentially rejective multiple test procedure. *Scand J Stat* 1979; **6**: 65–70.

30. Benjamini Y, Hochberg Y. Controlling the false discovery rate: a practical and powerful approach to multiple testing. *JRSS B* 1995; **57**: 289–300.

31. Bauer P, Röhmel J, Maurer W, and Hothorn L. Testing strategies in multi-dose experiments including active control. *Statist Med* 1998; **17**: 2133–46.

32. Dmitrienko A, Tamhane AC, Wang X, *et al*. Stepwise gatekeeping procedures in clinical trial applications. *Biometrical Journal* 2006; **48**: 984–91.

33. O'Brien PC and Fleming TR. A multiple testing procedure for clinical trials. *Biometrics* 1979; **35**: 549–56.

Chapter

6

Approaches to data analysis

William R. Clarke

Introduction

The goal of this chapter is to provide an introduction to several fundamental methods for analyzing data from clinical trials, including a brief overview of two very important and related concepts: confidence intervals and tests of hypotheses. The chapter begins with a few basic statistical ideas that will be needed in the rest of the chapter. Subsequently there is a brief introduction to descriptive statistics and a discussion of concepts of populations and samples. This is important because statistics provides methods for making inferences about populations from samples from those populations. A discussion of the normal and t distributions follows and the concepts of a confidence interval and hypothesis testing are then discussed, along with illustrations of their use. Finally two important issues in the analysis of clinical trial data are discussed: the Intention to Treat Principle and methods for handling missing data.

Descriptive statistics

Some methods for summarizing data are reviewed here. It is very brief and the reader is urged to review more detailed presentations that are provided in all introductory statistics texts.

First we provide an example. In a preliminary study, investigators selected a sample of ten subjects who would have been eligible for their study and measured their systolic and diastolic blood pressures. The data for this sample are displayed in Table 6.1. While the data provide all of the information that is available from this study, it is difficult to draw any conclusions from this presentation of the data.

In order to better understand the data, we calculate summary values called statistics. A statistic is just a value that is calculated from a collection of data. The usual summary or descriptive statistics describe two characteristics of the data: its centrality (the location of the 'middle' of the data) and its variability (how much the data vary about the 'middle'). In this chapter we will let the symbol x_i represent a data item and the series $\{x_1, x_2 \ldots x_n\}$ represent the data set.

The sample mean is a common descriptive statistic that locates the 'middle' of the data. It is defined as the arithmetic mean of the data set and is usually denoted by the symbol $\bar{x}$ (pronounced x-bar). In summation notation, the mean is defined as:

$$\bar{x} = \frac{\sum_{i=1}^{n} x_i}{n}$$

For the blood pressure data, the mean systolic blood pressure is given by:

$$\bar{x} = \frac{\sum_{i=1}^{10} x_i}{10}$$

$$= \frac{\left(138 + 150 + 160 + 143 + 160 + 159 + 150 + 156 + 135 + 159\right)}{10}$$

$$= \frac{1510}{10} = 151.0$$

The median is another measure of central tendency. It is defined as the middle item of the data set. If the number of data points is odd then there is a unique middle data item and the median is defined as that middle item. If the number of data points is even then the median is defined as the average of the two 'middle' items. If we order the systolic blood pressures in the sample data set we get the ordered data set:

$$\{135, 138, 143, 150, 150, 156, 159, 159, 160, 160\}.$$

Clinical Trials in Neurology, ed. Bernard Ravina, Jeffrey Cummings, Michael P. McDermott, and R. Michael Poole. Published by Cambridge University Press. © Cambridge University Press 2012.

Table 6.1 Blood pressure data

Subject	1	2	3	4	5	6	7	8	9	10
Systolic BP (mmHg)	138	150	160	143	160	159	150	156	135	159
Diastolic BP (mmHg)	94	97	100	98	99	104	106	105	93	112

Because there are ten data items, the two middle items are items 5 and 6 in the ordered list. The median is defined as the average of these two items. In this case the median systolic blood pressure is $(150 + 156)/2 = 153$. If the data set consisted of only the first nine items in the list then the median would be the 5th item or 150. By definition, half of the data items are less than or equal to the median and half of the data items are greater than or equal to the median. The mean and the median for these data are close but they are not the same. If the data are symmetrically distributed about the mean then the median and the mean will be approximately the same. However, if the data are not symmetrically distributed or if there are extreme items then the mean and median can be substantially different. The median is not affected by extreme values so when the data are not symmetrically distributed the median is the preferred descriptive statistic.

There are also a number of ways to describe the variability in a data set. Statisticians frequently report the minimum and the maximum values. The difference between the minimum and the maximum is called the range. For the systolic blood pressure data the minimum is 135, the maximum is 160, and the range is $(160–135) = 25$.

The variance and standard deviation are other commonly used statistics. They are used to describe the variability in a data set. The variance is defined as the average squared difference of each observation from the mean of the data set. Statisticians usually use the symbol s^2 for the variance. In summation notation, the variance is defined as:

$$s^2 = \frac{1}{n-1}\sum_{i=1}^{n}\left(x_i - \bar{x}\right)^2.$$

Note that we divide by $(n-1)$ not n. As it turns out, dividing by n will tend to underestimate the true variance. Statisticians have shown that by dividing by $(n-1)$, we obtain an unbiased estimator of the true variance (i.e., one that is on average close to the true value). We will discuss this concept more below.

The variance of the systolic blood pressure data is computed as:

$$s^2 = \left(\frac{1}{9}\right)\left\{\left(138 - 151\right)^2 + \left(150 - 151\right)^2 + ... + \left(159 - 151\right)^2\right\}$$

$$= \frac{\left(-13\right)^2 + \left(-1\right)^2 + \left(9\right)^2 + \left(-8\right)^2 + \left(9\right)^2 + \left(8\right)^2 + \left(-1\right)^2 + \left(5\right)^2 + \left(-16\right)^2 + \left(8\right)^2}{9}$$

$$= \frac{806}{9} = 89.56.$$

The variance is in squared units or, in this case, $(\text{mm Hg})^2$. The standard deviation is defined as the square root of the variance and in this case is $s = 9.46$ mm Hg. The standard deviation is in the same units as the underlying data.

This is a very brief discussion of descriptive statistics. We provide computational details about the mean and variance because we will be using them repeatedly in the following sections.

Populations and samples

A population is a group of individuals that are of interest. In clinical trials the inclusion and exclusion criteria define the population of interest. For example, the Intraoperative Hypothermia for Aneurysm Surgery Trial IHAST study was conducted to determine the efficacy of hypothermia during surgery to repair ruptured intracranial aneurysms [1]. Specifically, the aim of the IHAST study was to determine whether mild intraoperative hypothermia results in improved neurological outcome in patients with an acute subarachnoid hemorrhage undergoing an open craniotomy to clip their aneurysms. The population could be roughly defined as all such individuals. The inclusion and exclusion criteria for IHAST specifically defined this population as follows:

> Eligible patients were at least 18 years of age, were not pregnant, had had a subarachnoid hemorrhage from a radiologically demonstrated intracranial aneurysm within 14 days before surgery, and had a World Federation of Neurological Surgeons score of I, II, or III ('good grade') at the time of enrollment, which was verified on arrival in the operating room. Patients were required to have had a Rankin score of 0 (no neurological disability) or 1 (mild disability) before hemorrhage. Patients were excluded if

they had a body-mass index of more than 35, had a cold-related disorder, or had an endotracheal tube in place.

It is important to define the population because results from a clinical trial will only strictly apply to the population from which the study patients were selected. For statistical purposes, we are usually interested in measurable attributes of the population: height, weight, blood pressure, gender, age, etc. We can consider the collection of the values of each of these variables as a population of values. So, for example, we might be interested in the population of blood glucose levels in the IHAST-eligible population.

A sample is defined as a subset of the population. The IHAST sample consisted of 1001 patients that satisfied all inclusion and exclusion criteria and were randomized to receive either hypothermia or normothermia during surgery to clip their ruptured aneurysms.

When we consider a population, we are usually interested in a particular characteristic or characteristics of that population. For example, we might be interested in the blood glucose levels at baseline in the IHAST population. Individual members of the population will have different baseline blood glucose levels. The population of glucose levels can be considered to have a distribution of values. Because we can never observe every member of a population, we must make inference about the population from a sample from that population. Statistical analysis provides methods for making informed estimates or decisions about population characteristics based on statistical summaries prepared from data collected on a sample of the population. Most statistical techniques require that samples are collected in such a way that the probability that each individual from the population is included in the sample is known. The well-known simple random sample requires that the probabilities of being selected are the same for all members of the population. Clearly, it is very unlikely that this is the case for most clinical trials where the sample is a convenience sample and the probabilities of being selected are not known. However, randomizing subjects to treatments will ensure that the statistical analyses are valid [2]. The probability of being assigned to each treatment is known.

Just as each sample has a mean and a variance, each population has a mean and a variance. Characteristics of populations are called parameters. Population parameters include the population mean, the population variance, and the population standard deviation. These values would be calculated in much the same way that statistics are calculated from samples. These population parameters are the real characteristics

Table 6.2 Distribution of race/ethnicity in the IHAST population

Race/ethnicity	Relative frequency
White	80%
Black	7%
Hispanic	6%
Other	7%

of interest. For example, we might be interested in the mean or variance of baseline blood glucose levels in patients with ruptured intracranial aneurysms. Because there are a very large number of these individuals, it is impractical to measure them all.

Our inability to measure the entire population requires that we make inference about the population from a sample selected from that population. The discipline of statistics provides methods for making 'good' estimates of population parameters (e.g., mean or variance) from samples. It also provides methods for quantifying the degree to which statistical estimates are likely to deviate from the population parameters. Several of these techniques will be illustrated in this chapter.

We speak of the distribution of a certain characteristic in a population. The population distribution is the set of all possible values that a characteristic can assume and the frequencies with which those values occur in the population. We use the mean and variance to describe the distribution of a characteristic that is measured with a device like a ruler, scale, or thermometer. These characteristics are said to be continuous. Height, weight, blood pressure, and serum glucose are continuous variables. For characteristics like race and gender that can have only a small number of distinct values, the distribution is usually described by a listing of the values and the frequency that members of the population take on each value. These variables are called discrete. For example, the distribution of race in the IHAST sample is described in Table 6.2. This table lists all possible values and the relative frequencies with which those values occur in the sample of study participants.

One could ask how we know that this is the distribution of race/ethnicity in this population. The short answer is that we don't. This table was compiled from a sample of 1001 individuals from that population. Because the sample is so large, we can be confident that the population frequencies will be very close to these values. However, we will never be sure because we will never determine the characteristics the entire population. The value of statistics is that if we choose the sample in an appropriate way and if the sample size is sufficiently large then we can be confident that the estimated frequencies will be close to the true values. We can also make probability statements about how close the observed values are to the true values.

Some useful population distributions

The normal and *t* distributions

The normal distribution is commonly used in statistics. It has the well-known bell shape. Figure 6.1 provides a graph of a normal distribution. Note that it is symmetric about its mean (if we folded it on a line through the middle the two halves would coincide). The normal distribution is completely determined by its mean and variance. The mean is usually denoted by the Greek letter μ and the standard deviation is denoted by the Greek letter σ. The variance is denoted by σ^2. Figure 6.1 also illustrates some useful properties of the normal distribution. First, 68% of the distribution lies within 1 standard deviation of the mean. This means that if one randomly draws an observation from this distribution, the probability is 0.68 that the observed value will be within 1 standard deviation of the population mean. If the sample is large enough, 68% of the sample will fall within 1 standard deviation of the mean. Similarly, the probability is 0.95 that the observation will be within 2.0 standard deviations. (Note that the actual values are ±1.96 but this is commonly rounded to 2.0.) The probability is 0.025 that a randomly selected observation will be more than 2.0 standard deviations below the population mean and the probability is 0.025 that

a randomly selected observation will be more than 2.0 standard deviations above the population mean.

Figure 6.1 displays normal distributions with mean zero but different standard deviations. Note that a larger standard deviation (variance) means that the distribution has more variation (spread) about the mean.

Another useful distribution is the Student's t distribution. It looks very much like the unit normal distribution (mean zero and variance one); it is symmetric and is centered at zero but has greater variability (see Figure 6.2). The t distribution depends on one parameter called the degrees of freedom. For small degrees of freedom the distribution has much more spread than the unit normal distribution. As the number of degrees of freedom increases, the t distribution approaches the unit normal distribution. Note that with increasing degrees of freedom, the t distributions have higher maximum values and less probability in the tails.

Given the mathematical properties of distributions, we can compute probabilities associated with drawing observations from normal and t distributions. One very useful set of probabilities is the set of probabilities that a randomly drawn observation will be less than or equal to a given value. For a unit normal distribution (usually denoted by Z) these probabilities can be written as $P\{Z < z\}$. So for example, $P\{Z < 0\} = 0.5$ and $P\{Z \leq -1.96\} = 0.025$.

It is also useful to find values of z that have particular probabilities. These are called percentiles of the distribution and are denoted by the symbol z_α. A useful percentile is denoted $z_{.975}$. This number has the property

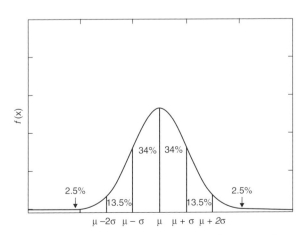

Figure 6.1. A normal probability distribution with mean μ and standard deviation σ.

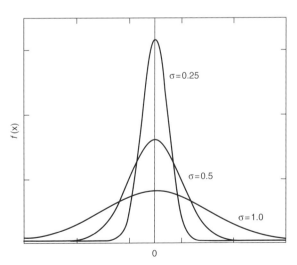

Figure 6.2. Normal probability distributions with mean zero but different variances.

55

Table 6.3 Selected percentiles for normal and t distribution

	Student's t distribution				Unit normal (df = ∞)
Percentile	df = 10	df = 15	df = 20	df = 30	
0.001	−4.144	−3.733	−3.552	−3.385	−3.09
0.01	−2.764	−2.602	−2.528	−2.457	−2.33
0.025	−2.228	−2.131	−2.086	−2.042	−1.96
0.05	−1.812	−1.753	−1.725	−1.679	−1.645
0.10	−1.372	−1.341	−1.325	−1.310	−1.282
0.90	1.372	1.341	1.325	1.310	1.282
0.95	2.228	1.753	1/725	1.679	1.645
0.975	1.812	2.131	2.086	2.042	1.96
0.99	2.764	2.602	2.528	2.457	2.33
0.999	4.144	3.733	3.552	3.385	3.09

that $P\{Z \le z_{.975}\} = 0.975$. We already know that 1.96 has this property so that $z_{.975} = 1.96$. This also means that $P\{Z > z_{.975}\} = 0.025$.

Table 6.3 provides percentiles for the unit normal distribution and the t distribution for selected degrees of freedom. Note that as the degrees of freedom (df) increase, the percentiles of the t distribution approach the corresponding percentiles of the unit normal distribution. We will use these percentiles in the sections on confidence intervals and testing of hypotheses.

The distribution of the sample mean

In making statistical inference, one draws a sample from a population and computes one or more statistics. Frequently, these include the sample mean and the sample standard deviation. Each sample has its own sample mean and sample variance. If the population is large, there are a large number of possible samples. Repeated sampling will lead to a distribution of sample means and sample variances. By drawing a large number of random samples from the population and computing a sample mean for each, the distribution of the collection of observed sample means will approximate the distribution of the population of all possible sample means. Statisticians have shown that if repeated samples are drawn at random from a normal distribution with mean μ and standard deviation σ then the distribution of the sample means (called the sampling distribution of the sample mean) will also be normal. The mean of this distribution will be the population mean μ and the

variance of this distribution will be the population variance σ² divided by the sample size n. We write:

$$\text{mean}(\bar{x}) = \mu$$
$$\text{variance}(\bar{x}) = \frac{\sigma^2}{n} \qquad (6.1)$$

Statisticians say that the sample mean is an unbiased estimator of the population mean because the mean of the sampling distribution of the sample mean is the population mean. If we use the sample mean to estimate the population mean then on average (over repeated samples) the calculated estimate will be close to the population value. Also note that as the sample size increases the variability of the sample mean gets smaller. If we select a very large sample then the variance of the sampling distribution of the sample mean will be very small and our repeated estimates will cluster closely about the true population mean. By taking a large enough sample, we can guarantee with high probability that our estimate is as close as we want to the true population value.

If the population distribution is normal then the sampling distribution of the sample mean will also be normal. Indeed, if the underlying distribution has a finite mean and variance and if the sample size is large enough, the sampling distribution of the sample mean will be normal regardless of the true underlying population distribution. This result is called the central limit theorem.

The standard deviation of the sampling distribution of the sample mean (the distribution of all possible sample means) is $\sqrt{\sigma^2/n} = \sigma/\sqrt{n}$. This quantity is also called the standard error of the mean. Note that it is smaller than the population standard deviation. We will use an estimator of this quantity $\sqrt{s^2/n} = \frac{s}{\sqrt{n}}$ in many of the methods for confidence interval estimation and hypothesis testing described below.

Confidence intervals

Confidence intervals for a single normal population mean

Using the facts about the sampling distribution of the sample mean from above ('The distribution of the sample mean') and a few simple algebraic calculations, one can show that the following probability statement is valid for any normal distribution:

$$\Pr\left\{\overline{x}-1.96\left(\sigma/\sqrt{n}\right)<\mu<\overline{x}+1.96\left(\sigma/\sqrt{n}\right)\right\}=0.95$$

This means that if we repeatedly draw samples of size n from a normal distribution with mean μ and standard deviation σ and if we calculate the interval

$$\left(\overline{x}-1.96\left(\sigma/\sqrt{n}\right),\overline{x}+1.96\left(\sigma/\sqrt{n}\right)\right)$$

for each of those samples, then 95% of those intervals will include the true population mean. This also means that 5% of the intervals will not contain the true population mean. We call the interval $\left(\overline{x}-1.96\left(\sigma/\sqrt{n}\right),\overline{x}+1.96\left(\sigma/\sqrt{n}\right)\right)$ a 95% confidence interval for the true population mean. If we use another percentile of the normal distribution instead of 1.96, say $z_{1-(\alpha/2)}$, then we know that

$$\Pr\left\{\overline{x}-z_{1-\alpha/2}\left(\sigma/\sqrt{n}\right)<\mu<\overline{x}+z_{1-\alpha/2}\left(\sigma/\sqrt{n}\right)\right\}=1-\alpha \tag{0.2}$$

We say that we are $100\times(1-\alpha)\%$ confident that the true population mean is in the interval:

$$\left(\overline{x}-z_{1-\alpha/2}\left(\sigma/\sqrt{n}\right),\overline{x}+z_{1-\alpha/2}\left(\sigma/\sqrt{n}\right)\right). \tag{0.3}$$

So, if $\alpha=0.05$ (and $z_{1-(\alpha/2)}=1.96$) then we are 95% confident and if $\alpha=0.10$ (and $z_{1-(\alpha/2)}=1.645$) then we are 90% confident.

These intervals require that we know the population standard deviation σ. Clearly, if we don't know the population mean then we don't know the population standard deviation. Fortunately, statistical theory states that if we use the t distribution in place of the unit normal distribution, the following probability statement is true:

$$\Pr\left\{\overline{x}-t_{1-\alpha/2,n-1}\left(s/\sqrt{n}\right)<\mu<\overline{x}+t_{1-\alpha/2,n-1}\left(s/\sqrt{n}\right)\right\}=1-\alpha$$

where s is the sample standard deviation. The degrees of freedom used to find the appropriate percentile of the t distribution is the sample size minus 1 ($n-1$). In general, we can be $100\times(1-\alpha)\%$ confident that the true population mean is in the interval:

Table 6.4 Blood glucose levels in a sample of IHAST eligible patients

Statistic	Computed value
N	16
Mean	134.1
Standard deviation	29.6

$$\left(\overline{x}-t_{1-\alpha/2,n-1}\left(s/\sqrt{n}\right),\overline{x}+t_{1-\alpha/2,n-1}\left(s/\sqrt{n}\right)\right). \tag{0.4}$$

In practice we only collect data on a single sample then we calculate the sample mean $\overline{x}$, the sample standard deviation s, and the single confidence interval $\left(\overline{x}-t_{1-\alpha/2,n-1}\left(s/\sqrt{n}\right),\overline{x}+t_{1-\alpha/2,n-1}\left(s/\sqrt{n}\right)\right)$. The probability is either 0 or 1 that this interval contains the true population mean μ; because there is only one interval. However, if we assume that the true population mean is in the interval then over many such computations we know we will be wrong only $100\times\alpha$ % of the time. By calculating intervals in this way, we have controlled the frequency that we will be wrong (the interval will not contain the true value μ).

Example:
An investigator is interested in estimating the mean blood glucose level in subjects who would be eligible for participation in the IHAST study. She collects a random sample of 16 subjects from the population and measures their glucose levels. The results of that experiment are summarized in Table 6.4.

She wants to compute a 95% confidence interval for the true population mean. The appropriate t distribution is determined by the sample size. If the sample size is n then the appropriate distribution is the t distribution with $n-1$ degrees of freedom. Because there are 16 observations in the sample, the standard error has $(16-1)=15$ degrees of freedom. If we want a 95% confidence interval then we would use the 97.5 percentile of the t distribution with 15 degrees of freedom. From Table 6.3 we see that this percentile is $t_{.975,15}=2.131$. A 95% confidence interval for the true mean glucose level in this population is given by:

$$\begin{aligned}
&\left(\overline{x}-t_{1-\alpha/2,n-1}\left(s/\sqrt{n}\right),\overline{x}+t_{1-\alpha/2,n-1}\left(s/\sqrt{n}\right)\right)\\
&=\left(134.1-2.131(7.40),134.1+2.131(7.40)\right)\\
&=\left(134.1-15.77,134.1+15.77\right)\\
&=\left(118.3,149.9\right)
\end{aligned}$$

We are 95% confident that the true mean glucose level in this population is between 118.3 and 149.9. The true mean may not be in this interval. However, we do know that if we were to repeat this experiment a large number of times (say 10,000,000) we would know that 95% of intervals computed in this way will contain the true population mean and 5% will not.

If we want to be 90% confident then the 95th percentile of the t distribution with 15 degrees of freedom is $t_{.95,15} = 1.753$. Using this percentile in our computation we find the 90% confidence interval:

$$\left(\bar{x} - t_{1-\alpha/2,n-1}\left(s/\sqrt{n}\right), \bar{x} + t_{1-\alpha/2,n-1}\left(s/\sqrt{n}\right)\right)$$
$$= \left(134.1 - 1.753(7.40), 134.1 + 1.753(7.40)\right)$$
$$= \left(134.1 - 12.97, 134.1 + 12.97\right)$$
$$= \left(121.1, 147.1\right)$$

Because the confidence coefficient is smaller (90% compared to 95%) the confidence interval is narrower. As we raise the required level of confidence we must widen our confidence interval.

Most confidence intervals use similar methods. In general, a confidence interval is made up of a *point* estimate (like $\bar{x}$), the standard error of that estimate, and a tabular value like the z or t values that were used in the previous sections. We will now describe methods for computing confidence intervals for several other situations.

Confidence interval for the difference between two independent normal population means

In a two-arm clinical trial we are usually comparing a new or innovative intervention to a standard or control intervention. If the outcome of interest is a characteristic that is approximately normally distributed then the parameter of interest is usually the difference in the population means, say $(\mu_x - \mu_y)$. Subjects are randomly assigned to treatments and we say that the two samples are independent. We might represent the sample from the innovative population as $\{x_1, x_2,...,x_m\}$ and the sample from the standard population as $\{y_1, y_2,...,y_n\}$. The data from the two samples are usually summarized as sample means and variances, say $\bar{x}$, s_x^2 and $\bar{y}$, s_y^2 respectively. The natural estimator of the difference between the two population means is the difference between the two sample means $\bar{x} - \bar{y}$.

If we want to construct a confidence interval then we will need the standard error of the difference in the sample means. If the two populations have the same variance then the variance of the difference in the sample means is given by $\sigma^2\left(\frac{1}{m} + \frac{1}{n}\right)$. Unfortunately, this variance has an unknown quantity σ^2. If we can assume that the variances in the two populations are approximately the same then we estimate this quantity from the observed standard deviations with the weighted average $s_p^2 = \dfrac{(m-1)s_x^2 + (n-1)s_y^2}{(m-1)+(n-1)}$ called the pooled estimate of the variance or the pooled variance. The standard error of the difference between the two treatment means is estimated by substituting this estimate for the unknown variance and then taking the square root. That is, the standard error of the difference in sample means is estimated by $s_p\sqrt{\dfrac{1}{m} + \dfrac{1}{n}}$. A $100(1-\alpha)$% confidence interval for the difference in the means is provided by the quantity:

$$\left(\left(\bar{x} - \bar{y}\right) - t_{1-\alpha/2,m+n-2}\, s_p\left(\sqrt{\frac{1}{m} + \frac{1}{n}}\right), \left(\bar{x} - \bar{y}\right)\right.$$
$$\left. + t_{1-\alpha/2,m+n-2}\, s_p\left(\sqrt{\frac{1}{m} + \frac{1}{n}}\right)\right)$$

where the degrees of freedom for the tabular t-value is $(m-1)+(n-1) = m+n-2$.

Example:
Investigators are interested in estimating the difference in mean glucose levels in two populations: subjects who receive a new intervention and subjects who receive a control intervention. The data from this study are summarized in Table 6.5.

In this case the estimate of the true difference in the population means (Standard minus Innovative) is $(138.40 - 119.00) = 19.40$ mg/dL. The pooled estimate of the variance is given by:

$$s_p^2 = \frac{(30-1)(31.82)^2 + (30-1)(29.46)^2}{(30+30-2)} = 940.20$$

$$s_p = \sqrt{940.20} = 30.66$$

The standard error of the difference is therefore:
$s_p\sqrt{\dfrac{1}{30} + \dfrac{1}{30}} = 30.66\sqrt{\dfrac{2}{30}} = 7.91$. The appropriate tabular value comes from the t distribution with $30 + 30 - 2 = 58$ degrees of freedom. For a 95% confidence interval we would use the 0.975 percentile of the t distribution

Table 6.5 Statistical summary of blood glucose levels in two samples

	Blood glucose levels (mg/dL)	
	Standard treatment	Innovative treatment
N	30	30
Mean	138.40	119.03
Standard deviation	31.82	29.46

with 58 degrees of freedom or $t_{0.975,58} = 2.002$ (not presented in Table 6.3). This yields the 95% confidence interval:

$$\left(19.37 - 2.002(7.91), 19.37 + 2.002(7.91)\right)$$
$$\text{or } \left(19.37 - 15.84, 19.37 + 15.84\right)$$
$$\text{or } \left(3.53, \ 35.21\right).$$

We are 95% confident that the true difference in mean glucose levels between the Innovative intervention and the Standard intervention lies between 3.53 and 35.21 mg/dL. Note that we are 95% confident that the true difference is greater than zero and, hence, that the true difference is in favor of the Innovative intervention.

Confidence interval for a single population proportion

When the outcome is a binary outcome like success or failure then we are usually interested in the success rate (or failure rate). That is, we are interested in the proportion of subjects who experience one of the two possible events. In the IHAST study, the primary measure of efficacy was a Glasgow Outcome Scale (GOS) score at 90 days after surgery. A subject was defined as a success if her/his GOS was 1 (no neurological deficit). In that study 301 of 501 normothermia subjects had a GOS 1 at 90 days after surgery. The success rate for normothermia subjects is:

$$301 / 501 = 0.601.$$

We would like a confidence interval for the true proportion of successes in this population. We can use a variant of the method that we used for the sample mean. If we collect a sample of m subjects and code the data as $x_i = 1$ if subject i had a success and $x_i = 0$ if subject i had a failure then the data are just a collection of 1s and 0s. The mean for this sample of m subjects is $\bar{x} = \dfrac{1}{m}\sum_{i=1}^{m} x_i = \dfrac{\text{the number of successes}}{m}$. But this is

the observed proportion of subjects who experience a success. We will denote this (sample) proportion by $\hat{p}$. We can use this sample proportion to estimate the population proportion but we would also like to compute a confidence interval for the true proportion.

We have already said that if the sample size is large enough then the sample mean will be approximately normally distributed even if the underlying distribution is not normal (as in this case where the underlying distribution is discrete, with outcomes taking on the values 0 or 1). Statisticians have shown that the variance of the sampling distribution of the sample proportion can be estimated by: $\dfrac{\hat{p}\left(1 - \hat{p}\right)}{m}$. A $100(1-\alpha)\%$ confidence interval can therefore be computed using the formula:

$$\left(\hat{p} - z_{1-\alpha/2}\sqrt{\frac{\hat{p}\left(1 - \hat{p}\right)}{m}}, \hat{p} + z_{1-\alpha/2}\sqrt{\frac{\hat{p}\left(1 - \hat{p}\right)}{m}}\right)$$

Example:
An investigator is interested in studying the ability of a new drug to lower the rates of hyperglycemia during the acute treatment of stroke. She conducted a study to compare the rates for her new treatment to those of the standard treatment. The results of this study are described in Table 6.6.

For her initial analyses she computes 95% confidence intervals for the rates of hypoglycemia in each of the two treatment groups. The calculations are provided in Table 6.7. These calculations indicate that we can be 95% confident that the true rate of hypoglycemia in the standard treatment group is between 0.1229 and 0.3021. Similarly, we can be 95% confident that the true rate of hypoglycemia in the innovative therapy groups is between 0.0601 and 0.2179. Because these two intervals overlap we should probably not expect that the true means are different in the two populations. We will discuss this more later.

Confidence interval for the difference in two independent population proportions

At this stage, the investigator would like to evaluate the difference in the rates of hyperglycemia for the two treatments. The obvious estimate of the difference is the observed difference in the rates $\hat{p}_S - \hat{p}_T = (.2125 - .1250)$.

Another alternative to intention to treat is called the **as treated** analysis. This analysis assigns subjects to their treatment at the end of the study. A subject who crosses over from the innovative drug to placebo is analyzed as a placebo subject and a subject who crosses over from placebo to the innovative drug is analyzed as an innovative drug subject. There are logical problems with this strategy because a subject receives one treatment for part of the follow-up period and another for the remainder of follow-up. Variations of this method will analyze a subject in the group that they were in the longest. In any case it should be clear that any results from this analysis will have potential for bias.

Regulatory organizations such as FDA and the International Conference on Harmonisation (ICH) [6] recommend that the primary efficacy analysis be based on the intention to treat principle. However, many studies report a compliers analysis and/or an as treated analysis. If these analyses agree then the overall conclusions will have more credibility since the results are likely to not strongly depend on compliance. If they do not agree, then both FDA and ICH recommend that the most valid conclusions are those based on the intention to treat analysis.

Other considerations in analyzing clinical trial data: Missing data and imputation

The intention to treat principle requires that **all** subjects be analyzed according to the treatment that they were assigned by the randomization. This means that subjects who drop out of the study or are lost to follow-up must be included in the analysis. In typical studies this means that we must impute (guess) the value that a subject would have provided had they not dropped out. Imputation can lead to bias in many of the same ways that crossover does. If drop-out is related to toxicity or tolerability then subjects in a more intensive intervention will be more likely to not finish the study. Any method used to impute missing values must address the potential bias that could result from 'guessing' the value that would have been observed had the subject completed the trial. One method may be good if the data are missing for one set of reasons while another might be preferred if there are other reasons for the data being unobserved.

Types of missing data

Rubin [5] has proposed a list of different classes of reasons for missing data. His first class is called 'missing

completely at random' or **MCAR**. In this case, the reason that the value was not observed is completely independent of the data observed for that subject as well as the value that would have been observed. This is the 'subject was run over by a bus' category. The reason that the observation is missing depends in no way on characteristics of the subject (e.g. severity of disease) or the true level of the potential observation. This is the best case because one can analyze the complete data and still obtain unbiased results.

The next class of missing data is called 'missing at random' or **MAR**. In this case, the reason why an observation is missing may depend on the observed data but the reason is not related to other processes once the observed data have been taken into account. All of the information about the reasons for the data being missing is contained in data that has already been observed. For example, a subject drops out and no longer continues in the study if her/his disease deteriorates to a level where the subject can no longer continue in the study. In this case, the reason for a subsequent value being missing only depends on the data that have already been observed but not on the unobserved (future) outcomes.

The third class of missing data is called 'missing not at random' or **MNAR**. Sometimes this is referred to as informative missingness. In this case the processes that cause observations to be missing are related to the values that would have been observed but are not. Think of the case of an Alzheimer's patient who is doing very well cognitively but, all of a sudden, 'falls off the cliff' in terms of becoming demented. This event happens after having observed the patient's 'good' cognitive scores but the patient drops out after this event and no 'bad' cognitive data are ever observed. In this case, the reason for missing data depends more on what is not observed, and not so much on what is observed. Methods for analysis of data that are MNAR are still being developed and will not be discussed here.

Methods for accounting for missing data

The best way to account for missing data is to vigorously manage the conduct of the study in ways that avoid missing data. If there are no missing data then one does not need to worry about how to account for it in the analysis. If the proportion of missing data is small then the results of the analysis probably will not depend strongly on how you account for the missing data. Unfortunately, this is not always possible.

Multiple methods have been used to impute missing data [7]. A method that was very commonly used in the past is called 'last observation carried forward' or **LOCF**. In this case, the last value that was observed on the subject earlier in the study is substituted for the missing value. This requires that the outcome be measured repeatedly during follow-up so that a value is available in case a subject drops out. Depending on the situation, this method can result in conservative conclusions that underestimate the true treatment effects or anticonservative conclusions that overestimate the true treatment effects. LOCF will be conservative if, for example, people in the placebo group have worse responses than people in the treatment group and drop out more frequently or earlier. LOCF will be anticonservative if, for example, the disease is progressive and people in the treatment group drop out more frequently or earlier than people in the placebo group. LOCF has been used extensively in the past but is no longer recommended. It is typically associated with bias regardless of the missing data mechanism (even if it is MCAR) and has generally very poor properties relative to other methods.

Other imputation methods are based on developing regression models that predict the value that would have been observed based on data that were observed (e.g., observed outcomes at earlier time points and baseline characteristics) and use the predicted value for the missing value. Clearly, these methods are only valid if the data are missing at random. Regression analyses estimate the mean of values that would have been observed for a subject with a given set of predictor values. The value that would have been observed would also have a random deviation about the predicted value. Ignoring this random component would result in underestimating the true variability in the data. This, in turn, results in inappropriately narrow confidence intervals and inappropriately large test statistics and small p-values. This is a problem with all so-called 'single imputation' methods such as those described above, including LOCF.

The method of multiple imputation was developed to overcome the deficiencies of the single imputation methods. It uses likelihood methods to impute missing values but incorporates additional features that account for the uncertainty in the imputation, which is related to the random variability of the individual's observed value. Many authors have proposed methods for imputing missing values. Some are based on likelihood methods such as the Estimation/Maximization (EM) algorithm. Others rely on regression models to predict the missing data for data that are observed. The procedures that are implemented in statistical packages allow the user to select from a menu of methods. We will not discuss these methods in detail but will briefly discuss the general ideas behind multiple imputation briefly.

The method of multiple imputation

The method of multiple imputation is described in many articles in the literature [8, 9]. The article by Enders [10] provides a useful primer on its use. One advantage of the MI method is that it has been implemented in several statistical software packages (for example both SAS and SPSS support multiple imputation). The basic strategy is to create multiple complete data sets with missing values imputed usually using a regression approach. The idea, in layman's terms, is that you impute not the predicted value, but the predicted value plus an appropriate amount of random 'jitter' that reflects the uncertainty associated with that predicted value. The multiple data sets are identical for the values that were observed; they only differ with respect to the values that are imputed, which depend on the random 'jitter' that is added to each predicted value. For a more detailed description of the process, see the Enders primer article cited above.

These data sets are each analyzed separately using the same statistical methods and the results for each analysis are recorded. Each analysis yields a parameter estimate and a standard error of that estimate. These individual estimates are combined to provide the final estimate of treatment effect and its associated standard error.

The MI method has several advantages. First, it uses observed data to develop the imputed values. Each predicted value is based on a regression analysis using observed data. Variables should be included in the prediction models that are either related to the variable being imputed or to the missing value process. The assumption is that data are MAR and so all of the information necessary for this process should be available. Another major advantage of the MI method is that it properly accounts for the uncertainty of the imputed (predicted) values and thus provides better estimates of the true variance of the treatment effects.

Conclusion

This chapter provides a very brief discussion of selected techniques for analyzing data from clinical trials. The methods presented here are both useful and are applicable in many real situations. The literature is rich with other statistical methods that can also be applied to these studies, including methods for analyzing time-to-event data, methods that incorporate covariate information, and methods that are less sensitive to assumptions (e.g., non-parametric methods). The reader is urged to consult appropriate sources to expand on the material presented here [2].

References

1. Todd MM, Hindman BJ, Clarke WR, *et al.* Mild intraoperative hypothermia during surgery for intracranial aneurysm. *New Engl J Med* 2005; **352**(2): 135–145.

2. Piantadosi S. *Clinical Trials: A Methodologic Perspective* (second edition). Hoboken, New Jersey: John Wiley and Sons, Inc, 2005.

3. Peduzzi P, Wittes J, and Detre K. Analysis as-randomized and the problem of non-adherence: an example from the veterans affairs randomized trial of coronary artery bypass surgery. *Stat Med* 1993; **12**: 1185–1195.

4. Lachin JM. Statistical considerations in the intent-to-treat principle. *Control Clin Trials* 2000; **21**: 167–189.

5. Rubin DB. Inference and missing data. *Biometrika* 1976; **63**; 581–592.

6. International Conference on Harmonisation, (n.d.). www.ich.org.

7. Liu M, Wei L, and Zhang J. Review of guidelines and literature for handling missing data in longitudinal clinical trials with a case study. *Pharm Stat* 2006; **5**: 7–18.

8. Fraset G and Ru Y. Guided multiple imputation of missing data: using a subsample to strengthen the missing-at-random assumption. *Epidemiology* 2007; **18**: 246–252.

9. Kenward MG and Carpenter J. Multiple imputation: current perspectives. *Stat Methods Med Res* 2007; **16**: 199–218.

10. Enders CK. A primer on the use of modern missing-data methods in psychosomatic medicine research. *Psychosom Med* 2006; **68**: 427–436.

Chapter

7

Selecting outcome measures

Robert G. Holloway and Andrew D. Siderowf

Introduction

The selection and proper use of outcome measures is of vital importance in clinical trials in neurology. Poorly developed and chosen outcome measures can result in missing true effects of a treatment (type II error) or may capture weak signals of effects that are not clinically significant (type I errors). These errors can result in missed opportunities, wasted resources, and patient harm. The field of translational research is providing us with an ever-increasing number of biomarker targets for early-phase clinical trials. Clear verdicts on therapeutic advances will not occur without a reasoned approach to outcomes measure selection based in a sound conceptual framework. The development of methodologically sound outcome measures is a critical step but is outside of the scope of this chapter which will focus on the use of measures rather than on their development. Here we provide an overview of outcome measures in neurology clinical trials, including developing a conceptual endpoint model, role and use of biomarkers, and considerations on how to select, use and interpret them in the context of early-stage clinical trial design.

Outcome measures in neurology clinical trials

The domains of outcomes used in neurology clinical trials range from biomarkers and lab correlates, signs and symptoms of disease, safety endpoints, functional scales, disability scales, survival endpoints, patient-reported outcomes, health-related quality of life measures, and economic endpoints. Each subspecialty in neurology has a growing portfolio of outcome measures [1]. Figure 7.1

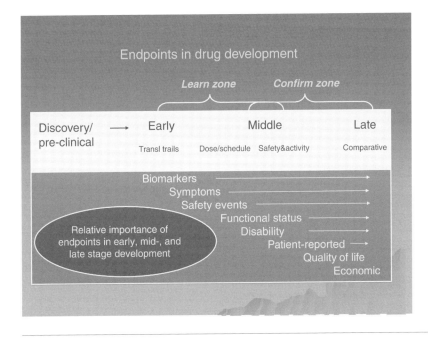

Figure 7.1. The relative importance of outcome measures and clinical trial endpoints in drug development.

Clinical Trials in Neurology, ed. Bernard Ravina, Jeffrey Cummings, Michael P. McDermott, and R. Michael Poole. Published by Cambridge University Press. © Cambridge University Press 2012.

Table 7.1 Endpoint models: treatments of various neurological disease

Concept	Outcome	Endpoints
Friedrich's ataxia and reduction in frataxin expression	Increasing frataxin expression	**Primary** Change from baseline in frataxin expression levels **Secondary** Symptom diary (ataxia rating scale) Physical performance (activities of daily living scale)
Stroke	Decrease in stroke rate	**Primary** Reduction in the proportion of patients with stroke over a 3-year period **Secondary** Recanalization of an occluded artery Stroke functional scale (e.g., NINDS)
ALS functional status	Slow functional decline	**Primary** Change in ALS Functional Status Rating Scale over 6 month period **Secondary** Health-Related Quality of Life Adverse event profile Biomarker outcome (e.g., proteonomic profiling of CSF)

shows relative importance of clinical trial endpoints in early, mid, and late stage therapeutic development.

Early stage clinical trials (phase 1–2) often employ biomarker targets for proof of concept or therapeutic validation. These trials are sometimes referred to as the 'learn zone' of drug development (see Chapters 1–3). A growing number of biomarkers are available for early stage clinical trial development and are explained below. Safety endpoints are of critical importance in all stages of development. Functional status and disability rating scales are commonly employed in neurology to capture the multi-dimensional concept and manifestations often associated with neurological conditions. These scales are often the primary outcome measures used in the 'confirm zone' of therapeutic development. Health-related quality of life (HRQL) and patient reported outcome measures are becoming increasingly important in clinical development programs. For example, the FDA issued its finalized guidance on the use of Patient Reported Outcome (PRO) measures to support new drug applications and labeling claims in product development [2]. The NIH Toolbox initiative is utilizing state-of-the-art psychometric and technological approaches to develop brief yet comprehensive assessment tools for measuring motor, cognitive, sensory, and emotional function [3]. The NINDS funded Neuro-QOL project aims to develop a clinically relevant and psychometrically robust HRQL assessment tool for adults and children that will be responsive to the needs of researchers in a variety of neurological disorders [4]. These trends toward 'patient-centeredness' are also being motivated by payers of medical care who will reward providers based on patient experiences and satisfaction with their care. Finally, economic endpoints will be an increasing consideration as the comparative cost and cost-effectiveness of competing interventions are evaluated.

Endpoint model

The choice of an outcome measure is one of the most important decisions in designing a clinical trial. Selection of a primary endpoint and secondary endpoints should be driven by the clinical trial objectives, the trial design, the target population enrolled, and the conceptual framework of disease mechanism and the hypothesized effect of treatment. The result of this process should be a rationale measurement sequence based on biological effects, concepts being measured, outcomes being used, and the appropriate selection of clinical trial endpoints. Table 7.1 shows examples of endpoint models from various neurological diseases and therapeutic programs. These examples include the important domains of measurement, the physiological markers (i.e., biomarkers), the clinical outcome measures, and the clinical trial endpoints used in the statistical analysis. The endpoint model is important to help focus on the primary endpoints, the secondary endpoints, and exploratory endpoints by explaining the exact demands placed on the endpoints to meet the clinical trial objectives.

Therapeutic development programs can be viewed as in the learn zone and confirm zone, with confirmation occurring in the phase 3 trial designed to test clinical efficacy against a standard or placebo [5]. The learn zone includes those studies in development that contribute to the necessary information to ultimately conduct confirmatory clinical trials. These are usually within traditionally grouped phases 1 and 2 clinical trials (see Chapter 17). Since many early stage (learn zone) clinical trials use physiological measures or biomarker endpoints in therapeutic development, we review the role and use of biomarkers and surrogate endpoints in various neurological disease programs.

Biomarker in clinical trials

There is consensus that better biomarkers are needed in almost every area of neurology. Biomarkers can assist in improved diagnosis of patients with neurological disorders. Perhaps more importantly, biomarkers may facilitate more rapid and reliable development of new therapeutics.

This account will focus on the role of biomarkers in clinical trials. The first part will review definitions of terms such as biomarker and surrogate endpoint, place them in a theoretical context, and review some reasons that biomarkers may not succeed as surrogate outcomes. Then the role of biomarkers in the progressive phases of clinical trials will be addressed and finally some examples of some classes of biomarkers currently or potentially available for assessment of neurological disorders will be discussed.

Biomarker definitions and conceptual framework

The NIH Biomarkers Definitions Working Group has produced a standard set of definitions for biomarkers and related concepts, and placed them in an overall theoretical framework [6]. The key definitions from this panel are as follows:

A biological marker (biomarker): A characteristic that is objectively measured and evaluated as an indicator of normal biological processes, pathogenic proc-

esses, or pharmacologic response to a therapeutic intervention.

A clinical endpoint: A characteristic or variable that reflects how a patient feels, functions, or survives. In a clinical trial, changes in a clinical endpoint may reflect the effect of a therapeutic intervention. For the purpose of understanding the usefulness of a drug in a clinical setting, clinical endpoints are the most credible measure that can be assessed in a clinical trial.

A surrogate endpoint: A biomarker that is intended to substitute for a clinical endpoint. A surrogate endpoint is expected to predict clinical benefit or harm or lack of benefit or harm based on epidemiologic therapeutic pathophysiologic or other scientific evidence. Surrogate endpoints are a subset of biomarkers. The term surrogate literally means 'substitute of' therefore the NIH working group discourages the use of the term surrogate marker because it suggests the substitution is for a marker rather than for a clinical endpoint.

The greatest interest in biomarkers in clinical trials is when they can be used as surrogate outcome measures. However, finding a valid surrogate outcome measures can be very difficult. According to Prentice [7], a surrogate endpoint must both correlate with the true clinical outcome and fully capture the net effect of treatment on the clinical outcome. A schematic showing this relationship is shown in Figure 7.2.

Excellent examples of valid surrogate outcome measures exist in some areas of medicine. Cholesterol as a marker for subsequent cardiovascular events is one example. However, there are also many notable examples of biomarkers that have not been successful surrogates. One of the most notorious examples of a failed biomarker is the use of electro-cardiogram in the Cardiac Arrythmia Supression Trial (CAST). In this case, ECG showing more regular heartbeats was *inversely* correlated with survival. Although results from trials with clinical measures as the primary outcome are generally required for drug approval, in some cases, the FDA may accept accelerated marketing approval based on effects on a surrogate endpoint.

The Biomarkers Definitions Working Group conceptual model (Figure 7.3, adapted from [6]) shows the relationship between biomarkers, surrogate markers, and clinical outcomes. In this model, surrogate outcome measures represent a fraction of biomarkers, since only some biomarkers will meet the additional

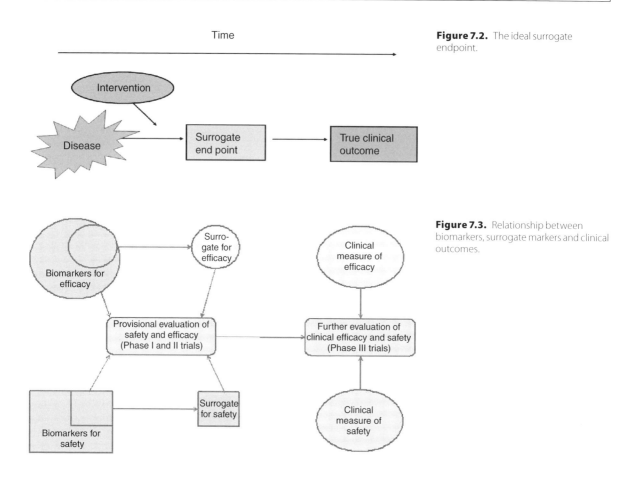

Figure 7.2. The ideal surrogate endpoint.

Figure 7.3. Relationship between biomarkers, surrogate markers and clinical outcomes.

The surrogate is not in the causal pathway of the disease process

Of several causal pathways of disease, the intervention affects only the pathway mediated through the surrogate

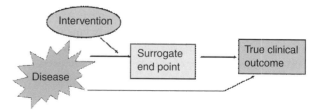

The surrogate is not in the pathway of the intervention's effect or is insensitive to the effect

The intervention has mechanisms of action independent of the disease process

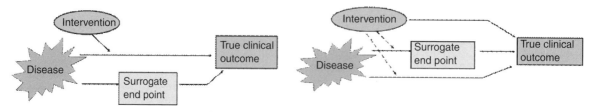

Figure 7.4. Reasons why biomarker endpoints may fail as surrogate endpoints (adapted from [8]).

Table 7.2 Types of biomarkers used in therapeutic development

Role	Description	Examples
Disease biomarker	Indicate the presence of likelihood of a particular disease	apoE 4 for Alzheimer's risk
Mechanism biomarker	Suggest a drug has its effect through a specific mechanism or pathway	Reduction in inflammatory markers in MS
Pharmacodynamic biomarker	Used to determine the dose that has the highest response to treatment	Dosage showing greatest reduction in platelet aggregation in patients with stroke risk
Target biomarkers	Show that a drug interacts with a particular target in in vitro studies, or in vivo imaging studies	PET study showing serotonin displacement by anti-depressant
Toxicity biomarkers	Indicate potentially harmful effects	Abnormal hepatic enzyme profile in novel anti-convulsant drug

conditions to be called a surrogate outcome measure. Biomarkers are particularly useful in early stages of drug development, including pre-clinical studies to determine the biological activity of a therapeutic agent. Surrogate endpoints become more useful in early clinical studies to predict whether an agent may have an effect on clinical outcomes. Ultimately, studies that employ clinical outcome measures are needed to determine whether an intervention should be adopted in clinical practice.

For the purposes of drug development, biomarkers may be characterized in several other ways depending on how the marker is used and the characteristic that it measures (See Table 7.2). One common schema is to classify biomarkers as measures of disease **state** or **trait**. A state biomarker measures the current status of disease, and may change over time as disease status changes. Examples of state biomarkers are imaging studies like MRI after a stroke, which would show a picture of the anatomic lesion that is producing clinical stroke symptoms. Trait biomarkers measure a characteristic that does not change over time, such as a genetic mutation. Trait biomarkers are more likely to be measures of disease risk. In the context of clinical trials, such markers, like a positive gene test for Huntington's disease, may be entry criteria for trial participation, but are not suitable outcome measures for clinical trials. Additional classification schemes to describe biomarkers have also been defined. Some examples of these categories are shown in Table 7.2, below.

As described by Fleming and DeMets [8], biomarkers may fail to be valid surrogate endpoints in four general ways. Reasons that a potential surrogate may fail are shown in Figure 7.3. The first is that the surrogate outcome is not in the causal pathway

between the disease and the true clinical outcome. The second, related, possibility is that there is more than one causal pathway and the potential surrogate is only relevant to one of these pathways. The third possibility is that the surrogate is not in the pathway of the intervention, or is insensitive to it. Finally, the intervention may have a mechanism of action that is independent of the disease process. This last scenario may be most commonly observed in the case of (potentially harmful) side effects of treatment. A fifth possibility proposed by Frank and Hargreaves is that the biomarker may be overly sensitive and not correlated with a meaningful clinical phenotype [9]. In this case, improvements in the biomarker may be demonstrated, but would not be associated with health benefits.

Role of biomarkers in clinical trials

The enthusiasm for using biomarkers in clinical trials is driven by the need to quicken the pace of clinical drug development, as well as the proliferation of new technologies. Using biomarkers has the potential to accelerate the pace of drug development. Novel clinical trial designs, including adaptive designs, are increasingly used with these novel endpoints [10]. This is particularly true in chronic and degenerative neurological disorders where true clinical outcomes evolve very slowly over time. In addition, biomarkers have the potential to provide complementary information about drug mechanisms that may be useful throughout the phases of testing a novel therapeutic.

The Code of Federal Regulations (CFR) defines clinical trials as belonging to three distinct phases (1–3) [11]. Phase 2 is sometimes divided into two subphases 2a and 2b. Phase 4 trials are not defined in the CFR, but are often included in discussions of development of pharmaceuticals (see Chapter 2). Biomarkers can be useful in furthering the goals of clinical trials at each stage; however, they may be particularly useful in phase 1 and phase 2 trials.

Biomarkers have a clear role in phase 1 clinical trials. The purpose of these trials, in addition to determining pharmacokinetics and metabolism is to identify early evidence for biological activity. In this context, biomarkers may be particularly useful, and do not necessarily need to be valid surrogate outcome measures, since the purpose is not to predict a clinical outcome, necessarily, but to detect signs of biological activity. This has led to a need for objective endpoints that allow clinical trial sponsors to quickly evaluate whether an exploratory drug is at least 'reasonably likely' to succeed and to help sponsors make a 'go-no go' decision. Despite the challenges of using biomarkers as true 'surrogates' in confirmatory trials for registrational purposes they have increasingly been used for learning purposes and to assist sponsors in making decisions [12].

Biomarkers continue to play a primary role in phase 2 trials. The purpose of phase 2a trials is to identify preliminary evidence of efficacy. Biomarkers, particularly those that are reliable surrogates for true clinical outcomes provide a means to accomplishing these objectives. Phase 2 trials can gain substantial efficiency from valid, reliable surrogate outcome biomarkers. However, for the biomarker to be useful, it must change more rapidly and/or be measured more precisely than the clinical outcome of interest. Relying on a surrogate biomarker rather than a clinical outcome measure also avoids the problem of performing underpowered efficacy studies in phase 2. These studies are generally difficult to interpret or inconclusive and, in the worst case, may create ethical barriers to conducting subsequent, definitive efficacy trials.

Biomarkers are also useful in phase 2b studies. The goal of phase 2b studies is to identify the best dose of a medication to use in definitive studies. Often, this dose may be chosen based on the dose that produces the greatest response in a surrogate biomarker.

In phase 3 and 4 studies, biomarkers generally play a secondary role relative to valid clinical outcomes. While there are examples in medicine where medications can receive FDA approval based on changes on a biomarker (i.e., change in blood pressure), this situation is the exception in neurology. Nonetheless, biomarkers may provide complementary information

about drug mechanism in a phase 3 trial, and add to the credibility of the changes observed in the primary, clinical outcome measure. Use of MRI lesion burden as a secondary outcome in clinical trials of immune modulating therapies for multiple sclerosis (MS) provides an example of this application [13].

Examples of biomarkers in neurology

Biomarkers have been used in studies of a wide variety of neurological disorders with varying degrees of usefulness. Some of these biomarkers address cellular or microscopic features of disease, examples of this group include biochemical biomarkers and the newer '-omics' markers. Other biomarkers address system level physiology, including electrophysiology or imaging studies. Clearly, however, overlap exists in these categories. For example, imaging is used with increasing frequency to probe cellular mechanisms.

Biochemical biomarkers

Biochemical biomarkers are chemical constituents of bio-fluids or tissue that reflect either disease pathophysiology or response to treatment. Biochemical biomarkers are attractive because they can potentially be measured in central laboratories with relatively low expenses. They may provide a more direct measurement of the biology of disease than other types of biomarkers.

Biochemical biomarkers are ubiquitous throughout medicine, ranging from measurement of serum electrolytes to the latest high-tech bioassay. Biochemical biomarkers are also common in neurological disorders including measurement of antibodies in inflammatory neuropathies or spinal fluid constituents in meningitis.

Work in biochemical biomarkers is well represented by efforts to translate knowledge about pathology in Alzheimer's disease (AD) into useful clinical markers to follow disease progression during life. The most frequently studied potential biochemical biomarkers for AD are beta-amyloid ($A\beta1-42$), total tau (t-tau) and phospho-tau (p-tau). These biomarkers are attractive because they reflect the plaque and tangle pathology characteristic of AD. $A\beta1-42$ has been studied frequently as a biomarker for AD. In the CSF of patients with AD, concentrations of $A\beta1-42$ are reduced by 40–50%. However, $A\beta1-42$ concentrations do not correlate with dementia severity, and levels remain essentially unchanged over intervals up to one year. By contrast, tau levels are increased in spinal fluid from patients with AD, but tend to decline over time and with disease progression. Because neither Aβ1–42 nor tau correlate with disease duration of severity, they are not valuable as natural history biomarkers. They may prove to be useful biomarkers of therapeutic effect if a drug can be shown to normalize levels. However, the roles of Aβ1–42 and tau as markers of therapeutic effect in clinical trials are not established [14].

'Omics' biomarkers

The combination of emerging high-throughput assay techniques and increased bio-informatics computing power has ushered in a new class of biomarkers including genomics, proteomics and metabolomics. The common links among these groups of biomarkers is that they are derived from unbiased sampling of very large amounts of biological data and that the read-out obtained is a pattern of changes in multiple constituents. This pattern of changes is sometimes referred to as a profile. Metabolomic approaches quantify large quantities of small molecules collectively known as metabolites using techniques such as mass spectroscopy. Computational methods capable of interpreting very large amounts of data are used to identify patterns of metabolites present in patients with a given disease that are not present in controls. Metabolomic studies have shown promise in identifying metabolomic profiles for motor neuron disease [15] and Parkinson's disease (PD) [16]. It remains to be determined whether these technologies may be useful in clinical trials. Proteomics takes a similar approach, dealing with large numbers of proteins sampled from biological specimens. Exploratory proteomics studies have identified panels of proteins that distinguish patients with degenerative disorders including AD and PD from each other and from normal controls [17]. Such biomarkers identified through unbiased approaches must be validated in independent samples before they can be widely accepted. Genomics studies data generated from studies of genes and gene expression and again requires intensive bio-informatic analyses. Although these -omics approaches show promise, to date they have primarily been studied as diagnostics. In the future, they may prove to be useful markers of response to therapy, and be integrated into clinical trials.

Imaging biomarkers

Imaging biomarkers are ubiquitous in neurology. These modalities include CT, MRI and metabolic imaging. In particular, metabolic imaging with PET or single photon emission computerized tomography (SPECT), are widely used as diagnostics and to follow disease progression in neurodegenerative disorders. Dopaminergic degeneration is clearly central to the pathological process in PD, and changes can be measured with imaging in a way that corresponds well to accepted ideas regarding PD pathology. PET and SPECT techniques are available to measure pre- and post-synaptic neurons in the nigro-striatal pathways. In particular, [123]iodine-labeled 2β-carbomethoxy-3β (4-iodophenyl)tropane ([^{123}I] β-CIT) SPECT, and [^{18}F] fluorodopa (Fdopa)-PET have been used as measures of the integrity of the nigro-striatal system. Both have proven to be useful natural history biomarkers, showing consistent declines in binding of approximately 10% per year. However, there have been significant problems with using these markers in clinical trials. In three trials where they have been used as biomarkers, the changes observed in the imaging biomarkers have been inconsistent with changes observed in clinical measures [18–20]. In all cases, the purpose of the biomarker study was to provide complementary evidence showing physiological changes consistent with clinical observation, thus bolstering the clinical data. However, the disconnect between clinical and biomarker results produced controversy regarding the validity of dopaminergic imaging biomarkers and the way that clinical disease severity is assessed in trials. The difficulty in interpreting these studies demonstrates challenges in validating biomarkers for use as surrogate outcome measures in interventional studies.

Recently, PET imaging studies using ligands that bind to β-amyloid have demonstrated the potential for this imaging modality as a biomarker for AD. Pittsburgh Compound-B (PiB) was the first of these compounds to be reported [21]. However, a number of other similar compounds are in development; in vivo studies show an excellent relationship between in vivo amyloid measurement in brain slices and amyloid imaging. Clinical studies have shown excellent capacity for amyloid imaging to differentiate between patients with AD and normal controls. Longitudinal studies are needed to determine the ability of amyloid imaging to predict progression of AD and to identify which patients with mild cognitive impairment will go on to develop AD. While compounds like PiB are beginning to be incorporated into clinical trials, there is too little experience with them as biomarkers in trials to judge their usefulness.

Structural imaging with MRI or CT has been used as both an entry criteria into clinical trials and as an outcome measure. For example, CT has been used to define entry criteria for thrombolysis trials in acute stroke [22].

MRI has frequently been used as a measure of treatment response of MS patients. The presence of multiple brain lesions in patients with an isolated clinical event is the best predictor of a subsequent diagnosis of relapsing-remitting MS. MRI monitoring has been recommended to screen new therapies [23], and is used as an outcome measure in MS clinical trials [13]. Although, the relationship between T2 lesions and long-term disability has been controversial [24, 25], one recent study reporting 13 years of clinical follow-up showed a strong relationship between T2 lesion burden and a number of important long-term clinical and imaging measures of disease progression [26]. These findings support the use of MRI as a biomarker for MS clinical trials, and possibly its use as a surrogate endpoint to predict important clinical outcomes.

Practical considerations in endpoint selection

Researchers should define the role each endpoint is intended to play in the clinical trial (e.g., primary, secondary, or exploratory endpoint). This is important so that instrument development and performance can be reviewed in the context of its intended role and to properly plan for the appropriate statistical analysis. Each endpoint should be fit to purpose and be cohesively part of the endpoint model (see Chapters 20–26). A less is more approach rather than a value-added approach to endpoint selection often helps focus on those critical domains needing measurement and helps avoid the temptation to collect too much information.

Characteristics of instruments and selection of endpoints includes an extensive review of the literature and detailed consideration of the proposed clinical trial. Issues needing review include the concepts being measured, the number of items for each instrument, the conceptual framework of the instrument, the medical condition for the intended use, the population for intended use, the data collection method, the administration mode, the response options for each measure (e.g., visual analog scale, likert scale, rating scale, checklist, recording of events as they occur), the recall period in question, the scoring of the instrument, the weighting of items or domains, the format, the

respondent burden, and the availability of culturally adapted versions. Each instrument should have a demonstration of adequate measurement properties (reliability, validity, and ability to detect change, content and score distributions, and information about method of administration and user acceptability. Factors that can contribute to respondent burden include length of questionnaire/interview, formatting, font size, literacy level, need for privacy, and need for physical help in responding. Modifications to existing instruments should be avoided unless additional qualitative work is proposed to document consistent measurement properties. Depending on the endpoint or measure being used, raters will need sufficient training to standardize procedures, reduce random error, and improve measure reliability. This will not only improve study quality but ultimately lower sample size requirements through precision of measurement.

Much of the above information may not be available for newer physiological measures proposed for use as biomarkers in early translational trials. Therefore, early stage translational trials are also helping to establish the measurement properties of biomarkers in an iterative process. This may lead to a situation where biomarker validation lags behind the drug development program it is intended to support. Therefore, when using a newly developed physiological measure consultation with the appropriate sponsor is critical for planning and implementing the measure into the clinical trial.

Pitfalls to avoid in selecting outcome measures

There are several pitfalls to avoid in selecting outcome measures in clinical trials. These include choosing an endpoint or instrument with little known information about its validity, reliability, and ability to detect change. In addition, one should not use a new measure without proper pilot testing or use a measure differently than recommended, including altering questions or response options. One should use outcome measures judiciously. For example, outcome measure development may occur in early stage clinical trials to refine measurement properties to support their use in confirmatory clinical trials. Alternatively, exploratory outcome measures and endpoints may be used in confirmatory clinical trials for a variety of purposes, including selecting sub-populations who may demonstrate greatest clinical benefit (e.g., 'patient-selection' biomarkers).

References

1. ProQolid Database. http://www.proqolid.org/. (Accessed June 11, 2010.)

2. Guidance for Industry. Patient-reported outcome measures: Use in medical product development to support labeling claims. 2009. http://www.fda.gov/downloads/Drugs/GuidanceComplianceRegulatoryInformation/Guidances/UCM193282.pdf. (Accessed June 17, 2010.)

3. Gershon RC, Cella D, Fox NA, *et al.* Assessment of neurological and behavioural function: the NIH Toolbox. *Lancet Neurol* 2010; **9**: 138–39.

4. Neuro-QOL. Quality of Life in Neurological Disorders. http://www.neuroqol.org/default.aspx. (Accessed June 17, 2010.)

5. Sheiner LB. Learning versus confirming in clinical drug development. *Clin Pharmacol Ther* 1997; **61**: 275–91.

6. Biomarkers Definitions Working Group. Biomarkers and surrogate endpoints: preferred definitions and conceptual framework. *Clin Pharmacol Ther* 2001; **69**: 89–95.

7. Prentice RL. Surrogate endpoints in clinical trials: definitions and operational criteria. *Stat Med* 1989; **8**: 431–40.

8. Fleming TR and DeMets DL. Surrogate end points in clinical trials: Are we being misled? *Ann Int Med* 1996; **125**: 605–13.

9. Frank R and Hargreaves R. Clinical biomarkers in drug discovery and development. *Nature Rev* 2003; **2**: 566–80.

10. Coffey CS and Kairalla JA. Adaptive clinical trials: Progress and challenges. *Drugs* 2008; **9**: 229–42.

11. The Food and Drug Modernization Act of 1997. Title 21 Code of Federal Regulations Part 312 Subpart H Section 314.500.

12. Spinella DC. Biomarkers in clinical drug development: realizing the promise. *Biomarkers Med* 2009; **3**: 667–69.

13. Jacobs LD, Beck RW, Simon JH, *et al.* Intramuscular interferon beta 1a therapy initiated during the first demyelinating event in muliptle sclerosis. *New Engl J Med* 2000; **343**: 898–904.

14. Sonnen JA, Montine KS, Quinn JF, *et al.* Biomarkers for cognitive impairment and dementia in elderly people. *Lancet Neurol* 2008; **7**: 704–14.

15. Rozen S, Cudkowicz ME, Bogdanov M, *et al.* Metabolomic analysis and signature in motor neuron disease. *Metabolomic* 2005; **2**: 101–8.

16. Bogdanov MB, Beal MF, McCAbe DR, *et al.* Metabolomic profiling to develop blood biomarkers for Parkinson's disease. *Brain* 2008; **131**: 389–96.

17. Abdi F, Quinn JF, Jankovic J, *et al.* Detection of biomarkers with a multiplex quantitative proteomic platform in cerebrospinal fluid of patients with neurodegenerative disorders. *J Alzheimer's Dis* 2006; **9**: 293–348.

18. Parkinson Study Group. Dopamine transporter brain imaging to assess the effects of pramipexole vs levodpa on Parkinson disease progression. *JAMA* 2002; **287**: 1653–61.

19. Fahn S, Oakes D, Shoulson I, *et al.* Levodopa and the progression of Parkinson's disease. *New Engl J Med* 2004; **351**: 2498–508.

20. Whone AL, Watts RL, Stoessl AJ, *et al.* Slower progression of Parkinson's disease with ropinirole versus levodopa: The REAL-PET study. *Ann Neurol* 2003; **54**: 93–101.

21. Klunk WE, Engler H, Norberg A, *et al.* Imaging brain amyloid in Alzheimer's diease with Pittsburgh Compound B. *Ann Neurol* 2004; **55**: 306–19.

22. NINDS Stroke rt-PA Stroke Study Group. Tissue plasminogen activator for acute ischemic stroke. *N Engl J Med* 1995; **333**: 1581–88.

23. Miller DH, Albert PS, Barkhof F, *et al.* Guidelines for the use of magnetic resonance techniques in monitoring the treatment of multiple sclerosis. *Ann Neurol* 1996; **39**: 6–16.

24. Sormani MP, Bozano L, Roccatagliata L, *et al.* Magnetic resonance imaging as a potential surrogate for relapse in multiple sclerosis: a meta-analytic approach. *Ann Neurol* 2009; **65**: 270–77.

25. Li DKB, Held U, Petkau J, *et al.* MRI T2 lesion burden in multiple sclerosis. A plateauing relationship with clinical disability. *Neurology* 2006; **66**: 1384–89.

26. Rudick RA, Lee J-C, Simon J, *et al.* Significance of T2 lesions in multiple sclerosis: A 13 year longitudinal study. *Ann Neurol* 2006; **60**: 236–42.

Selection and futility designs

Bruce Levin

Introduction

Selection designs and futility designs offer investigators a way to screen potential therapies in early phase clinical research in a relatively rapid manner with fewer patients than would be required for a traditional phase 3 trial for each candidate. To do so requires changing the standard phase 3 paradigm in some substantial way. In a futility design, the paradigm is still that of hypothesis testing, but the traditional null hypothesis of no effect and the two-sided alternative hypothesis of unequal efficacies are reformulated in such a way as to better screen out unpromising therapies. In a selection design, there is a radical shift away from the hypothesis testing paradigm altogether, with a different goal – to select the best from among several competing treatments. In this chapter we explain the rationale for these changes and the basic methods required, starting on more familiar ground with the futility design.

The logic of the futility design

The futility design has appeal for phase 2 clinical trials which seek to obtain a preliminary indication of promising efficacy of an experimental treatment, or the lack thereof, i.e., an indication that further research with the treatment would be futile. The motivation for a futility study arises from a familiar context encountered in cancer research and currently facing neurodegenerative disease researchers: there are many possible treatment candidates but each has only a low a priori probability of having worthwhile efficacy. In such circumstances it would be impractical to demand a definitive phase 3 study for each of those high-cost, low-expectation endeavors. A better strategy is to screen candidate therapies using relatively fewer patients in each case, to be sensitive to suggestions of efficacy, but to stand ready to weed out candidates that lack sufficient promise.

Resources may then be saved to bring only the non-futile treatments forward for definitive testing. The futility design was adopted by the National Institute of Neurological Disorders (NINDS) supported NET-PD network to screen out unpromising neuroprotective agents in Parkinson's disease (PD), and was introduced in the neurological literature by this group in a series of reports and didactic publications [1–6]. The design has also been proposed, discussed, and/or used in stroke research [7], amyotrophic lateral sclerosis (ALS) [8–11], and Huntington's disease [12].

To gain some insight into the characteristics that a useful screening program would have, consider what impact errors of omission and commission have. Suppose a treatment which is truly superior to a placebo fails by chance to show promise in early phase human trials. If the development program for this treatment were terminated as a result, the loss to humanity could be tremendous. But if a treatment which is truly no better than a placebo looks promising by chance in early tests and is brought forward for definitive testing as a result, the costs could be measured in time, money, and perhaps risks for the patients involved, yet the disappointing truth will ultimately be revealed. Assuming that the first type of error is the more serious, and given that we so desperately need safe and effective neuroprotective agents with precious few resources to find them, it makes sense to design the screening program to be less specific than phase 3 testing traditionally requires in exchange for greater sensitivity to promising treatments. This implies that we should be willing to tolerate a low positive predictive value – after all, good therapies will be hard to find under any circumstances – in exchange for a high negative predictive value, such that candidate treatments which fail the screen are quite likely to be truly without merit. These conclusions are consistent with a public health and

Clinical Trials in Neurology, ed. Bernard Ravina, Jeffrey Cummings, Michael P. McDermott, and R. Michael Poole. Published by Cambridge University Press. © Cambridge University Press 2012.

economic perspective: it is important not to overlook potentially useful drugs but carrying forward agents with a low probability of success is not economically sustainable.

The futility design has the above desired properties. It is more properly designated a *non-superiority* design because the null hypothesis which it tests states that the experimental treatment possesses a *pre-specified degree of superiority*, while the alternative hypothesis, which generally confers a design its name, states that the experimental treatment does not possess the required degree of superiority, i.e., is non-superior.[1]

To formalize the statement of the design, let θ denote a population parameter measuring, for example, the true average clinical progression of disease over a period of time, with larger values indicating greater disease progression. For example, θ might denote the average increase in the Unified Parkinson's Disease Rating Scale (UPDRS) over a given time period for a population of PD patients, or the average decline in the revised ALS Functional Rating Scale (ALSFRS-R) over a given time period for a population of ALS patients.[2] The key step is to define the criterion of superiority, which can be specified in several ways depending on other design elements. In a *single-arm design*, a value of θ, say θ_0, is pre-specified such that an experimental treatment will be defined as 'superior' if $\theta_E \leq \theta_0$ and will be defined as 'non-superior' if $\theta_E > \theta_0$, where θ_E denotes the true value of θ for patients on the experimental treatment. Note that θ_E is unknown,

so statistical methods must be used to infer whether the superiority or non-superiority hypothesis is true. Note also that θ_0 should represent an average disease progression *better* than that of untreated patients or patients on placebo. In fact, in order for the alternative hypothesis of non-superiority to imply that it would be futile to conduct further testing, the value of θ_0 should represent an agreed upon *minimum worthwhile efficacy* (or maximum allowable progression). This must be done with care, and a consensus of expert judgment is essential, as is careful education of, and buy-in by, key trial participants and patients. In order to qualify as superior, then, an experimental treatment must lead to a certain *minimum slowing* of disease progression, which we represent by the positive quantity $\Delta_0 = \theta_P - \theta_0 > 0$, where θ_P denotes the true average disease progression for patients on placebo. If $\theta_E > \theta_0$ the experimental treatment is deemed non-superior or 'futile' even if it represents a true average disease progression better than that of a placebo, i.e., even if $\theta_P > \theta_E > \theta_0$, because it does not achieve the minimum worthwhile efficacy.

We may now formally state the null and alternative hypotheses for a single-arm futility design, as follows:

$$H_0: \theta_E \leq \theta_0 \text{ (superiority) versus}$$
$$H_1: \theta_E > \theta_0 \text{ (non-superiority).}$$

Note that in this formulation we do not need to know what the true placebo progression θ_P might be exactly, only that $\theta_P > \theta_0$. If a value of θ_P is known, the hypotheses can be restated equivalently in terms of the *slowing* of disease progression $\Delta_E = \theta_P - \theta_E$ and $\Delta_0 = \theta_P - \theta_0$ as:

$$H_0: \Delta_E \geq \Delta_0 \text{ (superiority) versus}$$
$$H_1: \Delta_E < \Delta_0 \text{ (non-superiority).}$$

This is an *additive* formulation of treatment effect. Sometimes a multiplicative formulation may be preferred. In that case the definition of superiority would be stated in terms of the quantity $R_E = 100(1 - \theta_E/\theta_P)\%$, which is the *percentage reduction* in the true average disease progression of the experimental treatment relative to placebo, and $R_0 = 100(1 - \theta_0/\theta_P)\%$, which is the minimum worthwhile percentage reduction:

$$H_0: R_E \geq R_0 \text{ (superiority) versus}$$
$$H_1: R_E < R_0 \text{ (non-superiority).}$$

In the *two-arm* design with concurrent placebo controls, both θ_E and θ_P are unknown. The hypotheses of the futility design are then defined in terms of the

---

[1] The non-superiority design should not be confused with the non-inferiority design which is often used in the pharmaceutical industry. In a non-inferiority design, the null hypothesis states that a new treatment has a pre-specified degree of *inferiority* compared to a standard active treatment, and the goal is to reject that hypothesis in favor of the alternative hypothesis of non-inferiority, i.e., acceptable comparability with the standard treatment. Thus the goals (demonstrating non-superiority versus non-inferiority) and the types of comparators (placebo versus active) make these designs quite distinct. See Chapter 16 for further discussion of the non-inferiority design. The futility design should also be distinguished from phase 3 monitoring plans that allow early stopping for lack of efficacy, called 'futility stopping' in that context. See Chapter 19.

[2] We sidestep here the question of whether θ truly measures a characteristic of the actual mechanism underlying disease progression, includes merely symptomatic features, or both. We wish to let θ refer to representative changes in the usual clinical measures of disease severity.

slowing of disease progression due to the experimental treatment compared to placebo, $\Delta_E = \theta_P - \theta_E$, and a pre-specified positive *minimum worthwhile slowing* of disease progression, which we also denote by $\Delta_0 > 0$:

$$H_0: \Delta_E \geq \Delta_0 \text{ (superiority) versus}$$
$$H_1: \Delta_E < \Delta_0 \text{ (non-superiority).}$$

In a multiplicative formulation, it is easiest to state the hypotheses as follows:

$$H_0: \theta_E - \pi_0\theta_P \leq 0 \text{ (superiority) versus}$$
$$H_1: \theta_E - \pi_0\theta_P > 0 \text{ (non-superiority),}$$

where $100(1 - \pi_0)\%$ is the minimum worthwhile percentage reduction in the true average disease progression. For example, if a treatment would be deemed superior if it caused a 20% decrease in the decline of the ALSFRS-R over a nine month follow-up period, then $\pi_0 = 0.80$ and we would test $H_0: \theta_E - 0.8\theta_P \leq 0$ versus H_1: $\theta_E - 0.8\theta_P > 0$. Such a formulation was used in the futility trial of coenzyme Q_{10} in ALS (the QALS trial [8, 9]).

Are there any practical differences between a futility design and a traditional one-sided hypothesis test? Why not just use a traditional test using a more liberal type I error rate to reduce the sample size? The answer is somewhat surprising: the practical difference between the designs is *not* a matter of statistical power or sample size. Indeed, as discussed below, a traditional one-sided design and a futility design have parallel operating characteristics. Rather, the practical difference appears in terms of what can be said and how to proceed in the event that we fail to reject the null hypothesis in one design or the other. For the traditional test we make statements such as 'we cannot rule out that the experimental treatment is no better than placebo with 95% confidence' and exhibit the disappointing confidence intervals which include the parameter $\Delta_E = 0$. Even if the trial results are truly inconclusive concerning the efficacy of the treatment and the confidence interval includes rather promising values, the pall of insignificance has been cast over the results and 'spin' statements are ultimately post hoc. With the futility design, however, failure to reject the null hypothesis of superiority leads to statements such as 'with 95% confidence we cannot rule out that the experimental treatment is superior,' and thus the research should continue to definitive phase 3 testing. This difference may be philosophical, but the latter statement represents a huge advantage. It is consistent with a screening program, and it has the strength of having been planned a priori. Moreover, given that sample sizes in phase 2 trials

are generally smaller than in phase 3 trials, use of the traditional formulation can easily produce an underpowered study, even more so if a traditional two-sided design is used, with all of the consequent logistical uncertainties when one fails to reject the null hypothesis of no benefit.[3]

Another difference is revealed by considering type I and type II errors and the corresponding sensitivity and specificity of the screening program. In a futility design, a type I error occurs when a truly superior treatment by chance produces sufficiently unpromising results as to cause a declaration of futility. Our premise is that this would be a serious error whose rate of occurrence is controlled by specifying a reasonably low alpha level at the criterion of superiority, $\Delta_E = \Delta_0$. A type II error occurs when we fail to declare a truly non-superior treatment futile. It is natural to assess the power of the test at the particular parameter value of placebo efficacy in the alternative hypothesis. For a single-arm trial we consider the design alternative to be $\theta_E = \theta_P$; for an additive two-arm trial the design alternative is taken to be $\Delta_E = 0$; and for a multiplicative two-arm trial the design alternative is taken to be $\theta_E - \pi_0\theta_P = (1 - \pi_0)\theta_P$ for some assumed value of θ_P.[4] Let us define 'sensitivity' to mean the probability that we declare a truly superior treatment 'non-futile' and 'specificity' to mean the probability that we declare a truly non-superior treatment 'futile'. Then sensitivity is equal to the probability of failing to reject the null hypothesis of superiority with a truly superior treatment, i.e., $1 - \alpha$, at the criterion for superiority (or greater if the treatment is even better), while specificity is equal to the power of the test. In the traditional design, sensitivity would correspond to the power of the test (the probability of rejecting the null hypothesis of no benefit with a superior treatment at a given level of efficacy) while specificity would correspond to the probability of failing to

---

[3] It is worthwhile to point out here that, as always in hypothesis testing, failure to reject H_0 is not equivalent to accepting H_0 as true. In the futility design if we fail to reject the null hypothesis of superiority, we do *not* conclude the experimental treatment is superior to placebo. *That inference must await an adequate and well-controlled phase 3 clinical trial.* We must only conclude that the evidence was insufficient to rule out true superiority.

[4] As always, it is best to examine the entire power curve for all values of θ_E (or Δ_E or $\theta_E - \pi_0\theta_P$) rather than just at the specific design alternative, in order to fully perceive the operating characteristic of the trial under all possible parameter values.

reject the null hypothesis of no benefit given that the efficacy of the treatment is the same as that of placebo, or $1 - \alpha$. Insofar as it is typical to set the type I error probability α lower than the type II error probability β in a traditional trial, it follows that sensitivity will be greater than specificity for the futility design compared to the traditional design. For example, if $\alpha = 0.05$ and $\beta = 0.20$ (for 80% power) at the design alternative, the futility design will have 95% sensitivity and 80% specificity, whereas the traditional design would have 80% sensitivity and 95% specificity.

What does this say about the predictive values of the screening program? Suppose we interpret 'futility' as a negative outcome and 'non-futility' as a positive outcome. Then the negative predictive odds of a futility outcome is given by the prior odds on a non-superior treatment times the likelihood ratio of specificity over one minus sensitivity, or $(1 - \beta)/\alpha = .80/.05 = 16$. This likelihood ratio means that a futility outcome is at least 16 times more likely under the non-superiority hypothesis at the design alternative of no benefit than under the null hypothesis of criterion superiority. On the other hand, the positive predictive odds of a non-futile outcome is given by the prior odds on a superior treatment times the likelihood ratio of sensitivity over one minus specificity, or $(1 - \alpha)/\beta = 0.95/.20 = 4.75$ (meaning a non-futile outcome is 4.75 more likely under the superiority hypothesis than under the design alternative of no benefit).[5] Thus a futility outcome multiplies the prior odds on non-superiority – which must be quite high, given the rarity of neuroprotective agents – by a factor of 16 or more, yielding a posterior odds on non-superiority yet an order of magnitude greater than the prior odds, whereas failure to declare futility increases the prior odds on superiority – which must be quite small – by a factor of only 4.75.[6] Consequently,

---

[5] Strictly speaking, these likelihood ratios consider only the evidence of having declared a treatment futile or non-futile but nothing more. More informative likelihood ratios can generally be constructed using the observed data from the experiment.

[6] For instance, if the prior odds on non-superiority is 10 to 1 (corresponding to a prior probability of superiority of 1/11), then increasing the prior odds by a factor of 10 yields posterior odds on non-superiority of 100 to 1 (corresponding to a posterior probability of superiority of $1/101 \approx 0.01$). On the other hand, increasing the prior odds on superiority of 1 to 10 by a factor of 4.75 yields posterior odds on superiority of 4.75/10 = 0.475 (corresponding to a posterior probability of superiority of only $0.475/(1 + 0.475) = 0.322$).

the futility design does a reasonable job of producing negative weight of evidence for unpromising therapies, though enthusiasm should be tempered when a borderline non-futile result is obtained. If a therapy passes the screen of non-futility, it still must undergo subsequent definitive phase 3 testing before it can be considered efficacious.

Conducting a futility test and sample size considerations

A futility analysis is conducted depending on the precise formulation of the hypotheses and the statistical distribution of the primary endpoint. For brevity, we shall only consider the case of a normally distributed variable with mean θ_E and standard deviation σ, and illustrate with the primary endpoint of the NET-PD futility studies described in [5], namely, the increase in the UPDRS total score between baseline and either the time at which there was sufficient disability to warrant symptomatic therapy for PD or 12 months, whichever came first. The threshold value was defined as an increase in the UPDRS that was 30% less than the mean progression observed on the total UPDRS score in a historical control group. In this case, the historical control group was chosen to be the group receiving either placebo or α-tocopherol in the Deprenyl and Tocopherol Antioxidative Therapy of Parkinsonism (DATATOP) trial ($n = 401$), and the mean increase in total UPDRS score was 10.65 units with a standard deviation of 10.4 units [14]. Taking θ_P as 10.65 and σ as 10.4, θ_0 was defined as 0.7×10.65 or $\theta_0 = 7.455$.

First consider a single-arm study. Let Y_i denote the observed decline for the ith patient ($i = 1,\ldots,n$), let $\bar{Y}$ denote the average of these values, and let s be the sample standard deviation. The pivotal test statistic is then Student's t statistic, $t = (\bar{Y} - \theta_0)/s/\sqrt{n}$. We reject the null hypothesis of superiority in favor of the alternative hypothesis of non-superiority and declare futility if $t \geq t_{n-1;\alpha}$ where $t_{n-1;\alpha}$ is the critical value of Student's t distribution with $n-1$ degrees of freedom cutting off probability α in the upper tail. Equivalently, we reject the null hypothesis of superiority if the one-tailed p-value (computed from the t distribution with $n-1$ degrees of freedom) is less than α. The power of this test is given by $P[t_{n-1}(\lambda) > t_{n-1;\alpha}]$, where $t_{n-1}(\lambda)$ has a non-central t distribution with non-centrality parameter $\lambda = (\theta_E - \theta_0)/(\sigma/\sqrt{n})$. At the design alternative of treatment efficacy equal to that of placebo, the non-centrality parameter is

$\lambda = \Delta_0/(\sigma/\sqrt{n})$. Standard software for computing power for a one-sample t-test can be used with specification of the difference to be detected as $\Delta_0 = \theta_P - \theta_0$, the standard deviation as σ, the significance level as α (one-tailed), and the sample size as n.

In the NET-PD studies the type I error probability was chosen as $\alpha = 0.10$ with a sample size of $n = 58$.[7] This sample size provided 85% power to detect futility if the efficacy of the treatment was the same as that of placebo ($\theta_E = \theta_P = 10.65$) assuming $\sigma = 10.4$ and $\theta_0 = 7.455$.

For an additive two-arm design, the t statistic is: $t = (\bar{Y}_p - \bar{Y}_E - \Delta_0)/(s_p\sqrt{n_p^{-1} + n_E^{-1}})$, where $\bar{Y}_p$ and $\bar{Y}_E$ are the sample means in the placebo and treatment groups, respectively, n_p and n_E are the respective sample sizes, and s_p is the usual pooled standard deviation estimate. The null hypothesis $H_0:\Delta_E \geq \Delta_0$ is rejected in favor of the alternative hypothesis $H_1:\Delta_E < \Delta_0$ and futility is declared if $t \leq -t_{v;\alpha}$, where the degrees of freedom are $v = n_p + n_E - 2$. Equivalently, futility is declared if the one-tailed p-value (computed from the t distribution with $n_p + n_E - 2$ degrees of freedom) is less than α. The power of this test is given by $P[t_v(\lambda) < -t_{v;\alpha}]$, where the non-centrality parameter is now $\lambda = (\theta_P - \theta_E - \Delta_0)/(\sigma\sqrt{n_E^{-1} + n_p^{-1}})$. At the design alternative $\theta_E = \theta_P$, the non-centrality parameter for equal sample sizes $n_E = n_P = n$ is the quantity $-\Delta_0/(\sigma\sqrt{2/n})$. Standard software for computing power for a two-sample t-test can be used with specification of the difference to be detected as $-\Delta_0$, the standard deviation as σ, the significance level as α (one-tailed), and the sample size (per group) as n.

If the NET-PD studies had been designed as two-arm studies with concurrent placebo groups having equal sample sizes, $\Delta_0 = 10.65 - 7.455 = 3.195$, and $\sigma = 10.4$, they would have required $n = 115$ per group to achieve the same power of 85%, essentially quadrupling the total number of patients compared to the single-arm study.

For a multiplicative formulation in the two-arm design, some saving in sample size is possible. For H_0: $\theta_E - \pi_0\theta_P \leq 0$, the pivotal test statistic is:

$$t = (\bar{Y}_E - \pi_0\bar{Y}_P)/(s_p\sqrt{n_E^{-1} + \pi_0^2 n_P^{-1}}),$$

which again has Student's t distribution with $v = n_p + n_E - 2$ degrees of freedom under H_0. The null hypothesis $H_0:\theta_E - \pi_0\theta_P \leq 0$ is rejected and futility is declared

if $t \geq t_{v;\alpha}$. Equivalently, futility is declared if the one-tailed p-value (computed from the t distribution with $n_p + n_E - 2$ degrees of freedom) is less than α. The power of this test is given by $P[t_v(\lambda) > t_{v;\alpha}]$, where the non-centrality parameter is now given by:

$$\lambda = (\theta_E - \pi_0\theta_P)/(\sigma\sqrt{n_E^{-1} + \pi_0^2 n_P^{-1}}).$$

At the design alternative $\theta_E = \theta_P$, the non-centrality parameter for equal sample sizes $n_E = n_P = n$ is the quantity:

$$\lambda = (1-\pi_0)\theta_p / \left(\sigma\sqrt{(1+\pi_0^2)/n}\right).$$

In our example with equal sample sizes of n per group and $\pi_0 = 0.70$, corresponding to a 30% improvement in disease progression, the non-centrality parameter is $\lambda = (0.30\cdot10.65) / [10.4\cdot\{(1+0.7^2)/n\}^{1/2}] = 2.334$ at the design alternative $\theta_E = \theta_P = 10.65$. Now a sample size of $n = 86$ patients per group or 172 in total would be needed to achieve 85% power, about triple the sample size of the single-arm design and a saving of 58 patients over the two-arm additive formulation. The saving is due to the reduced variability of $\bar{Y}_E - \pi_0\bar{Y}_P$ compared with $\bar{Y}_E - \bar{Y}_P$, by the factor $(1 + \pi_0^2)/2$.

It should be noted that the power of the multiplicative futility test depends on the true value of the placebo parameter θ_P. For given sample sizes, if θ_P is at least as large as assumed in the design, the power will be at least as large as planned at the design alternative $\theta_E = \theta_P$, but if the true placebo decline is smaller than assumed, power will decrease because the non-centrality parameter at the design alternative decreases as its numerator $\theta_E - \pi_0\theta_P = (1 - \pi_0)\theta_P$ decreases. This phenomenon does not occur with the additive formulation if Δ_0 is chosen independently of the assumed placebo decline, although if Δ_0 is expressed as a fraction of the assumed placebo decline, the power will again depend on it. This phenomenon is also analogous to the effect of overestimating θ_P in the single-arm design. There, if the historical control value of θ_P is greater than the true concurrent placebo value and θ_0 is set at π_0 times the historical control value, an experimental treatment with only the true concurrent placebo efficacy may fail to be declared futile with high probability. This is why it is important to have consensus that a therapy with disease progression no worse than θ_0 would indeed be a superior treatment. We discuss this point further below.

To summarize, the factors that determine the sample size needed for a futility design are, in roughly

---

[7] The actual target enrollment was set at $n = 65$ in order to allow for losses to follow-up.

82

decreasing order of importance: (i) the number of arms in the study; (ii) the standard deviation of the primary endpoint, σ; (iii) the non-centrality parameter at the design alternative, which in turn depends on Δ_0 in the single arm design and the additive two-arm design, as well as θ_P in the multiplicative two-arm design; and (iv) the type I error probability, α, and desired power $1 - \beta$.

Potential pitfalls

There are a few pitfalls to be avoided when planning a futility study. The first is that if the sample size is too small, a rather awkward situation can arise. Consider Figure 8.1, which schematically portrays a properly designed two-arm additive futility study with equal sample sizes. The vertical axis portrays the difference in the mean disease progression between the placebo and experimental arms. Positive values towards the top of the diagram indicate better efficacy for the experimental treatment than placebo and negative values towards the bottom indicate worse efficacy for the experimental treatment. On the left side of the diagram, the scale portrays true population parameter values and identifies the regions in the parameter space corresponding to the null hypothesis of superiority and the alternative hypothesis of non-superiority. On the right side of the diagram the scale portrays the sample average values of $\bar{Y}^{(P)} - \bar{Y}^{(E)}$ and identifies the critical region $\bar{Y}^{(P)} - \bar{Y}^{(E)} \le \Delta_0 - t_{2n-2;\alpha} s_p \sqrt{2/n}$, where the null hypothesis of superiority is rejected and its complement where superiority cannot be ruled out at level α. The distance $t_{2n-2;\alpha} s_p \sqrt{2/n}$ between Δ_0 and the critical

region depends on the sample standard deviation s_p and the group sample sizes, n. As n increases this distance narrows, implying a greater demand on the experimental treatment to demonstrate promising efficacy in order to avoid a declaration of futility. Conversely, as n decreases, the demand is lessened.

However, one wants to avoid the awkward situation portrayed in Figure 8.2. Here n is so small that the critical value is actually negative. This means that if the observed average disease progression in the experimental group falls into the circled region, actually looking *worse* than that in the placebo group, it would nevertheless fail to cause a rejection of superiority. The same result could occur if σ were seriously underestimated, such that the value of $s_p \sqrt{2/n}$ that results is too large. It would be awkward indeed to argue in favor of bringing the experimental treatment forward for phase 3 testing as a promising therapy when it looked worse than placebo in the futility trial. There is nothing logically inconsistent here – the statement that the data are insufficient to rule out superiority at level α is still correct, but the data possess such small evidentiary weight that the statement has little value. This is analogous to the situation with an underpowered phase 3 design. The key is to be sure to have an adequate sample size (to have a high probability of declaring futility when the experimental treatment is truly ineffective) and not to underestimate σ.

An interesting case arises that is intermediate between Figures 8.1 and 8.2, portrayed in Figure 8.3. Here the critical value for $\bar{Y}^{(P)} - \bar{Y}^{(E)}$ is exactly zero, as would occur if Δ_0 happened to equal $t_{2n-2;\alpha} s_p \sqrt{2/n}$. In

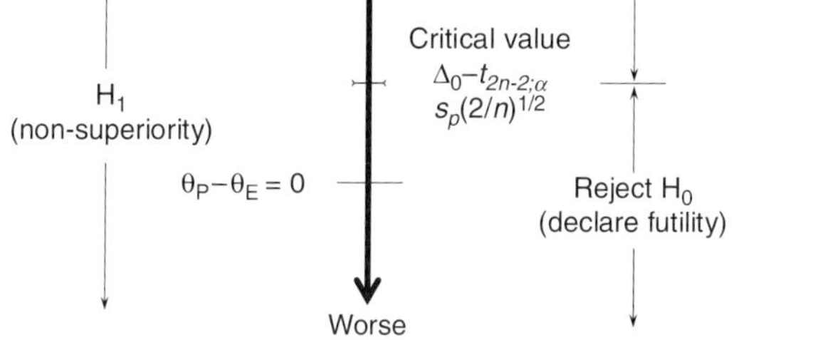

Figure 8.1. Schematic diagram of a well designed futility study.

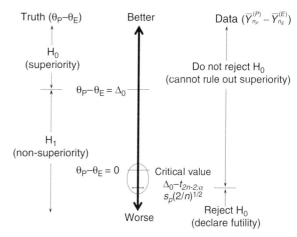

Figure 8.2. Schematic diagram of a poorly designed futility study. The oval indicates the awkward region.

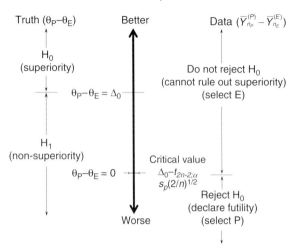

Difference in endpoint means

Truth $(\theta_P - \theta_E)$ Better   Data $(\bar{Y}_{n_P}^{(P)} - \bar{Y}_{n_E}^{(E)})$

H_0
(superiority)

Do not reject H_0
(cannot rule out superiority)
(select E)

$\theta_P - \theta_E = \Delta_0$

H_1
(non-superiority)

Critical value
$\Delta_0 - t_{2n-2;\alpha}$
$s_p (2/n)^{1/2}$

$\theta_P - \theta_E = 0$

Reject H_0
(declare futility)
(select P)

Worse

Figure 8.3. Schematic diagram of a futility design equivalent to a selection design.

this case the decision rule is identical to that of a symmetric *selection procedure*: declare futility if and only if $\bar{Y}^{(E)} \geq \bar{Y}^{(P)}$, i.e., we select the experimental treatment as potentially preferable to the placebo if and only if it does better, no matter by how small an amount. The power of this test is 50% at the design alternative of treatment efficacy equal to that of placebo. Different views are possible here, but some would argue that in this case a one-half chance of proceeding to phase 3 may be reasonable because in such close cases, where the treatment looks better than placebo, a phase 3 trial ought to be done to settle the question. The QALS trial came close to this case [8]. We discuss selection procedures below.

We mentioned above that a futility test and a one-sided test of the traditional null hypothesis that $\theta_E \geq \theta_P$ versus the alternative hypothesis that $\theta_E < \theta_P$ have parallel operating characteristics. That is because, in the additive two-arm design, for example, if the type I error rate is α in each case, the critical values for $\bar{Y}^{(P)} - \bar{Y}^{(E)}$ lie the same distance away from the respective null hypothesis values, the distance in each case being $t_{2n-2;\alpha} s_p \sqrt{2/n}$. It follows that the non-centrality parameter λ and the power function, $P[tv(\lambda) > t_{v;\alpha}]$, are identical for the two designs. Thus it is incorrect to view the futility design as inherently more efficient than a traditional design (another pitfall). If futility designs are more efficient than those used for phase 3 trials, it is because futility designs may use one arm rather than two, one-tailed rather than two-tailed testing, and $\alpha = 0.10$ or more rather than $\alpha = 0.05$ or less.

The last pitfall relates to the use of historical control data in the single-arm design. The problems of interpreting studies using historical control data are well-known and need not be repeated here. It will suffice to point out that if θ_0 (or π_0) represents a superiority criterion based not on an absolute judgment of how well a superior treatment should perform in the current patient population but instead represents a value that would have been superior in the historical patient population, the single-arm futility study may not rule out even a true placebo as futile. This is what occurred in the early NET-PD futility studies, where θ_0 was determined based on a 30% improvement in the DATATOP placebo/tocopherol group, observed about 15 years earlier. It turned out that θ_0 was too large relative to the current patient population, such that even the placebo-treated patients recruited concurrently in the futility studies as 'calibration controls' [13] could not be rejected as futile. This required a series of sensitivity analyses that ran counter to the notion of a pre-specified definition of superiority. For further discussion, see [5–7]. The lesson to be learned is that the additional resources needed for a two-arm study with concurrent controls may well be worth the cost to preserve internal validity. Later NET-PD futility studies have used concurrent controls.

Selection designs

Not every research goal calls for a hypothesis test. There are times when the primary goal is to *select* a treatment or a dosage of a treatment to bring forward for the next phase of clinical testing or the next study, which need not be phase 3, or to select a subset of candidate treatments from amongst a larger set of competitors. When a choice *must* be made – because constrained resources do not allow phase 3 testing of all competitors, or, in other circumstances, because an optimal dosage of the experimental drug is unknown – it is natural to use a selection procedure to assist in the decision-making. At such times setting up a null hypothesis and controlling the probability of committing a type I error may be entirely irrelevant. Indeed, if all of the competitors have equal efficacy, we might be completely indifferent as to which treatment we select.[8] If, however, there is

---

[8] Other things like cost and side effects being equal. We shall assume 'other things equal' here in order to focus on basic principles. In practice, if there is only weak evidence supporting a selected treatment against a competitor, other factors will of course play a role in the final decision.

a truly superior treatment among the competitors, we shall want our selection procedure to select that one correctly with high probability. Selection procedures thus offer an attractive approach to the problem of screening potentially good treatments.

Selection procedures have been in the statistical literature for more than a half century [15–19]. They first appeared in the clinical trials literature in the 1980s [20–22] and are enjoying a resurgence due to current interest in adaptive clinical trial designs [23–24]. When an optimal dosage of a drug is unknown, for example, it is very appealing on grounds of trial efficiency to consider selecting a good dose as part of the same experiment that will evaluate the drug's promise (in the context of an adaptive phase 2 trial) or its actual efficacy (in the context of an adaptive phase 3 trial). The QALS trial [8, 9] was a two-stage adaptive phase 2 trial that used a selection procedure in its first stage to choose which of two high doses of coenzyme Q10 (1800 mg/day versus 2700 mg/day) to bring forward for a futility test in the second stage. It was adaptive in the sense that the same data used for the selection decision were used again in the futility test to compare the selected dose with the concurrent placebo control data. As another example, the Combination Drug Selection Trial had as its primary goal the selection between two combination therapies (celecoxib and creatine versus minocycline and creatine) for further study in ALS [25].

When a relatively rapid endpoint is available, sequential selection procedures are especially useful [18, 26–33]. The TNK-S2B phase 2B/3 trial of tenecteplase vs. alteplase in acute stroke used a sequential selection procedure with a rapid endpoint to choose between three doses of the experimental drug tenecteplase (0.1, 0.25, or 0.4 mg/kg). The rapid endpoint was a three-category variable for outcomes of major neurological improvement (defined as at least an eight-point improvement at 24 hours on the NIH Stroke Scale or a score of zero), symptomatic intracerebral hemorrhage on CT scan at 24 hours, or neither. This trial was also designed adaptively. See [34] for details of this trial and Chapter 9 for further discussion of adaptive clinical trial designs.

The indifference zone approach and simple selection with fixed sample sizes

Suppose we have two active treatments labeled 1 and 2 and our goal is simply to select the better treatment

to bring forward for further testing. In the so-called *indifference zone approach,* which we follow here, one pre-specifies a minimally worthwhile difference in efficacy, denoted by Δ_0. As in our discussion of the futility design, and with the same notation, we assume a normally distributed measure of disease progression Y with mean θ_1 or θ_2 and common standard deviation σ. If the true difference between θ_1 and θ_2 is less than Δ_0 in magnitude, then one should be indifferent as to which treatment is selected, precisely because the difference is not worthwhile. If, however, the true difference between θ_1 and θ_2 is at least Δ_0 in magnitude (falling into the 'preference zone'), then the selection procedure should provide a correct selection with probability no smaller than some pre-specified value P^* such as 0.80. Thus, if $\theta_1 = \theta_2$, we are completely indifferent (in terms of efficacy) as to which treatment is selected, and a one-half chance of selecting either is perfectly acceptable. As θ_1 and θ_2 diverge, we want the probability of correct selection (which we abbreviate PCS) to grow, approaching P^* as $|\theta_1 - \theta_2|$ approaches Δ_0. For even larger differences, the PCS should surpass P^* and approach certainty for large $|\theta_1 - \theta_2|$.

To achieve these goals with fixed sample sizes we may randomize n patients on each treatment and select the treatment with the smallest observed average disease progression. The probability of a correct selection is then given by $P[\bar{Y}_1 < \bar{Y}_2]$ if $\theta_1 < \theta_2$ or $P[\bar{Y}_2 < \bar{Y}_1]$ if $\theta_2 < \theta_1$.[9] In either case, the PCS equals the probability to the left of $\sqrt{n}\,|\theta_1 - \theta_2|/(\sigma\sqrt{2})$ in the standard normal distribution. For example, in the QALS trial a sample of size $n = 35$ patients in each of the two high-dosage coenzyme Q10 groups was sufficient to guarantee $PCS \geq 0.80$ if there were a difference of 1.7 points between the true average declines in the nine-month ALSFRS-R, assuming a common standard deviation of $\sigma = 8.4$ for the individual declines.[10] This is because $\sqrt{35}\cdot1.7/(8.4\cdot\sqrt{2}) = 0.847$, which has probability 0.80 to its left in the standard normal distribution.[11]

---

[9] Tied averages do not occur for normally distributed random variables. In practice, disease progression measures with finitely many possible values could result in tied averages with very small probability, in which case a tie-breaking device is used to choose between treatments.

[10] The difference of 1.7 represents a 20% improvement in the assumed average placebo group decline of 8.5 units, which was used for planning purposes.

[11] When there are more than two groups, tables or special software are required to derive the PCS. See, e.g., the tables in [19].

By comparison, a traditional test of the null hypothesis H_0: $\theta_1 = \theta_2$ versus the alternative hypothesis H_1: $\theta_1 \neq \theta_2$ with $\alpha = 0.05$ (two-tailed) and power of 80% at the design alternative $|\theta_2 - \theta_1| = 1.7$, assuming $\sigma = 8.4$, would require samples of size $n = 384$ per group! The selection procedure requires so many fewer patients because there is no need to control for type I errors to make a good selection. One way to see this is to view the selection design as a hypothesis test that rejects the null hypothesis of equal efficacy in favor of $\theta_1 < \theta_2$ if $\bar{Y}_1 < \bar{Y}_2$ or rejects H_0 in favor of $\theta_2 < \theta_1$ if $\bar{Y}_2 < \bar{Y}_1$. Under H_0 then, by symmetry, the probability of a type I error is controlled only at 0.50 (not 0.05). *However, no type I errors will be made at all if we do not attempt any declarations of statistical significance upon making the selection.* This is the fundamental difference between hypothesis testing and selection; in a simple selection design, the primary task at hand is to choose one treatment or the other, not to make any formal declaration of statistical significance. Note that post hoc statements of statistical significance at $\alpha = 0.05$ would be seriously underpowered, so failure to achieve traditional levels of significance would not be considered meaningful.

Sequential selection procedures

There are many different procedures for more general ranking and selection goals such as selection from among more than two treatments, selection of best subsets of treatments (e.g., the best two treatments), ranking treatments in order of efficacy, etc. For brevity we discuss just one, the Levin-Robbins-Leu (LRL) family of sequential selection procedures [28–33]. These procedures are convenient to implement, provide blocking for control of differences by site or prognostic covariates, and allow sequential elimination of inferior treatments as the trial progresses, sequential recruitment of superior treatments, or both. For variety, we now assume a rapid *binary* endpoint, such as major neurological improvement (MNI), yes/no. We want to choose the best from among $c \geq 2$ treatments, where 'best' means the one with highest success probability p_i ($i = 1,\ldots,c$) for MNI. The data will now consist of c binomially distributed success tallies after n patient outcomes per group are observed. In the response-adaptive LRL elimination procedure, one pre-specifies a reference integer $r \geq 1$ and sequentially observes single binary (yes/no) outcomes on each of the c treatments, one vector of c binary outcomes at a

time.[12] After any number of rounds n, if the running success tally of one or more treatments falls r successes behind the tally or tallies currently in the lead, the trailing treatments are *eliminated* from further consideration, and no further patients are randomized to them. The procedure continues randomizing patients in blocks to the remaining treatments, resuming the success tallies at their current values. The entire process iterates until finally only a single treatment is left, which is then selected as best.[13]

This selection procedure has the following important property. Let $w_i = p_i / (1 - p_i)$ denote the unknown odds on success for the binary outcome on treatment i. Then for any odds $w_1,\ldots,w_c$ the *PCS* is bounded from below by a simple formula:

$$ PCS \geq \frac{w_{[1]}^r}{\sum_{i=1}^{c} w_i^r}, $$

where $w_{[1]}$ denotes the largest odds corresponding to the best treatment. This result can be used to choose the integer r, as follows. Suppose we want the probability of correct selection to be at least P^* whenever the odds ratio $w_{[1]} / w_{[2]}$ between the best and second best treatment success probabilities is at least some pre-specified value Δ. In that case:

$$ \frac{w_{[1]}^r}{\sum_{i=1}^{c} w_i^r} \geq \frac{\Delta^r}{\Delta^r + c - 1}, $$

So if we choose r to be the smallest integer greater than or equal to:

$$ \frac{\ln\left\{\dfrac{(c-1)P^*}{1 - P^*}\right\}}{\ln \Delta}, $$

then for *any* set of success probabilities with $w_{[1]} / w_{[2]} \geq \Delta$:

---

[13] This is an "open" sequential procedure, meaning there is no pre-specified upper limit to the number of patients randomized. The procedure will terminate using a finite number of patients with probability one, but in practice one imposes an upper limit to the number of patients enrolled, such that if the criteria for selection are not yet met, the trial will be truncated and a special terminal decision made for the selection.

$$PCS \geq \frac{w_{[1]}^r}{\sum_{i=1}^{c} w_i^r} \geq \frac{\Delta^r}{\Delta^r + c - 1} \geq P^*.$$

For example, to select the best treatment from among $c = 3$ competitors with an odds ratio of $\Delta = 2$ defining the boundary between the indifference and preference zones, the criterion value $r = 3$ suffices to guarantee a PCS of at least $P^* = 0.80$ for any $p_1, \ldots, p_c$ in the preference zone.

The number of patients randomized in a sequential design is a random variable. The expected number of patients depends on r and the specific values of the success probabilities. To illustrate the above example, if $p_1 = \frac{1}{2}$ while $p_2 = p_3 = \frac{1}{3}$, so that $w_{[1]}/w_{[2]} = 2$, the expected number of rounds is 17.4, the expected total number of patients randomized is 43.6, and the expected total number of failures (non-MNIs) is 26.3. By comparison, a fixed sample size binomial procedure would require 24 patients per arm or 72 patients in total, and the expected number of failures would be $24 \cdot (1/2 + 2/3 + 2/3) = 44$, illustrating the expected efficiency gain of the sequential design. Note also that the expected total number of patients with the LRL procedure in this example, 43.6, is less than three times the expected number of rounds ($52.2 = 3 \times 17.4$) and the expected number of failures, 26.3, is less than the expected number of rounds times the total failure probability, or $17.4 \times (1/2 + 2/3 + 2/3) = 31.9$, thanks to the sequential elimination of inferior treatments. This feature strongly appeals on ethical grounds.[14]

The LRL family of procedures can also be used to select best subsets of pre-specified size b ($1 \leq b < c$). To select the best b treatments from c competitors with sequential elimination of inferior treatments and sequential recruitment of superior treatments, one proceeds as follows. Randomize patients a vector-at-a-time, and pause the first time that either of the following events occurs: (i) $S_{[b]}^{(n)} - S_{[c]}^{(n)} = r$, where $S_{[b]}^{(n)}$ denotes the bth largest success tally after n patient observations per treatment and $S_{[c]}^{(n)}$ denotes the cth largest, i.e., worst success tally. This is an elimination event, and any treatment with the worst tally is eliminated. If several treatments are tied with the worst tally, eliminate

them all. (ii) $S_{[1]}^{(n)} - S_{[b+1]}^{(n)} = r$, where $S_{[b+1]}^{(n)}$ denotes the $(b+1)^{\text{st}}$ largest tally. This is a recruitment event, and any treatment with a leading tally is recruited, meaning we select it immediately for further development. If several treatments are tied with the best tally, recruit them all. No further patients are randomized to recruited treatments.[15] After an elimination or recruitment or both events occur, the procedure continues with the remaining treatments at their current tallies, and the entire process iterates with the reduced number c' of remaining treatments and a possibly reduced number b' of treatments yet to be recruited. The procedure stops when exactly b treatments have been recruited and $c - b$ treatments have been eliminated.

The probability of correctly selecting the best b-tuple of treatments with highest success probabilities is bounded from below by:

$$PCS \geq \frac{w_{[1]}^r \cdots w_{[b]}^r}{\sum_{(b)} w_{(b)}^r},$$

where the summation is over all b-tuples of the form $(b) = (i_1, \ldots, i_b)$ with $1 \leq i_1 < \ldots < i_b \leq c$ and where $w_{(b)}^r = w_{i_1}^r \cdots w_{i_b}^r$. For example, if there are $c = 4$ treatments and it is required to select the best $b = 2$ treatments, the PCS is bounded from below by $w_{[1]}^r w_{[2]}^r / (w_1^r w_2^r + w_1^r w_3^r + w_1^r w_4^r + w_2^r w_3^r + w_2^r w_4^r + w_3^r w_4^r)$. The preference zone now contains all sets of success probabilities for which $w_{[2]}/w_{[3]} \geq \Delta$. The value of r is chosen large enough so that:

$$PCS \geq \frac{w_{[1]}^r w_{[2]}^r}{w_1^r w_2^r + w_1^r w_3^r + w_1^r w_4^r + w_2^r w_3^r + w_2^r w_4^r + w_3^r w_4^r}$$
$$\geq \frac{\Delta^{2r}}{\Delta^{2r} + 4\Delta^r + 1} \geq P^*.$$

---

[14] The exact PCS in this example is 0.814. If the open procedure is truncated after $n = 35$ rounds, the PCS is 0.80, still large, while the expected number of rounds, patients, and failures decrease slightly to 16.5, 41.8, and 25.2, respectively.

[15] It may seem odd to remove the leading treatment from competition in the case $b > 1$. It should be noted, however, that there is no claim that the first treatment to be eliminated is the truly worst treatment, only that its record is sufficiently poor that it should not be selected. Similarly, there is no claim that the first treatment to be recruited is truly the best treatment, only that its record is good enough to be among the best b treatments to be selected. Since it is not known that the best treatment has been removed, it is ethical to continue randomizing patients to the other treatments, assuming at the outset there are good reasons to select more than one treatment.

Additional properties of these procedures are discussed in [31–32].

Selection bias

If a selection procedure is used as the first stage of an adaptive trial where the selection data will be used in the final evaluation of the whole trial, an adjustment for selection bias is required due to the potential for capitalizing on chance (see Chapter 5 for more on bias). Suppose, for example, that we will select one of two active treatments in a first selection stage and then use the selected treatment's data to compare with a concurrent placebo. Suppose further that all three treatments have the same true efficacy. In replications of the experiment, whichever treatment is selected will have a systematic advantage over the placebo because its very selection requires it to look better than its competitor. If patients are not too scarce, a simple method to avoid selection bias is to conduct the selection as a separate experiment from the subsequent evaluation. An adjustment for selection bias was used in the QALS trial because the investigators considered ALS patients relatively rare and wanted to use their selection data in the second-stage futility test. Formulas for correcting the selection bias are given in [8].

Comparative selection trials

Although selection procedures efficiently achieve their goal of selecting best treatments, the desire to 'test something' with an accompanying statement of statistical significance seems irresistible. There is the following issue to consider too: if a selection trial is conducted with only active treatments, i.e., without including a placebo as eligible for selection in the contest, then it is possible that all of the active treatments under consideration may be worse than placebo, so that none 'should' be selected. Of course, when a placebo is excluded from consideration in a selection trial, consideration of whether or not the selected treatment is better than a placebo is simply outside the goal of the selection trial and additional testing must address that comparative question. Therefore it should be emphasized that just because an active treatment has been selected in a head-to-head comparison with other active treatments, there is no direct evidence that the one selected need be efficacious (compared to placebo). These considerations suggest that a selection design with a concomitant hypothesis test would be of great practical interest.

A new design called the 'comparative selection trial' combines selection and hypothesis testing with no need for selection bias adjustments [33]. Briefly, the trial compares c_0 placebo arms to c_1 active treatment arms, for a total of $c_0 + c_1 = c$ arms. The goal is to select a subset of pre-specified size b ($1 \leq b \leq c_1$) of all 'better-than-placebo' (BTP) treatments, assuming one or more exists, or if not, to declare that no such subset exists. The null hypothesis H_0 is that there exists no BTP b-tuple of treatments (because at least one placebo arm is better than the bth best active arm in terms of efficacy). The alternative hypothesis H_1 is that a BTP b-tuple exists (wherein all b active arms are better than the best placebo arm in terms of efficacy). We wish to test H_0 controlling the type I error rate at level α and in so doing, we will control the probability that we will make a false declaration that a BTP b-tuple exists when H_0 is true. If H_1 is true, we want to have a high probability P^* of correctly declaring that a BTP b-tuple exists and correctly selecting one. For example, if there are $c_1 = 2$ active treatments and $c_0 = 1$ placebo treatment and we want to select the best $b = 1$ treatment, we will test the null hypothesis that there is no better-than-placebo active treatment. If true, we will want to declare this to be the case with probability at least $1 - \alpha$. If either or both of the active treatments are better than the placebo, we will want to declare the existence of a BTP treatment and select the best one with probability at least P^*.

The LRL family of selection procedures can be used for this problem. The idea is to use data augmentation to 'handicap' the placebo treatments' outcome tallies while selecting a best b-tuple. If the selected b-tuple contains a placebo treatment, we do not reject H_0 and we declare that there is no BTP b-tuple of treatments. If the selected b-tuple contains only active treatments, then we reject H_0 and declare that the selected b-tuple is a BTP b-tuple. The LRL lower bound formula for the probability of correct selection is used both to select r and to determine how to augment the placebo data in order to control both the type I error rate and the probability of making a false declaration. The type I error rate can be controlled because the data augmentation adds successes to the placebo arms in a carefully specified manner so as to make the placebo arms look better than the active treatments, thereby yielding a high probability of selecting at least one placebo arm under the null hypothesis, avoiding a type I error. The choice of r then guarantees a high probability of correctly rejecting the null hypothesis when it is false and simultaneously selecting a BTP b-tuple when there is a sufficiently large separation between the success probabilities of the best *b* active and placebo treatments. See [33] for details on how to do this.

References

1. Palesch Y, Tilley BC, Sackett DL, *et al.* Applying a phase II futility study design to therapeutic stroke trials. *Stroke* 2005; **36**: 2410–4.

2. Levin B. The utility of futility (editorial). *Stroke* 2005; **36**: 2331–2.

3. Elm JJ, Goetz CG, Ravina B, *et al.* A responsive outcome for Parkinson's disease neuroprotection futility studies. *Ann Neurol* 2005; **57**: 197–203.

4. Tilley BC, Palesch YY, Kieburtz K, *et al.*, on behalf of the NET-PD Investigators. Optimizing the ongoing search for new treatments for Parkinson's disease: using futility designs. *Neurology* 2006; **66**: 628–33.

5. The NINDS NET-PD Investigators. A randomized, double blinded, futility clinical trial of creatine and minocycline in early Parkinson's disease. *Neurology* 2006; **66**: 664–71.

6. The NINDS NET-PD Investigators. A randomized clinical trial of coenzyme Q10 and GPI-1485 in early Parkinson disease. *Neurology* 2007; **68**: 20–8.

7. Tilley BC and Galpern WR. Screening potential therapies: Lessons learned from new paradigms used in Parkinson disease. *Stroke* 2007; **38**: 800–3.

8. Levy G, Kaufmann P, Buchsbaum R, *et al.* A two-stage design for a phase II clinical trial of coenzyme Q10 in ALS. *Neurology* 2006; **66**: 660–3.

9. Kaufmann, P, Thompson, JLP, Levy, G, *et al.*, for the QALS Study Group. Phase II trial of CoQ10 for ALS finds insufficient evidence to justify phase III. *Ann Neurol* 2009; **66**: 235–44.

10. Czaplinski A, Haverkamp LJ, Yen AA, *et al.* The value of database controls in pilot or futility studies in ALS. *Neurology* 2006; **67**: 1827–32.

11. Cudkowicz M, Katz J, Moore DH, *et al.* Toward more efficient clinical trials for amyotrophic lateral sclerosis. *Amyotrophic Lateral Scler* 2010; **11**: 259–65.

12. The Huntington Study Group DOMINO Investigators. A futility study of minocycline in Huntington's disease. *Mov Disord* 2010; **25**: 2219–24.

13. Herson J and Carter SK. Calibrated phase II clinical trials in oncology. *Stat Med* 1986; **5**: 441–7.

14. The Parkinson Study Group. Effect of deprenyl on the progression of disability in early Parkinson's disease. *New Engl J Med* 1989; **321**: 1364–71.

15. Bechhofer RE. A single-sample multiple decision procedure for ranking means of normal populations with known variances. *Ann Math Stat* 1954; **25**: 16–39.

16. Gupta SS. *On a decision rule for a problem in ranking means.* Mimeograph Series 150, Institute of Statistics. Chapel Hill, University of North Carolina, 1956.

17. Gupta SS. On some multiple decision (selection and ranking) rules. *Technometrics* 1965; **7**: 225–45.

18. Bechhofer RE, Kiefer J and Sobel M. *Sequential Identification and Ranking Procedures.* Chicago, University of Chicago Press, 1968.

19. Gibbons JD, Olkin I and Sobel M. *Selecting and Ordering Populations: A New Statistical Methodology.* Wiley, Hoboken, 1977; corrected, unabridged version Society for Industrial & Applied Mathematics, Philadelphia, 1999.

20. Simon R, Wittes RE and Ellenberg SS. Randomized phase II clinical trials. *Cancer Treat Rep* 1985; **69**: 1375–81.

21. Thall PF, Simon R and Ellenberg SS. Two-stage selection and testing designs for comparative clinical trials. *Biometrika* 1988; **75**: 303–10.

22. Schaid DJ, Wieand S and Therneau TM. Optimal two-stage screening designs for survival comparisons. *Biometrika* 1990; **77**: 507–13.

23. Stallard N and Todd S. Sequential designs for phase III clinical trials incorporating treatment selection. *Stat Med* 2003; **22**: 689–703.

24. Bischoff W and Miller F. Adaptive two-stage test procedures to find the best treatment in clinical trials. *Biometrika* 2005; **92**: 197–212.

25. Gordon PH, Cheung Y-K, Levin B, *et al.*, for the Combination Drug Selection Trial Study Group. A novel, efficient, randomized selection trial comparing combinations of drug therapy for ALS. *Amyotrophic Lateral Scler* 2008; **9**: 212–22.

26. Buringer H, Martin H and Schriever, KH. *Nonparametric Sequential Selection Procedures.* Birkhauser, Boston: 1980.

27. Bechhofer RE, Santner TJ and Goldsman DM. *Design and Analysis of Experiments for Statistical Selection, Screening, and Multiple Comparisons.* Wiley, New York: 1995.

28. Levin B and Robbins H. Selecting the highest probability in binomial or multinomial trials. *Proc Natl Acad Sci USA* 1981; **78**: 4663–6.

29. Leu CS, Levin B. On the probability of correct selection in the Levin-Robbins sequential elimination procedure. *Stat Sinica* 1999; **9**: 879–91.

30. Leu CS and Levin B. Proof of a lower bound formula for the expected reward in the Levin-Robbins sequential elimination procedure. *Sequent Anal* 1999; **18**: 81–105.

31. Leu CS and Levin B. A generalization of the Levin-Robbins procedure for binomial subset selection and recruitment problems. *Stat Sinica* 2008; **18**: 203–18.

32. Leu CS and Levin B. On a conjecture of Bechhofer, Kiefer, and Sobel for the Levin-Robbins-Leu binomial subset selection procedures. *Sequent Anal* 2008; **27**: 106–25.

33. Leu CS, Cheung YK and Levin B. Subset selection in comparative selection trials. In: Bhattacharjee M, Dhar SK, Subramanian S, eds. *Recent Advances in Biostatistics,*

False Discovery, Survival Analysis and Other Topics. Series in Biostatistics, Volume 4. World Scientific, 2011.

34. Haley EC, Thompson JLP, Grotta, JC, *et al.*, for the Tenecteplase in Stroke Investigators. Phase IIB/III trial of tenecteplase in acute ischemic stroke: Results of a prematurely terminated randomized clinical trial. *Stroke* 2010; **41**: 707–11.

Adaptive design across stages of therapeutic development

Christopher S. Coffey

Introduction to adaptive designs

During the planning phase, an investigator must make important decisions that affect the design of a clinical trial (e.g., patient population, primary outcome, and primary hypothesis). Unfortunately, there may be limited information to guide these initial choices. Since more knowledge will accrue as the study progresses, one attractive suggestion is to incorporate an adaptive design that modifies one or more characteristics of the trial based on interim information. This greater flexibility has the potential to require the use of fewer patients within trials, allow a more efficient use of resources, and provide the ability to make effective treatments available to patients more quickly or stop ineffective treatments earlier. Accordingly, there has been substantial recent interest, and a number of concerns, associated with the use of adaptive designs. This chapter will attempt to clarify the definition of an adaptive design, summarize some of the commonly proposed types of adaptive designs, summarize the use of adaptive designs in published neurological trials, and describe some logistical barriers that will need to be addressed in order to more fully achieve the benefits of promising adaptive designs in the future. The reader interested in more details regarding the subject should consult one of a number of excellent review articles [1–6] or recent guidance publications by regulatory agencies [7–8].

Definition of an adaptive design

The rapid proliferation of interest in adaptive designs, and inconsistent use of terminology, has created confusion about similarities and differences among the various techniques. For example, the definition of an 'adaptive design' itself is a common source of confusion. The term has been used rather ambiguously in the literature and there are a large number of potential study adaptations. There is clearly a need for a standardized definition of an adaptive design.

The Pharmaceutical Researchers and Manufacturers of America (PhRMA) Adaptive Designs Working Group (ADWG) was formed in 2006[1]. One of the earliest contributions of the working group was the publication of a white paper that provided one of the first formal definitions of an adaptive design: 'By adaptive design we refer to a clinical study design that uses accumulating data to modify aspects of the study as it continues, without undermining the validity and integrity of the trial' [1]. The white paper went on to stress that changes should be made '…by design, and not on an ad hoc basis' and that adaptive designs are '…not a remedy for inadequate planning'. A similar definition appeared in the recent FDA draft guidance document on adaptive designs: '…a study that includes a prospectively planned opportunity for modification of one or more specified aspects of the study design and hypotheses based on analysis of data (usually interim data) from subjects in the study' [8]. However, the definition in the FDA draft guidance document uses a more relaxed definition for what is meant by prospectively planned: 'This can include plans that are introduced or made final after the study has started if the blinded state of the personnel involved is unequivocally maintained when the modification plan is proposed.'

Much of the research on adaptive designs has been driven by drug development within the pharmaceutical industry. Although many basic principles remain

---

[1] The AD working group has established an external webpage: http://biopharmnet.com/doc/doc12004.html. This webpage provides a central location for publications, training courses, and other documents created by the working group to facilitate the sharing of knowledge.

Clinical Trials in Neurology, ed. Bernard Ravina, Jeffrey Cummings, Michael P. McDermott, and R. Michael Poole. Published by Cambridge University Press. © Cambridge University Press 2012.

the same regardless of the venue or funding source, some of the specific advantages and disadvantages of adaptive designs differ when considering the use of such designs in trials funded by the NIH, foundations, or non-profit organizations. To address this issue, a 2009 workshop was held on 'Scientific Advances in Adaptive Clinical Trial Design.' The workshop definition of an adaptive design was very similar to that of the ADWG: 'A protocol that allows certain design features to change from an initial specification based on evolving trial information while maintaining statistical, scientific, and ethical integrity.'

Hence, all three definitions clearly state that only studies with pre-planned adaptations would be considered adaptive designs. For the purposes of this chapter, we take the same approach and consider valid adaptive designs to be only those that consider pre-planned changes.

Types of adaptive designs

Based on the above definitions, it is clear that there are an infinite number of adaptive design possibilities and any number of aspects of the study can be changed. Design features that can change include, but are not limited to, the maximum sample size, the stopping time, the allocation of patients, dosing, the number of treatment arms, the endpoints, or the hypotheses. Clearly, changes to some of these elements are more controversial than others.

In all instances, the objectives of the adaptations should be clearly defined and the operating characteristics should be well understood. For example, before utilizing any adaptive design that involves hypothesis testing, researchers should assess the impact of the increased power on the overall type I error rate and make steps to adjust for any inflation that might be introduced. Such assessments are crucial because adaptive designs are not always better than standard fixed designs. One important assessment when considering an adaptive design is to compare its properties with those obtained from a standard fixed design. The need for such evaluations underscores the need for adaptations to be planned in advance. In order to enable a full simulation of any proposed adaptive design, the extent to which adaptation is planned should be described a priori in detail. As stated by Hung *et al.*: 'At the very least, the regulatory agencies need to know every detail of how the trial proceeded during the conduct and adaptations' [9].

In this chapter, we focus on some specific adaptive designs that have received the most attention to date. Although many adaptive designs employ the use of Bayesian statistical techniques, it is important to consider both Bayesian and Frequentist approaches to adaptive designs.

Adaptive designs for early stage exploratory development

Early exploratory (phase 1) trials generally represent the initial introduction of an investigational new drug into humans. These studies are generally small (15–30 subjects) with an objective of determining the maximum tolerated dose (MTD) – the largest dose of the drug that can be given before patients start to experience a dose limiting toxicity (DLT) at an unacceptably high rate. These trials help to guide the decision whether to continue a drug development program and, if so, which dose(s) to select for further development. If additional development is planned, an accurate determination of the MTD is very important to the planning and conduct of trials in later phases. Selecting too low a dose may not allow future studies to show efficacy of a potentially useful drug. Similarly, selecting too high a dose may put patients in future trials at unnecessary risk. Traditional approaches for designing phase 1 clinical trials include up-and-down designs or model-based designs where the MTD is treated as a quantile that can be estimated [10]. The most common approach is the '3+3 design', which treats three subjects at each dose level of interest. If no subjects experience a DLT, the dose is increased to the next level. If two or more subjects experience a DLT, the process stops and selects the lower dose as the MTD. If one subject experiences a DLT, then three additional subjects are treated at the given dose. If none of the three additional subjects experiences a DLT, the dose is increased to the next level. Otherwise, the process stops and the dose below is selected as the MTD. This approach is easily understood by clinicians and requires no complex computer program to implement, but tends to treat many subjects at low, ineffective doses and may provide poor estimates of the MTD in neurological settings where DLTs of interest occur less frequently than in the oncology settings where this design originated. Recently, more sophisticated approaches for adaptive dose ranging have been proposed. The most common of these approaches, the continual reassessment method (CRM), is discussed below [11].

Continual reassessment method

The CRM assumes that the probability of both efficacy and toxicity increase with dose and that toxicity can be defined as a binary outcome. The 'acceptable' level of toxicity must be explicitly defined by the investigators. The MTD is then defined as the highest dose with a toxicity level at or below the specified acceptable level of toxicity. In its original formulation, the method begins with an assumed a priori dose-toxicity curve and a chosen target toxicity level. The first enrolled subject is assigned the dose most likely to be associated with the target toxicity level, based on the initial curve. After the outcome for this patient has been observed, the estimated dose-toxicity curve is refitted (i.e., the posterior distribution of the model is shifted slightly up or down depending on whether the patient experienced a DLT). The next subject is assigned the dose closest to the MTD based on the updated dose-toxicity curve. This process continues until some pre-defined stopping criteria are met. There are two general strategies for defining the stopping rules: 1) Continue until a specified number of patients are treated at the same dose and the next patient would also be treated at that dose; or 2) Continue until the dose-toxicity curve changes by less than some pre-specified threshold. Regardless of the stopping rule chosen, once the stopping criteria are achieved, the final dose is selected as the MTD. To address some of the concerns raised with the initial CRM proposal, several modified CRM approaches have been developed and implemented. These modifications include always starting at the lowest dose level under consideration, enrolling 2–3 patients in each cohort, proceeding as a standard 3+3 dose escalation design until the first DLT occurs, and specifying that dose escalation cannot increase by more than one level at any time during the study. As compared to the 3+3 design, the CRM typically treats more subjects at the target dose and fewer subjects at ineffective doses. However, the implementation of a CRM requires a substantial collaboration between an investigator and statistician. The method is also rather computationally intensive, although there are documented software packages available for the implementation of the technique. A free package can be downloaded from:

- M.D. Anderson Cancer Center (http:// biostatistics.mdanderson.org/Software Download)

Adaptive designs for late stage exploratory development

Late exploratory (phase 2) trials typically have a number of different goals [12]. These include establishing that the response changes with the dose (proof of concept) and selecting a target dose to take forward into the confirmatory phase. Traditional approaches to such trials involve random allocation to multiple fixed doses with multiple comparison adjustments. A number of adaptive model-based approaches have been proposed, including a D-optimal approach, a normal dynamic linear model (NDLM) [13], and a general adaptive dose allocation. A PhRMA adaptive dose-ranging studies working group was formed in 2006 to address the concern that a poor understanding of dose response is a leading cause of high attrition in late development. One of the initial objectives of this group was to conduct a comprehensive simulation study comparing adaptive model-based approaches to other dose-finding methods [14]. The group concluded that the sample sizes typically used for traditional approaches to dose-finding studies are too small for accurate dose selection and estimation of the dose-response curve. The adaptive model-based methods had increased power to detect dose-response and better precision with respect to selecting a target dose. However, they caution that there is a need to balance gains associated with adaptive dose-ranging designs against the greater methodological and operational complexity currently associated with the use of these designs. In particular, there are very few public software packages available for implementing these methods. As new software is developed, the use of these methods will become much more practical.

Adaptive designs for confirmatory clinical trials

Adaptive designs are generally well accepted and encouraged for early phases of drug development. For a variety of reasons, including the potential for type I error inflation, the use of adaptive designs in confirmatory (phase 3) trials is a bit more controversial. However, it is clear that unplanned adaptations have been utilized for many years in clinical trials. For example, most trials involve changes related to logistical issues, such as recruitment criteria, that do not affect the inferences of interest. Furthermore, in order to determine the required sample size to ensure a desired level of statistical power, an investigator must specify a clinically meaningful treatment difference and values for any 'nuisance' parameters. A nuisance parameter represents any value that must be specified in order to perform a sample size calculation that is not directly related to the effect of the treatment (e.g., the standard deviation of a continuous measure, the overall event rate for a binary outcome, and the accrual rate for a time-to-event outcome). The uncertainty associated with the estimation of most key nuisance parameters at the beginning of a trial, perhaps due to complications from using natural history data to plan a clinical trial, has led to unplanned sample size adjustments in a number of ongoing studies. As an example, the Secondary Prevention of Small Subcortical Strokes (SPS3) study recently increased the overall planned sample size from 2500 to 3000 in order to account for a lower than expected overall event rate.

The biggest change in recent years is that such unplanned design changes are starting to receive greater scrutiny. This is actually a good thing because it forces researchers to give more thought to possible adaptations earlier in the planning process. As a result, investigators are being proactively encouraged to consider adaptation in the original development of a study protocol. However, the use of adaptive designs in the confirmatory setting requires researchers to proactively assess the operating characteristics of any proposed adaptations via simulation. This has the potential to require more resources for study planning, but can lead to great benefits during the conduct of the trial. Below, we briefly summarize the possible adaptations for confirmatory trials that have received the most attention in the literature to date. Although many can also be used in earlier studies, they are most often used for confirmatory trials and that will be our focus.

Group sequential methods

Sequential monitoring of interim data has become integral to modern clinical trials (see Chapter 14). A Data Safety Monitoring Board (DSMB) is usually given the responsibility for monitoring the accumulating data in a clinical trial. In general, DSMBs can be charged with stopping trials for: 1) safety, 2) efficacy or lack of efficacy, or 3) futility (insufficient power). Appropriate statistical methods for interim monitoring exist [15] and are implemented in a number of statistical software packages. Importantly, given the definitions above, group sequential designs are one of the most commonly used adaptive designs in clinical trials.

Adaptive randomization

An adaptive randomization design allows the randomization schedule to be modified during the course of an ongoing trial. There are a number of different types of adaptive randomization procedures. With response adaptive randomization, the allocation probability for assigning patients to treatment groups is determined by the responses observed in previous patients. Examples include the randomized play-the-winner model [16] and the use of a Bayesian bandit allocation rule [17]. Covariate adaptive randomization uses the covariate values of previously enrolled subjects to determine the allocation probabilities for future subjects. For example, a minimization algorithm can be used to assign subjects to treatments in a way that maximizes the balance among treatment groups with respect to the distributions of several covariates [18]. Although adaptive randomization methods are one of the oldest proposed adaptations, the use of response-adaptive randomization in confirmatory trials remains the source of much controversy due to concerns that the approach may lead to imbalances in important covariates and has the potential to add complexity to the final analysis. For example the recent FDA draft guidance document states that 'Adaptive randomization should be used cautiously in adequate and well-controlled studies, as the analysis is not as easily interpretable as when fixed randomization probabilities are used' [8].

Sample size re-estimation

The traditional approach to study design involves a substantial effort on the part of the investigators to ensure an adequate sample size is determined before the trial is initiated. Once all required design features have been specified, and a clinically meaningful treatment difference and values for any nuisance parameters have been specified, the investigators can compute the sample size required to achieve the desired power. This approach can be quite complicated since the specification of a 'clinically meaningful' treatment difference may not be straightforward or a great deal of uncertainty may exist with respect to the specified values for nuisance parameters. If the assumptions used for the sample size calculations are not correct, the study may have a sample size that is too small or too large. If the sample size is too small, the study will be underpowered and may lead to discarding a potentially useful treatment. Such underpowered studies lead to great confusion in the literature since they are often perceived as negative studies, but would properly be interpreted as inconclusive. Similarly, overpowered studies collect larger sample sizes than required and waste investigator resources that might have been directed elsewhere. A sample size re-estimation design refers to an adaptive design that allows for a sample size adjustment based on a review of interim data.

Historically, there has been a great deal of controversy surrounding designs that utilize sample size re-estimation. In general, the acceptance of such methods depends greatly on whether the sample size is being modified based on a re-estimated treatment effect or only on re-estimated values for the nuisance parameters. Methods have been proposed that allow the use of sample size re-estimation methods based on a revised treatment effect without inflating the type I error rate [19–23]. However, such methods have proven to be controversial due to concerns as to whether there is any benefit above and beyond that which can be achieved with a standard group sequential design [24]. Generally, a sample size re-estimation method based on a revised estimate of the treatment effect is nearly always less efficient than a group sequential approach [25–26]. That being said, the flexibility involved with such designs may be attractive because it allows starting a smaller study with an option of increasing if interim results seem promising. This could be very attractive to a small company or investigator with limited resources. However, it is vitally important that the rules for modifying the sample size be stated prior to any unblinding of the data. Thus, although methods exist to adjust for potential type I error inflation, the adjustments only apply conditional upon the specific decision that was made. Importantly, if the adaptation was made on an ad-hoc basis, these methods cannot guarantee unconditional control of the type I error rate because it is impossible to simulate the entire study design since one can never go back and clearly state all different decisions that might have been made had different interim results been observed. As a consequence, researchers should avoid post-hoc modifications of the sample size based an observed interim treatment differences.

With internal pilot designs, modifications are based only on re-estimated nuisance parameters [27]. With moderate to large sample sizes, there is minimal (if any) inflation of the type I error rate associated with the use of such designs [28–30]. Thus, internal pilot designs can be used in moderate to large randomized clinical trials to assess key nuisance parameters and make appropriate modifications with little cost in terms of an inflated type I error rate. The fact that internal pilot designs can be used in large trials, with little to no inflation of

the type I error rate, suggests that the protocols for all large trials should include re-assessments of nuisance parameters at some interim time point. However, such designs have not been routinely implemented to date.

Adaptive seamless designs

Seamless designs attempt to accomplish, within a single trial, objectives that are normally achieved through separate trials. The goal is to eliminate the downtime between trials. An adaptive seamless design combines phases and uses data from patients enrolled before and after the adaptation for the final analysis. Most interest to date has involved seamless phase 2/3 designs that transition an adaptive dose-finding study into a standard confirmatory trial. However, there are also opportunities for adaptive seamless designs in early development (phase 1/2a) or biomarker adaptive designs that allow design modification (dose selection, dropping arms, etc.) to be based on a short-term biomarker, while using a longer-term clinical endpoint for the confirmation stage.

The use of an adaptive seamless design will result in a more complicated statistical analysis at the end of the trial. When an adaptive seamless design is used, statistical methods must account for the fact that data from the second stage are combined with data from the first stage for the final analysis. The data from both stages must be combined in a way that guarantees control of the overall type I error rate, produces unbiased parameter estimates, and produces confidence intervals with the correct coverage probability. For example, Kaufman et al [31] conducted an adaptive seamless trial of coenzyme Q10 (coQ10) for the treatment of amyotrophic lateral sclerosis (ALS). The primary outcome was the nine month decline in the ALS Functional Rating Scale-revised. The first stage used a selection design (see Chapter 8) to select one of two dosages of coQ10 (1800 or 2700 mg/day) to carry forward into stage 2. The second stage compared the selected dose from stage 1 against placebo using a futility design [32] (see Chapter 8). If no adjustment is made to the final test statistic, the type I error rate may be increased due to the positive bias introduced by the fact that the test statistic does not account for the fact that the dose being compared to placebo was chosen as the best dose in stage one. To address this issue, the investigators used simulations to develop and validate a bias correction. This bias correction was then incorporated into the final test statistic in order to preserve the overall type I error rate at the desired level.

The added flexibility of an adaptive seamless design may be offset by the added complexity associated with such designs. Investigators should carefully consider the feasibility of implementing an adaptive seamless design within a given project. Some projects might be better suited to seamless development than others. The length of time needed to make a decision should be small relative to the time for enrollment. If a biomarker will be used for dose selection, it should be validated and well understood. Drug supply and packaging may be more challenging in the seamless design setting because the number of treatment groups may change during the trial. Finally, at the end of each phase in the traditional approach, all analyses are carefully studied by the investigators and sponsors. As a consequence, the 'go' or 'no go' decision is made by the investigator and sponsor based on a careful review of all data. Adaptive seamless designs raise particular concerns at the end of the first phase because there is the need to keep the investigators and sponsors from knowing any interim findings. To alleviate this concern, the DSMB may play an important role in the decision-making process between phases. As a consequence, the roles and responsibilities of the DSMB are becoming more complex. In general, there should be a clear advantage for implementing a seamless transition before such designs should be utilized. Although important for any adaptive design, the importance of advanced study planning, adequate statistical support, and the need for simulation studies to assess operating characteristics is magnified in an adaptive seamless design.

Examples in neurology

Because this is a rapidly expanding area of research, outside of group sequential designs, there are few published examples of neurology clinical trials using an adaptive design. Some of the published neurological trials that utilized an adaptive design will be discussed here. We stress that this is in no way meant to be an exhaustive list. There are many trials for which some type of adaptation may take place that are not clearly reflected in the published paper. One of the goals of ongoing education efforts is to more clearly delineate exactly what should be described in any publication that utilizes an adaptive design.

As reflected in the recently released FDA draft guidance on the topic [8], adaptive designs are currently better accepted in the 'learn' phase of drug development where investigators are generally freer to

consider novel designs. Correspondingly, the majority of the published examples describing the use of adaptive designs in neurology fit into this category.

- Krams *et al* [33] described a dose-response study with randomized adaptive allocation to 1 of 15 doses of UK-279,276 or placebo for the treatment of acute ischemic stroke (AIS). The primary outcome was the change from baseline to day 90 on the Scandinavian Stroke Scale. During the trial, an NDLM continuously reassessed the dose-response curve in order to estimate the dose-response relationship. The NDLM fitted a linear regression model to each dose in order to obtain posterior estimates and 95% posterior credible intervals of the dose-response curve, the minimal dose that yields near maximal efficacy (ED_{95}), and the effect over placebo at the ED_{95}. After each evaluation of the dose-response curve, a termination rule specified that the trial would stop for efficacy if the lower 80% boundary of the credible interval for the effect over placebo at the ED95 was >2 or stop for futility if the upper 80% boundary of the credible interval was <1. This termination rule was used to recommend cessation of the study after futility had been established.

- Ho *et al* [34] described a two-stage adaptive dose-ranging design to determine an effective and tolerable dose of a novel oral calcitonin gene-related peptide receptor antagonist (MK-0974) for the acute treatment of migraine. The primary outcome was pain relief, defined as a reduction to mild or none two hours after dosing. During the first stage, subjects were randomized to one of seven MK-0974 levels or matching placebo. After 192 patients were randomized, an interim analysis was performed to determine the lowest dose with at least 70% conditional probability of being nominally significant at the end of the trial based on a comparison with placebo. Only the MK-0974 groups with dose levels at least as high as the dose level identified at the end of stage 1 were carried forward into stage 2. When the design was implemented, the study led to the discontinuation of the four lowest doses at the end of the first stage. The results at the end of the second stage suggested that the remaining doses of MK-0974 were generally effective and well tolerated for the treatment of migraine.

- Whelan *et al* [35] described an outcome-adaptive dose-finding design that will be used in a dose-finding trial for tissue plasminogen activator (tPA) in childhood AIS. The design uses both efficacy (angiographic recanalization or restoration of flow past the area of occlusion on follow-up magnetic resonance angiography) and toxicity (fatal or symptomatic intracranial or systemic hemorrhage) to determine doses for successive patient cohorts. The investigators argue that by integrating both efficacy and toxicity in the selection of doses, the design avoids the additional costs in terms of time and money associated with the usual approach of first assessing toxicity alone, followed by a separate assessment of efficacy. The results of this study have not yet been published.

- Elkind *et al* [36] conducted an adaptive dose-finding study using the CRM. The study demonstrated that 8 mg/kg/day is the maximum tolerated dose of lovastatin for the treatment of AIS, and demonstrated that the CRM method could be successfully utilized in early phase stroke trials.

- As previously described, Kaufman *et al* [31] performed an adaptive seamless trial (selection design in stage one, futility design in stage two) of coQ10 for the treatment of ALS. The first stage selected the 2700 mg/day dosage. The second stage established that the effect of coQ10 was not of sufficient magnitude to justify the cost and effort associated with undertaking a confirmatory trial. For this reason, the trial should be considered a success. By using an adaptive seamless design, the investigators were able to select a preferred dose and conclude that further study would not be worthwhile using a sample size of only 185 participants.

- Haley *et al* [37] described an adaptive seamless trial of intravenous tenecteplase versus standard-dose rtPA in patients with AIS. The trial began by comparing three doses of tenecteplase with standard 0.9 mg/kg rtPA in patients within three hours of stroke onset. The initial phase used a selection design (see Chapter 8) to establish the 'best' dose of tenecteplase for further study based on a 24-hour assessment of major neurological improvement balanced against the occurrence of symptomatic intracranial hemorrhage. The trial would then proceed with a futility assessment between the selected dose and rtPA, on the basis of the three month modified Rankin scale, to determine whether or not to proceed with a phase 3 trial. The trial was terminated for slow enrollment after only 112 patients had been randomized, so the advantages of the adaptive design could not be realized.

There are currently very few published examples describing the use of adaptive designs in confirmatory, randomized clinical trials (excluding the common use of group sequential methods for interim monitoring). Olesen *et al* [38] described a group sequential adaptive randomization design to assess whether a calcitonin gene-related peptide might be effective in the treatment of migraine attacks. The primary outcome was the reduction from severe or moderate migraine at baseline to mild or no migraine at 2 hours after treatment. Subjects presenting with severe to moderate migraine were treated in groups of six, with two subjects in each group assigned to placebo and the other four subjects assigned to one of six doses (0.25, 0.5, 1, 2.5, 5, or 10 mg administered intravenously over 10 minutes). The dose assignment to the next group of patients depended on the responses observed in all previous patient groups. Based on a total enrollment of 126 patients, the design selected the 2.5 mg dose and found that it was effective in treating acute attacks of migraine ($p = 0.001$ when comparing the response rate to that observed with placebo). Unfortunately, the design did not lead to early stopping, so the advantage of the adaptive design is not easily apparent.

Although there are few published examples of the use of adaptive designs in confirmatory trials, the use of adaptive designs has become more common in recent years. Because of the lag between study initiation and the publication of final study results, it will take a few years before the impact of an increasing use of adaptive designs is seen in the literature. Hence, the number of published confirmatory randomized controlled trials using an adaptive design in neurology is expected to dramatically increase over the next few years. There is a need for further discussion regarding what aspects of an adaptive design should be included in publications in order to give the reader a clear sense of how the adaptations were planned and implemented.

Barriers to adaptive designs

While the development of additional statistical methodology is needed, this chapter illustrates that appropriate statistical methods currently exist for implementing a number of well-accepted adaptive designs. However, before any adaptive design can be practically implemented, there are a number of logistical barriers that need to be overcome [39–40]. A few of the most pressing issues are discussed below. However, the reader is cautioned that this is far from an exhaustive list and the barriers may change as progress is made to address some of the barriers and/or new barriers are introduced.

Funding

Current funding mechanisms make it difficult to include an adaptive design since the final sample size may not be known at the outset. This causes logistical problems associated with setting up an overall trial budget and contracting with potential study sites. Discussions will need to take place among sponsors to determine how to gain the advantages of adaptive design within the current funding framework.

Transparency

Adaptive designs require a high degree of transparency with respect to the decisions that will be considered throughout the trial. The extent to which adaptation is planned should be described a priori in detail. However, if all possible adaptations are clearly specified in the protocol, a great deal of information can be inferred once a decision is implemented. This has the potential to unblind researchers and other individuals regarding any observed interim trends in the data. Discussions are needed to resolve this issue. For example, should the details of the adaptation be defined a priori in a separate document for which a limited number of individuals have access?

Computational complexity

Methods for the design and analysis of adaptive designs are often computationally complex. As a result, getting the clinical trials community to accept any particular type of adaptation is merely the first step to utilizing the method. Achieving widespread implementation of accepted methods will require the creation of high quality software packages with validated codes and well-documented examples.

Impact on the Data and Safety Monitoring Board

The DSMB may be required to play a major decision-making role in an adaptive design protocol. This greatly expands the responsibilities of the DSMB. There must also be a good sense of trust between the investigators and DSMB members, since the use of a seamless adaptive design may involve some loss of control on the part of the investigators. Discussions are needed as to whether this should be a responsibility of the DSMB or an external group. If the DSMB is to be involved in this process, it is likely that the time demands on DSMB members will be increased. In addition, at the beginning of the study a number of different possible scenarios should be discussed with the investigators, since this will be the only time that the DSMB will be able to solicit investigator input on how to react at the time of an important design decision. Removing the investigator from discussions surrounding these key design decisions reinforces the need for investigators to pre-specify all adaptations in the protocol so that the DSMB (or other third party) has a clear set of rules to follow for implementing the adaptations.

Summary

The term 'adaptive design' creates much confusion since it has been used to refer to a variety of situations. As a result, many incorrectly perceive all adaptive designs as controversial. In fact, regulatory agencies generally encourage the use of adaptive designs for early phases of research. For confirmatory trials, regulatory agencies will accept some adaptive designs but are cautious about others. A number of adaptive designs have been classified as 'generally well understood adaptive designs with valid approaches to implementation' in the recently released FDA guidance document on adaptive designs [8]:

- Adapting study eligibility criteria based on analyses of baseline data
- Sample size re-estimation based on blinded interim analyses of aggregate data
- Adaptations based on interim results of an outcome unrelated to efficacy (e.g., discontinuing doses with unacceptable toxicity)
- Adaptations using group sequential methods for early study termination due to demonstrated efficacy or lack of benefit
- Adaptations in the data analysis plan that are not dependent on within study, between group outcome differences.

The list above does not imply that these are the only types of adaptations that should be considered. A number of other adaptive designs may be appropriate, provided that the investigators have adequately addressed the operating characteristics of the design for the scenario in which it will be utilized. In general, the concept of 'adaptive by design' is crucial. By specifying all adaptations in advance, researchers have the ability to simulate the study in order to gain a clear understanding of the operating characteristics of the design. It is extremely important to ensure reliable, well-planned, and thorough simulation studies are employed during the planning phase of an adaptive clinical trial [41]. A common misconception is that an adaptive design requires less planning than a standard trial design. In actuality, the opposite is true. An adaptive design typically requires much more time for the upfront planning and simulation studies that must be done to ensure the validity and integrity of the trial.

The major barriers to the implementation of adaptive designs in future clinical trial protocols are primarily logistical, rather than statistical. A recent publication by members of the adaptive designs working group describes current thinking on good practices for adaptive clinical trials in pharmaceutical product development [42]. However, there is an immediate need for further educational efforts to clarify the strengths and weaknesses of the different types of adaptations that have been proposed. There is also a need for discussions among study sponsors and investigators regarding how to address the logistical barriers associated with the use of adaptive designs within current funding frameworks, and to address whether major changes are needed to the funding models in order to accommodate the use of adaptive designs.

Greater usage of adaptive designs for neurology trials should be encouraged. This will require a better understanding of the strengths and weakness of the different types of adaptations that have been proposed. Because this is a rapidly expanding area of research, more practical experiences and case studies are needed in the literature.

References

1. Gallo P, Chuang-Stein C, Dragalin V, et al. Adaptive designs in clinical drug development – An executive summary of the PhRMA working group. *J Biopharm Stat* 2006; **16**: 275–83.

2. Krams M, Burman CF, Dragalin V, et al. Adaptive designs in clinical drug development: Opportunities, challenges, and scope reflections following PhRMA's November 2006 workshop. *J Biopharm Stat* 2007; **17**: 957–64.

3. Chow SC and Chang M. Adaptive design methods in clinical trials – A review. *Orphanet J Rare Dis* 2008; **3**: 11.

4. Coffey CS and Kairalla JA. Adaptive clinical trials: Progress and challenges. *Drugs RD* 2008; **9**: 229–42.

5. Bretz F, Branson M, Burmann CF, et al. Adaptivity in drug discovery and development. *Drug Dev Res* 2009; **70**: 169–90.

6. Bretz F, Koenig F, Brannath W, et al. Adaptive designs for confirmatory clinical trials. *Stat Med* 2009; **28**: 1181–1217.

7. EMEA. Reflection paper on methodological issues in confirmatory clinical trials with flexible design and analysis plan. EMEA (European Medicines Agency) 2007.

8. Food and Drug Administration. Guidance for Industry: Adaptive Design Clinical Trials for Drugs and Biologics Draft Guidance. http://www.fda.gov/Drugs/GuidanceComplianceRegulatoryInformation/Guidances/default.htm (Accessed May 2010.)

9. Hung HMJ, O'Neill RT, Wang SJ, et al. A regulatory view on adaptive/flexible clinical trial design. *Biometrical J* 2006; **3**: 1–9.

10. Gaydos B, Krams M, Perevozskaya I, et al. Adaptive dose-response studies. *Drug Inf J* 2006; **40**: 451–61.

11. Garrett-Moyer E. The continual reassessment method for dose-finding studies: A tutorial. *Clin Trials* 2006; **3**: 57–71.

12. Bretz F, Hsu J, Pinheiro J, et al. Dose finding – A challenge in statistics. *Biometrical J* 2008; **50**: 480–504.

13. West M and Harrison PJ. *Bayesian Forecasting and Dynamic Models*. Springer-Verlag: New York, 1997.

14. Bornkamp B, Bretz F, Dmitrienko A, et al. Innovative approaches for designing and analyzing adaptive dose-ranging trials. *J Biopharm Stat* 2007; **17**: 965–95.

15. Proschan MA, Lan KKG, Wittes JT. *Statistical Monitoring of Clinical Trials: A unified approach*. Springer: New York, 2006.

16. Rosenberger WF. Randomized play-the-winner clinical trials: Review and recommendations. *Control Clin Trials* 1999; **20**: 328–42.

17. Hardwick JP and Stout QF. Bandit strategies for ethical sequential allocation. *Control Clin Trials* 1991; **23**: 421–24.

18. Taves DR. The use of minimization in clinical trials. *Contemp Clin Trials* 2010; **31**: 180–84.

19. Bauer P and Kohne K. Evaluation of experiments with adaptive interim analyses. *Biometrics* 1994; **50**: 1029–41.

20. Proschan MA and Hunsberger SA. Designed extension of studies based on conditional power. *Biometrics* 1995; **51**: 1315–24.

21. Lehmacher W and Wassmer G. Adaptive sample size calculations in group sequential trials. *Biometrics* 1999; **55**: 1286–90.

22. Cui L, Hung HMJ and Wang S. Modifications of sample size in group sequential clinical trials. *Biometrics* 1999; **55**: 853–57.

23. Muller HH and Schafer H. Adaptive group sequential designs for clinical trials: Combining the advantages of adaptive and classical group sequential approaches. *Biometrics* 2001; **57**: 886–91.

24. Mehta CR and Patel NR. Adaptive, group sequential, and decision theoretic approaches to sample size determination. *Stat Med* 2006; **25**: 3250–69.

25. Tsiatis AA and Mehta C. On the inefficiency of the adaptive design for monitoring clinical trials. *Biometrika* 2003; **90**: 367–78.

26. Jennison C and Turnbull BW. Efficient group sequential designs when there are several effect sizes under consideration. *Stat Med* 2006; **25**: 917–32.

27. Wittes J and Brittain E. The role of internal pilot studies in increasing the efficiency of clinical trials. *Stat Med* 1990; **9**: 65–72.

28. Proschan MA. Two-stage sample size re-estimation based on a nuisance parameter: A review. *J Biopharm Stat* 2005; **15**: 559–74.

29. Friede T and Kieser M. Sample size recalculation in internal pilot study designs: A review. *Biometrical J* 2006; **48**: 537–55.

30. Proschan MA. Sample size re-estimation in clinical trials. *Biometrical J* 2009; **51**: 348–57.

31. Kaufman P, Thompson JLP, Levy G, *et al.* Phase II trial of CoQ10 for ALS find insufficient evidence to justify phase III. *Ann Neurol* 2009; **66**: 235–44.

32. Ravina B and Palesch Y. The phase II futility clinical trial design. *Prog Neurother Neuropsychopharmacol* 2007; **2**: 27–38.

33. Krams M, Lees KR, Hacke W, *et al.* Acute stroke therapy by inhibition of neutrophils (ASTIN): An adaptive dose-response study of UK-279,276 in acute ischemic stroke. *Stroke* 2003; **34**: 2543–48.

34. Ho TW, Mannix LK, Fan X, *et al.* Randomized controlled trial of an oral CGRP receptor antagonist, MK-0974, in acute treatment of migraine. *Neurology* 2008; **70**: 1304–12.

35. Whelan HT, Cook JD, Amlie-Lefond CM, *et al.* Practical model-based dose finding in early-phase clinical trials: Optimizing tissue plasminogen activator dose for treatment of ischemic stroke in children. *Stroke* 2008; **39**: 2627–36.

36. Elkind MSV, Sacco RL, MacArthur RB, *et al.* High-dose lovastatin for acute ischemic stroke: Results of the phase I dose escalation neuroprotection with statin therapy for acute recovery trial (NeuSTART). *Cerebrovasc Dis* 2009; **28**: 266–275.

37. Haley EC, Thompson JLP, Grotta JC, *et al.* Phase IIB/III trial of tenecteplase in acute ischemic stroke: Results of a prematurely terminated randomized clinical trial. *Stroke* 2010; **41**: 707–711.

38. Olesen J, Diener H, Husstedt IW, *et al.* Calcitonin gene-related peptide receptor antagonist BIBN 4096 BS for the acute treatment of migraine. *New Engl J Med* 2004; **350**: 1104–10.

39. Quinlan JA and Krams M. Implementing adaptive designs: Logistical and operational considerations. *Drug Information Journal* 2006; **40**: 437–444.

40. Quinlan J, Gaydos B, Maca J, *et al.* Barriers and opportunities for implementation of adaptive designs in pharmaceutical product development. *Clin Trials* 2010; **7**: 167–73.

41. Burton A, Altman DG, Royston P, *et al.* The design of simulation studies in medical statistics. *Stat Med* 2006; **25**: 4279–92.

42. Gaydos B, Anderson KM, Berry D, *et al.* Good practices for adaptive clinical trials in pharmaceutical product development. *Drug Inf J* 2009; **43**: 539–56.

Crossover designs

Mary E. Putt

Introduction

This chapter describes crossover trials and their applications in neurology. In a typical crossover trial, each subject receives more than one experimental intervention or placebo during the different periods of the trial. This chapter discusses conditions in neurology suitable for this design, the efficiency that is possible with a crossover trial, and the benefits and limitations of the design. Considerable thought is given to the thorny issue of carryover. This chapter will also review study design, provide guidance regarding the logistics of carrying out a crossover trial and briefly describe some of the issues with missing data. Bioequivalence studies, which typically use crossover designs, are not discussed: the interested reader is referred to [1] for an excellent discussion and to [2] for an illustration in neurology.

Applications in neurology

Table 10.1 lists several recently published crossover studies. Chronic neurological conditions, where the outcome of interest is stable over the duration of a study, are excellent candidates for the design. Crossover trials, in principle, could be used to study aspects of many common neurological disorders including Parkinson's disease, Alzheimer's disease, stroke, multiple sclerosis, pain and headache, epilepsy, traumatic brain and spinal cord injury, psychiatric disorders such as social anxiety disorder or generalized anxiety disorder, and developmental disabilities such as attention deficit hyperactivity disorder (ADHD) or autism spectrum disorders.

We briefly describe the trials in Table 10.1; later we revisit these studies to illustrate our discussion. Headache is ideally suited to the crossover design as the condition is chronic and frequently stable over

time; our example showed high-flow oxygen to be more effective than placebo for treating cluster headaches [3] (see also [4, 5]). To treat pain, Gilron et al. [6] showed that gabapentin combined with nortriptyline was a more effective analgesic than either alone. For stroke patients in rehabilitation, several assistive walking devices improved functional mobility [7]. Symptoms of restless leg syndrome improved after treatment with ropinrole [8]. In studies of methylphenidate, children with pervasive developmental disorder responded with decreased hyperactivity while a child with ADHD more often completed homework independently [9,10]. Lastly, in an example of a trial reporting a negative finding, patients with Parkinson's disease showed no significant improvement in the primary outcome, ADAS-cog, during periods on donepezil compared to placebo [2]. Table 10.1 shows that the sample size for each study was small to moderate. While sample size must be calculated carefully for any particular study of interest, Table 10.1 introduces the idea that successful crossover studies are often carried out with modest sample sizes. This has obvious benefits in terms of study cost and accrual; if resources are limiting and/or if eligible patients are difficult to come by, the crossover may be the only feasible design for a clinical trial. Reasons for the design's efficiency are discussed next.

Efficiency

Crossover designs are efficient. To illustrate, we present sample size estimates for two placebo-controlled parallel and one crossover design for a trial examining the efficacy of donepezil in treating dementia in patients with Parkinson's disease. We note that a somewhat different design was ultimately used in the published study [11,12]. We estimated that 26 subjects were needed for the simplest crossover design, a 2-treatment 2-period

Clinical Trials in Neurology, ed. Bernard Ravina, Jeffrey Cummings, Michael P. McDermott, and R. Michael Poole. Published by Cambridge University Press. © Cambridge University Press 2012.

Table 10.1 Examples of crossover trials. N is the number of subjects in the study

Study	Condition	Treatment	Design	N Enrolled	N Analyzed (Percent)
Cohen et al. [3]	Cluster headache	High-flow oxygen vs. placebo	ABAB:BABA[1]	109	76(70%)
Gilron et al. [6]	Neuropathic pain	Morphine vs. gabapentin vs. combination vs. placebo	Balanced Latin square	57	44(77%)
Tyson and Rogers [7]	Walking impairment post-stroke	Four assistive walking devices and control during rehabilitation	Randomized order of receipt of devices	20	20(100%)
Adler et al. [8]	Restless leg syndrome	Ropinorole and placebo	2 x 2	22	22(100%)
Research units on Pediatric Psychopharmacology Autism Network [10]	Hyperactivity in children with pervasive developmental disorder	3 doses of methylphenidate versus placebo	Placebo followed by 3 randomized doses of methylphenidate	66	58(88%)
Proschan 2008 [9]	ADHD	Methylphenidate versus nothing	N of 1	1	1(100%)
Ravina et al. [11]	Parkinson's disease	Donepezil versus placebo	AABB:BBAA[2]	22	19(86%)

[1] Four-period design with alternating treatments beginning with A in the first sequence and B in the second sequence

[2] Four-period design analogous to the 2 x 2 design except with two consecutive periods of each treatment

Sequence	Period	
	1	2
AB	A	B
BA	B	A

Figure 10.1. 2 × 2 design.

(2 × 2) design (see Figure 10.1) to detect a difference in the mean of ADAS-cog, the cognitive subscale of the Alzheimer's Disease Assessment Scale, of 3.5 units. A standard deviation of 10 units, and an intra-class correlation coefficient, ρ, of 0.8 was assumed with a type I error rate of 0.05 and a power of 80%. In contrast, a parallel design with a single outcome and a baseline measurement would need 103 patients if the difference between baseline and response was used as the outcome; if analysis of covariance was used for the same data, the estimated sample size is 93 patients [13]. The dramatic savings in patients for the crossover trial reflects the assumed large intra-class correlation coefficient of $\rho = 0.8$. The intra-class correlation is the ratio of the between-subject variance to the total variance, the sum of the within and between-subject variance, with values closer to 1 indicating that subjects demonstrate substantial heterogeneity in response. The treatment effect in the 2 × 2 design is usually estimated largely, if not wholly, from a within-subject comparison. A value of ρ near 1.0 indicates that variability among patients is large compared to variability within patients. Thus eliminating between-subject variability and basing the estimate on within-subject comparisons yields large savings in patients for the crossover design. Figure 10.2 shows the same calculations for a range of ρ, suggesting that even for more modest ρ substantial savings in patients are achieved. With such efficiency it is natural to ask why crossover studies are not more common. There are perhaps three reasons. First, crossover trials are generally limited to chronic conditions where the endpoint is stable and can be repeatedly measured (but see [14]). Second, bias in the estimated treatment effect may arise from unequal carryover or period by treatment interactions; in my experience this is the primary concern limiting the use of crossover trials (see below). The last part of this chapter describes some logistical challenges involved in successfully completing a crossover trial.

The simplest crossover design

In the simplest crossover design, a 2 × 2 or AB:BA design, subjects are randomized to either the AB

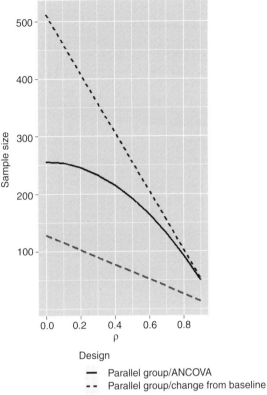

Figure 10.2. Sample size as a function of the intra-class correlation, ρ, for a parallel group design or a 2 × 2 crossover. For the parallel group a single outcome and baseline are collected and analyzed either by subtracting the baseline from each subject's outcome or by analysis of covariance (ANCOVA). Calculations are for a difference in mean outcome of 3.5 units, a standard deviation of 10 units with 80% power for a two-sided Type I error of 0.05 assuming normality as described in [12, 13]; similar results were obtained in PASS 2008 using a more conservative T-distribution for the test statistic.

sequence, where they receive treatment A in the first period followed by treatment B in the second period, or to the BA sequence, where the treatment order is reversed (Figure 10.1). Of interest is the treatment effect, in the case where the outcome is continuous, the mean difference in outcome that is due purely to differences between treatments. To develop a procedure for estimating the treatment effect we describe an approach based on a model to account for a number of 'nuisance parameters', changes in mean outcome that are not of direct interest in the trial because they are due to factors other than treatment. We then describe approaches for data analysis for several types of outcome variables.

Table 10.2 Expected outcomes expressed as combinations of nuisance and treatment parameters in a 2 x 2 crossover trial. Sequence effects which behave similarly to subject effects are omitted to simplify the explanation.

Sequence	Period 1 (P1)	Period 2 (P2)	Sequence-specific period difference (P1 − P2)
No Carryover (Figure 10.3A,B)			
AB	$\pi_1 + \delta_j + \mu_A$	$\pi_2 + \delta_j + \mu_B$	$(\pi_1 - \pi_2) + (\mu_A - \mu_B)$
BA	$\pi_1 + \delta_j + \mu_B$	$\pi_2 + \delta_j + \mu_A$	$(\pi_1 - \pi_2) + (\mu_B - \mu_A)$
Overall Effect[a]			$\mu_A - \mu_B$
With Carryover (Figure 10.3C,D)			
AB	$\pi_1 + \delta_j + \mu_A$	$\pi_2 + \delta_j + \mu_B + \lambda_A$	$(\pi_1 - \pi_2) + (\mu_A - \mu_B) - \lambda_A$
BA	$\pi_1 + \delta_j + \mu_B$	$\pi_2 + \delta_j + \mu_A + \lambda_B$	$(\pi_2 - \pi_1) + (\mu_A - \mu_B) + \lambda_B$
Overall Effect[a]			$(\mu_A - \mu_B) - \dfrac{1}{2}(\lambda_A - \lambda_B)$

[a] *(P1-P2) for AB less (P1-P2) for BA, divided by 2*
π = period mean; δ_j = the effect of the *j*th subject; μ = added effect of treatment; λ = added effect of carryover

Modeling

Nuisance parameters commonly considered in crossover trials include:

a. Subject effects: Individual differences in response.
b. Period effects: Differences in the mean outcome of interest between different periods that would occur irrespective of treatment in those periods.
c. Carryover: The lingering effect of a treatment given in one period into the subsequent period (or periods) of the crossover trial.
d. Treatment by period interactions: Changes in the effect of treatment at different periods of the study. For example, if a treatment is only effective with minimally or moderately affected patients, and the condition of the subjects deteriorates rapidly, a treatment may be effective in the first period(s) of the study and ineffective in subsequent period(s).
e. Sequence effects: Differences in the mean outcome that reflect differences in the response to treatment for subjects assigned to different groups. Sequence effects are essentially aggregated subject effects. For example a sequence effect would occur if patients assigned to one sequence are older and older subjects on average have worse responses.

Period by treatment interactions and carryover are conceptually distinct. A treatment by period interaction is a component of outcome that depends on the treatment administered in the same period where the outcome is measured; in contrast, carryover is a component of outcome due to the treatment administered in the previous period(s). However treatment by period interactions and carryover effects are mathematically indistinguishable in the 2×2 trial. Treatment by period interactions are not considered further here. We note that using relatively short trials may reduce the chance of a period by treatment interaction. Additionally there are designs that distinguish carryover and treatment by period interactions if the latter are a potential problem in the study (e.g., see [15]).

Table 10.2 illustrates two models, first without, and then with carryover. The equation form used by statisticians includes sums of nuisance and treatment parameters; the combination of parameters for any one period, or combination of periods is the expected outcome, sometimes called simply the 'expectation'. This expectation is the mean response expected for the population represented by the sample of patients used in the study.

The model without carryover

Referring to Table 10.2, we hypothesize a situation where we measure the outcome of interest in each period in the absence of experimental treatments; with parameters for period 1 (π_1) and period 2 (π_2) and an added effect of subject, δ_j in each period. Layered onto these parameters are treatment parameters where μ_A is the added effect of treatment A; μ_B is the added effect of treatment B.

Table 10.3 Numerical values of parameters used in Figure 10.3

			Parameter	
			λ	λ
π	δ_j	μ	(Fig. 10.3A,B)	(Fig. 10.3C,D)
$\pi_1 = 8$	$\delta_j = 2$	$\mu_A = 5$	$\lambda_A = 0$	$\lambda_A = 5$
$\pi_2 = 3$		$\mu_B = 1$	$\lambda_B = 0$	$\lambda_B = 5$

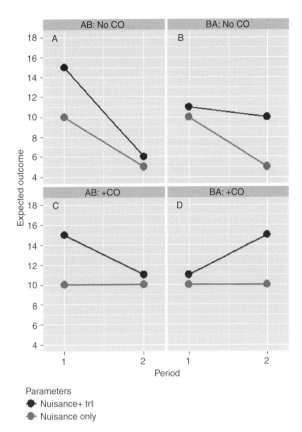

Parameters

◆ Nuisance+ trt
● Nuisance only

Figure 10.3. Examples of expected outcomes for the AB and BA sequences without (A,B) and with (C,D) carryover (see Table 10.3).

Without carryover, the combined data from the two periods can yield an unbiased estimate of the treatment effect, $\mu_A - \mu_B$. The column 'Period difference (P1 – P2)' shows the difference in expected outcome for periods 1 and 2 for each sequence. Note that taking the period difference eliminates subject effects. This is the basis of the efficiency described above ('Efficiency'); the estimate of the treatment effect and, importantly, its variance reflects only a within-subject difference. In contrast, in a parallel group trial, the variance of the estimated treatment effect contains both between and within-subject components. Next consider the overall estimate, which is determined by taking the mean difference in outcome P1 – P2 for each sequence, and dividing by 2. The expectation of this estimate, the 'Overall effect', shows that period terms cancel, leaving the desired treatment effect.

Figures 10.3A and 10.3B illustrate these effects for a hypothetical trial using the parameters in Table 10.3, where the only nuisance parameters are period and subject effects. The total of the nuisance parameters ($\pi_1 + \delta_j$ for Period 1 and $\pi_2 + \delta_j$ for Period 2) is shown in grey and the total of all parameters appears in black. At first glance, Figures 10.3A and 10.3B suggest that the response on the AB and BA sequence is very different. For the AB sequence the total for Treatment A versus Treatment B is superior by nine units; for the BA sequence the total for Treatment A versus Treatment B is inferior by one unit. This type of pattern can be disconcerting. However the average difference of the sequence-specific period differences (P1 – P2) from Table 10.2, $\frac{1}{2}[(8-3+5-1)-(8-3+1-5)]=4$, is exactly the treatment effect. For the AB sequence the difference in expected outcome for the two periods appears pronounced because the treatment effect layered over a substantial period effect; for the BA sequence the difference in expected outcome between treatment conditions appears muted because it is opposite in direction to the period effect and the trends almost cancel. When the effect of treatment is constant across periods, when there is no carryover, and the design is balanced so

that each treatment is represented in each period, the data yield an unbiased estimate of the treatment effect despite pronounced period effects such as those in Figure 10.3.

The model with carryover

Consider an identical model, but allow carryover in Period 2, as seen in Table 10.2. The expectation of the mean of the difference of the sequence-specific period differences is $(\mu_A - \mu_B) - \frac{1}{2}(\lambda_A - \lambda_B)$ (Overall effect in Table 10.2). The data combined from the two periods no longer yield an unbiased estimate of the treatment effect; the overall estimate is biased from the treatment estimate by a term that is half of the 'carryover effect'. This problem occurs only when the two carryover terms differ. Carryover itself does not cause bias; differences in carryover yield bias in the estimated treated effect. We illustrate equal and unequal carryover using Figure 10.3.

Equal carryover

Figure 10.3C and 10.3D show a trial where the two treatments have equal, albeit large, positive carryover terms. Because carryover from treatments A and B into the next period is identical, the sum of the nuisance parameters changes by an identical amount in period 2. For these data, the mean of the two P1 − P2 differences yields an unbiased estimate of the treatment effect.

Unequal carryover

Now imagine a trial where treatment A carries over into period 2 for the AB sequence (Figure 10.3C) but treatment B does not carry over in the BA sequence (Figure 10.3B). In this case the expectation of the estimated treatment effect is $\frac{1}{2}[(8-3+5-1-5)-(8-3+1-5)]=1.5$, a substantial underestimate of the true treatment effect of 4. Because the positive effect of treatment A lingers into period 2 in the AB sequence, the difference between treatments A and B is attenuated.

In this example, carryover from treatment A is large, identical to the original treatment effect of A while treatment B has no carryover. This results in a huge carryover effect. In practice carryover can be reduced using washout periods (see below), leading to the question: `If my washout period reduces but does not completely eliminate carryover, how serious is the bias in the estimated treatment effect?' [12,16]. Here it can help to think of the carryover effect as a proportion of the treatment effect, i.e.:

$$k = \frac{\lambda_A - \lambda_B}{\mu_A - \mu_B} \tag{1.1}$$

The expected bias in the estimated treatment effect is the ratio of the treatment effect estimated with and without carryover effects less the desired value of 1. Substituting using Equation 1.1 gives:

$$
\begin{aligned}
Bias &= \frac{(\mu_A - \mu_B) - \frac{1}{2}(\lambda_A - \lambda_B)}{\mu_A - \mu_B} - 1 \\
&= 1 - \frac{1}{2}k - 1 \\
&= -\frac{1}{2}k
\end{aligned}
\tag{1.2}
$$

So for example if k from Equation 1.1 is 20%, indicating that the carryover effect is 20% of the treatment effect, the expectation of this contaminated treatment estimate will underestimate the true treatment effect by 10% (Bias = −10%). The treatment effect is underestimated when k is positive, often because the positive effect of

a treatment lingers into the subsequent period. For example, in the study to improve walking post-stroke, a device could have a positive impact on strength, that continues into a subsequent period where no device is used, leading to an underestimate of the effect of the device. The treatment effect is overestimated when k is negative, for example when there is a rebound effect, and say a treatment yields a negative effect in the subsequent period. This type of carryover may have occurred in a study where a child had insomnia after taking methylphenidate possibly leading to depressed performance on the subsequent day and an inflated estimate of the true improvement on homework performance [9].

Analysis

Under the null hypothesis, there is no treatment effect while under the alternative there is a treatment effect, i.e.:

$$
\begin{aligned}
H_0 &: \mu_A - \mu_B = 0 \\
H_A &: \mu_A - \mu_B \neq 0
\end{aligned}
\tag{1.3}
$$

We briefly describe the analysis of data arising from continuous or discrete outcomes, as well as censored time-to-event data [15,17]. These methods are described for the 2×2 trial but extend readily to more complex designs.

Continuous outcomes

For continuous outcomes the observations on each subject can be reduced to a single observation by constructing paired differences between periods for each subject [18]. The treatment effect is estimated from half the mean of the difference of these paired differences as described above ('The model without carryover', 'The model with carryover'). Under the null hypothesis, the P1 − P2 differences have identical means (Table 10.2). Under the alternative hypothesis, the expected mean difference is twice the treatment effect. If it is reasonable to assume normality, or if the sample size is large, a two-sample t-test can be used for hypothesis testing.[1] When the sample size is small a permutation test, generally in the form of the Wilcoxon-rank sum test, should be used to maintain a valid test. If the distribution of the outcome is believed

---

[1] A paired t-test can be used if the number of subjects on each sequence is identical; a paired t-test will be biased if there are period effects and the number of subjects per sequence differs.

to deviate from normality, either because of outliers or skewness, a Wilcoxon-rank sum is again the test of choice irrespective of sample size. In addition to being a valid test, the Wilcoxon has better power for heavy-tailed or skewed distributions.

Equivalently, for the 2 × 2 design, and for some of the more complicated designs described below, a model that accounts for the repeated measures on each subject can be constructed to provide both estimates and hypothesis tests. When the outcome is approximately normally distributed, the model may be a simple linear regression, or equivalently an analysis of variance, including terms for treatment and period as well as a fixed effects term for subject, or a mixed effects model where treatment and period are included as fixed effects and subject is included as a random effect. In crossover trials with small sample sizes, normality is difficult to evaluate. Chen and Wei provide guidance for robust methods for analysis when sample sizes are small [19].

Binary outcomes

The approach is similar for binary outcomes (e.g., any vs. no improvement). It is simplest to reduce the data to one of two outcomes, i.e., improvement on one of the periods compared to the other, or no difference between periods. Under the null hypothesis, results should be similar across sequences. These data can be analyzed using an exact test, either by dropping the outcomes where the results are tied and using Mainland-Gart's approach, essentially Fisher's exact test, or by Prescott's extension of Fisher's exact test to incorporate information from ties into the 2 × 3 contingency table [20]. A more general approach models the binary or categorical outcome as a function of treatment and period, and can be carried out using a marginal approach implemented with generalized estimating equations (GEE) or a model where the subjects effects are considered random [21, 22]. These approaches both account for correlation among repeated responses on the same individual, but they answer subtly different questions. The marginal approach makes inference about response averaged across the population where the question of interest is: 'on average do the odds of response differ for patients receiving different treatments?' In contrast the mixed effects model is used to ask: 'Is the odds of response different among treatments for patients receiving both treatments?' Random effects models are fitted using either conditional logistic regression, which eliminates any between-subject effects, or using a generalized linear mixed effects model [22].

Censored data

As a hypothetical example, in a study of treatments to prevent seizures, the primary outcome could be time to first seizure in each (fixed-length) period. The observation is censored if no seizure occurs in a period. Hypothesis tests for censored data are constructed using a modified version of the Wilcoxon rank sum test taking into account whether censoring is absent or present in one or both periods [23]. Estimates and confidence intervals can also be derived.

Reducing the impact of carryover

Unwanted bias in the estimated treatment effect attributable to a carryover effect has already been described ('Unequal carryover'). Here we describe approaches to mitigate carryover effects.

Washout periods

'Sufficient washout periods' are often recommended to reduce or eliminate carryover effects. In practice it can be difficult to define sufficient. For a pharmacologic intervention, knowledge of kinetics can be valuable in the planning stages. For example, after seven half-lives less than 1% of the agent remains; at this time point meaningful pharmacologic carryover is removed for many drugs. If the effect of the agent is reasonably rapid and the outcome is closely related to physiological concentration then this might be all of the information that is needed. Other situations might be more complicated if pharmacodynamic effects persist beyond the physical elimination of the drug. The trial of donepezil on cognitive function in Parkinson's disease used a washout equivalent to 17 half-lives of donepezil effectively eliminating a pharmacologic carryover [11]. Here the primary outcome was ADAS-cog and we were concerned about carryover related to a training effect, i.e., improved performance over repeated administration of the ADAS-cog instrument. We anticipated period effects reflecting improvement across periods related to the training effect. However if donepezil were effective, outcomes would be better on donepezil than placebo in the first period, and the donepezil effect might carry over into the second period as an enhanced training effect. Using the model described in Table 10.2 the treatment effect would be underestimated. In this trial we used a long washout period primarily to mitigate non-pharmacologic carryover. We note that if donepezil were ineffective (null hypothesis in Equation 1.3 true) any carryover for donepezil and placebo would likely be identical, and under the model in Table 10.2, the test would be valid [24]. In practice there are many scenarios where it is reasonable to assume that hypothesis tests are valid under the null hypothesis even when the possibility of carryover may bias the estimate under the alternative hypothesis.

The two-stage approach

It was once common to base the analysis of a crossover trial on a preliminary test for carryover effects; to this day investigators sometimes report that a test for carryover proved negative [25]. In the two-stage approach the analysis proceeded as described above ('Continuous outcomes') when the test for carryover was negative; if unequal carryover was detected the analysis used the data from the first period of the study, essentially turning the study into a parallel group design and discarding the information from the second period of the study. This approach has numerous problems. First, it is essentially a sequential testing approach, but without proper adjustment for the multiple testing, leading to inflated type I error rates for the test of the treatment effect [26]. Second, the test for unequal carryover is based on a between-subject comparison and the power to detect even large carryover effects is dismal, often comparable to the type I error rate of the test [24]. Declaring the carryover effect absent generally reflects nothing more than lack of statistical power. Lastly, in the unlikely event that unequal carryover is detected, the subsequent test for the treatment effect using only the first period data generally has little power. Instead of the two-stage approach, the study should be carefully designed to reduce potential carryover effects. Moreover in planning the study, a sensitivity analysis can be performed using Equation 1.2 to determine how carryover effects of different magnitudes might impact the estimated treatment effect. Similarly power can be calculated for the combined treatment and carryover effect (Table 10.2, last line 'Overall effect') and compared to the power determined using the desired treatment. If treatment effects may be underestimated as a result of carryover effects but the magnitude of the possible bias in the estimate is acceptable to the investigator, sample sizes may be adjusted upward to achieve the desired power for a study.

Baselines and carryover effects

Baselines are measurements collected post-randomization but prior to the start of treatment. Baselines may be collected once at the start of the study or prior to each treatment period. Investigators sometimes use the difference between the baseline and outcome as the primary outcome for the analysis. This procedure may have unexpected consequences [27]. Let $\lambda_A^{(Bsl)}$ and $\lambda_B^{(Bsl)}$ be the carryover of treatments A and B into the baseline measurement for period 2. Following Table 10.2, taking the difference of the outcome during the active period less its baseline values yields an expectation for the estimated treatment effect of:

$$\left(\mu_A - \mu_B\right) - \frac{1}{2}\left(\lambda_A - \lambda_B\right) + \frac{1}{2}\left(\lambda_A^{(Bsl)} - \lambda_B^{(Bsl)}\right) \quad (1.4)$$

As in Equation 1.1

$$k^{(Bsl)} = \frac{\lambda_A^{(Bsl)} - \lambda_B^{(Bsl)}}{\mu_A - \mu_B}, \quad (1.5)$$

And the bias in the expected outcome is:

$$Bias = \left[1 + \frac{1}{2}\left(k^{(Bsl)} - k\right)\right] - 1 = -\frac{1}{2}\left(k - k^{(Bsl)}\right) \quad (1.6)$$

This analysis produces a biased estimate of the treatment effect unless $\lambda_A - \lambda_B = \lambda_A^{(Bsl)} - \lambda_B^{(Bsl)}$ or equivalently $\lambda_A - \lambda_A^{(Bsl)} = \lambda_B - \lambda_B^{(Bsl)}$. The analysis eliminates bias only if differences in carryover between outcome and baseline are identical for the two treatments. Otherwise collecting baselines just alters the bias. In a more realistic scenario, if treatment B is a placebo with no carryover and carryover from treatment A decreases in the interval between baseline and outcome, then subtracting off baseline values changes the sign of the bias, e.g., if $k^{(Bsl)} = 40\%$ and $k = 20\%$, the treatment effect is overestimated by 10% (Bias = 10%), compared to 'Unequal carryover' (above) where, without baselines, the treatment effect was underestimated by 10%.

Study design

Alternatives to the 2×2 design are used to increase efficiency, provide unbiased estimates in the presence of carryover effects, and to compare more than two treatments. These topics are reviewed along with several recent innovations in design including response adaptive designs, matching and N of 1 trials.

Designs to address carryover effects

An extensive literature describes ways of choosing the number of periods and treatment sequences to maximize statistical power while simultaneously allowing unbiased estimates of the treatment effect in the presence of carryover effects [28]. Much thought has gone into realistic models of carryover in these studies, for example allowing carryover to depend on the treatment that induces carryover as well as the treatment administered in the period where the carryover occurs. For example, carryover from an active treatment, say A, for headache, may differ depending on whether the subsequent period involves treatment with placebo or a second period of treatment A at a different dose. This type of carryover, called a mixed carryover effect, replaces the less realistic 'simple carryover' model that assumes that carryover from treatment A is unaffected by treatment in the subsequent period.

Designs that yield unbiased estimates of the treatment effect in the presence of carryover effects tend to have power that is intermediate to the 2 × 2 design and the parallel group design. While washout periods can eliminate or dramatically reduce carryover, they may be ruled out either for ethical or logistical reasons. Patients may not tolerate the washout, or an effective washout would lengthen the study to the extent that extensive loss to follow-up might occur in the later periods. Here these alternative crossover designs can provide an efficient alternative to the parallel group design.

Baselines and efficiency

Kenward and Roger [29] thoroughly reviewed the use of baselines in crossover trials recommending analysis of these data using ANCOVA and concluding that baselines may improve efficiency, particularly when there is information about the treatment effect that can be gained from between-subject information (see also [30]). Specifics of the ANCOVA analysis are described in [29]. The less desired alternative uses the change from baseline as the outcome in the analyses described above ('Continuous outcomes'). The efficiency of this approach depends on the decay in the correlation between repeated measurements over time. The method may have better efficiency when the baselines are collected relatively close in time to that of the outcome, and the washout period is long. Under these conditions the baseline and outcome measurement within a period are more highly correlated than say the baseline and outcome from the subsequent period. However the analysis of change from baseline may have worse efficiency than an analysis without baselines if the baseline measure is equally correlated

with outcomes from multiple periods. Here ANCOVA should be used.

Matched crossover designs

Modern genomic techniques allow the possibility of individualizing treatments to patients based on their genetic profile. More generally there is interest in tailoring treatments to individual subjects. For example, in asthma, patients with Arg/Arg at the 16th position of the beta-agonist receptor gene may respond differently to inhaled albuterol than those with the Gly/Gly genotype [31]. Similar scenarios are easily envisioned for neurological phenotypes associated with complex underlying genotypes. In the asthma study, individual crossover studies for each group are sufficient if it is of interest to know whether albuterol is more effective than placebo for each group [30]. A design where patients are matched based on their genotype and baseline function, and then randomized to a crossover sequence is usually preferred if the question of interest is whether albuterol is more effective for Arg/Arg than Gly/Gly. The matched design is more efficient than individual studies as long as correlation of the paired subjects on the same treatment is greater than their correlations on different treatments.

Response adaptive designs

Balaam's design is a two-treatment, four-sequence design which adds two sequences, one with two periods of A and one with two periods of B to the 2 × 2 design (Figure 10.4). Balaam's design can be the basic design for an appealing response adaptive design where patients are initially randomized to one of the four sequences but over time the probability of allocation to a sequence is altered by the relative success of the treatments. For example if treatment A is consistently superior to B, patients over time are increasingly allocated with higher probability to the AA sequence.

Sequence	Period	
	1	2
AB	A	B
BA	B	A
AA	A	A
BB	B	B

Figure 10.4. Balaam's design: Re-randomization or response adaptive design.

More information on response adaptive designs as they relate to crossover studies appears in [32,33]. Response adaptive designs are appealing because they ultimately allocate more patients to the better treatment sequence. However, they are more complicated to administer and potentially less efficient than a fixed allocation scheme.

N of 1 trials

Most clinical trials answer questions about mean differences in response to treatment for patients eligible to enroll in the trial, with little information to guide the clinician on how individual patients may respond. Matching (see above, 'Matched crossover designs') addresses one approach to individualizing the information from a trial, but still asks questions about the mean response in subsets of patients. N of 1 trials are designed to determine which of two treatments is more effective for a particular individual of interest [9,34]. Generally this design involves assigning treatment pairs to an individual in random order. For example in [9] the study design specified methylphenidate and no intervention be assigned in random order to a child with ADHD on Monday and Tuesday, Wednesday and Thursday. The study duration was 7 weeks and the primary outcome was independence in homework completion assessed by a blinded observer. This study could be analyzed using the two-sample t-test or Wilcoxon rank sum test on the P1–P2 differences as described above ('Analysis') if the outcome were continuous, or using Fisher's exact test for a binary outcome (e.g., a binary indicator of whether homework was completed independently). Here each Monday/Tuesday and Wednesday/Thursday pair is considered an observation on period 1 and 2 of a single sequence[2].

Designs for more than two treatments

Crossover designs in neurology often involve more than two experimental conditions (see Table 10.1). To treat pain, investigators compared placebo to two agents individually and in combination. To study hyperactivity in subjects with pervasive developmental disorders, a number of doses of methylphenidate were of interest [10]. Table 10.1 includes studies with two approaches to design when the number of periods available for study is equivalent to the number of treatments: using a Latin square design or simply randomizing patients to a treatment order. A Latin square is a block with t columns corresponding to periods and t rows corresponding to treatment sequences where t is the number of treatments (Figure 10.5). Each treatment appears in each row and each column exactly once. The 2×2 design is the simplest example of a Latin square. As we showed for the 2×2 design, Latin squares give unbiased estimates of treatment effects in the presence of period effects. When the order of treatments is simply randomized care must be taken in the analysis to avoid introducing bias due to period effects.

Designing a crossover trial with more than two treatments is more complicated when either carryover effects need to be considered or when the number of periods differs from the number of treatments. Simple carryover depends only on the treatment in the period prior to when carryover occurs. Senn has written extensively about the irrelevance of simple carryover to clinical research [18]. While these arguments have merit, the simple carryover assumption yields a mathematically tractable model leading to the use of 'balanced' Latin square designs where not only does a treatment appear in each period and sequence once, but where each treatment follows every other treatment the same number of times (see Figure 10.6). These designs are intricate involving multiple sequences. Jones and Kenward [15] provide a detailed description of the issues involved in designing such studies.

Sequence	Period		
	1	2	3
ABC	A	C	B
CAB	C	A	B
BCA	B	C	A

Figure 10.5. Latin square: Three treatment design.

Sequence	Period			
	1	2	3	4
ABDC	A	B	D	C
BCAD	B	C	A	D
CDBA	C	D	B	A
DABC	D	A	C	B

Figure 10.6. Balanced Latin square: Four treatment design.

---

2 For this study a 5th observation was also collected each week on Friday. For this reason, instead of analyzing paired differences the analysis was carried out on the unpaired data using only a two-sample t-test, an approach which maintains Type I error as long as the intra-class correlation is non-negative.

Logistics

Crossover trials have logistical challenges beyond the careful planning and implementation that accompanies any successful clinical trial. The design requires repeated contact with patients, possibly over a prolonged period of time, with increased risk of drop outs. Recruitment can be slow if subjects with neurological conditions need to make repeated visits to a medical center, particularly if caretaker support is needed to make the visit. Patients must be randomized to a sequence of at least two treatments so the investigator must carefully plan how this will occur, particularly if it is a blinded study. In a blinded study, the risk for un-blinding increases when each patient can compare multiple treatments; careful attention to the preparation of the experimental treatment is needed if blinding is to be maintained. Lastly, the investigator must balance the desirability of a washout period (see above) with the risk that patients become non-compliant during the washout and seek alternative treatment, particularly if their condition deteriorates during the washout due to inactive treatment.

Missing or incomplete data

In Table 10.1, the sample size in the analysis was often smaller than the number of subjects who enrolled. Often this reflects loss to follow-up (See Chapter 5 for more on bias and random error). The study report should describe patients who enroll but contribute no observations to, at least qualitatively, understand how the missing data might influence the study's generalizability. The analysis can use information from patients with 'incomplete' observations, i.e., subjects who contribute at least one observation and are missing at least one observation with the analysis depending on the so-called missing data mechanism [21,22]. Data missing completely at random (MCAR) are missing without regard to either the observed or unobserved data in the study. For example if a machine randomly fails to measure an outcome, the missing data are MCAR. The observed data are a random sample of the complete data that would have been observed had the machine not malfunctioned. Information about data that are missing at random (MAR) is contained solely in the observed data. For example in the stroke rehabilitation study, a patient who felt success walking using the first device she tried and subsequently refused to try other devices would have MAR data [7]. Lastly, data that are not missing at random (NMAR) or non-ignorable, have a missingness mechanism that depends on information that is unobserved. For example, if a patient from a Parkinson's disease study had relatively intact cognitive function at all follow-up visits that he attended, but then withdrew from the trial due to a sudden and sharp deterioration in condition (and such deterioration was never observed), the subsequent missing data would reasonably be classified as NMAR [11].

The assumption regarding the missing data mechanism is critical for the analysis but in general these assumptions are untestable with the available data. Thus the investigator chooses a method based on best available knowledge about the trial. For data that are MCAR, dropping those cases with missing data in a 'complete case analysis' yields valid, albeit inefficient, inference. Data that are either MCAR or MAR both yield valid inference in likelihood-based models such as mixed effects models. For example in a 2×2 design, subjects with missing data in one period contribute to a between-subject component estimate of the treatment effect in this approach. The likelihood-based approach is preferred over the complete case analysis for MCAR because of the efficiency gained by using all of the data collected in the study. Likelihood-based approaches do require strong distributional assumptions that may not be justifiable; several more robust approaches are available [17]. One approach that should never be used is 'last observation carried forward' (LOCF). The very strong assumptions LOCF makes are rarely justified in practice and may introduce bias into the estimates [22]. Lastly, NMAR requires advanced statistical methods and is generally used as a sensitivity analysis rather than as the pre-specified analysis; Simon and Chinchilli [35] suggest one approach for using an NMAR analysis for the 2×2 paired crossover trial.

References

1. Chow S, Liu J. *Design and Analysis of Bioequivalence Studies.* 3rd ed. Boca Raton, FL: Chapman & Hall, 2007.

2. Constantinescu R, McDermott MP, Dicenzo R, *et al.* A randomized study of the bioavailability of different formulations of coenzyme Q(10) (ubiquinone). *J Clin Pharmacol* 2007; **47**: 1580–6.

3. Cohen AS, Burns B and Goadsby PJ. High-flow oxygen for treatment of cluster headache: A randomized trial. *JAMA* 2009; **302**: 2451–7.

4. Schytz HW, Birk S, Wienecke T, *et al.* PACAP38 induces migraine-like attacks in patients with migraine without aura. *Brain* 2009; **132**: 16–25.

5. Hauge AW, Asghar MS, Schytz HW, *et al.* Effects of tonabersat on migraine with aura: a randomised,

double-blind, placebo-controlled crossover study. *Lancet Neurol* 2009; **8**: 718–23.

6. Gilron I, Bailey JM, Tu D, *et al*. Morphine, gabapentin, or their combination for neuropathic pain. *N Engl J Med* 2005; **352**: 1324–34.

7. Tyson SF and Rogerson L. Assistive walking devices in nonambulant patients undergoing rehabilitation after stroke: the effects on functional mobility, walking impairments, and patients' opinion. *Arch Phys Med Rehabil* 2009; **90**: 475–9.

8. Adler CH, Hauser RA, Sethi K, *et al*. Ropinirole for restless legs syndrome: a placebo-controlled crossover trial. *Neurology* 2004; **62**: 1405–7.

9. Proschan M. Self-experimentation and web trials. *Chance* 2008; **21**: 7–9.

10. Research Units on Pediatric Psychopharmacology (RUPP) Autism Network. Randomized, controlled, crossover trial of methylphenidate in pervasive developmental disorders with hyperactivity. *Arch Gen Psychiatry* 2005; **62**: 1266–74.

11. Ravina B, Putt M, Siderowf A, *et al*. Donepezil for dementia in Parkinson's disease: a randomised, double blind, placebo controlled, crossover study. *J Neurol Neurosurg Psychiatry* 2005; **76**: 934–9.

12. Putt ME and Ravina B. Randomized, placebo-controlled, parallel group versus crossover study designs for the study of dementia in Parkinson's disease. *Control Clin Trials* 2002; **23**: 111–26.

13. Borm GF, Fransen J and Lemmens WA. A simple sample size formula for analysis of covariance in randomized clinical trials. *J Clin Epidemiol* 2007; **60**: 1234–8.

14. Nason M and Follman D. Design and analysis of crossover trials for absorbing binary endpoints. *Biometrics* 2010; **66**: 958–65.

15. Jones B and Kenward MG. *Design and Analysis of Cross-Over Trials*. 2nd ed. Boca Raton, FL: Chapman & Hall/CRC, 2003.

16. Willan AR and Pater JL. Carryover and the two-period crossover clinical trial. *Biometrics* 1986; **42**: 593–9.

17. Vonesh EF and Chinchilli VM. *Crossover Trials. Linear and nonlinear models for the analysis of repeated measurements*. New York: Marcel Dekker Inc, 1997; 119–201.

18. Senn S. *Cross-over trials in Clinical Research*. 2nd ed. Chichester, John Wiley & Sons, 2002.

19. Chen X and Wei L. A comparison of recent methods for the analysis of small-sample cross-over studies. *Stat Med* 2003; **22**: 2821–33.

20. Prescott RJ. The comparison of success rates in crossover trials in the presence of an order effect. *Appl Stat* 1981; **30**: 9–15.

21. Diggle P, Heagerty P, Liang KY and Zeger S. *Analysis of Longitudinal Data*. 2nd ed. New York: Oxford University Press, 2002.

22. Fitzmaurice GM, Laird NM and Ware JH. *Applied Longitudinal Analysis*. Chichester: John Wiley & Sons, 2004.

23. Feingold M and Gillespie BW. Cross-over trials with censored data. *Stat Med* 1996; **15**: 953–67.

24. Putt ME. Power to detect clinically relevant carry-over in a series of cross-over studies. *Stat Med* 2006; **25**: 2567–86.

25. Brimacombe J, Keller C, Eschertzhuber S and Hohlrieder M. The problem of cross-over design in airway studies: a reply. *Aneasthesia* 2009; **64**: 919.

26. Freeman PR. The performance of the two-stage analysis of two-treatment, two-period crossover trials. *Stat Med* 1989; **8**: 1421–32.

27. Fleiss JL. A critique of recent research on the two-treatment crossover design. *Control Clin Trials* 1989; **10**: 237–43.

28. Hedayat AS and Stufken J. Optimal and efficient crossover designs under different assumptions about the carryover effects. *J Biopharm Stat* 2003; **13**: 519–28.

29. Kenward MG and Roger JH. The use of baseline covariates in crossover studies. *Biostatistics* 2010; **11**: 1–17.

30. Liang Y and Carriere KC. On the role of baseline measurements for crossover designs under the self and mixed carryover effects model. *Biometrics* 2010; **66**: 140–8.

31. Simon LJ andChinchilli VM. A matched crossover design for clinical trials. *Contemp Clin Trials* 2007; **28**: 638–46.

32. Liang Y and Carriere KC. Multiple-objective response-adaptive repeated measurement designs for clinical trials. *J Stat Plan Inf* 2009; **139**: 1134–45.

33. Bandyopadhyay U, Biswas A and Mukherjee S. Adaptive two-treatment two-period crossover design for binary treatment responses incorporating carry-over effects. *Stat Meth Appl* 2009; **18**: 33.

34. Guyatt G, Sackett D, Taylor DW, *et al*. Determining optimal therapy – randomized trials in individual patients. *N Engl J Med* 1986; **314**: 889–92.

35. Simon LJ and Chinchilli VM. A pattern mixture model for a paired 2 × 2 crossover design. *IMS Collections* 2008, **1**: 257–271.

Two-period designs for evaluation of disease-modifying treatments

Michael P. McDermott

Introduction

Many pharmacologic agents have been developed in recent years for the treatment of certain progressive neurological diseases such as Alzheimer's disease (AD) and Parkinson's disease (PD). Cholinesterase inhibitors such as tacrine, donepezil, rivastigmine, and galantamine and the glutamate antagonist memantine have been US FDA-approved for treatment of the symptoms of AD. Vitamin E has also been suggested to be beneficial in AD [1]. A wider array of treatments is available for the motor symptoms of PD, including levodopa, dopamine agonists (e.g., pramipexole and ropinirole), monoamine oxidase type B (MAO-B) inhibitors (e.g., selegiline and rasagiline), amantadine, anticholinergics, and catechol-O-methyl transferase (COMT) inhibitors (e.g., entacapone and tolcapone). Surgical treatments such as deep brain stimulation and pallidotomy are also employed later in the disease course. While these treatments have been established as efficacious, none have been conclusively shown to modify the underlying course of the disease and most are believed to exert their effects only on disease symptoms.

There is great interest in the problem of designing clinical trials to establish the extent to which a treatment has disease-modifying effects, symptomatic effects, or both in neurodegenerative diseases. Indeed, discovering a treatment that either slows, halts, or even reverses underlying disease progression has been termed the 'highest priority in PD research' [2]. The issue of disease modification is of paramount importance to many constituencies, including: 1) people with the disease who are seeking improved quality of life for a longer period of time, if not a cure; 2) governments who will have to confront increasing drains on health care resources and increased health care costs as their populations age; 3) research scientists who seek clearer understanding of the mechanisms that underlie diseases and treatments; 4) pharmaceutical companies who seek product differentiation and an increasing market share; and 5) regulatory agencies such as the FDA and European Medicines Agency (EMA) who will need to make decisions concerning the necessary evidentiary standards to approve a new treatment for an indication of disease modification. All of these constituencies, of course, are also motivated by the desire to help people who have disease.

The term disease modification implies that the treatment has exerted an enduring effect on the course of the underlying disease. For example, in AD this may mean that a key pathological feature of the disease has been modified, such as tau and β-amyloid protein levels in the brain [3]. In PD, it may mean that the rate of loss of catecholaminergic neurons, primarily the dopaminergic projection from the substantia nigra to the striatum, has been altered [4]. Alternatively, it may reflect an alteration in the physiological compensatory mechanisms in PD [5–7]. In either case, for a disease modifying effect to be important, the impact on the underlying disease would have to be accompanied by a measurable benefit on the clinical course of the disease [8]. This is in contrast to treatments that ameliorate the symptoms of the disease without affecting the underlying disease process. When such a treatment is discontinued, the effect of the treatment disappears in a relatively short period of time.

In order to establish that a treatment has an impact on underlying disease progression, a clinical trial must clearly distinguish between the symptomatic and disease-modifying effects of the treatment. It would not be difficult to design such a trial if a valid marker of the underlying progression of the disease were available.

Clinical Trials in Neurology, ed. Bernard Ravina, Jeffrey Cummings, Michael P. McDermott, and R. Michael Poole. Published by Cambridge University Press. © Cambridge University Press 2012,

Although a considerable amount of research has been (and continues to be) devoted to establishing such markers, these efforts have, so far, been unsuccessful. As a result, special trial designs have been developed that attempt to distinguish the symptomatic and disease-modifying effects of treatment using clinical outcome measures. These designs, termed 'two-period designs' [9], include the so-called withdrawal and delayed-start (or 'staggered-start') designs and their variations. This chapter describes these study designs in terms of their rationale, assumptions, design features, implementation, statistical analysis, and sample size considerations. Important limitations of the designs are also discussed. To date, published results are available for only three trials in neurodegenerative disease (all in PD) that have used the two-period design. Additional experience with this design will ultimately determine its usefulness in discerning the mechanisms of treatment effects (symptomatic, disease-modifying, or both) in neurodegenerative disease.

Problems with single-period designs

One of the earliest examinations of disease modification took place in the Deprenyl and Tocopherol Antioxidative Therapy of Parkinsonism (DATATOP) trial, which was designed to test the hypothesis that selegiline and vitamin E slowed the progression of PD [10–11]. Eight hundred participants with early, untreated PD were randomized to receive selegiline, vitamin E, both treatments in combination, or placebo in a 2 × 2 factorial design. The primary outcome variable was the time from randomization until the development of disability sufficient to require treatment with dopaminergic therapy, as judged by the enrolling investigator. It was assumed that neither of the study interventions had a symptomatic effect, and that the study design, a standard parallel group trial, would be sufficient to demonstrate disease-modifying effects. Although a pronounced beneficial effect of selegiline on the primary outcome variable was demonstrated, an unanticipated short-term symptomatic effect of selegiline was also apparent [10], making the results difficult to interpret with respect to mechanism.

The DATATOP study is an example of a trial that attempted to use an important disease milestone as an outcome variable to measure the disease-modifying effects of an intervention. A virtually identical design was used in a trial of selegiline and vitamin E in AD in which the milestone was death, institutionalization,

loss of basic activities of daily living, or a diagnosis of severe dementia, whichever occurred first [1]. The difficulty with this strategy is that such endpoints can be influenced by symptomatic effects as well as disease-modifying effects. This is true even of mortality, which may be delayed by the beneficial consequences of symptomatic prevention of a decline in function.

Others have suggested that standard parallel group designs can be used to address the issue of disease modification by examining the pattern of mean responses over time on a suitable clinical rating scale [12–13]. Even if the pattern of change over time is linear in each treatment group, a group difference in the rate of change (slope) does not necessarily indicate an effect of treatment on the underlying progression of the disease. This pattern is also compatible with the interpretation of a very slow-onset symptomatic effect [14]. It may also arise if the symptomatic effect of the treatment changes as a function of time. For example, the magnitude of the symptomatic effect in a participant may increase as the underlying disease worsens, as the score on the clinical rating scale worsens, or as the participant ages. Indeed, such a pattern might be expected with some treatments in neurodegenerative disease. It is thus clear that a divergence in mean response over time cannot necessarily be attributed to a disease-modifying effect of the intervention.

As noted above, standard single-period parallel group designs could be used to establish a disease-modifying effect of a drug if valid measures of the underlying neurodegenerative process were available. In PD, two imaging outcomes have been explored in this regard. Striatal uptake of fluorodopa, as determined by PET imaging, has been investigated as a measure of the capacity of dopamine neurons to decarboxylate and store levodopa/dopamine [15]. Similarly, striatal uptake of β-CIT, as determined by single photon emission computerized tomography (SPECT), has been examined as a measure of the density of dopamine transporters on presynaptic dopamine terminals [16]. Both markers have demonstrated a characteristic pattern of asymmetric signal loss primarily in the posterior putamen in PD patients and appear to decline linearly over time [17], but have yielded ambiguous results in clinical trials comparing dopamine agonists with levodopa [15–16], possibly due to differential acute effects of these drugs on the dopamine transporter [17–18]. As a result, there remain concerns with these outcomes as measures of the underlying neurodegenerative process in PD. Several candidate biomarkers have been proposed in AD, including CSF levels of tau and β-amyloid protein, regional and whole brain atrophy on MRI, and imaging of amyloid plaques; these and other proposed markers remain to be established as valid measures of AD progression [8,13].

Two-period designs

Withdrawal design

In the context of AD, Leber [19] formally introduced the concept of the two-period design to investigate the disease-modifying effects of an intervention. One such design is the so-called *withdrawal design* in which participants are randomly assigned to receive either active treatment or placebo in the first period (Period 1) and followed for a fixed length of time. All participants are then given placebo in the second period (Period 2), i.e., those on active treatment are withdrawn from that treatment and switched to placebo, and those on placebo continue to receive placebo (Figure 11.1). The two periods do not have to be of equal length; Period 1 is chosen to be long enough to allow any disease-modifying effect of the treatment to become apparent, and Period 2 is chosen to be long enough to eliminate (or wash out) any symptomatic effect of the treatment from Period 1. Any group difference in mean response at the end of Period 2 in favor of the group receiving active treatment in Period 1 may then be attributed to a disease-modifying effect of the treatment. This design has been previously employed. For example, in the

DATATOP trial participants had study medications withdrawn after either reaching the study endpoint (disability sufficient to require dopaminergic treatment) or completing their final evaluation and were re-evaluated 1–2 months later [11].

The purpose of the withdrawal maneuver is to determine whether any portion of the treatment effect that is evident at the end of Period 1 persists after withdrawal of treatment, i.e., to distinguish between the short-term symptomatic effect and the disease-modifying effect. A key assumption is the adequacy of the length of the withdrawal period (Period 2). In the DATATOP trial, although the mean response on the Unified Parkinson's Disease Rating Scale (UPDRS) total score in participants originally receiving selegiline remained slightly better than that in participants not receiving selegiline, this may have been due to the relatively short duration of the withdrawal period (1–2 months) [11]. In the Early vs. Late L-dopa in Parkinson's Disease (ELLDOPA) trial, participants were randomized to receive one of three dosages of levodopa or matching placebo and followed for 40 weeks, after which they underwent a 2-week withdrawal of study medication [20]. Participants receiving levodopa continued to have substantially better mean UPDRS total scores than those receiving placebo after the withdrawal period, but this again may have been due to the short duration of the withdrawal period. It should be noted that the underlying hypothesis being tested in the ELLDOPA trial was that levodopa would be associated with a *worsening* of PD progression.

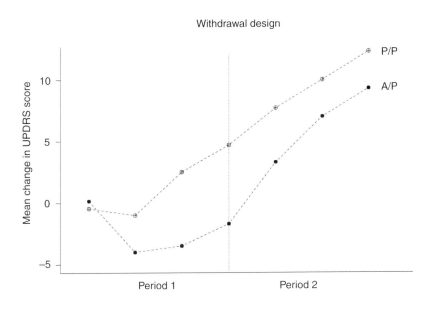

Figure 11.1. Illustration of the withdrawal design, in which trial participants are randomly assigned to receive either active (A) or placebo (P) treatment in Period 1 followed by placebo treatment for all participants in Period 2. The notation 'A/P' indicates the group that received active treatment in Period 1 followed by placebo treatment in Period 2. The outcome variable is the mean change in the Unified Parkinson's Disease Rating Scale (UPDRS) total score, where positive changes indicate worsening. Disease modification is supported by a persisting difference in mean response between the A/P and P/P groups at the end of Period 2.

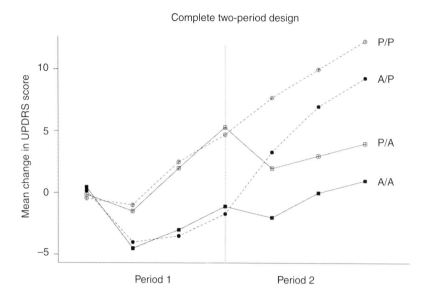

Complete two-period design

Figure 11.4. Illustration of the complete two-period design, in which trial participants are randomly assigned to receive either active (A) or placebo (P) treatment in Period 1 followed by either active or placebo treatment during Period 2. This may be viewed as the combination of the withdrawal and delayed start designs. The notation 'A/P' indicates the group that received active treatment in Period 1 followed by placebo treatment in Period 2; similar notation is used for the other three groups.

expected from a drug that had an effect with a disease-modifying component (Figure 11.3).

In the PROUD trial, participants were randomized to receive pramipexole 1.5 mg/day or matching placebo and followed for 9 months in Period 1. In Period 2, participants in the placebo group were switched to pramipexole 1.5 mg/day (delayed start group) and participants in the pramipexole group maintained their original treatment assignment for an additional 6 months. The trial demonstrated no evidence of a disease-modifying effect of pramipexole as the delayed start group caught up to the early start group in terms of mean response on the sum of the UPDRS motor and activities of daily living component scores during Period 2 [23].

The delayed start design shares with the withdrawal design the potential problem that there is no blinding with respect to the treatment received during Period 2. Again, one strategy to address this concern is to add a third randomized group to the study in which participants remain on placebo in both Period 1 and Period 2. This third group, however, has no value in distinguishing between the disease-modifying and symptomatic effects of the treatment; hence, efficiency is lost [9]. Relatively few participants can be allocated to this third group in order to minimize the loss of efficiency. A practical problem is that this third group, which would never receive active treatment, might make it less attractive for potential participants to enroll in the trial.

Simulation studies using disease progression modeling suggest that the withdrawal design may provide more power than the delayed start design to detect disease-modifying effects of a treatment [14]. The aforementioned concerns regarding participant recruitment and retention associated with the withdrawal design, however, significantly limit its use in practice.

Complete two-period design

A combination of the withdrawal and delayed start designs, termed the *complete two-period design* [9], was first presented by Whitehouse *et al.* [25] who described its use in a trial of propentofylline in AD. The trial had four treatment arms (Period 1/Period 2): placebo/placebo, placebo/propentofylline, propentofylline/placebo, and propentofylline/propentofylline. The results of this trial were apparently never published. The general design is depicted in Figure 11.4.

Under certain assumptions (discussed below), the complete two-period design would have the advantage of blinding without sacrificing efficiency, i.e., data from all treatment arms would provide information on the distinction between the symptomatic and disease-modifying effects of the treatment [9]. In essence, the information from the withdrawal component and the delayed start component of this design can be combined to produce an estimate of the disease-modifying effect of the treatment. As will be explained below, however, the assumptions required for this are somewhat strong.

A statistical model

A statistical model for data from a complete two-period design assumes that a normally-distributed outcome

Table 11.1 Statistical model for mean responses in the complete two-period design

Component	Group	End of Period 1	End of Period 2
Withdrawal	P/P	μ_1	μ_2
	A/P	$\mu_1 + \alpha_S + \alpha_D$	$\mu_2 + \alpha_D$
Delayed start	P/A	μ_1	$\mu_2 + \alpha'_T$
	A/A	$\mu_1 + \alpha_S + \alpha_D$	$\mu_2 + \alpha_D + \alpha''_T$

Group indicates the treatment assignments (Period 1/Period 2), with P = placebo and A = active.

α_S = Symptomatic effect acquired during Period 1.

α_D = Disease-modifying effect acquired during Period 1.

α'_T = Total incremental effect (symptomatic + disease-modifying) acquired during Period 2.

α''_T = Total incremental effect (symptomatic + disease-modifying) acquired during Period 2.

variable Y is measured on each participant at the end of Period 1 (Y_1) and at the end of Period 2 (Y_2). A typical analysis of data from this design might include certain covariates such as site and the baseline value of the outcome variable, but these will be ignored here for simplicity. Additional details regarding this model are presented by McDermott *et al* [9].

The model for the mean responses at the end of each period in each of the four treatment arms is provided in Table 11.1. The notation 'P/A', for example, indicates the group that received placebo (P) in Period 1 and active treatment (A) in Period 2. At the end of Period 1, participants receiving placebo (i.e., those in the P/P and P/A groups) have a common mean response termed μ_1, but participants receiving active treatment (i.e., those in the A/P and A/A groups) have a mean response that includes a treatment effect that is assumed to be a sum of two components: a symptomatic effect (α_S) and a disease-modifying effect (α_D). Of course, the data at the end of Period 1 cannot be used to distinguish between these two components. For example, in the withdrawal component of the design, the difference in mean response between the A/P and P/P groups would estimate $\alpha_S + \alpha_D$; the same is true for the delayed start component of the design (difference in mean response between the A/A and P/A groups). The data from Period 1 are used to estimate only the *total* treatment effect accrued during that period; the data from Period 2 are used to distinguish between the symptomatic and disease-modifying components of that effect.

At the end of Period 2, participants who received placebo in both periods (P/P) have a mean response

termed μ_2. The A/P group, which had active treatment withdrawn in Period 2, is assumed to retain the disease-modifying effect acquired from active treatment during Period 1, but any symptomatic effect acquired during Period 1 is assumed to disappear by the end of Period 2. Thus, the mean response in this group is $\mu_2 + \alpha_D$. The P/A and A/A groups both receive active treatment in Period 2, the total (symptomatic + disease-modifying) effects of which are denoted by the parameters α'_T (P/A group) and α''_T (A/A group). The A/A group is also assumed to retain the disease-modifying effect (α_D) and lose the symptomatic effect (α_S) acquired during Period 1.

This simple model for the mean responses illustrates several important assumptions that underlie the withdrawal and delayed start designs: 1) Period 1 is long enough for a detectable disease-modifying effect to become apparent; 2) the disease-modifying effect acquired over the duration of Period 1 (α_D) remains with the participant (at least through the end of Period 2, but presumably longer); 3) Period 2 is long enough for the symptomatic effect from Period 1 (α_S) to completely disappear by the end of this period; and 4) withdrawal of active treatment does not modify (e.g., hasten) the disease process in some way.

It is clear from Table 11.1 that the difference in observed mean response between the A/P and P/P groups (withdrawal component) at the end of Period 2 will provide an unbiased estimate of the disease-modifying effect α_D. In the delayed start component of the design, however, the difference in observed mean response between the A/A and P/A groups at the end of Period 2 will provide an unbiased estimate of α_D only if $\alpha'_T = \alpha''_T$, i.e., if the incremental effect of treatment acquired during Period 2 is the same for the P/A and A/A groups. Put another way, it must be assumed that the total (symptomatic + disease-modifying) effect of treatment received in Period 2 is independent of whether or not the participant received treatment during Period 1. This implies that Period 2 should be chosen to be long enough for the symptomatic effect of the treatment to become fully apparent (P/A group). This critical assumption for the delayed start design is often overlooked and is not testable in a trial that only has treatment groups P/A and A/A. It can be tested, however, using data from a complete two-period design. The parameter α'_T can be estimated by the difference in observed mean response between the P/A and P/P groups at the end of Period 2, and the parameter α''_T can be estimated by the difference in observed mean response between the A/A and A/P groups at the end of Period 2. The difference between these differences, therefore, would form the basis for a test of the null hypothesis that $\alpha'_T = \alpha''_T$. If this assumption is correct, then the disease-modifying effect α_D could be estimated by averaging the estimators obtained from the withdrawal and delayed start components of the complete two-period design [9].

The optimal allocation of trial participants to the four treatment arms in a complete two-period design was discussed by McDermott *et al* [9]. Equal allocation within the withdrawal component (i.e., between the P/P and A/P arms) and within the delayed start component (i.e., between the P/A and A/A arms) is optimal in terms of minimizing the variance of the estimator for α_D. The allocation of participants *between* these two components, however, can be arbitrary. Indeed, it may be best to allocate fewer participants to the withdrawal component to improve recruitment and retention in the trial. On the other hand, equal allocation between the withdrawal and delayed start components would maximize the power of the test of the assumption that $\alpha'_T = \alpha''_T$ [9].

Additional design considerations

Eligibility criteria

Trials in PD that have used two-period designs to address the question of disease modification have thus far involved participants with recently diagnosed PD who do not yet require treatment [2, 21, 24]. In ADAGIO, patients were eligible if they had been diagnosed within the previous 18 months. In PROUD, eligible patients needed to be diagnosed within the previous 2 years. A reasonable hypothesis is that a disease-modifying effect may be more readily detected if treatment is given earlier in the disease course. A potential problem is misdiagnosis in the early stages of a neurodegenerative disease such as PD or AD, although this is not an issue in Huntington's disease for which the genetic defect is known. Studies in participants with 'pre-manifest' disease may be even more attractive, although there are many issues that would need to be resolved in terms of defining a population at high risk for the development of the disease and of defining appropriate outcome measures before such trials could be recommended [26–27]. The study of potentially toxic treatments in individuals who have not yet developed a disease is also associated with practical

challenges [26]. The sample size requirements for trials in this population may also be larger than those for trials in a population with manifest disease.

The use of concomitant medications should ideally be minimized in trials of potentially disease-modifying agents, particularly if it is not firmly established that they do not have disease-modifying effects themselves. In ADAGIO, for example, use of levodopa, dopamine agonists, selegiline, rasagiline, or coenzyme Q_{10} (> 300 mg/day) was prohibited within 4 months of randomization. The difficulties involved in recruiting large numbers of (essentially) untreated subjects must be carefully considered when formulating eligibility criteria.

Eligibility criteria can be tailored to maximize retention since this is a major concern in two-period designs. For example, in ADAGIO only patients who were judged by the site investigator to not likely require symptomatic treatment in the subsequent 9 months were eligible. It may be helpful to exclude those with certain comorbid conditions as well. The concern has been raised that such restrictions on eligibility may yield a cohort of slowly progressive patients in whom a disease-modifying effect may be more difficult to detect [6, 28] or may significantly limit generalizability of the results [6].

Duration of follow-up periods

As summarized above, Period 1 should ideally be chosen to be long enough for a detectable disease-modifying effect to become apparent. Period 2 should be chosen to be long enough for the symptomatic effect from Period 1 to completely disappear by the end of Period 2 and, in the case of a delayed start design, for the symptomatic effect of the treatment to become fully apparent in Period 2. A practical consequence of this is that, in either the withdrawal design or the delayed start design, the group differences in mean response near the end of Period 2 should not be continuing to decrease over time. The duration of these periods, therefore, will depend on the nature of the treatment being studied. Practical aspects related to recruitment and retention also have to be carefully considered.

In PD, an initial treatment period of 9 months was used in both the ADAGIO and PROUD delayed start studies. The length of Period 2 was 9 months in ADAGIO and 6 months in PROUD. Given the inexorable progression of PD and the availability of dopaminergic treatments, a duration of Period 1 beyond 9 months is likely impractical. The current opinion among PD researchers seems to be that withdrawal designs are not feasible, a situation that may be magnified in trials of AD, although this could be reconsidered for treatments with symptomatic effects that might be expected to disappear relatively rapidly. In neurodegenerative diseases having no known effective treatment, such as Huntington's disease, longer period durations may be feasible.

Schedule of evaluations

The timing of evaluations needs to be carefully considered for the efficient design of two-period studies. There is the usual consideration of the balance between cost and participant burden versus the benefit of having more information and maintaining contact with participants to monitor safety and improve retention. Since participant withdrawal is a potential concern and some missing data are inevitable, it is important from an analysis perspective to have a reasonable amount of information on the trajectory of a participant's responses prior to withdrawal. Another important consideration is the evaluation of the assumption that the group differences in mean response near the end of Period 2 are not continuing to decrease over time. To adequately test this assumption, more frequent evaluations may be required in the latter part of Period 2. This aspect was carefully considered in the design of the ADAGIO trial [2, 22] but was not considered in the design of the PROUD trial [24].

Withdrawal due to worsening disease

A practical issue that arises in two-period designs is how to accommodate participants who require additional treatment due to a decline in their condition. This issue is of particular concern for trials in PD, for which there are many available effective treatments, but applies to AD as well. It is helpful to have a formal operational definition of the need for additional treatment to distinguish this situation from the case where the participant may be doing well but desires to receive additional treatment for reasons unrelated to accumulating disability; the primary endpoint in the DATATOP trial, for example, was declared when the investigator, in his/her clinical judgment, felt that the participant had reached a level of functional disability sufficient to warrant treatment with levodopa [10]. There are a number of options for dealing with this issue, including: 1) withdrawing the participant from the trial; 2) moving the participant directly into Period 2 (this only applies to participants who require treatment in Period 1 and would clearly only be a reasonable option in a trial with a delayed start design, in which all participants receive active treatment during Period 2); and 3) allowing the participant to receive additional treatment while continuing participation in the trial. The third option may be viewed as being consistent with strict adherence to the intention-to-treat principle and might be sensible in a trial with a very pragmatic aim. On the other hand, a trial with a two-period design that attempts to evaluate the disease-modifying effect of a treatment has a primary aim that is much more explanatory or mechanistic than pragmatic, making this option unappealing.

The delayed start trials conducted to date have all allowed participants who have been followed for a certain minimum duration in Period 1 (no minimum duration in TEMPO, 24 weeks in ADAGIO, and 6 months in PROUD) to proceed directly into Period 2 if judged by the enrolling investigator to require additional anti-parkinsonian medication. This allows information to be obtained in these participants on the mechanism of the effect of the treatment; however, the time scale for follow-up becomes compressed for these participants, the implications of which are not entirely clear. Also, if the active treatment has a beneficial effect (even if purely symptomatic), the early initiation of Period 2 may occur preferentially in those receiving placebo during Period 1, which may complicate interpretation of the results. In all of these trials, participants who required additional treatment in Period 2 were withdrawn from the trial at that time.

Statistical considerations

Primary analyses

The primary analyses for a two-period design typically focus on three issues: 1) comparison of the mean responses of those receiving active treatment and those receiving placebo at the end of Period 1; 2) comparison of the mean responses in the A/P and P/P arms (withdrawal design) or in the P/A and A/A arms (delayed start design) at the end of Period 2; and 3) evaluation of the assumption that the group differences in mean response near the end of Period 2 are not continuing to decrease over time.

Analyses for the first issue should involve simple comparisons of mean responses at the end of Period 1, as exemplified in the TEMPO [21] and PROUD [24] studies. In the ADAGIO trial, however, the analyses involved comparisons of the rates of change (slopes) between the rasagiline and placebo groups in Period 1, where the rates of change were based on data from Week 12 to Week 36 [2, 22]. The rationale for this strategy is not clear, particularly since it should only be of interest in Period 1 to determine whether or not the treatment groups differ with regard to mean response at the end of this period and not to try to make inferences about the mechanism of the treatment effect; if the latter were possible, there would be no need for a second period. Also, this analysis strategy requires the pre-specification of a time point beyond which the symptomatic effect of the treatment is fully apparent (Week 12, in the case of the ADAGIO trial), which may be problematic [29].

The key analyses are the group comparisons of the mean responses at the end of Period 2. These analyses should again be relatively straightforward. It may be advantageous to use data from multiple time points near the end of Period 2 to improve precision of the estimated mean responses, but this would require an additional assumption regarding the stability (constancy) of the treatment group difference at all of these time points.

Analyses to address the issue of whether or not the group differences in mean response near the end of Period 2 are continuing to decrease over time are somewhat more complex than those required to address the first two issues. First, a decision must be made prior to study initiation regarding which data to include in the analyses. For example, in ADAGIO the data from Weeks 48–72 were included because it was thought that the symptomatic effect of rasagiline would appear within 12 weeks of its initiation in the delayed start group at Week 36 [22]. Second, a decision must be made regarding how to quantify the evolution of the group difference in mean response over time. In ADAGIO, this was done using a rate of change (slope) that assumed linearity of the relationship between mean response and time during Weeks 48–72 [22].

A third complexity is that the goal of these analyses is to establish that the group differences in mean response are *not* continuing to decrease over time, a goal that translates into a hypothesis concerning *non-inferiority* (see Chapter 13 for a thorough explanation of this concept). Let $\beta_{P/A}$ be the slope (Weeks 48–72) in the delayed start (P/A) group and let $\beta_{A/A}$ be the corresponding slope in the early start (A/A) group. In ADAGIO the following statistical hypotheses were formulated:

$$H_0: \beta_{P/A} - \beta_{A/A} > \delta \text{ vs. } H_1: \beta_{P/A} - \beta_{A/A} \leq \delta,$$

where δ is the *non-inferiority margin*. This means that the slope in the P/A group would be considered to be not meaningfully larger than the slope in the A/A group if the difference between them can be demonstrated to be significantly less than the non-inferiority margin δ. As described in Chapter 13, the choice of the non-inferiority margin needs to be made with care to allow for proper interpretation of the trial results. In ADAGIO, the non-inferiority margin was chosen to be $\delta = 0.15$ UPDRS points/week, a value that was not justified in the trial publications [2, 22] and appears to be much too large. This value means that the group difference in mean responses could be shrinking by as much as 3.6 points over the 24-week time period (Weeks 48–72), *a value greater than the treatment effect observed during Period 1*, yet still be considered to be non-decreasing over time.

Despite the poor choice of non-inferiority margin in ADAGIO, the results for the 1 mg/day dosage indicated that the estimate of $\beta_{P/A} - \beta_{A/A}$ was 0.00 with a 95% confidence interval of (−0.04 to 0.04) [22]. The interpretation of the upper confidence bound of 0.04 is that differences between the slopes of more than 0.04 UPDRS points/week (or a convergence of the group means by more than ~ 1 point over 24 weeks) can be ruled out with a high degree of confidence. A choice of non-inferiority margin this small may make researchers more comfortable with the conclusion that the group difference in mean responses is not continuing to decrease appreciably over time.

It should be recognized that two-period studies that aim to investigate the ability of an intervention to modify disease course have an objective that is more explanatory than pragmatic in nature [30]. For this reason, carefully collected data on compliance with the intervention could potentially be quite valuable in the interpretation of the trial results. Statistical methods that attempt to account for participant compliance may be useful in this context [31–32], although these have not been applied to data from the TEMPO, ADAGIO, or PROUD trials.

A final point concerns multiple statistical testing. In order for an intervention to be considered disease modifying, it would likely have to be successful in each of the above three analyses (statistically significant benefit at the end of Period 1, continued statistically significant benefit at the end of Period 2, and non-decreasing group difference in mean response over time near the end of Period 2), not just one of them. If this were the case, correction for multiple statistical testing would not be required. In fact, this is an example of so-called *reverse multiplicity* [33] whereby the overall probability of a false-positive result will be *less* than the significance level used for each of the three tests (e.g., $\alpha = 0.05$). An exception is if it is desired to make a claim about a significant treatment effect during Period 1 alone, regardless of the mechanism of this effect. In this case, some multiplicity adjustment would be necessary [34].

Strategies for accommodating missing data

As in virtually any clinical trial, the problem of missing data (see Chapter 6) will arise in trials having two-period designs. The implications of missing data are arguably greater in a two-period design, however, due to the fact that information concerning the treatment mechanism (symptomatic vs. disease-modifying) is derived from the data acquired during Period 2. Studies with two-period designs also involve long duration of follow-up, which increases the probability of participant withdrawal. Several statistical methods have been developed to deal with the problem of missing data and are well summarized elsewhere [35–36].

Simple ad-hoc methods for dealing with missing data such as dropping cases with missing data ('complete case' analyses) or carrying forward the last available observation (LOCF imputation) have been widely criticized in the literature [37]. Analyzing data only from complete cases involves a comparison of subsets of treatment groups that are determined on the basis of outcome; hence, the benefits of randomization are lost and bias of unknown magnitude and direction can be introduced. LOCF imputation in the setting of a neurodegenerative disease is clearly problematic in terms of bias, particularly if the last observation for the participant is obtained relatively early during follow-up. Moreover, the use of single-imputation methods such as LOCF can artificially increase the precision of estimated treatment effects because the imputed data are treated in the analyses as if they were observed.

Better strategies for accommodating missing data include so-called 'mixed model repeated measures' (MMRM) analyses which treat time as a categorical variable and use maximum likelihood to estimate model parameters (e.g., mean treatment group responses at each individual time point) using all available data, including all observed data from participants who prematurely withdraw from the trial [38]. Linear or non-linear mixed effects models [37] that specify a functional form for the relationship between response and time can also be used for this purpose and may be more efficient than the MMRM strategy if the specified functional form is (approximately) correct. Multiple imputation is another technique that has been developed for inference in the setting of missing data [39–40]. It is superior to single-imputation methods because it accounts for the uncertainty associated with the model used for data imputation, i.e., it does not artificially increase the precision of estimated treatment effects. The primary analyses described above for a two-period design would be fairly easy to conduct using these strategies for accommodating missing data.

These methods rely on an important (and untestable) assumption concerning the missing data mechanism: that the data are 'missing at random' (MAR). This assumption specifies that the missingness depends only on observed outcomes in addition to covariates, but not on unobserved outcomes [35]. This may be a reasonable assumption under many circumstances, especially if data on participant response can be obtained at the time of withdrawal. One cannot determine, however, if the missingness mechanism is MAR vs. 'missing not at random' (MNAR), where missingness can depend on unobserved outcomes in addition to observed outcomes and covariates.

The TEMPO, ADAGIO, and PROUD trials all allowed participants who needed additional antiparkinsonian treatment in Period 1 to move directly to Period 2. The primary analyses in ADAGIO and PROUD, however, had minimum requirements for participation in Period 1 (24 weeks in ADAGIO and 6 months in PROUD) for this to be allowed. In all three trials, only participants who had at least one follow-up evaluation after the start of Period 2 were included in the primary analyses of Period 2 data. The bias introduced by the exclusion of randomized participants is of unknown magnitude and direction, although participant retention in these trials was generally excellent [21–23]. Methods such as propensity score adjustment [41] may be useful in reducing the bias resulting from such participant exclusion [34]. In TEMPO and PROUD, participants who withdrew in Period 2 had their last observed responses carried forward to the final visit for analysis. The ADAGIO trial used the MMRM strategy to deal with missing data in Period 2.

Sample size determination

There are several important considerations in determining the appropriate sample size for a trial with a two-period design. First, the minimally important effect size for disease modification needs to be specified. In ADAGIO, this was chosen to be 1.8 points for the UPDRS total score [22], and in PROUD, this was chosen to be 3 points [24]. These choices have been criticized by some to not represent clinically important effects [6]. One must bear in mind, however, that this group difference, if real, should be interpreted as the disease-modifying benefit that accrued over a very short period of time (9 months) relative to the duration of the disease and would be expected to continue to accrue over time, indeed possibly over many years. The ADAGIO investigators [22] noted that the observed effect of the 1 mg/day dosage of rasagiline (1.7 points over 36 weeks) represents a 38% reduction in the change from baseline which, if this truly represents disease modification, would be highly meaningful from a clinical standpoint. The choice of effect size for sample size determination should be based on a realistic expectation of the magnitude of a disease-modifying effect that could accrue over a relatively short follow-up period (e.g., 9 months) and may not be very large.

A second consideration is the sample size requirement for determining that the group difference in mean responses is not continuing to decrease appreciably over time near the end of Period 2. This was not a major consideration in the ADAGIO trial because of the large value chosen for the non-inferiority margin. A more appropriate (smaller) choice for the non-inferiority margin, however, may make this aspect of the design the most important determinant of sample size. Other problems such as participant withdrawal, non-compliance, and misdiagnosis also need to be carefully considered. In particular, clinical trial simulation can be highly useful in determining the impact of participant withdrawal, missing data, and the reverse multiplicity problem on the sample size requirements for the trial.

Alternative approaches to determining disease-modifying effects

There are alternative approaches to evaluating the disease-modifying effects of an intervention that require only a single treatment period. As mentioned above, a standard randomized, double-blind, parallel group trial with a valid biological measure of underlying disease progression as the primary outcome variable would be

the ideal approach. Such an approach, however, awaits the development of valid biomarkers of underlying disease progression. Another promising approach has been suggested that combines a model for disease progression with a pharmacodynamic model for drug effects [42–43], the latter facilitating inference concerning the mechanisms of the drug effect. These models have been applied to data from the DATATOP trial [44] and the ELLDOPA trial [29], providing evidence for disease-modifying effects of selegiline and levodopa. This approach was also used to provide independent validation (prediction) of the results of the ELLDOPA trial [45]. These methods are analytically complex and rely on several modeling assumptions, but they may overcome some of the limitations of two-period designs for this purpose and appear to hold great promise in facilitating understanding of the mechanisms of drug benefit [29].

Limitations of two-period designs

There are several limitations that accompany the use of two-period designs to determine whether or not an intervention has disease-modifying effects. Many of these have already been discussed, including the assumptions that: 1) Period 1 is long enough for a detectable disease-modifying effect to become apparent; 2) the disease-modifying effect acquired over the duration of Period 1 remains with the participant at least through the end of Period 2, but presumably longer; 3) Period 2 is long enough for the symptomatic effect from Period 1 to completely disappear by the end of Period 2; 4) withdrawal of active treatment does not modify (e.g., hasten) the disease process in some way (withdrawal design); and 5) the total (symptomatic + disease-modifying) effect of treatment received in Period 2 is independent of whether or not the participant received treatment during Period 1 (delayed start design), implying that Period 2 is long enough for the symptomatic effect of the treatment to become fully apparent. Many of these assumptions cannot be verified directly using the data from the two-period design and must rely on evidence external to the trial. Interventions with a very slow onset and/or offset of a symptomatic effect may not be well-suited for study using a two-period design [14, 29].

Other limitations previously mentioned include problems with acceptability of the withdrawal design by researchers and potential trial participants; a potential compromise of the blind if only two treatment arms are used; difficulties in recruiting large numbers of untreated subjects; potentially limited generalizability of the results if 'slow progressors' are preferentially represented in the trial; and difficulties with participant retention and the use of proper statistical methods to deal with the resulting missing data.

An additional limitation not previously mentioned includes the possibility of ceiling or floor effects of the clinical rating scale used to measure outcome that might limit the ability of the two-period design to assess disease modification. This might be particularly problematic if participants have very mild disease. A similar concern is that a two-period design might not be able to ascertain the mechanism of the effect of an agent with a very prominent symptomatic effect that overwhelms a disease-modifying effect in participants with very early disease [22, 24].

References

1. Sano M, Ernesto C, Thomas RG, *et al*. A controlled trial of selegiline, alpha-tocopherol, or both as treatment for Alzheimer's disease. *N Engl J Med* 1997; **336**: 1216–22.

2. Olanow CW, Hauser RA, Jankovic J, *et al*. A randomized, double-blind, placebo-controlled, delayed start study to assess rasagiline as a disease modifying therapy in Parkinson's disease (the ADAGIO study): rationale, design, and baseline characteristics. *Mov Disord* 2008; **15**: 2194–2201.

3. Kaye JA. Methods for discerning disease-modifying effects in Alzheimer disease treatment trials (editorial). *Arch Neurol* 2000; **57**: 312–14.

4. Clarke CE. A "cure" for Parkinson's disease: can neuroprotection be proven with current trial designs? *Mov Disord* 2004; **19**: 491–8.

5. Schapira AHV and Obeso J. Timing of treatment initiation in Parkinson's disease: a need for reappraisal? *Ann Neurol* 2006; **59**: 559–62.

6. Clarke CE. Are delayed-start design trials to show neuroprotection in Parkinson's disease fundamentally flawed? *Mov Disord* 2008; **23**: 784–89.

7. Olanow CW and Rascol O. The delayed-start study in Parkinson disease: can't satisfy everyone. *Neurology* 2010; **74**: 1149–51.

8. Cummings JL. Defining and labeling disease-modifying treatments for Alzheimer's disease. *Alzheimer's Dement* 2009; **5**: 406–18.

9. McDermott MP, Hall WJ, Oakes D, *et al*. Design and analysis of two-period studies of potentially disease-modifying treatments. *Controlled Clin Trials* 2002; **23**: 635–49.

10. The Parkinson Study Group. Effect of deprenyl on the progression of disability in early Parkinson's disease. *N Engl J Med* 1989; **321**: 1364–71.

11. The Parkinson Study Group. Effects of tocopherol and deprenyl on the progression of disability in early Parkinson's disease. *N Engl J Med* 1993; **328**: 176–83.

12. Guimaraes P, Kieburtz K, Goetz CG, *et al*. Non-linearity of Parkinson's disease progression: implications for sample size calculations in clinical trials. *Clin Trials* 2005; **2**: 509–18.

13. Vellas B, Andrieu S, Sampaio C, *et al*. Endpoints for trials in Alzheimer's disease: a European task force consensus. *Lancet Neurol* 2008; **7**: 436–50.

14. Ploeger BA and Holford NHG. Washout and delayed start designs for identifying disease modifying effects in slowly progressive diseases using disease progression analysis. *Pharm Statist* 2009; **8**: 225–38.

15. Whone AL, Watts RL, Stoessl AJ, *et al*. Slower progression of Parkinson's disease with ropinirole versus levodopa: the REAL-PET study. *Ann Neurol* 2003; **54**: 93–101.

16. Parkinson Study Group. Dopamine transporter brain imaging to assess the effects of pramipexole vs. levodopa on Parkinson disease progression. *JAMA* 2002; **287**: 1653–61.

17. Schapira AHV and Olanow CW. Neuroprotection in Parkinson disease: mysteries, myths, and misconceptions. *JAMA* 2004; **291**: 358–64.

18. Clarke CE and Guttman M. Dopamine agonist monotherapy in Parkinson's disease. *Lancet* 2002; **360**: 1767–69.

19. Leber P. Observations and suggestions on antidementia drug development. *Alzheimer Dis Assoc Disord* 1996; **10(Suppl 1)**: 31–5.

20. The Parkinson Study Group. Levodopa and the progression of Parkinson's disease. *N Engl J Med* 2004; **351**: 2498–2508.

21. Parkinson Study Group. A controlled, randomized, delayed-start study of rasagiline in early Parkinson disease. *Arch Neurol* 2004; **61**: 561–6.

22. Olanow CW, Rascol O, Hauser R, *et al*. A double-blind, delayed-start trial of rasagiline in Parkinson's disease. *N Engl J Med* 2009; **361**: 1268–78.

23. Schapira A, Albrecht S, Barone P, *et al*. Immediate vs. delayed-start pramipexole in early Parkinson's disease: the PROUD study. *Parkinsonism Relat Disord* 2009; **15**: S2–S81.

24. Schapira AHV, Albrecht S, Barone P, *et al*. Rationale for delayed-start study of pramipexole in Parkinson's disease: the PROUD study. *Mov Disord* 2010; **25**: 1627–32.

25. Whitehouse PJ, Kittner B, Roessner M, *et al*. Clinical trial designs for demonstrating disease-course-altering effects in dementia. *Alzheimer Dis Assoc Disord* 1998; **12**: 281–94.

26. Kieburtz K. Issues in neuroprotection clinical trials in Parkinson's disease. *Neurology* 2006; **66(Suppl 4)**: S50–S57.

27. Vellas B, Andrieu S, Sampaio C, *et al.* Disease-modifying trials in Alzheimer's disease: a European task force consensus. *Lancet Neurol* 2007; **6**: 56–62.

28. Ahlskog JE and Uitti RJ. Rasagiline, Parkinson neuroprotection, and delayed-start trials: still no satisfaction? *Neurology* 2010; **74**: 1143–8.

29. Holford NHG, Nutt JG. Interpreting the results of Parkinson's disease clinical trials: time for a change. *Mov Disord* 2011; **26**: 569–77.

30. Schwartz D and Lellouch J. Explanatory and pragmatic attitudes in therapeutical trials. *J Chronic Dis* 1967; **20**: 637–48.

31. Robins JM, Hernan MA and Brumback B. Marginal structural models and causal inference in epidemiology. *Epidemiology* 2000; **11**: 550–60.

32. Frangakis CE and Rubin DB. Principal stratification in causal inference. *Biometrics* 2002; **58**: 21–9.

33. Offen W, Chuang-Stein C, Dmitrienko A, *et al.* Multiple co-primary endpoints: medical and statistical solutions. *Drug Inf J* 2007; **41**: 31–46.

34. D'Agostino RB Sr. The delayed-start study design. *N Engl J Med* 2009; **361**: 1304–6.

35. Little RJA, Rubin DB. *Statistical Analysis with Missing Data.* Hoboken, NJ: John Wiley and Sons, Inc., 2002.

36. Molenberghs G and Kenward MG. *Missing Data in Clinical Studies.* Chichester: John Wiley and Sons, 2007.

37. Molenberghs G, Thijs H, Jansen I, *et al.* Analyzing incomplete longitudinal clinical trial data. *Biostatistics* 2004; **5**: 445–64.

38. Mallinckrodt CH, Clark WS and David SR. Accounting for dropout bias using mixed-effects models. *J Biopharm Statist* 2001; **11**: 9–21.

39. Little R and Yau L. Intent-to-treat analysis for longitudinal studies with drop-outs. *Biometrics* 1996; **52**: 1324–33.

40. Schafer JL. *Analysis of Incomplete Multivariate Data.* Boca Raton, FL: Chapman and Hall/CRC, 1997.

41. D'Agostino RB Jr. Propensity score methods for bias reduction in the comparison of a treatment to a non-randomized control group. *Statist Med* 1998; **17**: 2265–81.

42. Chan PLS and Holford NHG. Drug treatment effects on disease progression. *Annu Rev Pharmacol Toxicol* 2001; **41**: 625–59.

43. Holford NHG and Ludden T. Time course of drug effect. In: Welling PG, Balant LP, eds. *Handbook of Experimental Pharmacology.* Heidelberg: Springer-Verlag, 1994.

44. Holford NHG, Chan PLS, Nutt JG, *et al.* Disease progression and pharmacodynamics in Parkinson disease – evidence for functional protection with levodopa and other treatments. *J Pharmacokinet Pharmacodyn* 2006; **33**: 281–311.

45. Chan PLS, Nutt JG and Holford NHG. Levodopa slows progression of Parkinson's disease: external validation by clinical trial simulation. *Pharm Res* 2007; **24**: 791–802.

Chapter

12

Enrichment designs

Kathryn M. Kellogg and John Markman

Introduction

Enriched enrollment designs allow researchers to identify subjects for whom a proposed treatment is more likely to be beneficial and to include only those subjects in the randomized phase of a clinical trial. Since the introduction of enrichment approaches over three decades ago, this method is increasingly used to enhance assay sensitivity for study drug effects when only a subset of subjects in a population is expected to respond to an intervention. This chapter will examine the varied strategies involved in developing a trial using an enrichment design, the advantages and disadvantages of this method, and issues to be considered when planning a study using enrichment strategies. Clinical trials using this design have a variety of names in the literature, examples of which can be found in Table 12.1.

The enrichment design is a relatively new clinical trial method first described by Amery and Dony in 1975 [1]. These researchers identified a need for an alternative to the traditional randomized controlled trial (RCT) in pharmaceutical clinical development because of the high incidence of placebo response and the ethical implications of prolonged placebo exposure in half of the study participants who might benefit from alternative treatments. The run-in periods common in enrichment designs may have multiple objectives, some of which are clinically relevant such as tolerability, and others which are trial specific such as subject adherence to the protocol. Since its introduction, this design type has been adopted and refined in many areas of medicine, most notably in psychiatry and pain research. In these study populations, placebo response rates are often high and the complex trade-off of symptom relief for drug tolerability frequently leads to high dropout rates in clinical trials.

Table 12.1 Names for a two-stage clinical trial design using select patients from the first stage in the second stage

Enrichment design
Discontinuation design
Randomized discontinuation design
Enriched enrollment with randomized withdrawal
Study with a qualification period

Clinical trials using enrichment designs involve at least two periods (Figure 12.1). In the first period, the enrichment period, subjects are screened for their responsiveness according to predetermined criteria (e.g. a 30% reduction in baseline pain intensity). These criteria vary depending on the type of study being performed. Researchers often use the putative response to the treatment to be studied in the subsequent phase of the trial as a direct screening tool during the enrichment period. However, some researchers use other screening criteria such as biomarkers that may indicate potential response to the intervention. This may be particularly useful when there is a biomarker that can be identified in the short term that predicts response to long-term treatment [2].

Researchers use a variety of methods to perform the first stage of an enrichment design trial. In the simplest method, the test drug is given in the first phase and participant response is used to gauge advancement to the second stage (Figure 12.1). However, some studies examine more than one intervention in the first phase in order to find a subject's ideal treatment or dose to be used in the second phase or select subjects whose symptoms worsen upon withdrawal of study drug [3]. Other enrichment strategies aim to select for participants with specific traits, such as the ability to report acute pain consistently as evaluated by psychophysical screening. Other enrichment approaches feature

Clinical Trials in Neurology, ed. Bernard Ravina, Jeffrey Cummings, Michael P. McDermott, and R. Michael Poole. Published by Cambridge University Press. © Cambridge University Press 2012.

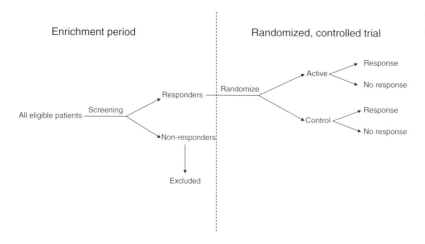

Figure 12.1. The steps for a clinical trial using the enrichment design.

pharmacogenomic testing, assessment of baseline characteristics such as a previous response to another treatment, or induction of a pain flare on withdrawal of study medication [4].

Further refinement of enrichment definitions has been proposed. For example, in their 2008 systematic review Straube *et al* defined 'complete enriched enrollment' as a study in which all participants are known to have been exposed to the test drug, either in clinical practice or in a clinical trial setting [4]. In this case, either the putative responders are advanced to the second phase of the study or the non-responders are excluded. They then defined 'partial enriched enrollment' as a study in which previous non-responders are excluded from the study, but those who had not been previously exposed may also have been included, such that not all participants are definitively known to have been exposed to the test drug [5].

Advantages of the enrichment design

If the treatment to be examined in the trial is administered during the enrichment period, observations from this period approximate how a general population may be expected to respond to the treatment in clinical practice. It is important to note that the extent to which the experience of subjects during this uncontrolled exposure is attributable to non-specific treatment effects, natural history, spontaneous resolution, placebo effects, and regression to the mean cannot be discerned. As such, the study period that follows the enrichment phase may be viewed as testing the hypothesis that the response observed in the subjects in the enrichment period is due to chance. In the most

commonly used enrichment design, subjects who are putative responders during the enrichment period are enrolled in the subsequent, randomized, controlled trial portion of the study [2].

While the clinical trial without an enrichment phase has long been viewed as the gold standard for clinical evidence, this traditional design has a number of weaknesses, particularly when studying certain disease processes. In a group of subjects with a common chronic pain etiology but heterogeneous underlying pain mechanisms and symptom patterns, the average treatment response in the group exposed to active drug may reveal little about the experience of most participants. The vast majority of subjects may endorse a very limited response while others experience significant benefit; it is the norm that few subjects experience the 'average' response [6]. In diseases for which a high proportion of subjects are expected to be non-responders, such as in chronic pain or depression, using group mean reduction as the primary endpoint may mask a clinically meaningful benefit in a subset of subjects due to degradation of assay sensitivity [7–8]. This liability of RCT-based evidence can be mitigated by using an enrichment design.

Another rationale driving the increasing use of the enrichment design is its close replication of clinical practice when compared to the traditional RCT. In the RCT, subjects are enrolled and maintained on the study treatment regardless of its effect. However, in clinical practice it is common for a treatment to be discontinued in subjects for whom no benefit is perceived during an initial treatment interval defined by the expected onset of action and kinetics of the agent. Only patients who tolerate a therapy and perceive benefit during an initial period of titration and observation are typically maintained on a treatment in actual clinical practice. It is in the population of study subjects that most resemble an intended patient population that clinicians are most concerned about the rates of positive and adverse effects [7, 9]. In actual practice, patients who failed to tolerate an antidepressant or analgesic due to intolerable side effects would be changed to an alternative therapy. The extent to which the results of the enrichment phase emulate clinical practice will vary in accord with the method used to define a responder.

For example, Ho *et al* performed a trial using gabapentin or tramadol for treatment of pain due to small fiber neuropathies in a group of subjects with biopsy-proven small fiber neuropathy [10]. The enrichment period in this study involved two single-blind phases. In the first single-blind phase, subjects were treated with gabapentin at their pre-study dose. Those whose pain scores were less than or equal to 7.5 were determined to be responders and were enrolled in the subsequent portion of the study. The included subjects were then treated with placebo in the second single-blind phase. Those subjects whose pain did not increase while on placebo were then excluded from the double-blind, randomized portion of the study. By using two stages in the enrollment period, the researchers were able to first eliminate non-responders, and potentially exclude placebo responders.

There are many strengths of the enrichment design that have been cited by its advocates. First, because a trial employing the enrichment design includes only subjects who have been shown to respond to the screening criteria and not the general subject population, these trials are configured to detect the treatment effect in a subpopulation with greater efficiency. That is, fewer subjects are required to be included in the randomization period than in a non-enriched RCT in order to show the separation from placebo thereby yielding higher assay sensitivity [4–5, 9]. Use of the enriched enrollment randomized withdrawal design has been associated with reduced variability and an increased effect size (mean treatment difference/SD) compared with parallel-group design in trials of post-herpetic neuralgia and painful diabetic neuropathy [11].

Kopec *et al.* used a computer model based on a variety of assumptions, to demonstrate this feature of the enrichment design. The model showed that with 80% sensitivity and 80% specificity for identifying treatment effect, the sample size required in an enrichment design could be reduced by 30% compared to that of an RCT [9]. This increase in sensitivity is particularly relevant when the anticipated effect size of the treatment is small and significant heterogeneity of treatment response is anticipated across subpopulations of subjects. Enrichment designs are not as efficient when only partial enrichment is used. When the effect size is large in the responsive subpopulation of subjects but enrichment is incomplete, the power of the enrichment design has been shown to be similar to that of the RCT [12].

The concept that an enrichment design can have increased sensitivity was demonstrated in a trial performed by Byas-Smith *et al* in 1995. The first portion of this study was a randomized, double-blind, placebo-controlled crossover trial that included 41 subjects with painful diabetic neuropathy. Subjects were randomly assigned to one of four 3-week treatment sequences including placebo (P) or clonidine (C): C-P-C, P-C-P, C-P-P, or P-C-C. In the first week of each treatment period, the clonidine patch dosage was titrated from the initial dosage of 0.1 mg/day in 0.1 mg increments up to 0.3 mg/day. Subjects kept a daily pain diary and the outcome measures for this portion of the study were ratings of pain intensity and a global relief assessment. Their results showed that there was little difference in pain relief between subjects using the clonidine or placebo patches [13].

The researchers then enrolled 12 subjects who appeared most responsive to clonidine treatment in Phase 1 of the study into a subsequent study. In the next phase, subjects were randomly treated with their maximum tolerated dose of clonidine, as established in Phase 1, in 2 of 4 consecutive 1-week periods as follows: C-P-C-P, C-P-P-C, P-C-P-C, or P-C-C-P. When only those subjects who responded to treatment in Phase 1 were examined in this way, the researchers found these subjects had significantly reduced pain with clonidine treatment when compared with placebo [13].

The mathematical model generated by Kopec also supported this finding [9]. The model showed that if the proportion of non-compliers and those who experience dose limiting adverse effects occurred in 20% of the initial population and these subjects could be excluded with both 80% sensitivity and specificity, the sample size requirement for the subsequent study would be reduced by greater than 30%. When this filtering was performed in conjunction with the exclusion of non-responders with similar accuracy, the overall reduction in sample size was 20% (rather than the 30% found previously) in comparison to an RCT without enrichment [9]. One important drawback of the enrichment design to be considered below is that such filtering undermines the controlled assessment of the safety of the active treatment.

Another advantage of the enrichment design is the opportunity to use the enrichment period to adjust drug dosing in a flexible fashion to achieve maximum treatment effect before comparing the treatment to placebo [6, 8, 14–15]. The subject may then be assigned to either the subject's own best dose or to placebo during the randomization period. This can serve to both increase the likelihood of a successful trial, and provide an ethical way to ensure that each subject is optimally disposed to treatment effect [14]. As many RCTs have fixed timetables for drug administration, the less rigid timetable of the enrichment period can also offer researchers more flexibility in dose finding for each subject [8].

The Cardiac Arrhythmia Suppression Trial (CAST) was one of the earlier large, multi-center studies to use an enrichment design. This study examined the hypothesis that the death rate in subjects with asymptomatic or mildly symptomatic ventricular arrhythmia after myocardial infarction would be reduced with arrhythmia suppression. During the enrichment period, the researchers strove to find the treatment that yielded a response for each subject by testing a variety of antiarrhythmics at different dose levels. Researchers defined response as either an 80% reduction in ventricular premature contractions or a reduction of at least 90% in runs of unsustained ventricular tachycardia as recorded on 24h Holter monitoring. Once a subject achieved this outcome, the titration was stopped and that drug and dose were used for the subject in the randomization sequence if the subject was in the treatment group. Specifically, subjects with an ejection fraction (EF) of ≥30% were randomly assigned to receive either encainide-morcizine-flecainide or flecainide-morcizine-encainide, and each drug was tested at two dose levels. Subjects with an EF <30% were not administered flecainide due to its negative inotropic properties but were administered either encainide-morcizine or morcizine-encainide [16–17]. By finding each subject's best dose, the researchers maximized the chances that the treatment would have a benefit over placebo in the RCT portion of the trial. Notably this trial was halted prematurely due to increased deaths in the treatment groups. This trial is now seen as an example of

the need for caution when using surrogate endpoints as outcomes in a clinical trial and shows the problem of enrichment based on a biomarker of unknown predictive value [18].

Focus on the average outcome in the traditional RCT may serve to mask efficacy in a subgroup by including other subgroups in which the treatment has poor efficacy. This may lead to a treatment with great utility for certain subjects failing to achieve regulatory approval and not going to market due to negative RCTs that are a reflection of study design failure rather than an intervention's lack of therapeutic efficacy. Because the enrichment design examines a subgroup in which the treatment was tolerated and perceived as effective during an initial exposure, the problem of effects being masked by averaged results among groups in a parallel design may be mitigated [6]. However, this design does not ensure that the optimal subgroup of responders was defined in advance of the randomized phase. The issue of heterogeneity is also seen at a molecular level in the field of oncology, and it has been suggested that enrichment strategies may be appropriate to increase the sensitivity of cancer treatment trials through means such as genotyping [19].

Disadvantages of the enrichment design

Despite its increasing use in multiple fields, the utility and merits of the enrichment design continue to be debated. Some researchers feel there are limitations of the design that cannot be overcome, such as placebo effect issues and problems with unblinding and carryover effects [20–21]. Others maintain that these issues can be overcome in the early stages of trial design or with the use of active comparators [7]. A frequently cited concern is the loss of generalizability (i.e., external validity) in selecting a specific subpopulation in the enrichment phase. It is important to note that in both an enriched trial and one lacking enrichment, subjects are randomized to study treatments. The key difference of course is that a group of putative responders rather than all comers are randomized with the enrichment design. To whom do the results of an enriched trial demonstrating a benefit of active therapy over placebo apply? These considerations will be discussed further below.

Some caveats do apply to the use of the enrichment design. This design is best utilized to study non-curative treatments, as subjects cannot be cured during the enrichment period and still be studied during the randomization period [1]. Nor can this design be used to study any irreversible treatment, such as surgery [9]. This design is most appropriate for chronic conditions such as chronic pain with target symptom endpoints that remain relatively stable. If a disease is progressive, as was found in a study with design in an Alzheimer's disease population, it can be difficult to ascertain which effects are due to the study treatment and which are attributable to disease progression [21]. Additionally, subjects may not return to baseline before the randomization period, which could also potentially affect results [1, 7]. This is similar to problems with other designs such as crossover trials (see Chapter 10), where a washout may be required. Despite these limitations, this design has been employed across a broad array of fields from neurology to oncology to cardiology to study conditions as varied as chronic pain, cancer, Alzheimer's Disease, and mortality after myocardial infarction [16, 22–24].

The limitation most often cited regarding the enrichment design is that of generalizability. Ascertaining the broader population of subjects to which the results of a clinical trial can be extrapolated is a key interpretative challenge for clinicians. Because this design uses an initial enrichment period during which subjects who do not putatively respond to the enrichment criteria are excluded, critics of this design argue that the results of a trial with an enrichment design have reduced generalizability than those without such a feature. These critics have argued that this screening method often magnifies the treatment benefit that may be realized when giving the therapy to the general population in routine clinical practice and that discretion is warranted when considering results of this trial type [21]. Equally important, controlled evaluation of the safety profile of the active treatment is truncated. It is likely that some subjects discontinuing the treatment during the enrichment phase due to adverse effects would potentially develop more severe adverse effects were they to continue on therapy. An RCT without an enrichment phase provides a controlled safety evaluation of the active therapy over a longer time period. This drawback is significant because many of these therapies are indicated for chronic diseases that will result in prolonged exposure. However, proponents of the design have countered that the examination of a subgroup makes deciphering benefits to subpopulations defined by treatment rather than pain etiology easier. Clinicians need to be advised that the evidence

supporting the use of therapies studied in this way applies to a more restricted population of patients [7].

It has been argued that the enrichment design decreases recruitment efficiency [25–26]. Because only a subset of subjects from the enrichment period of the trial will continue on to the randomized period, additional subjects need to be screened in the enrichment period to meet statistical power requirements. Lemmens *et al.* [26] discuss this concern, noting that as the proportion of subjects from the enrichment period who are randomized decreases, the power of the study decreases [25]. This is particularly concerning when: 1) the pool of available study participants is limited; 2) the designers have little guidance as to the relative proportion of subjects who will not be excluded after the enrichment phase; or 3) there is concern that the enrichment phase is not accurately identifying responders to specific treatment effects of the therapy in question. Conversely, Kopec's computer-simulated comparison of sample sizes indicated that the number of subjects enrolled in the enrichment period to achieve equivalent power in the randomization period was actually slightly lower than the number of subjects required in a conventional RCT. These results were based on an assumption of sensitivity and specificity of greater than 70% for identifying responders in the enrollment period of the enrichment design.

In addition to the above criticisms, there are a number of issues that must be considered by researchers planning a clinical trial using an enrichment design, many of which are not unique to this design. In a classic parallel group RCT without enrichment, participants are exposed to the treatment or the comparator, most often a placebo, and nothing more. In an enrichment design, however, the participant is often exposed to the study intervention during the enrichment period [21, 27]. Participants may therefore be better able to identify what they are receiving for the randomized portion of the study. If adverse events experienced in the enrichment period increase, the subject may assume that he or she is in the treatment group, and if the effects decrease the participant may believe him or herself to be in the placebo group. This unblinding could bias results in either direction, but the 'reverse placebo effect' is of particular concern. In this instance, the participant feels he or she has been switched to placebo and therefore reports more symptoms than he or she might in a completely blinded study [7]. These occurrences would be more likely in the case of a study drug with multiple adverse effects that would be obvious to the participant, or in trials that rely on subject reporting for outcome measures, such as pain scores in a study of analgesics [21].

These concerns have been cited in reference to studies such as the Tacrine Consortium study performed by Davis *et al* [21, 24]. In this study, otherwise healthy subjects with Alzheimer's disease were initially randomized to receive tacrine at a dosage of 40 mg or 80 mg or placebo in two-week blocks of varying order. The Alzheimer's Disease Assessment Scale (ADAS-cog) was used to assess the subjects during each phase of treatment. The subject's 'best dosage' of tacrine was defined as the dosage at which the ADAS was at least 4 points lower than during the two-week placebo baseline period following the dosage-titration period. Subjects who achieved a best dosage were then included in a six-week randomized, double-blind, placebo-controlled period [24]. This design has been criticized because it involved exposure of subjects to both the study drug and placebo during enrichment. Particularly in the case of a drug such as tacrine with adverse effects including nausea and vomiting, when participants experienced the switch to placebo it is possible that unblinding may have occurred. This effect may have influenced the outcome of the study [21].

Unblinding is a concern in many types of clinical trials. However, there are multiple methods that can be used to minimize this effect. By randomizing only subjects who experience minimal adverse effects in the enrichment period, a strategy most enrichment design trials employ, the chance that subjects will recognize a change in frequency in these adverse events may be reduced. Also, if the study drug is tapered for subjects in the placebo group prior to the start of the randomized portion, rather than stopped abruptly, the chance that subjects will identify their treatment may be reduced if using a class of therapy with known withdrawal syndromes such as opioids. The only manner to definitively assess the benefit of tapering vis-a-vis the issue of unblinding is to ask the subjects directly as to their beliefs about treatment allocation [28].

In order to identify the existence and extent of any unblinding, subject questionnaires can be directly used to query study participants about their belief as to when they received treatment or placebo [7]. These questionnaires may inquire about the treatment the subject believes she is receiving, as well as the reasons for this guess. The answers may be used to determine if there is a higher rate of unblinding than would be predicted by chance. Study results cannot be adjusted for unblinding and unblinding may make the study results difficult to interpret

Concern about the validity of the enrichment design also exists due to the potential for carryover effects. If the effects of this treatment take time to wane after the treatment is stopped, this time lag must be factored into the study design. If this washout time period is not considered, there is potential that effects seen in the placebo group could be attributable to study treatment given to those participants during the enrichment period [21, 29].

Issues related to washout periods were considered by Irving *et al.* in their trial using the enrichment design to examine the use of gabapentin for treatment of postherpetic neuralgia (PHN). This study was enriched by including only subjects who had previously demonstrated a response to ≥ 1200 mg of gabapentin and excluding those subjects with dose-limiting adverse events and subjects with hypersensitivity to gabapentin. Because most subjects with PHN continue to have issues with pain control, most available subjects were undergoing treatment with various agents when they were enrolled in the study. Therefore, the researchers included a pharmacokinetic washout period of > 5 times the half-life of typical treatments for PHN including benzodiazepines, tricyclic antidepressants, oral steroids, and others, and a 14-day washout of potent opioids. In the study design, a one-week dose tapering period was built in before subjects were begun on active treatment in the randomized portion of the study [30]. These types of washout periods are essential in an enrichment design to reduce carryover effects.

Conclusion

The enrichment design is relatively novel and its many permutations are still being explored. While most studies to date have used criteria in the enrichment period such as subject response to a drug or response to a screening test, in the future these screening criteria may come to more frequently include molecular markers. The distinction between enrichment by response and enrichment by expected mechanism of action is significant. This type of enrichment design study will likely be very important in fields such as neuro-oncology. As more assays are being developed with increasing sensitivity and specificity for different molecular markers, it becomes more realistic to use these markers to screen subjects in an enrichment design setting.

Table 12.2 Examples of enrichment strategies for identifying responders in an enrichment design trial

1. Utilize study drug to identify responders

Identify responders to study drug given in open fashion

Identify responders to study drug given in single-blind fashion

Identify responders to study drug given in double-blind fashion

Identify patients who have responded to study drug in clinical practice

Identify patients whose condition flares when study drug is withdrawn

2. Utilize alternate methods to identify responders

Identify responders to a drug similar to study drug

Identify patients in whom symptoms can be induced, e.g., induce pain with treadmill test

Identify patients whose symptoms worsen with study drug withdrawal

3. Identify and exclude placebo responders using a placebo run-in

4. Identify and exclude patients with poor compliance

Source: Ref [3, 4].

Enrichment designs are being increasingly used in fields such as chronic pain research because they may better reflect routine clinical practice than other study designs. This strategy has specific advantages for testing a non-curative treatment in a chronic, non-progressive condition [7]. An enrichment design is well suited to examine treatments with small effect sizes in a general population with increased efficiency, particularly those treatments with a greater expected effect in a particular subpopulation of subjects [9]. Issues such as carryover effects and planning for an appropriate washout period must be considered when designing a trial using enrichment design [21]. When used to study an appropriate condition, and with proper planning to avoid pitfalls facing this and other similar clinical trial designs, enrichment enrollment designs offer an efficient way to evaluate potential therapies.

References

1. Amery W and Dony J. A clinical trial design avoiding undue placebo treatment. *J Clin Pharmacol* 1975; **15**: 674–9.

2. Chow SC LJ. *Design and Analysis of Clinical Trials*, 2nd ed. Hoboken, NJ,:John Wiley & Sons, Inc, 2004.

3. Quessy SN. Two-stage enriched enrolment pain trials: a brief review of designs and opportunities for broader application. *Pain* 2010; **148**: 8–13.

4. Straube S DS, Derry S, McQuay HJ and Moore RA. Enriched enrolment: definition and effects of enrichment and dose in trials of pregabalin and gabapentin in neuropathic pain. A systematic review. *Br J Clin Pharmacol* 2008; **66**: 266–75.

6. McQuay HJ, Derry S, Moore RA, *et al*. Enriched enrolment with randomised withdrawal (EERW): Time for a new look at clinical trial design in chronic pain. *Pain* 2008; **135**: 217–20.

7. Katz N. Enriched enrollment randomized withdrawal trial designs of analgesics: focus on methodology. *Clin J Pain* 2009; **25**: 797–807.

8. Quitkin FM and Rabkin JG. Methodological problems in studies of depressive disorder: utility of the discontinuation design. *J Clin Psychopharm* 1981; **1**: 282–8.

9. Kopec JA, Abrahamowicz M and Esdaile JM. Randomized discontinuation trials: Utility and efficiency. *J Clin Epidemiol* 1993; **46**: 959–71.

10. Ho TW BJ, Froman S and Polydefkis M. Efficient assessment of neuropathic pain drugs in patients with small fiber sensory neuropathies. *Pain* 2009; **141**: 19–24.

11. Hewitt DJ, Ho TW, Galer B, *et al*. Impact of responder definition on the enriched enrollment randomized withdrawal trial design for establishing proof of concept in neuropathic pain. *Pain* 2011; **152**: 514–21.

12. Fu P, Dowlati A and Schluchter M. Comparison of power between randomized discontinuation design and upfront randomization design on progression-free survival. *J Clin Oncol* 2009; **27**: 4135–41.

13. Byas-Smith MG, Max MB, Muir J and Kingman A. Transdermal clonidine compared to placebo in painful diabetic neuropathy using a two-stage 'enriched enrollment' design. *Pain* 1995; **60**: 267–74.

14. Knipschild P, Leffers P and Feinstein AR. The qualification period. *J Clin Epidemiol* 1991; **44**: 441–4.

15. Chow SC, editor. *Encyclopedia of Biopharmaceutical Statistics*. New York, Marcel Dekker, 2000.

16. Echt DS Liebson PR, Mitchell LB, Peters RW, *et al*. Mortality and morbidity in patients receiving encainide, flecainide, or placebo. The Cardiac Arrhythmia Suppression Trial. *N Engl J Med* 1991; **324**: 781–8.

17. Chow S-C. *Encyclopedia of Biopharmaceutical Statistics*. New York, Marcel Dekker, 2000.

18. Fleming TR, DeMets DL. Surrogate end points in clinical trials: are we being misled? *Ann Intern Med* 1996; **125**: 605–13.

19. Betensky RA, Louis DN and Cairncross JG. Influence of unrecognized molecular heterogeneity on randomized clinical trials. *J Clin Oncol* 2002; **20**: 2495–9.

20. Staud R, Price DD. Long-term trials of pregabalin and duloxetine for fibromyalgia symptoms: how study designs can affect placebo factors. *Pain* 2008; **136**: 232–4.

21. Leber PD and Davis CS. Threats to the validity of clinical trials employing enrichment strategies for sample selection. *Controlled clinical trials* 1998; **19**: 178–87.

22. Lynch ME, Clark AJ and Sawynok J. Intravenous adenosine alleviates neuropathic pain: a double blind placebo controlled crossover trial using an enriched enrolment design. *Pain* 2003; **103**: 111–7.

23. Rosner GL, Stadler W and Ratain MJ. Randomized discontinuation design: application to cytostatic antineoplastic agents. *J Clin Oncol* 2002; **20**: 4478–84.

24. Davis KL, Thal LJ, Gamzu ER, *et al*. A double-blind, placebo-controlled multicenter study of tacrine for Alzheimer's disease. The Tacrine Collaborative Study Group. *N Engl J Med* 1992; **327**: 1253–9.

25. Lemmens HJM WD, Munera C, Eltahtawy A, *et al*. Enriched analgesic efficacy studies: an assessment by clinical trial simulation. *Contemporary Clin Trials* 2006; **27**: 165–73.

26. Freidlin B SR. Evaluation of randomized discontinuation design. *J Clin Oncol* 2005; **23**: 5094–8.

27. Staud R and Price DD. Role of placebo factors in clinical trials with special focus on enrichment designs. *Pain* 2008; **139**: 479–80.

28. Moore RA, Derry S and McQuay HJ. Response to: Long-term trials of pregabalin and duloxetine for fibromyalgia symptoms: how study designs can affect placebo factors. *Pain* 2008; **139**: 477–9; author reply 9–80.

29. Sonpavde G GM, Hutson TE and Von Hoff DD. Patient selection for Phase II trials. *Am J Clin Oncol* 2009; **32**: 216–9.

30. Irving G, Jensen M, Cramer M, *et al*. Efficacy and tolerability of gastric-retentive gabapentin for the treatment of postherpetic neuralgia: results of a double-blind, randomized, placebo-controlled clinical trial. *Clin J Pain* 2009; **25**: 185–92.

Non-inferiority trials

Rick Chappell

Introduction and definitions

The scope of this chapter

The traditional role of the randomized clinical trial is to determine if there is superiority of one treatment, diagnostic technique, or preventive measure over one or more others (See Chapter 2). This paradigm is reasonable when standard of care interventions are non-existent or, in situations when they do exist, have undesirable characteristics such as low efficacy and/or high toxicity rates. As medical progress creates more alternatives and ethical considerations prohibit the use of inactive interventions in many cases, active-control trials are becoming common. These are studies in which one or more experimental treatments are compared to a control treatment whose effectiveness has previously been established [1]. (For simplicity's sake, this chapter will refer to any intervention under study as a 'treatment', though all comments are generalizable to prevention and diagnostic trials.) Active-control superiority trials, each with the goal of trying to determine if a new treatment is better than an existing one with respect to the primary outcome, are possible and indeed common. But a control which shows clinical activity allows a type of question other than superiority to be answered: that of equivalence (also referred to, for reasons explained below, as non-inferiority). That is, we may wish to know if an experimental treatment is approximately as good as the control with respect to a given outcome. Thus active-control trials are not always equivalence studies although most equivalence trials are active-control. A possible exception to the latter statement is when a treatment is investigated as being equivalent to a placebo or other control using toxicity or other undesirable event as an outcome. See [2, 3] for non-technical summaries of

ethical, practical, and scientific aspects of equivalence trials.

Despite certain problems in implementation and interpretation, which are discussed below, equivalence trials have yielded useful clinical results. Table 1 of [3] lists examples of important therapeutic advances in which the treatment was not proven more effective than an established treatment – including selective serotonin reuptake inhibitor antidepressants, which, though not shown to be more effective than tricyclic antidepressants, are better tolerated; and the antipsychotic drugs risperidone, olanzapine, and quetiapine which also were found to have fewer side-effects than the existing phenothiazine and butyrophenone classes of drugs without being proven more effective. Therefore, for better or worse, equivalence is being used as evidence for approving and implementing new classes of treatments.

A little clarification regarding terminology may now be useful. First, this chapter only mentions multi-arm randomized trials in 'Multiple hypothesis testing and non-inferiority trials with more than two treatments' (below); however, all other discussion also applies to studies with three or more comparators. Also, please notice that the preceding paragraphs use descriptions such as 'approximately as good as' and 'equivalence' instead of 'equal to.' This is because equivalence does not imply mathematical equality and, indeed, the latter cannot be statistically proven. More concretely, it is impossible to prove one treatment's effect on an outcome to be exactly equal to another's if the outcome has random variation, as of course do all clinical endpoints. We can only show one treatment to be 'not much worse' than another, a point which is made in more detail in 'A false method of showing equivalence' and 'Formal definition of non-inferiority with respect to the equivalence margin and statement of hypotheses' (below). Another ambiguity is that

Clinical Trials in Neurology, ed. Bernard Ravina, Jeffrey Cummings, Michael P. McDermott, and R. Michael Poole. Published by Cambridge University Press. © Cambridge University Press 2012.

equivalence is sometimes used to mean non-inferiority combined with non-superiority. Therefore, equivalence trials are now commonly referred to with greater precision as non-inferiority trials as they are below.

Finally, it is useful to distinguish the terms 'equivalence' and 'bioequivalence' if only to limit our attention to the former. The term 'bioequivalence' is used to describe a study of pharmacokinetic similarity between two treatment formulations, often in healthy subjects [4]. Design and analytic considerations for such experiments are different than those used in non-inferiority trials with clinical outcomes such as the example (SPORTIF III) described below. I do not discuss bioequivalence trials further.

A brief summary of superiority trials' relevant properties

A few important aspects of superiority trials' conduct and analysis are now mentioned as background for subsequent development of non-inferiority trials and a comparison of the two types of studies in 'Key comparisons between superiority and non-inferiority trials'. These are perforce cursory and selected. See Chapter 5 in this volume for more information.

The role of randomization

Randomization is as central to the conduct of non-inferiority as it is to superiority trials. Fisher [5] argued that statistical inference (i.e., p-values and confidence intervals) is impossible without randomization. Even among those who consider that position to be extreme, a randomized controlled trial is the 'standard by which all other trials are judged' and 'the best method for achieving comparability' quoting [6], p. 61, but see also [7, 8]. This is because it is the only mechanism of assuring approximate comparability between the treatment groups with respect to both observed and unobserved predictors.

The role of intent-to-treat analysis

The intent-to-treat (or intention-to-treat; abbreviated ITT) principle states that patients who are randomized to a treatment group should be analyzed as part of that group even if they crossed over to a different treatment and requires that all outcomes be determined regardless of their purported relation to treatment. That is, the ITT analysis strategy uses all randomized patients along with all of their outcomes. It has been called 'the most fundamental principle underlying the analysis

from randomized controlled trials' and described as 'foundational to the experimental nature of randomized controlled trials' [9]. Bath [10], while describing approaches to clinical trials of stroke, noted that the definition of ITT is sometimes weakened to include only patients who receive one or more treatments (most trialists prefer this latter standard to be referred to in a qualified manner as 'modified intent-to-treat' or other similar term). A competing analysis strategy would be to only include those patients who comply closely enough with the protocol. These constitute a per protocol (PP) sample of patients and although a PP analysis is sometimes thought to be relevant for toxicity and other outcomes, it is almost universally considered less relevant than ITT. The role of ITT in non-inferiority trials is discussed further below ('Intent-to-treat in non-inferiority vs. superiority trials: which analysis population should be used?').

Other means of avoiding bias

Randomization and an ITT analysis are not the only ingredients of high-quality results in a clinical trial. Although a complete discussion is beyond the limits of the present chapter, I present three particularly important properties. The first is blinding or masking [11]. When a patient is unaware of his or her treatment, he or she is unable to attribute a clinical response to a specific treatment. Such an attribution, if it varied with the treatment group, would bias the estimated treatment effect. A general attribution of improvement without knowledge of the treatment group is certainly possible due to the well-known placebo effect; but if these subjective conclusions are unrelated to the treatment, as they must be in the presence of proper blinding, bias from this source is impossible. See Chapter 5 for details.

Well-defined endpoints, clearly prioritized and stated in advance, are important components of powerful trials yielding useful results. Lack of ambiguity is important in order for a study's conclusions to be clear. For example, suppose a treatment is hypothesized to reduce bone fractures due to falls. Of course the investigators could make the occurrence of any bone fracture following a fall the study's primary endpoint. However, even in high-risk populations this tends to be a rare occurrence with moderate follow-up and so a trial with this primary outcome would either be underpowered or very large. Alternative endpoints include: any bone fracture; the number of fractures; the number of separate incidents involving a fracture (this differs from the preceding when a single accident causes more than one fracture); the number of falls; the number of days on which a fall occurs (patients may not remember multiple falls in a single day); and various measures of balance and stability. These are just some examples of endpoints potentially assessing neurological interventions; trials of treatments which are thought to directly influence bone strength can have other outcomes such as measures of bone mineral density. Each endpoint and its associated hypothesis should be stated in advance, especially for the trial's primary question, and is often a trade-off between clinical relevance and the trial's ability to answer the question.

One important aspect of the research question for any outcome in which time plays a role (which is the majority of clinical outcomes) is length of patient follow-up. There are choices involved with even such an apparently unambiguous outcome as mortality: whether mortality is to be defined dichotomously as having occurred or not occurred over the course of the study; or whether time to death is to be the primary descriptor; whether all-cause mortality will be assessed; or, if not, which deaths due to intercurrent illnesses will be excluded; and, in all cases, how long each patient is to be observed. In all but the most pernicious illnesses some survivors will be seen and so their lack of events at the study's end, or right-censoring, will require special analytic techniques.

Statement of null and alternative hypotheses for superiority trials

Consider a superiority trial in which an endpoint is described with a quantity denoted, for simplicity's sake, as 'Effect'. This could be a mean or a median of a continuous outcome such as a stroke severity scale; a proportion of seizure-free patients; the hazard of or median time to death or other failure time outcome; or some other quantity of interest. Suppose also that the treatment groups are labeled 'Experimental' and 'Control', where the latter could refer to an active, placebo or other control, and are abbreviated E and C. Then assuming lower values of $Effect$ are better the null hypothesis of no difference is formulated as:

$$H_0: Effect_E - Effect_C = 0,$$

meaning that $Effect$ is identical in the experimental treatment and control groups, and the alternative hypothesis of superiority is:

$$H_A: Effect_E - Effect_C \leq 0,$$

implying that the treatment group betters the control as measured by $Effect$. Data from the superiority trial are used to either reject or not reject H_0 according to a pre-defined significance level (maximum false positive error rate, also called type I error rate or α) such as 0.05, 0.025, or 0.01. Rejecting H_0 and accepting H_A would imply that, subject to the possibility of error quantified by the p-value, E is superior to C. On the other hand failure to reject H_0 would not imply that H_A is false, rather that the trial does not contain enough information to support the conclusion that it is true. The inequality in H_A need not be strict – substituting $\neq$ for $\leq$ merely makes the hypothesis two-sided so that it tests superiority in either direction.

A false method of showing equivalence

The penultimate sentence of the previous part belies an informal, seemingly ubiquitous yet erroneous strategy for attempting to prove equivalence: performing a clinical trial then concluding superiority if H_0 is rejected and equivalence otherwise. Of course, a small clinical trial could fail to reject a false null hypothesis. In fact, if the goal of a trial is to show equivalence by not rejecting H_0, the chance of success would be maximized by a sample size of 0! No information yields no conclusive evidence of superiority, but of course should give no evidence of equivalence either.

An alternative has long been advocated by statisticians: computing a confidence interval for $Effect_E - Effect_C$ (using the notation of 'Statement of null and alternative hypotheses for superiority trials', again assuming large effects to be unfavorable) and using it to characterize the difference between treatment and control in terms of the effect of interest. A confidence interval may include zero, meaning that equivalence would not be ruled out, but it will also include a range of other possibilities for the difference in effects. This entire range must be compared to clinically interesting differences in order to be interpreted. (The considerations which go into defining 'clinically interesting' are discussed below in 'Choice of equivalence margin and scale'.) In particular, the upper endpoint of the confidence interval for $Effect_E - Effect_C$ gives the worst reasonable estimated performance of the experimental treatment compared to the control. 'Reasonable' reflects the coverage of the confidence interval and corresponding false positive error rate, often but not necessarily 97.5% and 2.5%, respectively.

Formal definition of non-inferiority with respect to the equivalence margin and statement of hypotheses

As with most aspects of the analysis of a randomized clinical trial, the standard to which the worst performance of the treatment vs. the control (the upper endpoint of the confidence interval just mentioned) is to be compared should be specified in advance. This standard is called a non-inferiority margin; the ICH Guideline E3 [12] requires the trial's protocol to state the margin to be a 'pre-specified degree of inferiority' often denoted as Δ. We can thus frame the hypothesis-testing paradigm in the usual fashion, where rejecting the null hypothesis H_0 gives a successful resolution of the trial's primary goal (a conclusion that the experimental treatment is non-inferior to the control treatment) and failing to reject it results in the opposite (that a conclusion of inferiority is reasonable). This requires a new pair of null and alternative hypotheses:

$$H_0: Effect_E - Effect_C > \Delta,$$

meaning that $Effect$ in the experimental treatment is inferior to $Effect$ in the control group by an amount exceeding Δ. Also

$$H_A: Effect_E - Effect_C \le \Delta,$$

meaning that the experimental treatment may be superior to the control, identical to it, or slightly inferior to it in terms of $Effect$ but, in the last case, the inferiority is no more than Δ. If we reject H_0 and accept the alternative hypothesis H_A we claim to have demonstrated E to be non-inferior to C with respect to a pre-specified margin Δ. If (and only if) so, the confidence interval for $Effect_E - Effect_C$ falls entirely below Δ. There are a variety of possible combinations of non-inferiority and superiority conclusions; these are discussed in the following part and shown in Figure 13.1.

Motivating example – SPORTIF III, a non-inferiority trial of ximelagatran vs. warfarin in stroke prevention

Brief description of study background and goals

The Stroke Prevention using Oral Thrombin Inhibitor in Atrial Fibrillation (SPORTIF) III trial was an open-label study of the efficacy of ximelagatran vs. warfarin

in the prevention of strokes and systemic embolic events in patients with atrial fibrillation. A blinded trial of otherwise similar design, SPORTIF V, was also conducted approximately concurrently. For simplicity's sake, this chapter will only mention SPORTIF III below although considerations discussed here apply to both studies. The trials' designs are described in more detail in [13] and their results in [14]. Ximelagatran was a new thrombin inhibitor under investigation as an alternative to warfarin because of the latter's side effects and intolerability in some patients. Because ethical considerations forbade a placebo arm in these high-risk patients, non-inferiority trials were conducted to determine whether or not ximelagatran is clinically equivalent to warfarin. SPORTIF III's salient characteristics are given in Table 13.1.

Statement of equivalence margin and hypotheses

Based on previous studies and assuming equality of effect, a primary event rate of 3.1% per year was estimated in advance of the study for patients in both treatment groups with additional patients or follow-up planned if necessary to guarantee at least 80 primary endpoints. The margin of equivalence was chosen to be 2% per year, inducing the following null and alternative hypotheses, denoted H_0 and H_A, respectively, where $Rate_E$ and $Rate_C$ refer to the annual rates of the primary endpoints in the two groups:

$$H_0: Rate_E - Rate_C > 2\%/year$$

and

$$H_A: Rate_E - Rate_C \le 2\%/year.$$

Thus ximelagatran ('E') is the experimental treatment and warfarin ('C') is the active control. The primary aim of SPORTIF III was to prove that ximelagatran does not cause an excess of 2%/year or more in strokes and systemic embolic events compared to warfarin. The logic behind the choice of a 2% margin is briefly discussed below ('Demonstrating superiority to placebo').

Interpretation of possible trial results

Figure 13.1, from Figure 2 of [13], summarizes an assortment of hypothetical SPORTIF III results with their interpretations. Point estimates (diamonds) with two-sided 95% confidence intervals are given for a variety of scenarios. Dotted lines show the 2% margins of clinical equivalence. The top two confidence intervals

Table 13.1 Design elements of SPORTIF III

Trial type	Randomized, parallel, two cohorts
Blinding status	Open-label, blinded assessment
Planned sample size	3407 patients at 259 sites in 23 countries
Patient population	Age ≥ 18 y.o., atrial fibrillation, high-risk (at least one of: hypertension; age ≥ 75 y.o.; previous stroke, TIA, or systemic embolism; left ventricular dysfunction; or age ≥ 65 y.o. and diabetes mellitus or coronary artery disease)
Timing	Enrollment 7/2000–12/2001
Planned average duration of treatment / followup	16 months
Treatment groups	Ximelagatran (*E*; experimental treatment) Warfarin (*C*; active control)
Primary endpoint	Stroke (ischemic or hemorrhagic) or systemic embolic event
Margin of equivalence	$\Delta = 2\%$/year
Size of test for equivalence	$\alpha = 0.025$
Power of test for equivalence	90% for primary event rate of 3.1%/year in each treatment group

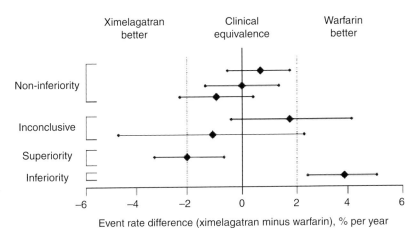

Figure 13.1. Hypothetical outcomes from the SPORTIF III trial with point estimates and 95% two-sided confidence intervals.

lie entirely within the region of clinical equivalence; for these cases, there is evidence that neither drug is superior to the other. The third interval indicates a possibility but no proof that ximelagatran is superior. For all three cases, non-inferiority of ximelagatran is demonstrated (H_0 in rejected in favor of H_A) because the confidence intervals do not overlap the right dotted line drawn at $\Delta = 2\%$/year. The next two confidence intervals are inconclusive, in that neither non-inferiority of ximelagatran nor superiority of warfarin can be demonstrated. The following interval shows a situation in which superiority (and thus, of course, non-inferiority also) of ximelagatran is concluded. The last possible case is that of ximelagatran's proven inferiority to warfarin.

Key comparisons between superiority and non-inferiority trials

Sample size

For a non-inferiority trial, the discussion above ('Formal definition of non-inferiority with respect to the equivalence margin and statement of hypotheses') shows that H_0 is rejected, and H_A accepted, if the confidence interval for the difference in treatment effects falls entirely below the non-inferiority margin Δ. Since confidence intervals narrow with increasing sample size, the chance of rejecting H_0 and concluding equivalence (the power of the trial) increases with sample size as long as H_0 is false. In this respect non-inferiority and superiority trials are identical: higher sample sizes give more information. It is also true that the sample size required for a superiority trial with a treatment effect ($Effect_E$ – $Effect_C$ in the notation above) of size Δ is the same as that needed for a non-inferiority trial with margin Δ assuming equality ($Effect_E$ = $Effect_C$). This holds exactly for normally distributed outcomes, approximately for other types of outcomes such as binary data, and assumes identical powers and critical p-values. See Chapter 4 by Bebchuk and Wittes for a description of sample size calculation in superiority trials.

The simplest binary sample size calculation, condensing Equation (11.5) of [15], gives the following formula for a two-arm non-inferiority trial with binary outcomes, non-inferiority margin Δ, and equality of proportions. The assumed proportion of events in the experimental and control groups (under the usual alternative hypothesis used for power/sample size calculation purposes, this is equal in the two groups) is denoted P. Then the *total* required sample size is

$$n = 4 \times P \times (1 - P) \times (Z_{Power} + Z_{1-\alpha})^2 / \Delta^2.$$

Z_{Power} is the normal quantile for the required power; for example, with 90% power $Z_{.9} = 1.28$. Also, $Z_{1-\alpha}$ is the normal quantile for one minus the significance level α; for a traditional significance level of 0.025, $Z_{.975} = 1.96$. Table 13.2 gives sample sizes for a two-arm non-inferiority trial with 90% power and a significance level of $\alpha = 0.025$ for a range of non-inferiority margins Δ and event proportions.

This table shows that if the event rate in both groups is 0.6 then 450 subjects (225 per group) are required to provide 90% power to demonstrate non-inferiority of the experimental group with respect to a 0.15 margin. Table 13.2 holds no matter whether events are successes or failures, but note that certain cells aren't applicable to both situations. For example if events are failures then the lower right corner isn't relevant: assuming proportions equal to 0.9 with a margin of 0.2 would allow non-inferiority to extend above a proportion of 1. An experimental treatment whose failure rate is 100% couldn't be usefully claimed to be non-inferior to anything. However if events are successes then the lower right corner *is* useful but the upper left is not.

Sample size formulas for proportions using a relative (multiplicative) instead of an absolute (additive) margin are given in [15], as are methods for time-to-event outcomes.

Fleming [16] claims the notion that non-inferiority trials with scientifically rigorous margins always

Table 13.2 Total sample sizes for two-arm non-inferiority trials with false-positive rate = 0.025 and power = 90% as a function of additive non-inferiority margin and event proportions.

Event proportion in both groups	$\Delta = 0.05$	$\Delta = 0.1$	$\Delta = 0.15$	$\Delta = 0.2$
0.05	800	200	90	50
0.1	1,514	380	170	96
0.2	2,690	674	300	170
0.3	3,532	884	394	222
0.4	4,036	1,010	450	254
0.5	4,204	1,052	468	264
0.6	4,036	1,010	450	254
0.7	3,532	884	394	222
0.8	2,690	674	300	170
0.9	1,514	380	170	96
0.95	800	200	90	50

require very large sample sizes is a common one, and correctly describes it as a myth. The logic varies with the situation; at times a large margin may be sufficient to show clinical equivalence and at other times a smaller one is required. Remember that all the sample size calculations above are carried out under the assumption of true equivalence, that proportions in each group are the same. It is certainly possible to perform these computations using the equations of [15] under a more optimistic assumption of superiority on the part of the experimental treatment. This procedure has been proposed [17] and indeed lowers the sample size. However, an investigator assuming superiority and testing only for non-inferiority can be accused of 'having his cake and eating it too' (or even her cake). On the other hand, pessimism – that is, assuming a slight inferiority of the new treatment compared to the standard treatment – could be a usefully conservative strategy in computing sample size.

How patient non-adherence influences results in the two types of trials

Consider a trial in which one drug is tested for superiority over another. Suppose the trial is successful in that the experimental treatment effect significantly improves upon the control's but that there is substantial non-compliance in each group. Although the results could be legitimately criticized on various grounds – including lack of generalizability, impracticality of extension to ordinary clinical practice, and underestimation of true efficacy and toxicity rates – the non-compliance would not contradict the basic conclusion of superiority. Non-compliance biases the 'true effect' (the difference achieved under the scenario of full drug exposure) towards the null and therefore the observed results would be conservative. The same cannot be said of non-inferiority trials: if nobody in either group of this type of study took their drugs then of course the treatments would appear to be equivalent. Thus it has been noted that 'One of the concerns that has been expressed regarding equivalence trials is that sloppiness in the conduct of the trial biases results towards no difference [18, 19].' But since nearly all trials are sloppy to some extent, this leads us to the question of what amount of non-compliance in a non-inferiority trial invalidates its results. No firm answer has been given so far; Chi *et al.* [1] have given a practical recommendation that 'One should design the current trial to be as similar as possible to the historical placebo control trials used in estimating the historical control effect.'

Intent-to-treat in non-inferiority vs. superiority trials: which analysis population should be used?

As stated above ('The role of intent-to-treat analysis'), the intent-to-treat strategy for analysis is crucial to the interpretation of superiority trials. The ICH Guideline E3 [12], in a section which neither specifically refers to nor excludes non-inferiority trials, states 'An analysis using all available data should be carried out for all studies intended to establish efficacy.' Most analysts agree with this statement. But per-protocol analyses, for reasons given above, are also particularly relevant for non-inferiority trials. The problem with the ITT strategy in non-inferiority trials is that it could bias results towards equivalence, making it an anti-conservative strategy. It can also bias results in the opposite direction if the patterns of non-compliance are different in the two groups. Since PP analyses can also be biased, we are left with a difficult choice. Wiens and Zhao [20] promote ITT, saying that 'The ITT analysis follows from randomization, and must be used to maintain the integrity of randomization.' They also point out that a non-inferiority trial should be conducted similarly to the trials which established efficacy of the control.

Since the latter were presumably superiority trials which used ITT, comparability is enhanced by using ITT in the non-inferiority trial. A practical compromise is to perform both ITT and PP analyses, hope that they are similar, and if so to use the former for the main results. If the two analyses differ then it may be a useful if laborious exercise to model the missing data/non-compliance mechanisms and perform sensitivity analyses on their effects upon the trial's results.

Practical issues in non-inferiority trials

Choice of equivalence margin and scale

Many authors have discussed the choice of margin in non-inferiority trials [21–25]. All agree that it should be made in advance and pre-specified in the protocol. A variety of guidelines have been put forth; although these are usually subjective, rational decisions can be made based on clinical factors and data from the historical study or studies which established the active control treatment's efficacy.

The margin Δ should clearly not exceed the benefit provided by the control treatment; otherwise the experimental therapy would not be shown superior to placebo (assuming that the control was tested against a placebo) even if non-inferiority by Δ was demonstrated. One rule of thumb is that the margin should be less than half the benefit ascribed to the control, i.e., the new treatment retains at least one-half of the benefit of the active control treatment. Even this '50% rule' is vague because it could use either the estimated control benefit or the lower bound of the 95% or other level confidence interval (the description of Figure 13.3 below uses estimated benefits but lower confidence bounds could be substituted without changing its message). One opinion, published in the aptly named 'The trials and tribulations of non-inferiority: the ximelagatran experience' [26], claimed that SPORTIF III had '… an unreasonably generous margin that was potentially biased toward non-inferiority'. The authors thus evinced '… a lack of confidence that ximelagatran retains at least 50% of warfarin's effect (a prerequisite to the establishment of non-inferiority)' and expressed a preference, based on a meta-analysis of warfarin's effect compared to placebo, for a margin of $\Delta = .68\%$/year. They did not mention their preference's consequence (because sample size is roughly inversely proportional to the square of the margin) that a change of the margin from 2% annually downward to .68% would have multiplied the sample size by a factor of 8.7, necessitating approximately 29,500 patients.

Another standard for setting the margin is that it should be clinically relevant. Even if the active control was shown to have a large effect, a margin of half that effect may be too large for judging non-inferiority between it and an experimental treatment. For example, if an active control antibiotic is known to cure about 90% of infections a margin of 45% is likely too large for comparing it to an experimental treatment. A successful trial may not yield clinically useful results even if it were to show a maximum 45% difference, allowing a cure rate as low as 45% for the new treatment. See [26] for an extensive discussion of the choice of margin for the SPORTIF III trial.

The choice of a margin's scale – e.g., should Δ constitute a difference between two means, proportions, or rates; or their ratio; or some other quantity such as an odds ratio – is less commonly mentioned but is also important. This is not an issue in superiority trials. For example, the null hypothesis of no effect on mean blood pressure could be expressed as a difference between means equaling 0 or a ratio equaling 1, but it wouldn't matter: the two are mathematically equivalent. In non-inferiority trials the scale used in the null hypothesis does matter because we need it in order to define the margin. The designers of the SPORTIF trial assumed for the sake of power calculations that event rates were 3.1%/year with an absolute, or additive, 2% margin (see Table 13.1). They could have chosen a relative, or multiplicative, scale to judge equivalence, for example 5.1/3.1 = 1.65. This would have resulted in a very different trial. The interpretation for patient populations with different risks would change: if we wanted to extrapolate SPORTIF's results to a higher-risk group with stroke/systemic embolic rate of 6%, a 2% absolute margin indicates that they would have a maximum rate of 8%; but a 1.65 relative margin gives a maximum rate of 9.9%. Power calculations produce different sample sizes for the two scales with a relative margin requiring a larger trial. Analytic methods would change as well – a relative margin relies on the well-known proportional hazards model, while an absolute margin requires the more rarely used additive hazards regression [27]. Note that although 'Formal definition of non-inferiority with respect to the equivalence margin and statement of hypotheses' (above) only shows hypotheses for absolute differences, they can also apply to relative differences when effects are logarithmically transformed.

Demonstrating superiority to placebo

The problem of invoking a non-randomized comparison

Temple and Ellenberg [3] state the fundamental problem of non-inferiority studies to be one of assay sensitivity: the ability of a trial to show that a new therapy is effective. This can be achieved by demonstrating it to be superior to a placebo control or, as discussed here, to not be inferior by some defined amount to a known effective treatment. However the inference that non-inferiority to the known treatment implies superiority to a placebo involves a crucial assumption, and Temple and Ellenberg point out that 'support for this assumption must come from sources external to the trial.' In the SPORTIF III example we must assume that warfarin is effective in the population under study in order for non-inferiority of ximelagatran to be clinically interesting. This is not provable by the trial because an inactive control group is not included in it. Thus inference between the experimental treatment and active comparator relies on historical evidence of sensitivity to drug effects (HESDE; see Section V of [28]), based on past trials. Figure 13.2a shows a schematic for this type of inference. A non-inferiority trial (right) yields a randomized comparison between the experimental and active control treatments in its patients while the historical superiority trial (left) gives a randomization-based estimate of the active control's effect compared to a control. But the inferential leap that the active control's effect in the non-inferiority trial is the same as in the historical trial is not based on evidence, or at least not on evidence of the same quality as that used for the other conclusions. Therefore HESDE, like all important truths, can be a nebulous thing [29]. This is illustrated by the International Conference of Harmonisation (ICH) Guideline E10 [30] which gives a variety of scenarios in which a well-run randomized controlled clinical trial's result may not be reproduced. HESDE is relevant only if it was achieved under conditions similar to those obtained by the new trials. These conditions include, but are not limited to, the patients under study, adjuvant treatments, and diagnostic standards. Note that comparisons conducted within a single trial have no such problems as shown by Figure 13.2b. Though their generalizability may be questioned, these conclusions' validity depends only upon all patients being drawn from the same population and their treatment randomly determined [31].

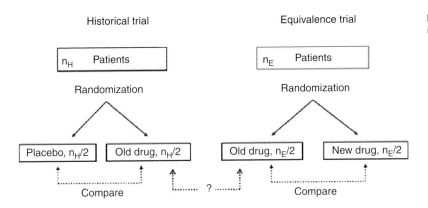

Historical trial   Equivalence trial

Figure 13.2a. Schematic for inference in non-inferiority trials.

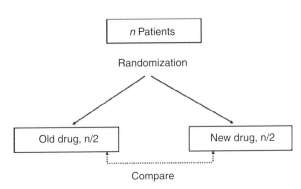

Figure 13.2b. Schematic for inference in superiority trials.

The problem of equivalency drift

Even if HESDE holds and the inference indicated by a question mark in Figure 13.2a is valid, other problems can interfere with non-inferiority studies' assay sensitivity. Suppose instead of an 'Old drug' and a 'New drug' we have a series of treatments denoted 'Drug 1' … 'Drug 4' and that Drug 1 was proven to be superior to a placebo by 4% in a historical trial. This is schematically illustrated in Figure 13.3, which depicts an artificial series of results via point estimates (these are less realistic than lower confidence interval endpoints but render a clearer example). For ethical or perhaps other reasons, Drug 2 was not compared to a placebo but to Drug 1 in a non-inferiority trial with a non-inferiority margin of 2%. We suppose that the null hypothesis was rejected in this trial and non-inferiority was concluded implying, in the presence of HESDE, that Drug 2's benefit exceeded 2%. In fact it was estimated to be 1.5% lower than Drug 1's, as 2.5%. Then, similarly, Drug 3 can be concluded to be non-inferior to Drug 2, with an estimated effect of 1.2%, say, and Drug 4 seen to be non-inferior to Drug 3. But Drug 4 has an estimated 0% benefit! This unpleasant feature, in which a series

of non-inferiority trials can make an active treatment appear equivalent to a placebo even in the presence of HESDE, has been termed 'bio-creep' [16]. It can be prevented by comparing Drugs 2, 3, and 4 all to Drug 1 and not to each other in an ever-more-imprecise sequence. This preventive may be impractical because Drug 1 could be off the market or undesirable due to considerations such as side effects.

The problem of an incentive to produce minimally significant results

In 'Practical issues in non-inferiority trials' (above) it was mentioned that the precision of the active control's estimated effect is relevant in choosing a non-inferiority margin for comparing it to an experimental treatment. If the active control's effect estimated from a historical trial was 10% with a confidence interval of ± 4% then we clearly don't want a non-inferiority margin in the new study to be 6% or higher. Under HESDE the active control's benefit in the new trial could be 6%, the lower end of the confidence interval, and so a 6% margin would allow an ineffective experimental treatment to be judged equivalent to it. This means that in a new age of active controlled non-inferiority trials a drug company could have an incentive to make demonstration of assay sensitivity as difficult as possible for its product's successors. One way to do so in the present example would be to aim, perhaps using interim stopping guidelines, for a confidence interval of ± 9.9% whereby the 50% rule could require a margin of 0.05%, half the control's minimum benefit. Are we headed for a future in which all confidence intervals just barely exclude 0 and all p-values are 0.049? A related point is that if there are several active controls available there is great incentive to choose the 'worst' active control as a comparator.

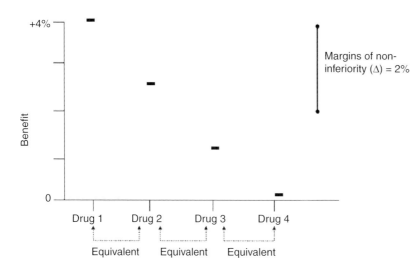

Figure 13.3. The problem of equivalency drift.

Multiple hypothesis testing and non-inferiority trials with more than two treatments

Designers of clinical trials which formally test two or more sets of hypotheses usually need to reduce the individual tests' p-values for significance in order to preserve the overall false positive error, also called type I error. This is true when the trial is declared a success if *any* null hypothesis is rejected, a common strategy in superiority trials with multiple endpoints (for example, when a treatment is hoped to reduce at least one of a number of symptoms). However, non-inferiority trials are often conducted to show equivalence on *all* sets of hypotheses. These hypotheses could reflect equivalence of two or more outcomes, in two or more patient subgroups, or among three or more treatments. In this case, setting the critical p-value for each comparison at the overall value (e.g., 0.025) has the result of making the tests of universal non-inferiority to be conservative. That is because every null hypothesis of inferiority must be rejected in order for this conclusion to be reached. Thus either the unadjusted p-values are used or each significance level could be increased to make the overall probability of erroneously rejecting all null hypotheses equal to a nominal value such as 0.025. The second choice is rarely made and involves specialized calculations. This scenario is a special case of the 'reverse multiplicity problem' [32].

Moving from a superiority to a non-inferiority hypothesis or vice-versa, after the results are in

Having failed to show superiority it may be tempting to switch to a 'salvage hypothesis' of non-inferiority or, having shown non-inferiority, to hope to successfully address the 'home-run hypothesis' of superiority. These strategies are theoretically possible but have the following practical pitfall. The caution concerning multiplicity of testing mentioned above can be waived in this specific instance. Dunnett and Gent [33] showed that because the hypothesis of non-inferiority is nested inside that of superiority (the latter always implies the former, for a given population), we can conduct both tests without adjusting for multiple comparisons. Wiens [34, informatively titled 'Something for nothing in non-inferiority / superiority testing: a caution'] pointed out that Dunnett and Gent's results crucially depend upon the same strategies (ITT vs. per-protocol) being used for each analysis. Although superiority trials usually use the ITT strategy for their primary analyses, 'Intent-to-treat in non-inferiority vs. superiority trials: which analysis population should be used?' (above) warns that both ITT and per-protocol strategies are relevant for non-inferiority trials. It is certainly possible for an ITT analysis to show superiority while a per-protocol analysis of the same data fails to demonstrate non-inferiority. How then would investigators interpret simultaneous superiority and inferiority?

Summary

In conclusion, non-inferiority trials can make useful scientific contributions when ethical considerations disallow a placebo or other inactive control. However, unlike the scenario of a superiority trial with a placebo, their assay sensitivity is not directly ensured by randomized comparison and so there are numerous cautions in their use. In particular, the measures of study quality mentioned in 'Key comparisons between superiority and non-inferiority trials' should be carefully examined. Finally, when interpreting results it is important to remember that non-inferiority can be shown only with respect to a given margin and is only as relevant as that margin.

References

1. Chi GYH, Chen G, Rothmann, M, and Li, N. Active control trials. In Chow SC, ed. *Encyclopedia of Biopharmaceutical Statistics* 3rd ed. London: Informa Health Care, 2010; 8–15.

2. Temple R, Ellenberg SS. Placebo-controlled trials and active-control trials in the evaluation of new treatments. Part 1: Ethical and scientific issues. *Ann Intern Med* 2000; **133**: 455–463.

3. Ellenberg SS, Temple R. Placebo-controlled trials and active-control trials in the evaluation of new treatments. Part 2: Practical issues and specific cases. *Ann Intern Med* 2000; **133**: 464–470.

4. Endrenyi, L. Bioequivalence. In *The Encyclopedia of Biostatistics*, 2nd ed. P Armitage and T Colton, eds. New York, Wiley, 2010.

5. Fisher RA. The arrangement of field experiments. *J Min Agric Great Britain* 1926; **33**: 503–513.

6. Friedman LM, Furberg CD, DeMets, DL. *Fundamentals of Clinical Trials*, 3rd ed. New York, Springer-Verlag, 1998.

7. Armitage P. The role of randomization in clinical trials. *Stat Med* 1982; **1**: 345–52.

8. Kempthorne O. *The Design and Analysis of Experiments*. New York, Wiley, 1952.

9. DeMets, DL, Cook, TD and Roecker, E. Selected issues in the analysis. In *Introduction to Statistical Methods for Clinical Trials*, DL DeMets and TD Cook, eds. Boca Raton, FL, Chapman & Hall/CRC, 2008.

10. Bath, P. Acute stroke. In *Textbook of Clinical Trials*, 2nd ed. D Machin, S Day, and S Green, eds. Chichester, John Wiley & Sons, 2006.

11. Day, S. Blinding or Masking. In *The Encyclopedia of Biostatistics*, 2nd ed. P Armitage and T Colton, eds. New York, Wiley, 2010.

12. International Conference of Harmonisation. Guideline E3: Choice of Control Group and Related Issues in Clinical Trials. 2000. http://www.ich.org/cache/compo/475-272-1.html#E3

13. Halperin JL. Ximelagatran compared with warfarin for prevention of thromboembolism in patients with nonvalvular atrial fibrillation: Rationale, objectives, and design of a pair of clinical studies and baseline patient characteristics (SPORTIF III and V). *Am Heart J* 2003; **146**, 431–8.

14. Hankey JH, Klijn CJM, and Eikelboom JW. Ximelagatran or Warfarin for stroke prevention in patients with atrial fibrillation? *Stroke* 2004; **35**: 389–391.

15. Julious, SA. *Sample Sizes for Clinical Trials*. Boca Raton, FL, Chapman & Hall/CRC, 2010.

16. Fleming, T. Current issues in non-inferiority trials. *Stat Med* 2008; **27**: 317–32.

17. Friedlin B, Korn EL, George, SL, Gray R. Randomized clinical trial design for assessing noninferiority when superiority is expected. *J Clin Onc* 2007; **25**: 5019–5023.

18. Temple, R. Government viewpoint of clinical trials. *Drug Inf J* 1982; **16**: 10–17.

19. Hauck, WW and Anderson, S. Some issues in the design and analysis of equivalence trials. *Drug Inf J* 1999; **33**: 109–118.

20. Wiens BL, Zhou W. The role of intention to treat in analysis of noninferiority studies. *Clinical Trials* 2007; **4**: 286–291.

21. Blackwelder W. Proving the null hypothesis in clinical trials. *Control Clinical Trials* 1982; **3**: 455–63.

22. Siegel JP. Equivalence and non-inferiority trials. *Am Heart J* 2000; **139**: S166–70.

23. Gould A. Another view of active-controlled trials. *Control Clin Trials* 1991; **12**: 474–85.

24. Hasselblad V, Kong DF. Statistical methods for comparison to placebo in active-control trials. *Drug Inf J* 2001; **35**: 435–49.

25. Snapinn SM. Alternatives for discounting in the analysis of noninferiority trials. *J Biopharm Stat* 2004; **14**: 263–73.

26. Kaul S, Diamond GA, and Weintraub, WS. Trials and tribulations of non-inferiority: the ximelagatran experience. *J Amer Coll Cardiol* 2005; **46**: 1986–95.

27. Klein, JP and Moeschberger, ML. *Survival Analysis*, 2nd ed. New York, Springer-Verlag, 2003.

28. Kwang IK. *Active-controlled noninferiority/equivalence trials: methods and practice*. In Buncher CR, Tsay JY,

eds. *Statistics in the Pharmaceutical Industry*. Boca Raton, FL, Chapman & Hall/CRC. 2006; 193–230.

29. Singer, IB. *A Crown of Feathers*. New York, Farrar, Straus and Giroux, 1973.

30. International Conference of Harmonisation. Guideline E10: Choice of Control Group and Related Issues in Clinical Trials. 2000. http://www.ich.org/cache/compo/475–272–1.html#E10.

31. Lachin J. Statistical properties of randomization in clinical trials. *Contr Clin Trials* 1988; **9**: 289–311.

32. Offen W, Chuang-Stein C, Dmitrienko, A *et al*. Multiple co-primary endpoints: Medical and statistical solutions. A report from the Multiple Endpoints Expert Team of the Parmaceutical Research and Manufacturers of America. *Drug Inf J* 2007; **41**: 31–46.

33. Dunnett CW, Gent M. An alternative to the use of two-sided tests in clinical trials. *Stat Med* 1996; **15**: 1729–1738.

34. Wiens BL. Something for nothing in noninferiority/superiority testing: a caution. *Drug Inf J* 2001; **35**: 241–245.

Chapter

14

Monitoring of clinical trials: Interim monitoring, data monitoring committees, and group sequential methods

Rickey E. Carter and Robert F. Woolson

Introduction

Accumulating data may be reviewed regularly in all phases of clinical development for decision-making based on safety or clinical benefit. In later phase clinical trials, especially phase 3 trials, this ongoing review ideally takes a comprehensive look at the trial's conduct, problems in clinical assessments, patient compliance, protocol adherence, patient safety, and patient response to therapy. For randomized controlled clinical trials, the review will also incorporate assessments of the integrity of the randomization and the maintenance of the treatment group assignment blind, in the event the trial is blinded, single or double. Clearly, these periodic evaluations are organized to meet the ethical obligations in conducting clinical research and protecting patients from undue harm. How these reviews are conducted, what is reviewed, and who conducts the reviews are critical features that impact the success in meeting these ethical obligations.

Randomized controlled therapeutic trials are often designed to compare two treatments, A & B, in an effort to decide which is superior. Randomization of a patient to treatment A or to treatment B can be defended ethically if clinical experts are truly uncertain which of the two is superior. This clinical uncertainty, *equipoise*, exists at the start of a trial, but accumulating data may alter this state as the trial proceeds. Therefore, a plan must be in place to review these data in a manner preserving the principles of sound research design. These research principles, at a minimum, include: an unbiased assessment of the two treatment groups, and the control of the statistical type I and type II error rates at the levels prescribed when the trial was launched. Simultaneously, this preservation of sound principles of research design can be secured while maintaining both individual patient safety, and the ethics of clinical practice.

This chapter discusses the process of reviewing accumulating clinical trial data in a formal manner. The presentation includes a discussion of the role of the Data Monitoring Committee (DMC), and a description of state-of-the-art statistical techniques of interim monitoring permitting ongoing review of these data. Together, these two elements of the DMC and interim monitoring contribute heavily to ethically and scientifically sound periodic reviews. In the next part, we provide an overview of the structure and the operations of a DMC. Following this the statistical issues and challenges of interim monitoring are elucidated; several commonly used approaches for interim monitoring are described. Applications to neurological clinical trials are considered; these illustrate the process and the challenge of monitoring efficacy data on an ongoing basis.

One example trial is the TOAST clinical trial. 'Trial of Org 10172 in Acute Stroke Treatment' (i.e., TOAST) was a phase 3 randomized, double-blind clinical trial examining the efficacy of a new antithrombotic drug for improving the outcome of persons with acute ischemic stroke [1]. The study was a joint effort of a number of academic medical centers, the National Institute Neurological Disease and Stroke (NINDS) and Organon, manufacturer of danaparoid (Org 10172), and this trial was organizationally complex with multiple components. The trial was funded primarily through formal grants from NINDS with additional support from Organon. Among the trial components were a clinical coordinating center, a statistical and data coordinating center, and a DMC. The total sample size was approximately 1200 participants and four interim analyses were planned and conducted over the course of the study. The study concluded with a non-significant efficacy difference between the ORG

Clinical Trials in Neurology, ed. Bernard Ravina, Jeffrey Cummings, Michael P. McDermott, and R. Michael Poole. Published by Cambridge University Press. © Cambridge University Press 2012.

10172 and placebo groups. In spite of the 'negative' finding of no difference in the primary efficacy outcome between the two treatment arms, important efficacy and safety information were gained. The complete study design was published [1], and the principal study findings have also been summarized [2]. The methods of this chapter will be illustrated using some information from these published papers.

Data monitoring committees and trial monitoring overview

Multi-center trials must be coordinated and administered efficiently. Often a set of committees is constituted to streamline this effort. While there is no single committee structure paradigm that fits every trial, there are several commonly used configurations. One such arrangement includes: a Steering Committee to govern overall study conduct; an Operations Committee to handle day-to-day decisions; a Publication Committee to form writing assignments and writing teams; and a DMC to monitor the trial on an ongoing basis.

With the exception of the DMC, members for these committees are selected primarily from the trial's clinical and scientific team. Thus, the trial's principal investigators, clinical investigators, biostatisticians, and other key trial leaders typically represent the pool from which committee members are chosen. In contrast, DMC members are frequently chosen from a group of individuals who are not actively involved in the trial, ideally limited to those individuals external to the trial and free from conflicts of interest. This degree of independence from the trial, investigators, and sponsors is a desirable attribute for the DMC to conduct its work in an unbiased manner. While a fully independent DMC is desired and should be viewed as a requirement for phase 3 registration trials, earlier phase clinical trials or clinical trials with particularly rare diseases may be unable to achieve complete independence. Furthermore, the degree of monitoring and independence of the committee should be commensurate with the risks of the interventions. These issues can be challenging to address and several groups provide guidance in this area, e.g., NIH Policy: http://grants.nih.gov/grants/guide/notice-files/not98–084.html.

Diverse membership is critical, since the DMC often will be the independent body responsible for monitoring the trial at intervals during the trial's conduct. The responsibility to perform independent review includes a review and evaluation of accumulated safety data as well as of key clinical efficacy data. Assessing the trial's performance and quality is also required, since a poorly conducted trial will be unable to test the trial hypotheses, and would therefore be unethical to continue. Clearly, expertise in clinical trial design and analysis is required in addition to clinical specialist knowledge of the disease. Specifically, from the scientific and clinical perspective it is important the DMC membership include experts in the clinical condition under investigation, experts in key related medical areas, biostatisticians with expertise in clinical trials and trial monitoring, and individuals in related areas specific to the trial. This last group might include bioethicists, basic science specialists, patient advocate representatives, and representatives from the public. The size and composition of the DMC should be commensurate with the risk and complexity of the study and the exact charge of the DMC.

For the DMC to provide effective safeguards for the human participants, the DMC must be fully informed of the trial's progress and have a mechanism for dialogue with the sponsor and investigators. This issue can be addressed by careful organization of the DMC meetings. Formal summary reports are prepared for the DMC's review or, in some cases, by members of the DMC itself. However, these reports only provide for one-way dialogue. A best practice is to have the reports distributed to the DMC sufficiently prior to the scheduled meeting so that a pre-meeting review of the materials can identify critical points that warrant clarification during the conduct of the DMC meeting. The conduct of this meeting should allow for dialogue with the investigative team while maintaining the scientific integrity of the trial. Typically, the meeting is conducted in at least two phases: an open session followed by a closed session. During the open session, representatives of the study team are invited to participate in the study's discussion, present an overview of the trial's current status and answer any questions that may have arisen during the pre-review of meeting materials. Often the summary reports prepared for the open session are called the Open Report. This summary report focuses on the overall study progress and does not provide any information about treatment group differences. This restriction is incorporated to minimize the risk of compromising the blind or otherwise jeopardize the scientific integrity of the study. After the open session draws to a close, the attendees not formally on the DMC are excused and a closed session begins. A Closed Report is prepared in advance for this session and is reviewed during the closed session. the closed session is when a formal confidential review of the entire trial occurs. The specific nature of both the open and closed sessions is detailed in writing in the form of a *DMC Charter*. This would include a detailed description of the planned open and closed reports.

A DMC is ordinarily constituted early in the life of a trial. Ideally, the committee is formed and has its initial meeting before the first patient is enrolled and randomized. As a first order of business the DMC must establish its template for its functioning. Many aspects of this template include the establishment and approval of a DMC Charter. This charter should be drafted by the trial organizers and the document is really a proposed protocol for the DMC's operations and functions. It is helpful if the trial organizers provide the first draft of this document, since they are among the most knowledgeable persons regarding what needs to be monitored for both safety and efficacy. The draft charter describes the DMC's responsibilities, identifies its members and chair, outlines the structure of tables and reports to be given to the DMC, describes the statistical plans for monitoring safety and efficacy, and includes a proposed set of times and intervals for DMC meetings. Most importantly, the DMC Charter identifies a clear delineation of the pathways of communication of the DMC with the trial investigators, sponsors and others. This last point requires careful consideration as the DMC must be mindful of its responsibility to protect confidentiality of trial results throughout the study. This draft charter is one that could be adopted by the DMC, or it might be revised and finalized by the DMC at this initial meeting. There is typically discussion regarding the statistical monitoring plan and the identification of threshold boundaries warranting special action should they be exceeded. This is one of the reasons it is best for this deliberation to take place before the trial's first patient is enrolled and randomized. Objectivity is essential in setting the monitoring and review guidelines. With no data available, this objectivity is easier to maintain and defend.

Once the charter is approved it becomes a central trial roadmap allowing others to see where the DMC will be going, and at the end where they have been. There are several excellent templates for a DMC Charter including Appendix A of Ellenberg, Fleming & DeMets [3] and NINDS provides templates for Open and Closed Reports on its website [4].

Composition and operations of a DMC

In TOAST the DMC was formed by the project's steering committee in consultation with, and with the approval of NINDS, the primary National Institutes of Health sponsor. The DMC members included individuals with no direct ties to the study and with no conflicts of interest. Hence, the DMC was constituted to be independent of the trial. After an initial DMC meeting at the trial's initiation, the DMC met face-to-face annually, and had multiple interim teleconferences. Each meeting began with an open session and key project investigators provided an overview of the trial's progress to date. This included an update on patient recruitment, data quality and study performance, and a summary of special issues requiring attention. The Statistical Center provided summary tables for the open session and for the closed session to follow. The open session attendees included the clinical principal investigators, the statistical investigators, project coordinators and additional appropriate staff, representatives from NINDS, representatives from Organon, and the DMC. In the open session no data were presented by treatment group; all data summaries were provided in the aggregate across the two treatment groups.

Following the open session, a closed session followed and those present included the DMC, the NINDS representative, and the study statisticians. (It is now more common for there to be a second statistical group preparing the DMC reports; this allows the study statistical group to remain blinded. This was not done in the TOAST trial.) Others were excused, but would be called back afterwards for a closing open session. Data presented at the closed session were separated by treatment group and depicted any differences in safety, efficacy, compliance, etc., between the two treatment groups. The DMC discussed any treatment group differences and interpreted the data to-date. In some cases additional analyses were requested by the DMC requiring the statistical center to do these and distribute these at a later date to the DMC. After the closed session the DMC met in executive session to form its recommendations. Following this, a final open session was held with the same attendees as the original open session. In this final session the DMC Chair delivered a set of recommendations and an evaluation of the trial to date. Following this the meeting adjourned. A meeting summary including overall recommendations of the DMC was prepared in writing following the meeting for distribution to the study investigators, sponsors and institutional review boards.

It is important to note that one of the major items to be reviewed in the closed DMC session was the accumulated efficacy data. The primary outcome in TOAST was favorable outcome at 3 months post-randomization. Patients were considered to have a favorable outcome if they had a good Glasgow Coma Score *and* a good Barthel Index (measure of activities of daily living). Thus, the favorable outcome assessment was a composite score. At each DMC meeting an interim analysis was done comparing the favorable outcome rates between the two treatment groups. A major challenge was to perform this comparison at each interim analysis while preserving the ability to do a valid comparison at the 5% significance level at the end of the trial. The rest of the chapter will deal with procedures for achieving these aims.

Mechanics/statistics of interim monitoring

A DMC's objectivity is in part due to independence of the members. A formal statistical framework can enhance the objectivity by providing a universal language to communicate the accumulating evidence. This part will introduce key terminology used in the statistical monitoring of clinical trials while motivating the need for this statistical framework.

Interim monitoring of efficacy and safety data & issues of multiple testing

Measuring an intervention's efficacy, for example, may require a complex battery of assessments in order to measure adequately the full scope of the disease or condition. Statistically, such a multi-faceted assessment introduces a set of hypothesis tests. The statistical implications of these multiple hypothesis tests can be characterized in the context of the well-known multiple comparisons problem. Added to this problem's complexity is the fact that modern clinical trials further introduce an additional dependency on this hypothesis testing problem. Namely, clinical trial data are routinely analyzed as the trial progresses (sequential analysis). This additional dependency dimension to the multiple testing setting is not as easily addressed by simple correction factors such as the Bonferroni adjustment. However, as this part will detail, statistical methodology has been developed to allow for the routine monitoring of a trial's accumulating data. This possibility enables the sound monitoring of the study. It

can be argued that *all* randomized clinical trials should consider some form of interim monitoring; the protocol should clearly detail how this monitoring will be accounted for in the final analysis. This part provides guidance for developing monitoring schemes.

Issue of multiplicity

Consider a setting where two or more measures are used to quantify the efficacy profile of an intervention. In the context of the TOAST trial, the Barthel Index and Glasgow Coma Scale were used to assess activities of daily living and level of consciousness, respectively. The NIH Stroke Scale was also used as a quantitative neurological exam, and finally, a supplemental motor exam was used to measure limb strength. In this scenario, there were four critical measures to assess an intervention's efficacy at improving post-stroke functioning. Intuitively, having four assessments increased the likelihood of declaring a treatment group difference. Thus, the power to detect a treatment group difference could be apparently increased, albeit at the cost of an increased type I error rate.

In usual statistical parlance, a type I error is a 'false positive' result. For example, when testing a single hypothesis, the probability of incorrectly concluding a significant effect (rejecting the null hypothesis) when in fact there is no effect is denoted as α. On the contrary, the probability of correctly failing to reject the null hypothesis when there is in fact no effect is $(1 - \alpha)$. When multiple statistical tests are performed, one obtains a set of hypothesis tests, each with a comparison-wise type I error rate. The family-wise error rate is the error rate for an entire collection of comparisons. Virtually any introductory biostatistics textbook describes many valid procedures for controlling one or the other of these rates. For interim testing the principle of a family-wise error rate applies to the notion of controlling the error rate for the entire collection of interim looks we take of the trial until its termination. We will return to this, but first we continue our general discussion of this concept of family-wise error rate.

To ensure the collection of hypothesis tests only contain α probability of any type I error (i.e., the family-wise error rate), the individual tolerance level for a type I error rate for each hypothesis test must be more rigorous ($\alpha' < \alpha$). Conceptually, a large number of tests each conducted at the 5% significance level is associated with a larger family-wise error rate than would a smaller number of tests each conducted at the 5% significance level [5]. This issue and approaches to managing the family-wise error rate have been fully discussed in clinical trial texts [6] and in the introductory biostatistics literature. With independent comparisons simple probability shows what can happen to the overall, i.e. family-wise, error rate. Suppose one intends to make two comparisons, each independent of one another, and suppose we plan to conduct each comparison at a type I error rate of 0.05. Under the hypothesis of no treatment group differences, the probability that one test does not reject the null is 0.95, (i.e., 1 – 0.05). If the two tests are independent, then the probability that *both* do not reject is (0.95) × (0.95) or 0.9025. Hence, the probability that at least one of the two tests rejects is 1 – 0.9025, or 0.0975. Thus, the family-wise error rate for this collection of two comparisons is not 0.05, but it is 0.0975. If you had c independent tests then the family-wise error rate would be $1 - (0.95)^c$. If $c = 5$, that is five independent tests, then the family-wise error rate can be calculated to be 0.2262. So, techniques to handle multiple comparisons evolved to allow us to lower the individual comparison rate to something smaller than 0.05 in order to keep the family-wise rate at 0.05. Interim testing in clinical trials builds on similar logic; although, the procedures are more involved since the interim comparisons are *not independent*, but are built on accumulating data (on the same endpoints) over time.

The probability of a false positive finding increases with repeated interim assessment of accumulating data from the same trial. This form of multiplicity presents special features because the probability of rejecting the null hypotheses is conditionally associated with previous examinations of the data. In fact, one could consider the probability of rejecting the null hypothesis at analysis K or earlier as

P(reject H_0 at Analysis K) $=$
P(reject at 1st look) $+ P$(reject at 2nd look |
did not reject at 1st)
$+... +$ (reject at K^{th} look | did not reject previously)

$$(14.1)$$

As with the regular multiple testing scenario, in order to control the overall type I family-wise error rate a higher degree of statistical evidence is required for rejecting the null hypotheses at each analysis (i.e., for the comparison at each analysis time) when this type of multiple testing is involved.

Contrary to the independent testing framework, however, an increased number of interim analyses does not inflate the type I error rate as appreciably as

one might expect (e.g., as it did in the preceding for independent tests). Ellenberg *et al.* illustrated the probability of a type I error based on the number of interim analyses for one-sided testing at $\alpha = 0.025$ [3]. With only one test, the type I error rate is the nominal 0.025, but with the addition of only one interim analysis halfway through the study, the error rate jumps to 0.041, a 64% increase. Adding additional interim analyses once one already has conducted one has a less pronounced effect on the inflation of the type I error rate. For example, with five total analyses, the type I error rate is 0.075, three times the nominal 0.025 rate, and with 10 analyses, the error rate is approximately four times the nominal rate (0.096). Thus, the greatest inflation in the type I error rate occurs when one moves from no interim analyses to *any* number of interim analyses. Thus, the relative 'penalty' for adding additional interim analyses is not as striking as adding additional hypothesis tests in the independent testing framework. Nonetheless, there is a significant inflation in the type I error rate when any interim analyses are performed. Therefore, there is a penalty and one must account for this when designing the study, if the intent is to keep the overall type I error for the trial at a prescribed level like 0.05 or 0.025, as is usually desired.

Two general approaches are available for specifying the required significance level for each of the successive evaluations of the data. The first method is a fully specified group sequential approach. This approach pre-specifies the stopping boundaries for all analyses. The second approach allows for more flexibility in the interim analyses in that unplanned analyses can be included while still providing appropriate control of the type I error rate. The presentation continues with a description of group sequential methods, followed by a more flexible design that increases practical utility.

Group sequential methods

Group sequential methods for determining the critical values to be used during interim analyses (i.e., 'stopping boundaries') represented a key advancement in the theory and application of sequential analyses. The design flexibility to allow for interim analyses fundamentally changed study design and provided a broad platform to monitor clinical trials. The group sequential foundation rests on two primary design considerations. The first consideration is that the number of analyses (interim analyses and the final analysis) is specified. Denote this number as k. The second consideration is

Table 14.1 Upper-limit critical values (stopping boundaries) for a Z-score required for termination due to efficacy at analysis point k, two-sided $\alpha = 0.05$

Planned analyses	Analysis number	Pocock	Haybittle-Peto	O'Brien-Fleming
1	1	1.95996	1.95996	1.95996
2	1	2.17827	3.00000	2.79651
	2	2.17827	1.96729	1.97743
3	1	2.28948	3.00000	3.47111
	2	2.28948	3.00000	2.45445
	3	2.28948	1.97510	2.00405
4	1	2.36129	3.00000	4.04862
	2	2.36129	3.00000	2.86281
	3	2.36129	3.00000	2.33747
	4	2.36129	1.98275	2.02431

the method in which the critical values will be selected. Clearly, these critical values for $k > 1$ need to be more stringent than the critical value if no interim analyses are to be conducted (i.e., $k = 1$). This is due to multiplicity in testing, which is the basis for the adjustment.

Specific stopping boundaries

While there are numerous stopping boundaries in the statistical literature, three are discussed here. The three methods differ in ease of implementation and intention, but all three are broadly applicable to clinical trials. They have been used widely. Pocock's method [7] is straightforward to implement since only one critical value is used through the study. A crucial limitation of this approach is that (relatively) little statistical evidence may be required to stop the trial early for efficacy but at the end of the trial, a p-value much less than the nominal error rate (α) is required to reject the null hypothesis. The Haybittle-Peto [8] method mirrors that of Pocock in that the same critical value is used for all interim analyses but a smaller critical value is used at the final analysis to bring the required level of significance more in line with the nominal error rate. To ensure overall control of the type I error rate, the stopping boundaries during the interim analyses are larger than that of Pocock's method, so this approach attenuates some of the concern with Pocock's method. A third group sequential method is due to O'Brien and Fleming [9]. Their approach allows for a gradation in the stopping boundaries with the first analysis requiring the largest amount of statistical evidence to reject the null hypothesis and concludes with the final analysis needing an observed level of significance very

near the nominal error rate. For analyses in the early study period, the required level of significance is much greater using the O'Brien-Fleming boundaries than the other two methods. Table 14.1 demonstrates the interrelationship of the number of analyses and the group sequential method. Note for $k > 2$, the Haybittle-Peto and O'Brien-Fleming approaches provide very similar final critical values. The key distinction between the two methods is the manner in which you reach the final critical value. O'Brien and Fleming's approach is such that a rejection of the null hypothesis is more likely during the mid-study period since a very conservative hypothesis test was conducted first early in the study. This judicious selection of the testing strategy is emphasized with the next part on α spending functions and flexible designs.

Flexible design methods

Clinical trials require rigor in the protocol to ensure consistency across multiple sites and reproducibility of the findings. However well-designed the protocol is, there is the likelihood that the study may progress in a manner that is generally unanticipated. This could be as straightforward as accrual being lower than anticipated, or there could be scientific concerns raised during the course of the study that warrant a more frequent examination of the study data. This could be driven in part by the needs of the DMC or by new literature that may affect the risk-to-benefit ratio. For all of these situations, having rigor in the analysis plan while balancing the ever present need to ensure human subject safety is essential. Flexible designs are well suited to meet this need. These designs relax the assumptions of the group sequential methodology. Specifically, these flexible designs allow the modification of k and the timing and spacing of the interim looks. Spending functions are the principal analytical tools permitting the flexibility in the study design. These spending functions are robust tools for dynamic application, and therefore are ideally applicable to large complex clinical trials. Spending functions primarily spend the α across the set of interim and final looks at the data. The general approach for 'spending' α over the course of a study is an important methodological advancement over the group sequential methodology.

Conceptually, the target α (say 0.05) is established a priori and each incremental analysis utilizes some of the available error. The rate of spending determines the overall stopping boundaries at any point during the study. Alpha spending functions have been developed to resemble a variety of group sequential stopping boundaries, with the O'Brien-Fleming-like boundaries being a highly attractive option for the reasons specified in the group sequential part above. A difference here is that we are now permitted to have unequally spaced evaluations or unplanned evaluations while still providing overall protection to the target α and β error rates. This protection requires complex conditional probability calculations, but greatly expands the capacity for trial monitoring.

Illustrative example

Prior to the formal introduction of the α spending functions, consider this scenario. Suppose a large phase 3 clinical trial has two formal efficacy interim analyses planned when 33% and 66% of the participants have the primary endpoint available for analysis. The protocol specifies that the O'Brien-Fleming group sequential stopping boundaries will be used to provide protection to the overall α level. According to Table 14.1, the three critical values (in absolute value for two-sided testing) required to have early stoppage of the trial due to efficacy are (3.47, 2.45, 2.00). Suppose during the review of the first interim analysis, the DMC determined that waiting until 66% of the participants have been enrolled would be unacceptable and that an interim analysis should be conducted when 50% of the participants have been enrolled instead. Using traditional group sequential methods, this type of modification is not possible. Specifically, the group sequential methods are based on equally-spaced *preplanned* analyses. Using the α spending approach, we will see that

we can re-estimate the remaining stopping boundaries on the basis of the amount of α already spent. This is not to suggest that one should be casual with respect to the original statistical analysis plan, but rather to reinforce the importance of design flexibility when needed.

Alpha spending functions

Such design flexibility was made possible with the advent of α spending functions. An α spending function [10–12], $\alpha(\tau)$, is a monotonically increasing function that regulates the amount of type I error spent during each interim analysis as the proportion of the information (τ) increases. At the start of the trial, the function equals zero reflecting that none of the type I error rate has yet been spent. At the conclusion, the α spending function should be α, the preplanned type I error rate. In a theoretical sense, when $\tau = 100\%$ this would represent the minimum variance-covariance obtainable for the given sample size (i.e., Fisher's information). Determining the fraction of this theoretical quantity may appear daunting at first; however, in practice, for the common clinical trial settings the fraction depends on either the planned total sample size and/or the planned total number of events in survival analysis. In particular, for normally distributed outcomes measured only once, the observed fraction of the total theoretical information is $\tau = n_{obs}/n_{planned}$. For survival analyses, the fraction of τ is approximated by $\tau \approx d/D$, where d represents the number of observed events at the interim analysis when a total of D events are anticipated. For repeated measures analysis, τ may represent the proportion of observed measurements of the dependent variable divided by all potential measurements, or $\tau \approx r/NM$, where r, N, and M represent the observed number of dependent measurements at the interim analysis, the total number of planned participants, and the number of repeated measurements per participant, respectively.

There is great flexibility of the shape of the monotonic spending function provided the constraints $\alpha(0) = 0$ and $\alpha(1) = \alpha$ are incorporated. For example, a function that is concave up would spend a small amount of the α early in the study. This may be desirable since there is imprecision in these early trial estimates. Conversely, a concave down function would increase the likelihood of stopping early but at the expense that a significant portion of the α would be spent early in the trial. This translates into a large critical value (or a requirement for a very small p-value) at the end of the study, something that may be undesirable. While there is in fact an infinite number of potential spending functions, framing a spending function around the familiar group sequential boundaries of Pocock or O'Brien-Fleming has proven to be a useful method of selecting a spending function.

An O'Brien-Fleming-like α spending function is:

$$\alpha_{O-F}(\tau) = 2 - 2\Phi\left[\frac{Z_{1-\alpha/2}}{\tau^{1/2}}\right], \qquad (14.2)$$

and a Pocock-like α spending function is:

$$\alpha_p(\tau) = \alpha \ln[1 + (e-1)\tau] \qquad (14.3)$$

[11]. Generation of the critical values for values of τ for the first interim analysis can be easily accomplished by hand, but generation of multiple stopping points (which are conditional on previous examinations) can be complicated. Use of specialized software is recommended in these settings. Before turning to this it is appropriate to comment on futility, or the lack of efficacy, which could be the basis for early study termination.

'Futility' analyses

The development of group sequential methods and α spending functions thus far has focused on early termination due to efficacy. When early termination for efficacy is considered, one has generally observed at interim analysis a test statistic value that exceeds the pre-determined stopping boundary. One could argue that a very strong reversal in the direction of the treatment effect would need to be observed for the effect to no longer be significant at the end of the trial, and based

on the most current information (the trial to date), the likelihood of this would be very low. Thus, *equipoise* is not present so early termination may be warranted. On the contrary, early termination due to a low probability of reaching a statistically significant conclusion is also justification for early termination. So called futility analyses address this concern. It is important to distinguish this type of interim analyses from the phase 2 futility design and analyses described in Chapter 8.

Futility analyses utilize the concept of stochastic curtailment to determine the likelihood of obtaining a statistically significant result based on the accumulating data obtained in the course of the study [13–14]. The rationale for early termination for futility mirrors that for early termination due to efficacy. In particular, based on the data accrued to date in the study, the likelihood of *crossing* the stopping boundaries is particularly low. Conditional power is used to determine the probability of concluding a statistically significant result. This power is calculated *conditionally* on the data observed to date. Figure 14.1 describes the interaction of conditional power with unconditional power (i.e., power estimated prior to the start of the study).

Lan and Wittes [15] provide formulas based on the 'B-value', a sample size independent quantity representing accumulating data, to calculate conditional power for a variety of settings. Ideally, one would want conditional power to remain in the range of the protocol's assumed power, but interpreting what is 'high' and what is 'low' is difficult, particularly if the decision is post hoc. Lan *et al.* [16] recommend a threshold for low to high conditional power in the range of 0.5 to 1.0, and specification of a lower limit for conditional power in the DMC Charter may prove useful in interpreting the

		Conditional power	
		Low	High
Unconditional power ('planned power')	Low	Early stoppage due to futility should be considered	Larger than anticipated effect or less variability observed, continue the trial
	High	If early in the study, need to consider imprecision in estimates but monitoring more closely is warranted. If in the mid- or late- stage of the study, consider early termination if safety profile is marginal. Consider maintaining the study if risks are acceptable so that a more informed conclusion regarding the alternative hypothesis can be made.	Continue study, but early termination due to efficacy may be possible.

Figure 14.1. Interrelationship of unconditional power with conditional power.

calculations. Note that at study completion, the null hypothesis will be either rejected or not, so high conditional power along the course of the study is generally desirable. Low conditional power, however, does not rule out the likelihood of rejecting the null hypothesis, so one must be aware of the potential inflation to the false negative error rate when considering early termination due to low conditional power.

A less formal method of estimating conditional power is to re-evaluate the sample size assumptions in the context of the accumulating data. Power can be re-estimated based on the minimum clinically significant difference defined in the protocol and the *observed* variation in the primary endpoint. It is not unreasonable to expect that changes in the assumed (within group) standard deviation may occur in a large phase 3 study, so reassessment of the necessary sample size may be warranted to allow for adequate power to detect the minimum clinically significant difference. Such considerations fall under the rapidly developing area of adaptive designs (see Chapter 9).

Fully sequential designs

While group sequential methods have broad applicability, there are sequential designs that involve examining the primary endpoint after *every* participant (or every two or three participants). For this approach, the endpoint needs to be available before the next participant is enrolled. For safety studies (e.g. phase 1 studies) with a clearly defined adverse event endpoint, this approach is often employed and the '3 + 3' or 'up/down' designs are examples of this more traditional sequential approach. For efficacy trials, particularly multicenter studies, this approach has numerous logistical issues to be overcome. That said, there are cases where the fully sequential designs could be appropriate, but in the context of neurology trials, which often require long-term follow-up to assess efficacy, their use will be less common. As such, the methods will not be covered further.

Use of statistical software for interim analyses

The statistical underpinnings of the methods discussed are complex computationally and are enabled through the use of specialized software. With recent additions to the SAS System and the increased popularity of R, the implementation of the methods is straightforward and broadly available. This part discusses three software approaches: R, SAS, and EAST. It is worth noting that the calculations often require polynomial approximations and numerical integration of approximated functions and are intense computationally. Practically, the use of approximation integrals can introduce trivial differences in the estimated stopping boundaries across statistical software. For this reason, it is important that the protocol specify the software used for calculations so that the stopping boundaries are reproducible and consistent over time.

This part does not provide comprehensive details regarding the use of each software, instead general features will be illustrated. To illustrate the calculations, a clinical trial with three planned analyses $\tau = \{0.33, 0.66, 1.00\}$ and the O'Brien-Fleming-like α spending function will be used. This scenario will be modified to include the addition of an unplanned analysis when 50% of the participants have the outcome measured ($\tau = \{0.33, 0.50, 0.66, 1.00\}$) as was illustrated earlier. The generation of the stopping bounds will be illustrated using R. The remaining two software approaches are described in the context of increased functionality over R, which is somewhat rudimentary.

The R-project is an open-source statistical computing environment, and users have contributed numerous modules ('packages') that contain programming code for specific analyses. There are several packages available within R to create the stopping boundaries, but for this presentation, the ldBounds package will be illustrated [17]. The ldBounds package is distributed through GNU-2 public license and comes with software documentation in the form of a help file [17]. Interface with the software is through command-line syntax in R. This implementation is most basic and only produces the stopping boundaries. Nonetheless, ldBounds may prove sufficient for many statisticians working on trials.

Generation of the stopping bounds for the illustrative scenario uses the 'bounds' command that is available once the ldBounds package is loaded. Figure 14.2 provides the necessary syntax to generate the original and modified study design. Note that the original stopping boundary ($|z|>3.7307$ @ $\tau = 0.33$) is unaffected by the addition of an extra interim analysis at $\tau = 0.50$. Furthermore, the final stopping boundary remained essentially identical ($|z|>1.9917$ vs. $|z|>1.9931$) with the addition of this one additional interim look. The same could be said for the originally planned second interim analysis ($|z|>2.5262$ vs. $|z|>2.5546$). This is an illustration of a point made earlier in the chapter;

Original (Planned) Study Design

R Syntax
```
> times1<-c(0.33,0.66,1.0)
> obf_original <-bounds(times1,iuse=c(1,1),alpha=c(0.025,0.025))
> summary(obf_original)
```

Output
```
Lan-DeMets bounds for a given spending function

n = 3
Overall alpha: 0.05

Type: Two-Sided Symmetric Bounds
Lower alpha: 0.025
Upper alpha: 0.025
Spending function: O'Brien-Fleming

Boundaries:
 Time Lower Upper Exit pr. Diff. pr.
1 0.33 -3.7307 3.7307 0.00019097 0.00019097
2 0.66 -2.5262 2.5262 0.01159656 0.01140558
3 1.00 -1.9917 1.9917 0.05000000 0.03840344
```

```
/*******************************************************/
```
Modified Study Design

R Syntax
```
> times2<-c(0.33,0.5, 0.66,1.0)
> obf_modified <-bounds(times2,iuse=c(1,1),alpha=c(0.025,0.025))
> summary(obf_modified)
```

Output
```
Lan-DeMets bounds for a given spending function

n = 4
Overall alpha: 0.05

Type: Two-Sided Symmetric Bounds
Lower alpha: 0.025
Upper alpha: 0.025
Spending function: O'Brien-Fleming

Boundaries:
 Time Lower Upper Exit pr. Diff. pr.
1 0.33 -3.7307 3.7307 0.00019097 0.00019097
2 0.50 -2.9692 2.9692 0.00305065 0.00285967
3 0.66 -2.5546 2.5546 0.01159656 0.00854591
4 1.00 -1.9931 1.9931 0.05000000 0.03840344
```

Figure 14.2. Command syntax and summary output from R using the ldBounds package.

namely, once a study is designed to include at least one interim analysis, the relative effect of a small number of additional analyses does not appreciably change the overall significance level.

SAS Version 9.2 for Windows incorporates new procedures for the design (PROC SEQDESIGN) and testing (PROC SEQTEST) of studies involving interim analyses. Prior versions of SAS utilized SAS MACROs to perform the necessary calculations. One of the more

informative set of MACROs are fully documented in an excellent general reference by Dmitrienko *et al* [18]. For the new SAS procedures, SAS provides thorough documentation in the software's help files with numerous examples.

In contrast to the ldBounds implementation in R, PROC SEQDESIGN includes provisions to estimate sample size during the design phase. This integration allows for estimates of expected sample sizes under the null and alternative hypotheses. In the context of study management and budget, these additional estimates could prove highly informative. Additionally, SAS provides computational routines for estimating conditional power. Since this is a new release, the level of sophistication and flexibility of the SAS offerings does not yet reach that offered by Cytel's EAST, but it may prove to be a very viable software package considering the widespread installation base for SAS.

EAST is a comprehensive design and analysis software tool and may be the most comprehensive of the three approaches described here. Like SAS, generation of the stopping boundaries coincides with the description of the distribution of the primary endpoint and the estimation of the sample size. For this reason, using EAST requires the largest amount of training, particularly if one is only seeking to generate general stopping boundaries. The interface, however, is intuitive and the software comes with comprehensive help files. This software is designed to be used throughout the course of the study. In doing so, estimates of conditional power, additions of unplanned analyses, and graphical displays of study estimates are readily available from within a single software. EAST is highly regarded as an excellent tool for interim monitoring of clinical trials; however, the other approaches do allow for application of the methods discussed in this chapter.

Recommendations and additional considerations

Selection of the stopping boundaries has been an active area of theoretical statistical research. Jennison and Turnbull [19] provide an excellent summary of this development in their comprehensive textbook on sequential methods for clinical trials. Each of the developed methods strives to balance several considerations. To present these considerations, a study will be divided into three coarse categories reflecting the amount of data and/or sample size accrued. The 'early' study category reflects the trial when a small fraction of the subjects have been enrolled (e.g., 30%). During this phase of the study, one would expect limited power for efficacy and imprecision in the estimates. The 'mid-study' category is when the treatment effects should be estimated with reasonable precision and informed decisions could be made regarding the protocol's assumptions (hypothesized effect size, sample size estimates, etc.). The 'late study' phase is when the final participants are being enrolled (perhaps 70–100%

of the planned sample size). One would expect during this phase that the treatment effects are estimated with desired precision and the final subjects will provide the additional observations to minimize the estimated standard errors so that the targeted power is obtained. Figure 14.3 presents a broader overview of these points.

Stopping boundary selection and interim analysis frequency

Using the framework presented in Figure 14.3, an interim analysis plan may ideally allow for an early study interim analysis with minimal impact on the overall type I error rate. One or more interim analyses during the middle period of the study would be viewed as critical to the ongoing management of the study. It is debatable as to whether interim monitoring is required late in the study. Thus, using equally spaced analyses (pure group sequential methods), $k = 2$ or 3 are attractive options.

When $k = 2$, one interim analysis will be conducted often when 50% of the study is complete. This approach is useful when the intervention has had numerous prior investigations so that the protocol assumptions are likely realistic. Virtually any of the group sequential methods discussed here would be appropriate when $k = 2$. When there is uncertainty with the assumptions, additional interim analyses are recommended. If using group sequential methods, it is recommended that only $k = 3$ and the O'Brien-Fleming stopping boundaries be used. This approach allows for interim analyses at 33% and 66% of the participant accrual. These time periods are included in the mid-study phase and a large treatment effect will be required to stop the trial with only 33% of the study data. When $k > 3$ and equally spaced analyses are planned, one or more interim analysis will be conducted late in the study. If more flexibility with testing is desired, particularly when we need flexibility to 'front load' the analyses in the early and mid-periods of the study, an α spending approach should be considered. The O'Brien-Fleming-like α spending function is an attractive choice, particularly if interim analyses will be conducted very early in the study's accrual. Finally, there may be practical issues governing the timing and spacing of interim analyses. For example, the DMC may plan to meet semi-annually and may also require a formal interim look at those times. Thus, the DMC Charter would provide this prescription governing the number and timing of the interim looks.

Clinical trial progress category	Efficacy considerations	Safety considerations
Early study: 30% or less of the sample size accrued	*Features:* • Unstable treatment effects • Wide confidence intervals *Implications:* • Only profound differences should warrant consideration for termination due to efficacy • Early study efficacy analysis could be viewed as a "practice run": ensure endpoint availability, data quality, etc.	*Features* • Only high incident events likely to be observed • Confidence intervals on event rates will provide little useful information *Implications:* • Unlikely trial could be stopped due to safety unless there is a vastly different risk profile or unanticipated complications are observed
Mid-study: 30–70% of the sample size accrued	*Features:* • Treatment effects can be estimated with reasonable precision • Point estimates can be compared to study/sample size assumptions *Implications:* • Critical period where efficacy and study assumptions should be validated • Termination due to efficacy and futility potential	*Features:* • Common, anticipated events observed in sufficient numbers to provide reasonable summaries • Rare and/or serious events may be observed, but probability of observation is still low *Implications:* • Critical to evaluate expected vs. unanticipated events to ensure study risks are appropriately communicated • Excessive unanticipated events may warrant early termination
Late study: 70% or more of the sample size accrued	*Features:* • Stable parameter estimates • Borderline to acceptable power for hypothesized clinical effect *Implications:* • Efficacy monitoring late in the study may be unnecessary and will result in lower than desired power due to increased "alpha spending" • Critical decisions regarding stopping for efficacy should have occurred previously	*Features:* • Maximum amount of safety data will be available • For large clinical trials (n>400), rare events (1%–5%) have reasonable probability of being observed; extremely rare (<1%) may not be observable *Implications:* • Adverse events rates between treatment groups can be quantified with acceptable precision

Figure 14.3. Statistical considerations related to the amount of study information available.

Sample size considerations

Whether group sequential methods or a flexible design approach is implemented, a result is that a greater amount of evidence (larger test statistic) is needed over the course of the study to reject the null hypotheses. Thus, the overall sample size required to test the same effect size is larger with planned interim analyses if the null hypothesis is true. On the other hand, if the alternative hypothesis is true, the expected sample size using interim analyses is actually lower [19].

Further, in practice, both forms of multiplicity (multiple endpoints/comparisons and sequential tests) readily occur and require attention in the statistical plan. A simple solution to addressing this is to first determine how the multiple endpoints will be addressed through the correction to the α level. This will determine the per-comparison level of significance for each endpoint. It is this adjusted level that can be used when planning the study for sequential analyses. It is comforting to note that the statistical literature suggests very little sample size inflation for the O'Brien-Fleming monitoring of a single endpoint. There is a slight increase, but given the massive uncertainties in other aspects of sample size estimation, the relative magnitude of this adjustment is of little practical importance and can often be disregarded.

Stopping is not always mathematically justified

Reaching conclusions regarding continuation or discontinuation of a study are rarely black and white. In the case an intervention lacks a sufficient safety profile and the dosage cannot be adjusted to improve the safety for the human participants, early termination of the study may be easily recommend. However, it is worth noting that this decision may not be from a statistically supported conclusion. Safety concerns do not equate with false positive results the same as in an efficacy scenario. In fact, a false positive result with safety (concluding the risk: benefit ratio is unfavorable) will likely slow the development of an intervention by suggesting that additional research is needed before the intervention moves forward. This is essential to the safety of the human participants and the population that may ultimately be a candidate for the intervention.

This part has focused on the statistical aspects of monitoring efficacy and safety data from a statistical and/or hypotheses oriented view. However, the reader should bear in mind that there are other aspects of routine trial monitoring. First, the study's data quality control process provides ongoing assessment of data quality. Good clinical practice provides recommendations for the data quality standard to which all studies should adhere [20]. If in the course of the study it is observed that data quality is poor (untimely, copious data entry mistakes, monitoring reports with numerous source document to case report form discrepancies, etc.) the trial may be stopped temporarily or permanently to account for these issues. Likewise, new information may become available that changes the risk: benefit ratio. These situations and many more are generally outside the purview of statistical decisions but are just as important to the scientific integrity of the study.

Comments

Statistically appropriate monitoring of a clinical trial by an independent DMC improves the safety to the participants while maintaining the scientific integrity of the study. All clinical trials should consider the need for interim analysis. While large phase 3 studies should include interim analyses, smaller studies will still benefit from the inclusion of an independent DMC and formal statistical monitoring.

References

1. Adams HP, Jr. Woolson RF and Clarke WR, *et al*. Design of the TRIAL of Org 10172 in Acute Stroke Treatment (TOAST). *Control Clin Trials* 1997; **18**: 358–77.

2. The Publications Committee for the Trial of ORG 10172 in Acute Stroke Treatment (TOAST) Investigators.

Low molecular weight heparinoid, ORG 10172 (danaparoid), and outcome after acute ischemic stroke: a randomized controlled trial. *JAMA* 1998; **279**: 1265–72.

3. Ellenberg SG, Fleming TR and DeMets DL. *Data Monitoring Committees in Clinical Trials: a practical perspective*. New York: John Wiley & Sons, LTD, 2003.

4. NINDS. Outline of DSMB Report. 2010. http://www.ninds.nih.gov/research/clinical_research/policies/dsmb_outline.htm (Accessed September 9, 2010.)

5. Carter RE. A simple illustration for the need of multiple comparison. *Teach Stat* 2010; **32**: 90–91.

6. Piantadosi S. *Clinical Trials: a methodologic perspective* (2nd ed.). Hoboken, NJ: John Wiley & Sons, Inc, 2005.

7. Pocock SJ. Interim analyses for randomized clinical trials: the group sequential approach. *Biometrics* 1982; **38**: 153–62.

8. Haybittle JL. Repeated assessment of results in clinical trials of cancer treatment. *Br J Radiol* 1971; **44**: 793–7.

9. O'Brien PC and Fleming TR. A multiple testing procedure for clinical trials. *Biometrics* 1979; **35**: 549–56.

10. Lan KKG and DeMets DL. Discrete sequential boundaries for clinical trials. *Biometrika* 1983; **70**: 659–63.

11. Lan KKG and DeMets DL. Changing frequency of interim analyses in sequential monitoring. *Biometrics* 1989; **45**: 1017–20.

12. Lan, KKG and DeMets DL. Group sequential procedures: calendar versus information time. *Statistics in Medicine* 1989; **8**: 1191–8.

13. Halperin M, Lan KK, Ware JH, *et al*. An aid to data monitoring in long-term clinical trials. *Control Clin Trials* 1982; **3**: 311–23.

14. Lan, KK, DeMets DL and Halperin M. More flexible sequential and non-sequential designs in long-term clinical trials. *Commun Stat* 1984; **13**: 2330–53.

15. Lan, KK and Wittes J. The B-value: a tool for monitoring data. *Biometrics* 1988; **44**: 579–85.

16. Lan KK, Simon R and Halperin M. Stochastically curtailed tests in long-term clinical trials. *Commun Stat* 1982; **C**(1): 207–19.

17. Casper C and Perez OA. Package 'ldbounds' 2006.

18. Dmitrienko A, Molenberghs G, Chuang-Stein C, *et al*. *Analysis of Clinical Trials Using SAS: a practical guide*. Cary, NC: SAS Institute Inc, 2005.

19. Jennison C and Turnbull BW. *Group Sequential Methods with Applications to Clinical Trials*. New York: Chapman & Hall/CRC, 2000.

20. ICH harmonised tripartite guideline: guideline for good clinical practice E6(R1), 1996.

Clinical approaches to post-marketing drug safety assessment

Gerald J. Dal Pan

Introduction

Monitoring and understanding the safety of drug and therapeutic biological products is a process that proceeds throughout the product's life cycle, spanning the period prior to first administration to humans through the entire marketing life of the product. Pre-approval drug safety assessment includes animal toxicology and pharmacology studies, clinical pharmacology studies (also known as phase 1 studies), proof-of-principle studies for the disease or condition under study (also known as phase 2 studies), and confirmatory studies of safety and efficacy (also known as phase 3 studies). In each of these stages of drug development, important drug safety information is obtained. These topics have been covered elsewhere in detail [1].

At the time a drug product is approved, there is a substantial amount of data regarding its safety profile. In the pre-approval review process, FDA reviews these data, along with data on the product's efficacy, to determine if the potential benefits of the drug exceed the potential risks for its intended use. As part of the approval process, FDA reviews the product's professional labeling (also referred to as the package insert), to insure that, amongst other things, the product's uses and its risks are explained. Risks of the products are presented in the following sections of the label: Highlights, Boxed Warnings, Contraindications, Warnings and Precautions, and Adverse Reactions [2,3].

Though the pre-approval testing of a drug is very rigorous, and the review of the data is very thorough, there are still some uncertainties about the complete safety profile of a drug when it is brought to market. Several factors contribute to these uncertainties. First, the number of patients treated with the drug prior to approval is limited, generally from several hundred to a few thousand. Second, patients in clinical trials tend to be carefully selected for inclusion in these trials, and are thus more clinically homogeneous than patients treated in the course of clinical practice once a drug is marketed. Compared to patients in clinical trials, patients treated in clinical practice may have a broader range of comorbidities, take a wider variety of concomitant medications, and have a wider spectrum of the underlying disease being treated. Third, additional populations of patients, such as children or the elderly, who may not have been studied in large numbers in clinical trials, may be treated with the product once it is marketed. In addition, marketed drug products are often used for diseases or conditions for which they are not indicated, or at doses outside of the approved range. Because of this 'off-label' use, patients treated in clinical practice are more diverse than those treated in clinical trials.

The goal of the post-marketing, or post-approval, safety program is to identify drug-related adverse events that were not identified prior to approval, to refine knowledge of the known adverse effects of the drug, and to understand better the conditions under which the safe use of the drug can be optimized.

The scope of this endeavor is broad. The core activity is usually the identification of previously unrecognized adverse events associated with the use of the drug. However, it is not sufficient simply to note that a drug can cause an adverse event. Rather, an investigation into not only the potential causal role of the drug in the development of the adverse event, but also into the conditions leading to the occurrence of the adverse event in one person or population and not in others should be the focus of any post-marketing drug safety effort. Factors such as dose-response relationships, drug-drug interactions, drug-disease interactions, drug-food interactions, and the possibility of medication error must be carefully considered.

Clinical Trials in Neurology, ed. Bernard Ravina, Jeffrey Cummings, Michael P. McDermott, and R. Michael Poole. Published by Cambridge University Press. © Cambridge University Press 2012.

A full understanding of the factors that can lead to a drug-related adverse event can, in some cases, lead to interventions that can minimize the severity or occurrence of the adverse event, and thus enhance the safe use of the drug. For this reason, the approach to understanding adverse events, especially serious adverse events, in the post-marketing period, must be as comprehensive as possible.

The identification of a new safety issue with a drug often begins with a single observation. Such observations may come from animal studies, chemical studies and assays, or observations of human experience with the drug. In the post-market period, such observations are usually clinical observations, often made at the point of care in the course of clinical practice. A practitioner or patient notes the development of symptoms or signs that were not present, or were present in less severe form, prior to the patient's using the medicine. If this sign or symptom is not listed in the product's approved labeling, patients and practitioners may not attribute it to the drug. If further evaluation reveals a clinically significant process (e.g., acute severe liver injury, rhabdomyolysis, agranulocytosis), it is important for the practitioner to keep a side effect due to a drug in the differential diagnosis of the event. If a medication side effect is not included in the differential diagnosis, a potential association between a drug and a previously unrecognized side effect will not be made, and the patient may not receive appropriate treatment. If, on the other hand, the practitioner believes the drug played a role in the development of the new clinical findings, he or she can forward relevant clinical information to either the drug's manufacturer or to a drug regulatory authority, such as the FDA in the US.

In the post-marketing period, the investigation of adverse events is a multi-disciplinary one. The analysis of a complex adverse event can involve the fields of medicine, pharmacy, epidemiology, statistics, pharmacology, toxicology, and others. A discussion of the role of each of these disciplines in drug safety assessment is beyond the scope of this chapter. This chapter will discuss the broad categories of clinical investigations used in post-market drug safety assessment.

This chapter will present an overview of the three main methods of clinical post-marketing safety assessment: case reports and case series, observational epidemiological studies, and clinical trials. As will be discussed, no one method is better than another. Rather, the choice of method depends on the particular safety question to be answered.

Case reports and case series

A core aspect of the post-approval drug safety system in the US is the reporting of adverse events to FDA. In the US, adverse events in individual patients are generally identified at the point of care. Patients, physicians, nurses, pharmacists, or anyone else at the point of care who suspects that there may be an association between an adverse event and a drug or therapeutic biological product can, but are generally not required, to report the adverse event to either the manufacturer or to the FDA.

The public – including health care professionals, patients, and consumers – can send reports directly to FDA via the MedWatch program (http://www.fda.gov/medwatch/), which was established in 1993 to allow health care providers and consumers to send a report about serious problems that they suspect are associated with any medical product (i.e., drug, biologic, device) directly to FDA. Members of the public can also report suspected adverse events to a product's manufacturer; the manufacturer, in turn, is then subject to regulations regarding the submission of these reports to FDA.

When the manufacturer of a product receives an adverse event report, it is required to report the event to the FDA. The specific reporting requirements depend both on the regulatory status of the product and on the nature of the event. In general, adverse events are defined as 'serious' if they result in any of the following outcomes:

> 'Death, a life-threatening adverse drug experience, inpatient hospitalization or prolongation of existing hospitalization, a persistent or significant disability/incapacity, or a congenital anomaly/birth defect. Important medical events that may not result in death, be life-threatening, or require hospitalization may be considered a serious adverse drug experience when, based upon appropriate medical judgment, they may jeopardize the patient or subject and may require medical or surgical intervention to prevent one of the outcomes listed in this definition. Examples of such medical events include allergic bronchospasm requiring intensive treatment in an emergency room or at home, blood dyscrasias or convulsions that do not result in inpatient hospitalization, or the development of drug dependency or drug abuse' [4].

Adverse events are also defined as 'unexpected' if they are:

> 'Not listed in the current labeling for the drug product. This includes events that may be symptomatically and pathophysiologically related to an event listed in the labeling, but differ from the event because of greater severity

or specificity. For example, under this definition, hepatic necrosis would be unexpected (by virtue of greater severity) if the labeling only referred to elevated hepatic enzymes or hepatitis. Similarly, cerebral thromboembolism and cerebral vasculitis would be unexpected (by virtue of greater specificity) if the labeling only listed cerebral vascular accidents. 'Unexpected,' as used in this definition, refers to an adverse drug experience that has not been previously observed (i.e., included in the labeling) rather than from the perspective of such experience not being anticipated from the pharmacological properties of the pharmaceutical product' [4].

From a public health perspective, adverse events that are both serious and unexpected are of the greatest concern, since information about such events may require regulatory action, such as a labeling change or dissemination of information to the public, on the part of FDA, the manufacturer, or both.

The above system of adverse event reporting is sometimes called a passive, spontaneous reporting system. It is called passive because FDA receives this information without actively seeking it out. It is called spontaneous because the persons who initially report the adverse events to either the FDA or to the manufacturer choose what events to report. Because this system of adverse event reporting is voluntary on the part of health care professionals, patients, and consumers, it is generally recognized that there is substantial underreporting of adverse events to FDA. Two survey-based studies conducted in the 1980s, one in Maryland [5] and the other in Rhode Island [6], examined physician reporting of adverse events to FDA, and concluded that fewer than 10% of adverse events were reported to FDA. These

studies were conducted prior to the development of the current MedWatch program in 1993, and do not consider the contribution of reporting from sources other than physicians. Calculating the proportion of adverse event reports that FDA actually receives requires that the true number of adverse events in the population be known. For most adverse events, this number is not known. In some cases, however, data are available that allow an estimate of the extent of reporting to be calculated. For example, the extent of reporting to FDA cases of hospitalized rhabdomyolysis associated with statin use was estimated using a projected estimate of the number of such cases in the US and comparing it to the number of reports of statin-associated hospitalized rhabdomyolysis in FDA's Adverse Event Reporting System, a database that houses FDA's post-marketing adverse event reports [7]. The projected national estimate was obtained by using incidence rates obtained from a population-based cohort study [8], and applying those incidence rates to national estimates of statin use. Across four statins (atorvastatin, cerivastatin, pravastatin, and simvastatin), the estimated overall extent of adverse event reporting was 17.7%. For individual statins, the estimated extent of reporting ranged from 5.0% (atorvastatin) to 31.2% (cerivastatin). Further analysis revealed that the high proportion of reporting of cerivastatin cases was driven by reports received after the dissemination of a Dear Health care Professional Letter noting physicians of the risks of cerivastatin-associated rhabdomyolysis. The estimated extent of reporting was 14.8% before the letter and rose to 35.0% after. It is important to note that the results of this study apply only to reporting cases of statin-

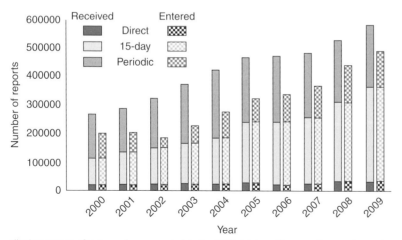

Figure 15.1. Number of direct, 15-day, and periodic reports received (solid bars) and entered (checkered bars) into the FDA Adverse Event Reporting System (AERS) from 2000 through 2009. FDA receives direct reports straight from the public; 15-day reports and periodic reports are submitted to FDA by industry. The 15-day reports describe adverse events that are both serious and unexpected (i.e., not in the product's approved labeling), as well as adverse events from post-approval clinical trials that are serious, unexpected, and judged to be reasonably associated with the drug. Industry submits all other adverse event reports as periodic reports. FDA enters all direct reports, 15-day reports, and all other reports of serious adverse events into the AERS database. Reports of non-serious adverse events are entered only for new-molecular entities in the first 3 years of marketing.

associated rhabdomyolysis. The extent of reporting for different drug-adverse pairs will be different, and can not be estimated from the results of this study.

FDA receives over 500,000 adverse event reports a year; approximately 94% are from manufacturers; the remainder are directly from the public via the MedWatch system. The number of reports has been increasing over the past decade (Figure 15.1). Many manufacturers submit reports to FDA electronically, using the standards set forth by the International Conference on Harmonisation (ICH) [9,10], which includes regulators and industry representatives from three regions, the US, Japan, and the European Union [9,10].

The adverse event reports that FDA receives from the public and from the manufacturers are entered into a database known as the Adverse Event Reporting System (AERS), which contains about 5 million adverse event reports. Adverse events in AERS are coded using a system called MedDRA, the Medical Dictionary for Regulatory Activities [11].

Other large databases of post-marketing adverse events are the European Medicine Agency's Eudravigilance and the World Health Organization's Vigibase. In large databases, datamining techniques can be applied to identify previously unrecognized potential drug-related adverse events [12,13].

The review of case reports of suspected adverse events is a complex process that has been described elsewhere [14]. It typically begins by identifying one or more case reports with the outcome of interest (e.g., aplastic anemia). Because the case reports that form a case series often come from several sources that do not report adverse events in a standardized way, it is usually necessary to develop a case definition. The case definition centers around the clinical characteristics of the event of interest, without regard to the causal role of the drug whose relationship to the adverse event is being investigated. Once a case definition is established, each report is reviewed to determine if the event meets the case definition and if the report is to be included in the case series. Depending on the specific question(s) to be answered by the case series, other exclusion criteria may also apply. For example, one would generally exclude a case in which the report provides no evidence that the patients ever took the drug of interest. In other cases, one may restrict the case series to only certain formulations of the drug if the drug safety question concerns some formulations but not others (e.g., include case reports in which an intravenous formulation, but not

an oral formulation, was used). In other cases, it may be appropriate to restrict case reports to certain age groups (e.g., limit the case series to only case reports describing the suspected adverse events in pediatric patients), or to certain indications for use (e.g., limit the case series to case reports in which the drug was used for a certain off-label indication). Exclusion criteria for a case series must be carefully considered so that potentially relevant cases are not excluded. In general, if the purpose of the case series is to examine the relationship between a drug and a suspected adverse event that has not been previously associated with the drug, it is best to include as many case reports as possible in the case series, and to minimize the number of excluded cases.

Once the case series has been developed, it is next necessary to review each case report individually in order to determine if there is a plausible causal relationship between the drug and the adverse event. At the level of the individual case report, it is often difficult to establish with certainty that the drug caused the adverse event of interest. For example, if the adverse event of interest is one that is common in persons with the disease or condition for which the drug is indicated when the drug is not used, establishing a causal role for the medicine in the development of the adverse event is generally not possible. For example, the incidence of Parkinson's disease is much higher in persons over age 60 years than it is in persons below that age [15]. In this situation, review of a report describing a myocardial infarction in a 70-year-old patient on an anti-parkinsonian agent will generally not be informative in determining if the anti-parkinsonian agent played a causal role in the development of the myocardial infarction, as myocardial infarction occurs commonly in this age group. Similarly, review of a case report is not likely to shed light on the causal relationship between a medicine and a suspected adverse event when the suspected adverse event is a manifestation of the underlying illness which the medicine is treating. For example, review of a case report of suicidal behavior in patients taking an antidepressant is not likely to be sufficient to establish a casual link between the suicidal behavior and the antidepressant. Review of a case series to establish a causal relationship between a drug and a suspected adverse event is most useful when the suspected adverse event is rare in the population when the medication is not used, is not a manifestation of the underlying disease, and is generally thought to be the result of exposure to a medicine. Examples of suspected adverse events in this category are acute hepatic failure, aplastic anemia, agranulocytosis, serious skin reactions such as Stevens-Johnson Syndrome and toxic epidermal necrolysis, and certain arrhythmias, such as torsade de points.

The approach to assessing the causal role of a medicine in the development of an adverse event has evolved over the past four decades [16,17]. In general, these approaches rely on a systematic review of each case report to ascertain the temporal relationship between drug use and the development of the adverse reaction, an assessment of any co-existing diseases or medications that could confound the relationship between the medicine and the adverse event, the clinical course after withdrawing the drug (de-challenge), and the clinical course after re-introduction of the drug (re-challenge). Naranjo and colleagues [18] have developed a quantitative method based on these general principles for estimating the probability that a drug caused an adverse clinical event. The World Health Organization [19] has developed a qualitative scale for categorizing causality assessments.

To help place reports of adverse events in a broader context, data on drug utilization are often incorporated into the analysis. Typically, these data provide information on the number of prescriptions dispensed for a given drug in a defined time period; in some cases data on the number of persons who have taken the drug may also be available. These data, which are obtained from commercial vendors, are used to calculate a reporting rate. The reporting rate is calculated by dividing the number of cases of an adverse event in persons taking a given drug reported in a defined time period by the number of prescriptions dispensed for that drug in a given time period. It is important to note that the reporting rate is not an incidence rate. The calculation of an incidence rate requires knowledge of the total number of cases of the adverse event in the population as well as knowledge of the total number of persons and the duration of drug exposure in the population taking the drug. Because the adverse event reporting systems only receive a small fraction of all drug-related adverse events occurring in the population, the total number of cases of the adverse event of interest is not available. In addition, the drug utilization data often report drug utilization in terms of number of dispensed prescriptions, not in terms of number of actual persons taking the medication. For these reasons, a reporting rate is not the same as an incidence rate. Nonetheless, despite some well-recognized limitations [20], reporting rates are useful for placing adverse event reports in a

population-based context, and for following trends over time.

The case of aplastic anemia associated with felbamate therapy illustrates the role that case reports can play in the assessment of a previously unknown adverse event in the post-approval period [21]. Felbamate is an antiepileptic agent approved for use in the US on July 29, 1993. Pre-approval studies showed no evidence of significant, non-reversible hematologic abnormalities [22]. Within about 1 year of approval, 20 cases of aplastic anemia, three of them fatal, had been reported in the US [21]. Review of the case reports suggested a causal role for felbamate. An estimated 100 000 patients had taken felbamate during this time [21]. While the true incidence of aplastic anemia in patients taking felbamate can not be calculated because case ascertainment may be incomplete, the estimated rate is 20/100 000/year, or 200/million/year. By contrast the population background rate of aplastic anemia is low, about 2/million/year [23]. Thus, the observed cases of aplastic anemia suggest that aplastic anemia is about 100 times more frequent in patients taking felbamate than in the general population. Based on this finding, the FDA and the manufacturer recommended that patients not be treated with felbamate unless the benefits of the drug were judged to outweigh the risk of aplastic anemia [21]. A subsequent review of 31 case reports of aplastic anemia in patients taking felbamate [23], using the criteria of the International Agranulocytosis and Aplastic Anemia Study (IAAAS), established that felbamate was the only plausible cause in three cases, and the most likely cause in eleven cases. For the remaining nine cases, there was at least one other plausible cause. The authors estimated that the 'most probable' incidence of aplastic anemia in patients exposed to felbamate was estimated to be to 127 per million. Because aplastic anemia is uncommon in the population and because it is generally the result of a medication or other toxin, a careful analysis of a case series can establish the relationship of felbamate to aplastic anemia.

Active surveillance

Active surveillance systems are also being explored to identify and examine drug safety issues. Drug safety active surveillance systems, which take advantage of large repositories of automated healthcare data, are now being developed and tested by multiple organizations. The common feature of these systems is that they do not rely on health care providers or patients to recognize and report adverse events that may be related to medication use. Rather, these systems often use sophisticated statistical methods to actively search for patterns in linked prescription, outpatient and inpatient utilization of care data that might suggest the occurrence of an adverse event related to drug therapy. This lack of reliance on healthcare providers or patients to detect the event, relate it to a drug and then report it to FDA, along with its prospective nature, is what makes these systems active rather than passive in their scope. However, one system is unlikely to address all drug safety problems or all patient populations. While there is much interest in developing these systems, there is also much work to be done in the validation of these systems.

Observational epidemiological studies

Observational epidemiological studies of drug safety, also known as observational pharmacoepidemiological drug safety studies, are widely used in the post-marketing period. Because these studies, like case reports and case series, rely on actual patient experience, they can provide an assessment of a drug's safety under actual conditions of use. Observational drug safety studies, which can be prospective or retrospective, can be used to make inferences about the safety of the drug, provided that they are carefully designed, conducted, analyzed, and interpreted. Unlike case reports and case series, observational epidemiological studies can include a control group. Unlike in clinical trials, the investigator in an observational epidemiological drug safety study does not assign treatment to patients; patient treatment decisions are made in the course of routine clinical care and are independent of the study.

The two most common observational epidemiological study designs are the case-control design and the cohort design [24]. In each type of study an 'exposure' is related to an 'outcome'. For drug safety studies, the exposure is usually the use of the drug being investigated, and the outcome is usually the adverse event of interest. Case-control studies of drug safety compare the frequency of exposure (i.e., the frequency of use of the drug being investigated) amongst cases (i.e., those with the adverse event of interest) to the frequency of exposure amongst controls (i.e., those without the adverse event of interest). Cohort studies follow persons with and without the exposure (i.e., those who use

and do not use the drug being investigated) over time for the outcome of interest.

In the design and analysis of observational pharmacoepidemiological studies, careful attention must be paid to the potential for bias and confounding, each of which can lead to an erroneous estimate of the effect of the exposure on the outcome. In drug safety studies, these factors would lead to an erroneous conclusion regarding the relationship of the use of a drug to the development of an adverse event [25]. One particular type of confounding, confounding by indication, is especially important to address in the design of observational epidemiological drug safety studies. Persons who take a given medication are different from those who do not take that medication in many ways. One important way in which they can be different is the reason, or indication, for which they are taking the medication. If the characteristics of those with this indication are also related to the development of the adverse event of interest, an observed association between the medication and adverse event may be confounded by the indication for treatment – that is, the association may be explained not by a direct effect of the drug on the outcome, but rather by the relationship of the indication for treatment to both use of the drug as well as to the development of the adverse outcome, which produces an indirect link between the drug and the adverse outcome. While analytic techniques may control for confounding by indication in some cases, it should not be assumed that such techniques will always eliminate the effect of confounding by indication. It is therefore important to consider carefully the potential impact of confounding by indication in the design of the study, in order to minimize the chance that this will occur.

Cohort studies

A cohort study is designed to determine if there is an association between an exposure and an outcome in a defined group followed over time [24]. In a drug safety cohort study, a group of persons treated with drug of interest and a comparable group of persons not treated with that drug are identified and followed over time. (The group of persons treated with the drug of interest can also be compared to a group of persons treated with an alternative treatment.) The incidence of the adverse event of interest is ascertained in each group. A relative risk is obtained by dividing the incidence in the group treated with the drug of interest by the incidence in the group not treated with the drug of interest. A relative risk of 1.0 implies that the incidence is equal in the two groups. A relative risk greater than 1.0 implies that those who receive the drug of interest have a higher risk of the outcome of interest than those who did not receive the drug of interest. Similarly, a relative risk less than 1.0 implies that those who receive the drug of interest have a lower risk of the outcome of interest than those not treated with the drug of interest. To determine if the relative risk is statistically significantly different from 1.0, it is customary to calculate and report p-values. To determine the precision of the estimate, 95% confidence intervals can be calculated and reported. Because cohort studies measure the incidence of the outcome in two groups, a risk difference can be calculated. This measure quantifies the excess risk attributable to the drug of interest, and is thus more suitable for considering the public health impact of the findings.

In a prospective cohort study, the investigator identifies the cohort members at the start of the study, ascertains drug exposure, and follows users and non-users of the drug contemporaneously over time to determine who develops the outcome of interest. This design may be particularly useful when the outcome of interest is common and is likely to occur within a reasonable time after drug treatment is initiated. A reasonable time after drug exposure is one in which a sufficient number of outcome events is likely to occur, but is not so long that it results in an unacceptable delay in obtaining study results.

When the outcome of interest is infrequent or when there is a long latency between exposure and the development of an outcome event, the prospective cohort study design may not be the most feasible approach, because it may take several years to complete the study. In addition, loss to follow-up may make the original study design inadequate to address the original question, especially in the case of very long follow-up periods. Similarly, the introduction of new treatments during the study period may make the results of the study uninterpretable, irrelevant, or both. Because of these limitations, the prospective cohort design is not often used in observational epidemiological drug safety studies.

In some situations, the cohort study design can be employed by using existing information on patient treatments and outcomes that have already occurred. If such data are available, mainly in administrative claims data or electronic medical records, cohorts can be constructed by identifying persons who took the drug of interest and those who did not take it. Similarly, outcomes of interest that occurred in patients after entry into the cohort can be ascertained in these datasets. This design is known as a retrospective cohort design. It is conceptually identical to the prospective cohort design, except that the use of the drug of interest and the development of the outcomes of interest occurred prior to the initiation of the study. By using already existing data, a retrospective cohort study can be conducted and completed much more rapidly than a prospective cohort study. Of course, if existing data are not available or suitable for a retrospective cohort study, this approach can not be used, and another approach must be sought.

The availability of large computerized administrative health care databases and electronic medical record systems provide a substantial source of data in which to examine drug safety questions. These databases contain information on medication exposure and health outcomes. Records of dispensed prescriptions and prescribed medications are the measure of medication exposure. Health outcomes are generally measured by diagnostic codes or procedure codes. Because diagnostic codes and procedure codes are recorded for administrative, and not research, purposes, it is important that their validity be understood when used in drug safety studies. To accomplish this, outcomes can be ascertained and adjudicated in a manner that is blinded to treatment received, in order to avoid bias in outcome ascertainment.

A retrospective cohort study using administrative claims data was used to examine the incidence of hospitalized rhabdomyolysis in patients treated with lipid-lowering agents [8]. Drug-specific inception cohorts of statin (atorvastatin, cerivastatin, fluvastatin, lovastatin, pravastatin, and simvastatin) and fibrate (fenofibrate and gemfibrozil) users were established by identifying new users (defined as no use within the 180 days prior to entrance into the drug-specific cohort). Hospitalization claims were reviewed for diagnosis codes indicative of possible rhabdomyolysis. Medical record review of hospitalizations by investigators blinded to statin or fibrate exposure status was performed to identify cases of rhabdomyolysis, according to a case definition. Incidence rates of rhabdomyolysis per 10 000 person-years of treatment were calculated. The incidence per 10 000 person-years for cerivastatin monotherapy was 5.34 (95% CI, 1.46–13.68). The corresponding rates were lower for monotherapy with atorvastatin (0.54, 0.22–1.12), pravastatin, (0, 0–1.1), and simvastatin (0.49, 0.06–1.76). Amongst the fibrates, the rate for gemfibrozil monotherapy was 3.70 (0.76–10.82) and the rate for fenofibrate monotherapy was 0 (0–14.58). Further analysis showed that the incidence rate for the combination of cerivastatin and gemfibrozil was markedly elevated (1036, 389–2117). This retrospective cohort study demonstrated that the risk of rhabdomyolysis was low for monotherapy with atorvastatin, pravastatin, and simvastatin, but higher for cerivastatin. Additionally, it demonstrated that statin-fibrate combination therapy increased this risk.

Case-control studies

Like cohort studies, case-control studies are designed to measure an association between an exposure and an outcome. While cohort studies follow defined groups based on exposure (i.e., cohorts) over time to ascertain the outcome of interest, case-control studies start with the identification of those who have the outcome of interest (cases) and an appropriately selected group that does not have the outcome of interest (controls). The frequency of exposure is then ascertained in each group and compared between groups.

In observational drug safety case-control studies, persons with the adverse event of interest (cases) are compared to persons without the adverse event of interest (controls). The proportion of cases that received the drug of interest is determined, as is the proportion of cases that did not receive the drug of interest. Similarly, the proportions of controls who did, and who did not, receive the drug of interest are determined. If the drug of interest is associated with the adverse event of interest, the frequency of the exposure amongst cases will be higher than that amongst the controls. The measure of this association in a case-control study is expressed as an odds ratio. The design of a case-control study does not permit calculation of incidence rates. A true relative risk, therefore, can not be calculated. However, when the outcome of interest is relatively rare, the odds ratio functions as an estimate of the relative risk. Like the relative risk obtained from cohort studies, an odds ratio of 1.0 implies no association between the drug of interest and the adverse event of interest. An odds ratio greater than 1.0 implies that those who receive the drug of interest have a higher risk of the outcome of interest than those who did not receive the drug of interest. Similarly, an odds ratio less than 1.0 implies that those who receive the drug of interest have a lower risk of the outcome of interest than those not treated with the

drug of interest. As with the relative risks obtained from cohort studies, p-values and 95% confidence intervals are customarily calculated and reported to determine statistical significance and precision of the estimate, respectively. A variant of the case-control study that is often used in pharmacoepidemiology is the nested case-control study, in which cases and controls are selected from a cohort.

Case-control studies are particularly useful when the outcome of interest is relatively uncommon, because such outcomes are not likely to be observed in a clinical trial or a cohort study. Similarly, if the outcome has a long latency relative to the exposure, a cohort study or a clinical trial may not be feasible. Designing a robust case-control study is complex. From a broad perspective, there are three features that must be carefully considered when designing a pharmacoepidemiologic case-control study: the definition of a case, the measurement of exposure to the drug, and the selection of a control group.

Case definitions must be carefully considered so that they insure that the outcome of interest is adequately captured. For example, an overly narrow case definition may result in failure to identify all clinically relevant events, while an overly broad case definition may result in inclusion of clinically irrelevant events. In either case, an imprecise definition can lead to an incorrect estimate of the association of the drug of interest to the adverse event of interest. An imprecise case definition can lead to failure to identify an association when one actually exists, or it can lead to an incorrect conclusion that an association exists when one actually does not exist. Case-control studies generally obtain data on drug exposure retrospectively. This can be accomplished either by examining medication records, such as medical records or administrative claims data, or by administrating questionnaires to patients, their health care providers, or other respondents. It is important to understand the method of medication exposure ascertainment in order to identify the potential limitations in their validity. Finally, selection of controls must be done in a way to minimize selection bias.

Despite these challenges, well-designed case-control studies can be useful sources of information about the adverse effects of medicines.

A nested case-control design was used to examine the relationship of dopamine agonists to cardiac-valve regurgitation [26]. Using the General Practitioner Research Database, a computerized medical records system containing information on approximately

6.3 million lives from about 350 general practices in the UK, the researchers identified a cohort of 11 417 patients who had at least two prescriptions for an anti-parkinsonian medication, were 40–80 years of age, and met other eligibility criteria. Anti-parkinsonian medications included levodopa, selegiline, bromocriptine, cabergoline, pergolide, lisuride, pramipexole, and ropinirole. From this cohort, they identified 81 patients with possible new valvular regurgitation. Fifty of these 81 patients were then excluded because they did not have a confirmed diagnosis ($n = 40$), because they had pre-existing valvular heart disease ($n = 2$), or because they had a myocardial infarction within the previous 3 years ($n = 8$). The remaining 31 patients formed the case group. For each case, up to 25 controls were selected from the patients in the cohort who did not have possible new valvular regurgitation, matched on sex, age (within 2 years) and year of entry into the study cohort. Patients with myocardial infarction within 3 years prior to the index date (the date that resulted in the same duration of follow-up for the control patients as the case patient) were excluded from the control group. The final case-control analysis included 31 cases and 663 controls. Exposure to a dopamine agonist was quantified in two ways. First, cumulative duration of use of a dopamine agonist was categorized as less than 6 months or more than 6 months. Second, for patients using pergolide or cabergoline, the total daily dose of the dopamine agonist was calculated and categorized as 3 milligrams (mg) or less daily or more than 3 mg daily. Conditional logistic regression, adjusting for multiple patient characteristics, was used to calculate odds ratios, which were used as estimates of incidence-rate ratios. The adjusted incidence-rate ratio of cardiac valve regurgitation was elevated amongst patients using pergolide (adjusted incidence rate ratio 7.1, 95% CI: 2.3 to 22.3) or cabergoline (adjusted incidence rate ratio 4.9, 95% CI: 1.5 to 15.6). No cases of new valvular regurgitation were found amongst users of the other dopamine agonists. This case-control study thus demonstrated that the use of pergolide or cabergoline was associated with the development of cardiac-valve regurgitation.

Clinical trials

Clinical trials play an important role in assessing the safety of medicine. The majority of clinical trials are performed primarily to assess the efficacy of a product. In these trials, safety assessments are routinely included, though there is usually not a specific safety hypothesis. As efficacy trials are powered to demonstrate the efficacy of a product, such trials are typically not well suited for detecting rare adverse events, nor are they generally of sufficient size to determine if there are clinically significant differences in the frequency of a specific adverse event between two treatments. In these settings, some of the most useful safety information gained from a clinical trial is an understanding of the frequency of the most common adverse events.

In the post-market period, clinical trials can play many important roles in the ongoing safety assessment of a medicine. The framework of a properly designed and carefully conducted clinical trial is well suited for assessing the safety of a medicine in selected circumstances. First, randomization assigns treatment independent of individual patient characteristics and physician preferences. Randomization thus avoids the problem of confounding by indication that can be present in observational studies. Second, patient data are collected in a standardized way defined in the clinical trial protocol. This method allows investigators to insure that all clinically relevant baseline and post-baseline data are captured, including detailed information on patient demographics, disease duration and severity, prior treatment, past medical history, and concomitant medications. Third, data on the dosage and duration of study treatment regimens are carefully recorded. Fourth, outcomes, including adverse events of interest, can be ascertained and recorded in a systematic and standardized way. Information on onset date or time, seriousness, clinical course and severity, response to treatment (including response to withdrawal of the test medicine), and extent of resolution can be obtained in a uniform way. For key adverse event outcome measures, the protocol can stipulate the additional clinical details that need to be recorded. If necessary, specific outcome events of interest can be adjudicated using pre-defined criteria by an independent group of experts not otherwise involved in the trial who can be blinded to treatment assignment. Finally, blinding of treatment assignment minimizes bias in assessing adverse events.

Despite the advantages of the clinical trial methodology for assessing adverse events, there are constraints to the set of clinical trials that are done prior to a drug's approval that limit knowledge of a drug's full safety profile. First, clinical trials are generally conducted in patients who are more homogeneous than the larger population of patients who will receive the drug once it is marketed. Patients in clinical trials may differ from those treated in clinical practice in terms of disease severity, concomitant and past illnesses, concomitant medication, and personal characteristics. These factors can each influence the development of an adverse event. Second, for medicines intended for chronic use, the duration of treatment in a clinical trial is generally relatively short compared to that used in clinical practice. Clinical trials are often not practical for the detection or characterization of adverse events that emerge only after prolonged exposure to a medicine.

Given the strengths and limitations of clinical trials for the detection of adverse events, what is the role of clinical trials in the assessment of safety in the post-approval period? There are actually many roles for clinical trials. First, clinical trials of efficacy often continue in the post-approval period. These trials are generally designed to expand the medicine's original indication, by studying different patient populations, different indications, and different dosing regimens. Though most post-approval clinical trials in these settings will be efficacy studies, each of these circumstances affords the opportunity to enhance knowledge of medicine's safety profile. For example, new patient populations may have a broader range of concomitant illnesses or a greater range of severity of the disease being treated. Similarly, studying the efficacy of a medicine in a new indication will often result in patient population that is different than the one previously studied. Careful collection of safety data in a clinical trial with a broader population or in a new indication may thus reveal new patterns of adverse events not previously recognized. Clinical trials with new dosing ranges or dose regimens may reveal dose-dependent toxicities not previously appreciated. For these reasons, careful collection of safety data in clinical trials is important in the post-approval period.

In some cases, a clinical trial is conducted specifically to test a safety hypothesis. The impetus for such a trial may be findings from case reports, observational studies, or previous clinical trials. In addition to general considerations for all clinical trials, there are certain features of clinical trials designed specifically to test drug safety hypotheses that must be considered carefully. First, while most clinical trials typically specify a primary efficacy endpoint, and collect adverse event data to characterize the general safety profile of a medicine, clinical trials designed to answer a specific safety question must clearly specify a defined safety endpoint. This endpoint may be a single outcome, or it may be a composite outcome.

Second, the design of a post-marketing clinical trial testing a safety hypothesis is often an active-controlled trial that uses a non-inferiority study design. If, in the post-marketing setting, effective treatments, in addition to the drug whose safety is being tested, exist for the condition being treated, it would generally be unethical to withhold treatment. Thus, placebo-controlled clinical trials to study a potential safety risk would likely not be possible, nor would they necessarily be relevant. In these cases, active comparators are used. In a clinical trial designed to test a drug safety hypothesis, the relevant demonstration of safety would be that the test drug of interest has no higher risk of the adverse event of interest than the comparator treatment (either an active comparator or a placebo), within a specified margin. To determine that the test drug has no higher risk of the adverse event of interest than does a comparator treatment, a non-inferiority clinical trial design is used [27,28]. The objective of a non-inferiority clinical trial is to show that the difference in the frequency of an outcome between two treatment groups is small (see Chapter 13). For non-inferiority trials with a primary safety outcome, the objective is to show that the frequency of the safety outcome between two treatments groups is small. Assuming that the frequency of the adverse event of interest in the comparator group is known, based on prior data, to be acceptable, the objective becomes showing that the frequency of the adverse event of interest in the test drug group is not clinically meaningfully higher than that of the comparator. To accomplish this goal, the investigators must determine the maximum clinically acceptable increase in the frequency of the adverse event of interest in the test drug group relative to the comparator group. This difference is known as the non-inferiority margin. With respect to the adverse event of interest, the test drug is non-inferior to the comparator drug if the upper limit of the 95% confidence interval around the measure comparing the two groups is below the pre-specified non-inferiority margin. Because the non-inferiority trial design seeks to demonstrate that the specified risk of the drug of interest is not greater than that of a comparator agent by a pre-defined, and usually small, amount, the magnitude of the non-inferiority margin is based on clinical judgment and must be carefully considered. Active-controlled, non-inferiority trials present a special set of challenges. The absence of a placebo arm results in loss of assay sensitivity, or the ability to distinguish between active and inactive treatments. If two treatments have the same frequency of an adverse event in an active-controlled clinical trial and the test drug is determined to be non-inferior to the comparator agent, it is still not known if that adverse event is related to treatment in each of the two arms, or if it is unrelated to treatment in the two arms [27,28].

Relative to observational epidemiological studies, clinical trials designed to answer drug safety questions are usually more costly and more time-consuming. One circumstance in which clinical trials are preferred for answering drug safety questions is when there is concern that the techniques used to adjust for confounding in observational epidemiological studies do not allow for complete controlling of the confounders. When the observed association is small (e.g., a relative risk of 1.5 or less) and there is concern that residual confounding is present, observational epidemiological studies will often not be able to sort out a causal effect from one driven by residual confounding. In this circumstance, if the drug safety question is important, and there is genuine uncertainty about the relationship of the drug to the adverse outcome of interest, a clinical trial may be the only acceptable option.

For example, the 'Prospective Randomized Evaluation of Celecoxib Integrated Safety versus Ibuprofen or Naproxen' (PRECISION) trial is designed to evaluate the cardiovascular safety of celecoxib, ibuprofen, and naproxen [29]. Celecoxib, a non-steroidal anti-inflammatory drug (NSAID), is a selective cyclooxygenase-2 inhibitor used in the treatment of osteoarthritis and rheumatoid arthritis. Prior data had indicated that another member of the class, rofecoxib, was associated with an elevated risk of cardiovascular morbidity [30]. A further review of the entire NSAID class revealed uncertainty about the relative cardiovascular effects of all drugs in the class. The PRECISION trial was designed to address this issue. The trial was designed to include 20 000 patients with symptomatic osteoarthritis or rheumatoid arthritis at high risk for, or with, established cardiovascular disease. Patients will be randomized to naproxen 375 mg bid, ibuprofen 600 mg tid, or celecoxib 100 mg bid in a 1:1:1 allocation. Subjects will be followed for 48 months. The primary safety outcome is the first occurrence of the Antiplatelet Trialist Collaboration (APTC) endpoint, which includes cardiovascular death, non-fatal myocardial infarction, or non-fatal stroke. The trial uses a non-inferiority design, with a statistical hypothesis that none of the treatments is inferior to either of the others. Three pairwise comparisons will be used to test each drug against the other two. The published non-inferiority definition for this trial specifies that two conditions must be met for the non-inferiority criteria

to be fulfilled: the upper limit of the one-sided 97.5% confidence interval for the hazard ratio can not exceed 1.33, and the point estimate of the hazard cannot exceed 1.12. The trial is ongoing.

A variant of the standard clinical trial that is sometimes used for drug safety studies is the so-called 'large simple trial'. This technique can be used when randomization is deemed to be the only way to control confounding completely.

In certain situations, prior data may suggest that the strength of an association between a drug and an adverse event is numerically small but clinically important. If the question is clinically important, a clinical trial may be the best way to address the issue, since in these situations observational studies may not completely control for confounding. However, numerically small associations require that clinical trial sample sizes be large. Such large trials might not be feasible if they were to collect all the detailed information that is typically collected in a standard clinical trial. The large, simple trial is an alternative approach that allows for large numbers of subjects to be studied by minimizing the volume and complexity of data collected, while maintaining the methodological rigor of a clinical trial. Protocols for large, simple trials are developed to insure that only data relevant for the specific question of interest is recorded at baseline and at follow-up, and that data on the specific outcome(s) of interest are captured. Because large amounts of detailed data are not collected, in a large, simple trial, the ideal outcome data in these trials are those that are objectively defined, such as hospitalization or death. Follow-up and outcome information may be obtained using epidemiological techniques not used in traditional clinical trials, such as vital records databases, or questionnaires administered to patients or caregivers not involving the investigator.

A large, simple trial was used to assess the safety of ibuprofen in children between 6 months and 12 years of age [31]. The investigators randomly assigned treatment with acetaminophen 12 mg/kg, ibuprofen 5 mg/kg, or ibuprofen 10 mg/kg to patients who were seen as outpatients for an acute febrile illness and who met other entry criteria. A total of 84 192 patients were recruited from the practices of 1735 pediatricians, family practitioners, and general practitioners. Outcome information was obtained via a self-administered questionnaire mailed to parents or guardians 4 weeks after enrollment. The questionnaire asked about the initial febrile illness, the amount of medication taken, supplemental treatments received, and the occurrence of serious adverse events in the four-week interval. If a hospitalization was reported, the investigators requested a copy of the hospital record. The principal outcomes of interest were acute gastrointestinal bleeding, acute renal failure, anaphylaxis, and Reye's syndrome. Follow-up data were obtained for all but 0.3% of enrolled children. The investigators found a risk of acute gastrointestinal bleeding of 7.2/100 000 children treated with either ibuprofen (95% CI, 2 to 18 per 100 000). The corresponding risk amongst acetaminophen-treated children was zero per 100 000 (95% CI, 0 to 11 per 100 000) ($p = 0.31$ for the difference). For acute renal failure, anaphylaxis and Reye's syndrome, the observed risk among children randomized to either dose of ibuprofen was zero per 100 000 (95% CI, 0 to 5.4 per 100 000). The authors concluded that the risks of hospitalization for gastrointestinal bleeding, acute renal failure and anaphylaxis were not increased following short-term use of ibuprofen in children.

Summary

There are many possible approaches to studying safety of drugs in the post-marketing period. These include review of individual case reports, case series, observational epidemiological studies, and clinical trials. Each approach has its own strengths and limitations, and no single approach is appropriate for all situations. Rather, the approach taken must consider what is already known about the adverse event and the knowledge gaps that need to be filled. Additional critical factors include the nature of the adverse outcome under study, its expected frequency, the availability of existing data, and the importance and urgency of answering the question. Regardless of the approach chosen, careful attention must be paid to selecting proper control groups and comparator agents, minimizing bias, and controlling for confounding.

References

1. Institutes of Medicine-Committee on the Assessment of the U.S. Drug Safety System. Natural History of a Drug. The Future of Drug Safety: Promoting and Protecting the Health of the Public. 2006.

2. US Food and Drug Administration. 21 CFR 201.56. 2009. http://www.accessdata.fda.gov/scripts/cdrh/cfdocs/cfcfr/CFRSearch.cfm?fr=201.56

3. US Food and Drug Administration. 21 CFR 201.57. 2009. http://www.accessdata.fda.gov/scripts/cdrh/cfdocs/cfCFR/CFRSearch.cfm?fr=201.57

4. US Food and Drug Administration. 21 CFR 314.80. 2009. http://www.accessdata.fda.gov/scripts/cdrh/cfdocs/cfcfr/CFRSearch.cfm?fr=314.80

5. Rogers A, Israel E, Smith C, et al. Physician knowledge, attitudes, and behavior related to reporting adverse drug events. Arch Int Med 1988; 148: 1596–1600.

6. Scott H, Rosenbaum S, Waters W, et al. Rhode Island physicians' recognition and reporting of adverse drug events. Rhode Island Med J 1987; 70: 311–6.

7. McAdams M, Staffa J, Dal Pan G. Estimating the extent of reporting to FDA: a case study of statin-Associated Rhabdomyolysis. Pharmacoepidemiol Drug Safety 2008; 17: 229–39.

8. Graham D, Staffa J, Shatin D, et al. Incidence of hospitalized rhabdomyolysis in patients treated with lipid-lowering drugs. JAMA 2004; 292: 2585–90.

9. US Food and Drug Administration. The ICH Guideline on Clinical Safety Data Management: Data Elements for Transmission of Individual Case Safety Reports. 2009. http://www.fda.gov/downloads/Drugs/GuidanceComplianceRegulatoryInformation/Guidances/ucm073090.pdf

10. US Food and Drug Administration. Guidance for Industry – E2B(M): Data Elements for Transmission of Individual Case Safety Reports. 2005. http://www.fda.gov/RegulatoryInformation/Guidances/ucm129428.htm

11. MedDRA MSSO. Medical Dictionary for Regulatory Activities Maintenance and Support Services Organization. 2010. http://www.meddramsso.com/

12. Almenoff J, Tonning J, Gould A, et al. Perspectives on the use of data mining in pharmacovigilance. Drug Safety 2005; 28: 981–1007.

13. Almenoff J, DuMouchel W, Kindman L, et al. Disproportionality analysis using empirical Bayes data mining: a tool for the evaluation of drug interactions in the post-marketing setting. Pharmacoepidemiol Drug Safety 2003; 12: 517–521.

14. Anonymous. Causality asssessment of adverse events following immunization. Weekly Epidemiol Rec 2001; 76: 85–9.

15. Bower J, Maraganore D, McDonnell S, et al. Incidence and distribution of Parkinsonism in Olmsted County, Minnesota, 1976–1990. Neurology 1999; 52: 1214–20.

16. Jones J. Determining causation from case reports. In: Strom B, ed. Pharmacoepidemiology. 4th edition. John Wiley & Sons, Ltd, 2005; 557–70.

17. Meyboom R, Hekster Y, Egberts A, et al. Causal or causal?: The role of causality assessment in pharmacovigilance. Drug Safety 1997; 17: 374–89.

18. Naranjo C, Busto U, Sellers E, *et al*. A method for estimating the probability of adverse drug reactions. *Clin Pharmacol Therap* 1981; **30**: 239–45.

19. The Uppsala Monitoring Centre. The Use of the WHO-UMC System for Standardised Case Causality Assessment. 2010. http://www.who-umc.org/

20. Rodriguez E, Staffa J, Graham D. The role of databases in drug postmarketing surveillance. *Pharmacoepidemiol Drug Safety* 2001; **10**: 407–10.

21. Nightingale S. Recommendation to immediately withdraw patients from treatment with felbamate. *JAMA* 1994; **272**: 995.

22. Pennell P, Ogaily M, Macdonald R. Aplastic anemia in a patient receiving felbamate for complex partial seizures. *Neurology* 1995; **45**: 456–60.

23. Kaufman D, Kelly J, Anderson T, *et al*. Evaluation of case reports of aplastic anemia among patients treated with felbamate. *Epilepsia* 1997; **38**: 1265–9.

24. Strom B. Study designs available for pharmacoepidemiology studies. In: Strom B, ed. *Pharmacoepidemiology*. 4th edition. John Wiley & Sons, Ltd, 2005; 17–28.

25. Csizmad I, Collet J and Boivin J. Bias and confounding in pharmacoepidemiology. In: Strom B, ed. *Pharmacoepidemiology*. 4th edition. John Wiley & Sons, Ltd., 2005; 791–809.

26. Schade R, Andersohn F, Suissa S, *et al*. Dopamine agonists and the risk of cardiac-valve regurgitation. *New Engl J Med* 2007; **356**: 29–38.

27. Temple R and Ellenberg S. Placebo-controlled trials and active-control trials in the evaluation of new treatments. Part 1. Ethical and scientific issues. *Ann Int Med* 2000; **133**: 455–63.

28. Ellenberg S and Temple R. Placebo-controlled trials and active-control trials in the evaluation of new treatments. Part 2: Practical issues and specific cases. *Ann Int Med* 2000; **133**: 464–70.

29. Becker MC, Wang TH, Wisniewski L, *et al*. Rationale, design, and governance of Prospective Randomized Evaluation of Celecoxib Integrated Safety versus Ibuprofen Or Naproxen (PRECISION), a cardiovascular end point trial of nonsteroidal antiinflammatory agents in patients with arthritis. *Am Heart J* 2009; **157**: 606–12.

30. Bresalier R, Sandler R, Quan H, *et al*. Cardiovascular events associated with rofecoxib in a colorectal adenoma chemoprevention trial. *N Engl J Med* 2005; **352**: 1092–102.

31. Lesko SM and Mitchell AA. An assessment of the safety of pediatric ibuprofen: A practitioner-based randomized clinical trial. *JAMA* 1995; **273**: 929–33.

Chapter

16

Ethics in clinical trials involving the central nervous system: Risk, benefit, justice, and integrity

Jonathan Kimmelman

Introduction

Drugs targeting the CNS have one of the highest rates of attrition during development [1]. Though there have been many spectacular successes in drug and biological development, the clinical course of many CNS disorders, like amyotrophic lateral sclerosis and Alzheimer's disease, has changed little in decades.

Development of safe and effective interventions against diseases of the CNS therefore remains an important goal. As with any clinical trials, those involving neurological disorders should cohere with the core principles underlying human research ethics: respect for persons, beneficence, and justice [2]. However, CNS trials often present particular challenges with respect to applying these principles. These relate to a cluster of factors: neurological disorders often implicate capacities necessary for informed consent, interventions in brain function involve significant degrees of uncertainty and risk, and many trials rely on subjective endpoints.

Here, we survey basic ethical principles and practices for human experimentation, and extend these to clinical trials of CNS interventions. This chapter only touches on the related subject of regulatory and legal issues in neurological research; we also refer the reader to other sources for specialized topics like advanced research directives [3], emergency studies [4], and neuroimaging. Finally, our discussion of informed consent is cursory; a more detailed account can be found in Chapter 17.

Basic principles of human research ethics

Research and clinical care as morally distinct activities

Why protect human subjects? Why is the consent process for research so much more laborious then it is in care settings? Why do clinical investigators have to get permission from third parties – institutional review boards (IRBs) – to give a drug to half their patients, while clinicians need not get permission from anyone to give the drug to all their patients?

The answers to these questions take us to the heart of human research ethics, which is founded on a recognition that research and care are morally distinct activities. One often cited reason for considering them distinct is risk: volunteers in human research endure higher degrees of uncertainty and risk than patients in clinical care. This is almost certainly the case for phase 1 clinical trials, in which interventions that have only been tested in animals are first applied in human beings. But research is not always riskier or more uncertain than care. As we will see below, principles like clinical equipoise are designed to ensure that the risks and benefits of research participation are equivalent to those in competent care settings. Moreover, some care interventions (e.g., surgical procedures) can be very risky, while some research procedures (e.g., a retrospective chart review) are minimally risky. Though risk

Clinical Trials in Neurology, ed. Bernard Ravina, Jeffrey Cummings, Michael P. McDermott, and R. Michael Poole. Published by Cambridge University Press. © Cambridge University Press 2012.

and uncertainty pose important challenges in clinical research, it seems difficult to argue that risks alone justify the extra ethical vigilance accorded to clinical research.

A more satisfactory explanation is that, in care settings, clinicians have obligations to consider only the best interests of their patients when making care decisions, whereas in research, clinical investigators legitimately endure divided loyalties. In particular, only in exceptional instances should caregivers consider external interests when making treatment decisions about a particular patient. In contrast, though researchers have well-established obligations to advance (or at least, not set back) the interests of their volunteers, they also have obligations to society by advancing medical knowledge. The latter obligations sometimes impose practices that, on their face, at least, seem to antagonize the interests of patients who volunteer for clinical trials. For example, most patients prefer to – and are indeed entitled to – know the identity of a drug they are receiving. In research, however, trialists often randomize study volunteers and then mask them to their treatment allocation. They perform such procedures to ensure the internal validity, and hence the social value, of the knowledge gained by the study. Other elements of research practice that help secure its social value, but that arguably are in tension with what patients might identify as in their own interest, include the use of comparators (especially placebos), subtherapeutic dosing in phase 1 trials, research procedures like blood draws that are not performed to inform care, exclusion criteria that prevent co-interventions, wash-out periods, and rigid protocols that prevent patients from selecting their dose, treatment schedule, or treatment.

It is clear, then, that medical research is morally distinct from clinical care. According to Immanuel Kant's celebrated categorical imperative, a person should never be instrumentalized, that is, used only as means to some other end. Medical research certainly uses people as means to another end. Research ethics offers a set of principles and practices to ensure that medical science does not *only* use human subjects for other ends.

The history of human protection: scandal and reaction

Contemporary research ethics practices emerged in response to a series of scandals and atrocities in human experimentation. Following the Nazi doctors trial, the Nuremberg Code established ten directives for human experimentation. Principal among these was an absolute requirement for the informed consent of subjects. In 1964, the World Medical Association relaxed this requirement with its Declaration of Helsinki, thus providing an ethical policy compatible with research on individuals lacking consent capacity. These policies were not widely honored in North America. A series of revelations, starting with Henry Beecher's 1966 exposé in the *New England Journal of Medicine* [5] and continuing past the Tuskegee Syphilis Study, led the US Congress to empanel a National Commission for the Protection of Human Subjects of Biomedical and Behavioral Research. The National Commission was the first body to articulate broad ethical principles for research in its Belmont Report. Their recommendations were largely taken up in regulations issued by the Department of Health Education and Welfare (45 CFR 46). In the years since, the Declaration of Helsinki has undergone several revisions, and various other countries and entities have developed their own policies. Policies of many professional societies, like the American Academy of Neurology [6], largely recapitulate themes in major policy documents like the Belmont Report and Declaration of Helsinki.

Core principles of major codes of research

Numerous policies, codes, and regulations have followed from this history. Though they take different positions on specific issues – for example, they differ about when the use of placebo controls is ethical – there is nearly universal consensus on certain principles and practices. All policies express the view that the autonomy and welfare of human subjects must be protected; that clinical studies should be designed to meaningfully advance medical knowledge; and that protocols should meet certain standards of justice. These principles are put into practice through a series of well-established frameworks and mechanisms. Autonomy is ensured through the provision of informed consent (for persons with capacity) or approximated through surrogate decision-making plus a restriction on research risk (for persons lacking capacity). The welfare of study volunteers is protected by ensuring that risks of clinical studies are justified by a credible appeal to direct benefits for study volunteers and benefits for society through knowledge. The latter establishes a requirement that all research meet a threshold of validity. The justness of clinical research is protected by ensuring that disadvantaged or vulnerable groups are not recruited in an opportunistic manner, that they do not disproportionately bear the burdens and risks of knowledge production activities, and that they are not denied the knowledge value of medical research through undue exclusion from trials. All major codes of research ethics agree that adherence to principles and practices outlined above should be prospectively and independently reviewed by an independent and competent body (in the US, these committees are IRBs).

The principles of research ethics are best thought of as conditions that must each be fulfilled for a study to proceed. There may be unusual circumstances where principles are in conflict, and it may be necessary balance competing objectives and principles. In general, however, one should avoid the temptation to think of principles as exchangable: the justice of a clinical trial cannot be 'purchased' by providing greater benefits to volunteers or their communities; an unfavorable risk-benefit balance in a protocol is not purchased by a particularly robust informed consent procedure.

Regulatory vs. ethical obligations

Regulations governing human protections aim at establishing a baseline level of ethical conduct. Researchers often assume, then, that unless an action is specifically excluded by regulations, it is ethical. Yet there are many examples of research conduct that clearly count as unethical, but are not specifically barred by regulations. For example, current human protections laws do not mandate full publication of negative or unfavorable findings in clinical trials. However, selective publication of clinical trial data is widely viewed as unethical.

In CNS research, the tensions between regulation and ethics are perhaps greatest around the use of placebo controls. As we will see below, many ethicists hold that clinical trials that violate the principle of clinical equipoise are unethical. Nevertheless, US regulations and FDA policy, as well as international policies aimed at harmonizing regulatory standards across jurisdictions, do not require clinical equipoise except where use of comparators present life-threatening and/or irreversible morbidity [7–8]. Another example where regulatory and ethical standards diverge is with the principle of justice: neither US nor ICH policy specifically address the fairness of locating trials in economically disadvantaged settings. Clearly, then, researchers should avoid conflating regulation and ethics.

With the above principles established, the sections below turn to how principles and practices surrounding risk, benefit, and justice play out in clinical trials involving CNS disorders.

Risk-benefit balance

Component analysis, clinical equipoise, and acceptable risk

A first step in establishing ethical design of a study is ensuring that risks are reasonable in relation to benefits. How are investigators and IRBs to make this judgment? The prevailing approach is through component analysis, which begins with the recognition that clinical trials often involve a mixture of different procedures, the risks of which will have different justifications [9–10]. When interventions are performed for scientific reasons (e.g., blood draws to monitor drug metabolites, or lumbar punctures to measure biomarkers), risks are only justified insofar as they are outweighed by knowledge benefits. There are restrictions on the level of risk for research procedures performed on patients deemed vulnerable or lacking consent capacity (e.g., children [11], prisoners [12]). The Declaration of Helsinki, for example, allows only minimal risk research procedures on incompetent subjects [13]. This thus establishes important limits on research risk in many realms of CNS research, including traumatic brain injury [14] and advanced neurodegenerative disease.

When interventions are performed with evidence sufficient to support belief that patients might benefit, the standard for deciding risk acceptability is clinical equipoise. Clinical equipoise establishes two conditions that must be met at the outset of a clinical trial. First, 'there must be honest, professional disagreement among expert clinicians about the preferred treatment.' According to this condition, patients should never be systematically disadvantaged by enrollment in a clinical trial by allocation to a study intervention that is demonstrably inferior to standard of care. As such, when trials administer drugs to patients with unmet medical needs, there should be uncertainty within the expert community as to the drug's comparative merits with other drugs provided within the study (e.g., in the control arm) or available outside the study in a care setting.

The second condition embodied in the principle of clinical equipoise is that studies should 'be designed in such a way as to make it reasonable to expect that, if it is successfully conducted, … the results should … be convincing enough to resolve the dispute among clinicians'

[15]. Because statistically underpowered or methodologically unsound trials only rarely resolve disputes among practitioners about the comparative clinical merits of drugs, such studies generally do not meet the principle of clinical equipoise, and are hence unethical.

The second condition of clinical equipoise builds on the principle that ethical research should fulfill a threshold condition of validity, and that the medical and social value of knowledge produced in clinical trials are important criteria in the ethical evaluation of clinical trials. The requirements of validity and value ground other ethical practices that have become well established in clinical research. For example, when results of clinical trials go unpublished, the broader clinical community cannot use such findings to inform practice. As such, failure to publish blocks a necessary step through which clinical research is translated into social value, and policies like the Declaration of Helsinki require prospective registration of clinical trials in a public database, and publication of positive, negative, and inconclusive research findings. CNS research has been subject to the same kinds of publication bias seen in other realms [16–17]. It should be noted here that, though FDA policy does not require prospective registration of phase 1 studies, the ethical rationale for prospective registration of early phase studies is similar to that for later phase studies.

Distinctive features of risk in studies involving brain interventions

There are many ways that risks presented by studies that involve brain interventions have a different character than those encountered in other therapeutic areas. First, the brain is *the* organ of personhood. Inadvertent disruptions to brain processes have the potential to diminish such essentially human capacities as language, cognition, identity, and sociality. In part because of the intricacy of brain circuitry, disruptions are extremely difficult to reverse.

A second challenging characteristic of risk in studies that involve the brain is the type of uncertainty about risk. Unlike most toxicities, impairments in human brain processes like cognition or sociality do not lend themselves to easy testing in animal models [18]. Uniquely human traits, like capacity for language, are, by definition, impossible to model in animals. Therefore, animal studies do not provide a reliable basis for anticipating many types of harms that can occur in CNS trials. They can also be difficult to monitor or detect.

These distinctive features each have several implications for the design and review of CNS trials. First, the greater uncertainty associated with brain interventions should be interpreted as higher risk. Greater uncertainty makes it more difficult to rule out the possibility of major adverse outcomes occurring. These adverse outcomes potentially implicate qualities that are essential to an individual's selfhood. Given that the primary aim of clinical research is the production of generalizable knowledge, investigators (and review committees) should proceed with extreme caution. Second, because distinctively human responses are impossible to anticipate in animal studies, human studies provide the first opportunity to monitor the effects of an intervention on the human mind. The principle of beneficence would favor study designs that carefully monitor subjects for changes in cognition, affect, and other brain functions as appropriate [19].

Human clinical experiments: role of preclinical studies

Phase 1 trials of new CNS interventions, as with all interventions, generally present a high degree of risk and uncertainty. The Nuremberg Code and the Declaration of Helsinki clearly articulate a requirement for preceding clinical testing with animal and/or laboratory experiments. A series of well-designed preclinical experiments can provide a sound ethical basis for initiating human clinical trials if they provide a reasonably reliable basis for estimating and avoiding risk, and sound reasons to expect that human testing will meaningfully inform the development of an intervention or a class of interventions.

A full discussion of design principles and ethics of preclinical research is well beyond the scope of this chapter. Nevertheless, there is a growing literature showing that many preclinical studies in neurology do not appear to take basic measures to ensure preclinical study validity. For example, various meta-analyses consistently show a minority of CNS preclinical studies address threats to internal validity through use of a priori statement of hypothesis, randomization, concealed treatment allocation, or masked outcome assessment (see, for example, [20–24]) Whether these methodological practices actually invalidate preclinical findings is unclear, though meta-epidemiological studies have found that failure to conceal treatment allocation [25] and to publish [26] led to larger effect sizes.

A lack of methodological rigor in preclinical studies raises concerns about risk-benefit balance in phase 1 studies. It is thus the responsibility of preclinical researchers to provide reasonably reliable evidence of an intervention's safety and promise, and it is the responsibility of clinical investigators to solicit study volunteers only after these standards have been met.

Phase 1 trials: planning for positive and negative results

One particularly vexing category of clinical research is the phase 1 trial (of which first-in-human trials are a special class). To these authors' knowledge, there are no reliable estimates of risks and benefits for phase 1 studies of any CNS disorders. Nevertheless, the very high attrition rate for CNS drugs would lead one to infer that direct benefits (that is, benefits attributable to receiving study interventions) are limited. In some circumstances, risks in phase 1 studies can be considerable. For example, recently completed clinical trials involving gene transfer of neurotrophic factors involved eight intraputaminal inoculations [27]. Assuming surgical risks in these studies are similar to those for electrode implantation in deep brain stimulation, delivery alone confers a 0.9% risk of mortality and a 4% risk of intracerebral hemorrhage leading to serious neurological deficits.

It is a matter of some controversy whether intervention risks can be ethically justified by the prospect of direct benefit for volunteers, or whether they are justified entirely by social knowledge. The present author finds the latter justification more plausible, especially for trials where enrollment requires withholding of validated interventions (in the case of Parkinson's disease, future trials might involve withholding deep brain stimulation from patients for whom it is indicated). Regardless of how one justifies risk in phase 1 trials involving surgical delivery, such trials are only justifiable insofar as laboratory and preclinical studies strongly support the initiation of human testing. To maximize the knowledge value of studies while minimizing the exposure of volunteers to risk, phase 1 trials should be designed with two objectives in mind: first, they should provide reliable evidence of optimal dose such that phase 2 trials can select the appropriate doses, route of administration, and, in some circumstances, patient population. Second, investigators should incorporate into trials research components that enable validation at key steps in the causal pathway of drug action.

These might include collection of biomarker data, imaging, histological studies, and a plan for autopsy in the event of volunteer death. Research components increase the likelihood that, in the event that desired responses are not observed in a trial, investigators can determine why a drug is failing, and whether modification of the approach might lead to successful translation [28–29].

Subject selection in early phase trials

CNS trials involving aggressive interventions often raise difficult ethical questions about which category of patients to include in initial tests. In realms like cancer or infectious disease, aggressive and novel approaches are most often tested in patients who are no longer responsive to standard therapies. This is because the risk-benefit balance of trial enrollment is more favorable for them: trial enrollment for patients with advanced disease entails less opportunity cost to them, because they are not imperiling adequate health status, and participation does not necessitate withdrawal of established effective care.

However, there are several reasons why patients in earlier stages of disease might be attractive candidates for early phase studies. One reason this author rejects is that, because interventions aim at halting progression of disease, patients with less advanced disease have a greater prospect of benefit. This argument necessarily subscribes to the position that risks in early phase trials are generally justified by an appeal to therapeutic benefit. Anyway, if other established effective forms of care are available for patients, it strains credibly to argue that a never before tested intervention, and for which appropriate dosing, scheduling, and delivery methods are not established, is in genuine clinical equipoise with one that is already validated. A more convincing rationale for enrolling patients with relatively recent disease onset is that such studies enable a more meaningful test of the intervention's properties. There is also less concern that, should adverse events occur, attribution of cause will be confounded by disease status. If later stage trials are to be pursued in patients with early disease, there may be validity advantages to performing earlier phase studies in a similar patient group. An additional factor that may make medically stable patients more attractive candidates from an ethical perspective is that they may be in a better position to provide valid and authentic informed consent, since their decisions are not impelled by perceived medical necessity [30]. However, this last advantage is tempered by the suggestion that patients with advanced disease might have advantages in decision-making as compared with patients with early disease, as the former are more likely to have adapted to their illness [31].

How this debate is resolved ultimately hinges on a utilitarian calculus that the risks of jeopardizing the adequate health status of patients in early disease stages are justified by the incremental gain in knowledge from enrolling them instead of patients who are treatment refractory. This author inclines toward the position that, if a study is primarily aimed at testing safety, feasibility, and defining conditions for testing in later stage trials, enrollment of patients with advanced disease is generally a more prudent course. However, reasonable people can disagree on this. We suggest that one way of resolving this controversy about risk and benefit is to seek advice from a representative cross-section of the disease community [30]. We will return to this point in our discussion of justice.

Placebo controls and clinical equipoise

At the opposite end of clinical development is the randomized controlled trial, in which new interventions are tested against a comparator drug. Few clinical trial design features have inspired as much debate as the use of placebo controls. Such debate has been further intensified by a proliferation of ethical standards, and tensions between regulatory standards and ethics bodies.

Many trials involving neurological disorders show evidence of placebo responses [32]. Controversy surrounding the use of placebo comparator arms has been especially pitched in clinical trials involving relapse-remitting multiple sclerosis [33–34]. On its face, relapse-remitting multiple sclerosis is precisely the type of condition for which placebo controls are methodologically desirable: its course is remitting, and outcome measurements often involve variables that are subjective or otherwise susceptible to bias. The rationale for including placebo comparators—plus randomized and masked treatment allocation—is to control for subjective report and assessment of study outcomes, expectancy effects triggered by perceived administration of therapy, and various factors that might cause spontaneous remission (e.g. regression to the mean).

The National Multiple Sclerosis Society twice issued policies specifying conditions where the use of placebo controls could be ethically acceptable in trials involving MS [33]. The most recently articulated conditions include (briefly): 1- forms of disease for which there is no established effective therapy; 2- participants refuse established effective therapy; 3- enrolling subjects are not responding to established effective therapy; 4- established effective therapy is not available to enrolling subjects because of resource constraints; 5- studies are short-term and aimed at proof of concept; 6- use of placebo controls will not cause serious or irreversible harm [33, 35].

In the opening of this part, we described the principle of clinical equipoise as the standard for justifying risk of drug administration in late phase clinical trials. To what extent are the conditions specified above consistent with the principle of clinical equipoise? Conditions 1 and 3 are uncontroversial and fulfill clinical equipoise. Condition 2 could, in principle, fulfill the principle of clinical equipoise provided that patient refusal of established effective therapy has a medical basis and occurs independently of the invitation to trial enrollment. Condition 4 could be consistent with clinical equipoise, though as we will see in the next part, it is constrained by concerns about justice. Provided that medications are withheld for a very short period, and that harms are carefully monitored, modest, and immediately treated, a nuanced reading of clinical equipoise could be compatible with condition 5. In such circumstances, the appropriate moral framework for evaluating risk under component analysis is to view the withholding of care as a research procedure. Condition 6 is more problematic for clinical equipoise: it would fall beneath the standards of competent care for clinicians to withhold medications from patients in a manner that led to moderate or long lasting (but not irreversible) morbidity. Moreover, even were such risk deemed ethically acceptable, placebo-controlled trials meeting the sixth condition would not enable the resolution of relevant clinical uncertainty: clinicians and their patients need to know whether a new drug works better than established effective drugs, not whether the new drug works better than no treatment. Proponents of clinical equipoise, then, would question condition 6, and instead urge the use of alternative trial designs, like placebo add-on or non-inferiority studies [36].

One last issue complicating the ethics of placebo use in clinical trials is the possibility that volunteers will become unmasked during the course of the study, as may happen if there are treatment-specific side effects. When unmasking occurs, interpretation of results is confounded by the possibility that outcome differences between arms represent a placebo effect rather than a pharmacologic response. Another confounding possibility is that unmasked subjects in the placebo arm are seeking co-interventions or dropping out of a study. To ensure valid interpretation of placebo-controlled trials, investigators should assess and report the quality of the blind at the completion of the study.

Sham controls

Further complicating ethical debates surrounding the choice of comparators is the use of sham surgical controls. Many cutting edge treatment strategies in neurology, like stem cell transplantation, gene transfer, and neurotrophic factors involve surgical delivery. Without active placebo controls—like sham surgical procedures—such studies are susceptible to confounding as a result of the placebo response.

This is because the strength of placebo responses tends to correlate with the degree of a procedure's invasiveness [37]. In addition, placebo responses tend to be greater when subjective outcomes are used. The methodological case for sham controls is therefore particularly strong for CNS disorder trials that involve both surgery and subjective endpoints. Parkinson's disease is one such example; in several instances, clinically significant and durable responses have been observed following sham procedures [38]. In this case, there is evidence to suggest that placebo responses are in part driven by disturbances in basal ganglia dopamine turnover [39–41].

Absent sham controls, then, inferences about causation for clinical response are likely to be unreliable, thus frustrating the ethical requirements of value and validity. Nevertheless, the use of sham controls is ethically contentious. Concerns divide into two categories. First, applying sham controls may expose patients to non-trivial risk and burden [42]. Sham interventions are, by definition, invasive and justified by an appeal to research warrant rather than therapeutic benefit for volunteers. The level of harm associated with sham interventions depends, of course, on the nature of the sham procedure. At one extreme is a study that performed sham implantations of catheters into the putamen of study subjects, thereby exposing volunteers to the full risk of brain surgery [43]. Some sham controls in movement disorder trials have involved exposing patients to a course of immunosuppression [44]. More typically, sham controls in brain intervention studies involve partial burr holes to the cranium without

penetration of the dura. Partial burr holes enable the masking of study volunteers to intervention, with only modest risk and burden. If sham interventions require extended withholding of established effective therapy from volunteers, they may also violate clinical equipoise. For instance, in trials involving Parkinson's disease, patients allocated to the sham arm may be asked to forgo otherwise medically indicated treatment like deep brain stimulation. This exposes patients with unmet medical needs to the burdens of unmanaged illness.

The second ethical critique of sham controls is their deceptive element. In studies that involve 'awake surgery,' sham procedures require that clinicians enact a theater of surgical delivery. Of course, there is an element of deception in any placebo controlled trial, as placebos are administered in part to elicit a level of expectation comparable to that for patients in the active arm. However, some commentators question whether it is ethical for clinical practitioners to actively mislead patients, even if they have been warned ahead of time about deceptive design elements [45].

Though use and design of sham controls continues to inspire debate [42, 46–47] even among volunteers themselves [31, 48], discussion appears to have moved well beyond simplistic and categorical opposition. As long as shams continue to be used, skeptics and proponents agree on three necessary conditions for use of sham controls. First, risks must be minimized: investigators should select sham procedures that reduce risk and burden for volunteers. As penetration of the dura exposes volunteers to a range of potential risks without being necessary for maintaining a blind, such invasive sham procedures should be avoided. Second, risks and burdens for sham procedures must be justified by the prospect of knowledge value. This means that there should be a very high degree of confidence that a study is addressing a significant and immanent question for the clinical community, and that the study is designed and likely to be executed in a way that will produce meaningful results that cannot be obtained through alternative study designs. Sham controlled studies therefore warrant particular attentiveness to supporting evidence and rigorous trial design. To that end, research teams should plan to query patients at the end of the study about whether they believe they have been allocated to the active arm. Third, research teams should ensure a careful informed consent process, making certain that patients understand that they may be allocated to sham interventions. Researchers sometimes substitute the word 'placebo' for 'sham' when discussing a trial. This substitution should be avoided during informed consent, as shams are considerably less benign than placebos. Research teams should also not attempt to entice wavering volunteers with the prospect of an open-label extension study in which patients in the sham arm can later receive active treatment, because this may not come to pass if the intervention shows unacceptable toxicity or activity. Finally, teams should provide a careful debriefing process for volunteers at the completion of the study.

Correlative studies

In realms like cancer research, the amount of tissue procured from patients for pharmacokinetic and pharmacodynamic studies has increased over the years [49]. Similarly burdensome or risky research procedures within clinical trials are likely on the rise in CNS research as well. Brain imaging and biomarkers in cerebrospinal fluid promise a way of measuring drug activity for conditions like amyotrophic lateral sclerosis [50], Alzheimer's, and MS before clinical responses are detectable. Imaging provides an opportunity to follow response in numerous brain diseases. Moreover, such studies provide an opportunity to test a drug's activity along key points in the causal pathway of drug action.

Correlative and marker studies raise two sets of issues. The first concerns the policies for storage and sharing of banked data and tissues. We direct the interested reader to other sources for a more complete discussion of privacy protections and data sharing policies. The second set of issues concerns the assessment and management of risk. Correlative and marker studies are neither designed nor expected to address a volunteer's unmet health needs. They therefore present volunteers with risks and burdens in the absence of a clinical rationale. Under component analysis, the risks of such study components must be justified by a credible claim about the value of the knowledge that will be produced. The assessment of research value requires that investigators and reviewers attend to three elements of burdensome studies embedded within clinical trials. First, investigators must demonstrate the validity of study design, including sampling and statistical methods. Because correlative studies are rarely the central focus of clinical trials, investigators may underestimate the ethical significance of ensuring statistically and methodologically valid design. Second, at the outset of the study, investigators should be able to establish the prognostic

or correlative value of markers that will be measured, including assay validity. The burdens of correlative studies are not justified if prognostic biomarkers have unproven predictive value. Third, researchers should demonstrate an intention to publish the results of their correlative studies. Trial registries tend not to list correlative study components within clinical trials, and there is generally little if any pressure to publish findings of correlative studies—especially when they produce negative or inconclusive results. This raises concerns that burdens that volunteers have submitted to will go unredeemed by a gain in generalizable knowledge.

Correlative studies embedded within drug trials also raise concerns about informed consent. Because correlative study procedures mingle with therapeutic activities, research subjects might not appreciate that the former are performed for research purposes only. One small study found that most patients receiving non-diagnostic serial tumor biopsies in the context of a phase 1 cancer study incorrectly perceived the procedure as aimed at disease management [51]. If this indeed shows failed comprehension (as the authors purport), it raises concerns that volunteers may not be providing valid informed consent. To thwart such misunderstandings, separate consent should be sought for burdensome research procedures like lumbar punctures, and research teams might assess the adequacy of a volunteer's understanding before accepting their informed consent as valid.

Brain imaging and incidental findings

Many CNS drug trials involve brain imaging; in one report, brain abnormalities, like malignancies or vascular malformations, were detected in as many as 18% of healthy volunteers [52]. Incidental findings are probably less common in the context of CNS trials, because many patients will have already received brain scans as part of their diagnosis. Nevertheless, trials involving brain imaging should plan for the management of incidental findings. Several guidelines for addressing incidental findings in brain imaging have been put forward [53–54]. These vary somewhat, but tend to concur on the following items: 1- researchers should submit a plan for managing incidental findings to the IRB, and disclose to subjects the possibility of incidental findings during informed consent; 2- researchers should obtain informed consent to report incidental findings to them should they occur; 3- research teams should consider whether professionals capable of interpreting the clinical relevance of neuroimaging scans should be included in the study personnel; 4- research teams should prioritize disclosure of incidental findings to subjects (or their surrogates) who have consented to receiving this information, and follow up with written communications [55].

Justice and fairness

Justice and a fair distribution of risks and benefits

Among the three canonical principles of research ethics, justice is probably the least familiar and celebrated within the clinical research community. The relative obscurity of this principle stems, at least in part, from the fact that considerations of justice do not implicate the kinds personal interests that clinicians routinely encounter with informed consent and risk. Despite the flagrant injustices behind early to mid twentieth century scandals that motivated research ethics policy, the principle of justice was articulated only belatedly with the Belmont Report. There, justice is conceived largely in terms ensuring that disadvantaged individuals do not disproportionately bear burdens and risks of clinical research.

Three historical developments have driven an expansion of what the principle of justice is thought to encompass in research. First is the globalization of research, and the increasing volume of high-income country-sponsored trials pursued in low and middle-income countries. Second is a recognition that certain classes of patients—namely, children, women (especially pregnant women), persons in low and middle-income countries, persons of color, the elderly—have been deprived of the benefits of medical knowledge in part because of their exclusion from clinical research. Third is the ascendancy of disease advocacy groups that have used justice-based arguments for greater access and inclusion not only to clinical trials, but also to experimental interventions outside of trials. All three expansions are apparent in contemporary CNS clinical research.

Research and disadvantaged populations

Patients disadvantaged by poverty, incarceration, confinement, lack of health care access, and/or marginal political status often present convenient research opportunities. Unchecked by the principle of justice, advancing the medical interests of relatively advantaged populations would build on unfair disadvantages of others.

Though first articulated by the National Commission in the 1970s, the principle of justice lay more or less dormant until its revival in the mid 1990s following a series of controlled trials in Africa and Thailand. In these studies, pregnant women were randomized to either an abbreviated course of AZT or placebo in order to test whether vertical transmission of HIV could be reduced. Critics alleged that, because a standard course of AZT had been shown to prevent vertical transmission, the studies violated clinical equipoise by depriving some patients of established effective care. Study defenders argued that because the standard course of AZT was not affordable for patients in impoverished settings, the study met a local standard of clinical equipoise.

Following this debate, major international codes of research ethics developed two policies for ensuring fair and non-exploitative research design. First, clinical trials should make provisions for post-trial access. The Declaration of Helsinki states that 'protocol[s] should describe arrangements for post-study access by study subjects to interventions identified as beneficial in the study or access to other appropriate care or benefits.' Study designers should therefore address the prospect that patients responding to a study intervention will not be withdrawn once the study ends. Though this policy applies to all trials, the issue of post-trial access is a particular concern where patients or health care systems are unable to afford continued treatment once a study ends.

The second policy is the principle of responsiveness: trials should always be part of a program of inquiry that will expand the capacity of health-related social structures in the host community to meet urgent health needs [56]. As such, studies should not actively recruit patients who are members of groups that are unlikely to be able to access or benefit from the knowledge that a trial produces.

Issues of justice arise with particular frequency whenever CNS trials involve placebos. Recall that, according to the MS Society of America, the use of placebo controls may be acceptable where established effective therapy is not available to enrolling subjects because of resource constraints. This policy can comply with the principle of justice if the study is testing an intervention for MS that is likely to be accessible despite the resource constraints of the local health care system. However, it violates the principle of justice where interventions are unlikely to be affordable or accessible to the types of patients recruited into the study [33]. Because patients unable to access established effective interventions are often unable to access new and cutting edge interventions, proposed placebo controlled trials in low-income settings will often falter on the principle of responsiveness. To address concerns about responsiveness, investigators should produce evidence that the intervention they are testing is likely to be affordable and deployable given the resource constraints of the host community.

Inclusivity, evidence needs, and inclusion

Exclusion of patients also has adverse consequence for society, because it deprives the health care system of evidence needed to provide effective care to certain classes of patients. Among the categories of patients that have been excluded historically are children, women, and people of color.

Though changes in research and patent policy have helped address some exclusions, various commentators point out that others—e.g. pregnant women [57] and the elderly—remain to be addressed [58]. For example, most epilepsy drugs are tested in younger populations; extending these results to elderly patients is made difficult by the presence of co-morbidities and altered metabolism associated with aging [59]

The design and review of clinical trials should determine whether eligibility criteria are fair and appropriate. On the one hand, trials should strive to test interventions in a population that is as diverse and heterogeneous as the ultimate target population for the drug. On the other hand, patients belonging to certain groups are expected to have biological differences that affect clinical responses. Inclusive eligibility criteria can antagonize validity aims if effects in one patient group 'dilute out' effects for another. Therefore, studies that recruit biologically diverse patients should adequately power and plan for a subgroup analysis. This is especially critical when recruiting members of vulnerable or disadvantaged groups.

The integrity of the research enterprise

A third salient along which the principle of justice has expanded concerns patient access to investigational agents. Organized patient advocates have pressed policy-makers to relax restrictions on access to investigational CNS drugs; they have also, at times, urged more permissive and inclusive standards for clinical trials [60–62]. These appeals—though often couched

in terms of patient autonomy—build on the intuition that, because patients ultimately bear the risks and burdens of trial participation, their perspectives should be incorporated into the design and review of trials.

Nevertheless, appeals for access should not be allowed to override the core objectives of clinical research. However much trials aim to protect the interests of subjects, they are ultimately designed to advance medical knowledge by producing generalizable knowledge. Greater access and inclusion present two threats to this objective. First, packaging trials as therapeutic vehicles potentially diverts attention from their scientific purpose. For example, clinicians are often tempted to fudge eligibility criteria in order to enable enrollment of otherwise excluded patients [63]. If these exclusions have a valid scientific justification, their violation can confound the interpretation of trial outcomes. Second, access and/or less restrictive risk standards can threaten the interests of other legitimate stakeholders in clinical research. For example, major adverse events in one trial can have cascading adverse effects on related lines of research [64], and poorly designed or executed studies potentially damage the credibility and standing of a broader research field.

The perspectives of potential research subjects and disease communities can and should inform the design and review of clinical trials—especially where contentious designs or levels of risk are involved. Nevertheless, the principle of justice also requires that investigators and reviewers safeguard the integrity of the research enterprise by maintaining appropriate standards of quality, safety, and methodology.

Beyond protecting human subjects

Clinical investigators and responsibilities to non-research subjects

The issues we have addressed thus far largely center on duties investigators (and by extension, IRBs) owe to human volunteers in CNS trials. However, investigators harbor duties to other stakeholders as well. With some exceptions, regulations and major ethical policies do not specifically address these other ethical duties. In this part, we briefly discuss several issues of particular relevance to CNS drug development.

Risks and burdens for third parties

Many neurological clinical trials require the participation not only of subjects, but also on their caregivers.

For example, Alzheimer's disease clinical trials often perform assessments of caregiver outcomes [65]. Even when they do not, the conduct of such studies involving patients with compromised or declining capacity may depend crucially on the cooperation of caregivers. Caregivers often do not fall within the definition of 'human subject,' and are hence not always accorded protections of informed consent and risk review under existing policy. Yet clearly, their interests are implicated in clinical trials, and they bear at least some burdens of the research. Elsewhere, I called implicated third parties 'research bystanders,' and argued that protections of some form should be extended to them in the form of risk review, burden minimization, and under some circumstances, informed consent [66–67].

The duty to initiate trials before diffusion of risky interventions

To a large degree, drug and biologics regulations bar clinicians from introducing non-validated interventions into medical practice without clinical testing. This helps protect the public from undue risk, while promoting the production of knowledge to enable evidence-based practice. Nevertheless, non-validated CNS interventions have occasionally been introduced into clinical practice before rigorous testing has established a favorable risk-benefit balance. For example, several overseas clinics market non-validated cell transplantation to patients with neurodegenerative diseases and spinal cord injury [68–69].

The Belmont report states that 'radically new procedures… should… be made the object of formal research at an early stage in order to determine whether they are safe and effective.' The Declaration of Helsinki makes a similar point in paragraph 35. Researchers thus have positive duties to subject their interventions to clinical testing—or, barring that, systematic study—regardless of whether an intervention falls within the remit of domestic drug regulatory bodies.

Fostering critical public engagement with findings

We began this chapter by noting the inexorable and morbid course of many neurodegenerative diseases. Patients and their families often invest significant energy in following and responding to cutting edge research developments. Patient expectations concerning an intervention's therapeutic possibilities shape their decision-making. Given that these expectations are often established prior to the consent encounter, the information patients and family members receive before being solicited for trial enrollment plays a crucial role in patient exercise of autonomy.

Researchers have obligations to interact with various publics in ways that foster critical engagement with the implications of their research findings. Specifically, they should avoid issuing press releases that do not provide context for evaluating the implications of a study. Thus, if an early phase study shows promising effects, researchers should emphasize that many interventions that show promising effects at this stage do not withstand larger, more rigorous testing. Researchers should also attend to various non-verbal or affective elements of communication that shape public expectations. For example, they should avoid presenting to the media patient testimonials from small, uncontrolled clinical trials.

Conclusion

Disorders of the CNS present a number of challenges for specifying core principles and practices of research ethics. Patients frequently have compromised consent capacities, and risks are often considerable: access to the brain can require invasive approaches, harms are potentially irreversible and difficult to model in animals, and they implicate functions necessary for personal identity and human interaction. The distinctive nature of neurological illnesses—and interventions designed to reverse them—lead to recurrent ethical tensions surrounding the initiation of translational clinical trials, subject selection, the use of placebo comparators in randomized controlled trials, and standards for acceptable risk.

Addressing unmet health needs of patients with CNS disorders will necessitate finding ways of adapting general principles and practices of research ethics to these circumstances. However compelling the need or objectives of clinical research, research ethics always begins with the premise that the rights and interests of human subjects are inviolable. The task of ethical research is both to work within these constraints, and to design studies that align knowledge production activities with patient care objectives. And where patient care and research objectives diverge in non-trivial ways (as they inevitably will), researchers should at least ensure that their subjects share with them a conviction in the value of the research.

Acknowledgments

This work was funded by the Canadian Institutes of Health Research (NNF 80045 and MSH 87725).

References

1. Pangalos MN, Schechter LE and Hurko O. Drug development for CNS disorders: strategies for balancing risk and reducing attrition. *Nat Rev Drug Discov* 2007; **6**(7): 521–32.

2. The National Commission for the Protection of Human Subjects of Biomedical and Behavioural Research. The Belmont Report: Ethical Principles and Guidelines for the Protection of Human Subjects of Research. Department of Health and Welfare, 1979.

3. Stocking CB, Hougham GW, Danner DD, *et al.* Speaking of research advance directives: planning for future research participation. *Neurology* 2006; **66**: 1361–6.

4. Schats R, Brilstra EH, Rinkel GJ, *et al.* Informed consent in trials for neurological emergencies: the example of subarachnoid haemorrhage. *J Neurol Neurosurg Psychiatry* 2003; **74**: 988–91.

5. Beecher HK. Ethics and clinical research. *N Engl J Med* 1966; **274**: 1354–60.

6. Ethical issues in clinical research in neurology: advancing knowledge and protecting human research subjects. The Ethics and Humanities Subcommittee of the American Academy of Neurology. *Neurology* 1998; **50**: 592–5.

7. International Conference on Harmonisation (ICH). Guidance for Industry. E10 Choice of Control Group and Related Issues in Clinical Trials: U.S. Department of Health and Human Services, Food and Drug Administration, Center for Drug Evaluation and Research (CDER), Center for Biologics Evaluation and Research (CBER), 2001.

8. Temple R and Ellenberg SS. Placebo-controlled trials and active-control trials in the evaluation of new treatments. Part 1: ethical and scientific issues. *Ann Intern Med* 2000; **133**: 455–63.

9. Weijer C and Miller PB. When are research risks reasonable in relation to anticipated benefits? *Nat Med* 2004; **10**: 570–3.

10. Freedman B, Fuks A and Weijer C. Demarcating research and treatment: a systematic approach for the analysis of the ethics of clinical research. *Clin Res* 1992; **40**: 653–60.

11. Protection of Human Subjects: Criteria for IRB approval of research 45 CFR 46.400 et seq. Department of Health and Human Services, 2005.

12. Protection of Human Subjects: Criteria for IRB approval of research 45 CFR 46.300 et seq. Department of Health and Human Services, 2005.

13. World Medical Association. Declaration of Helsinki, 1964.

14. Menon DK. Unique challenges in clinical trials in traumatic brain injury. *Crit Care Med* 2009; **37**(1 Suppl): S129–35.

15. Freedman B. Equipoise and the ethics of clinical research. *N Engl J Med* 1987; **317**: 141–5.

16. Rowbotham MC. The impact of selective publication on clinical research in pain. *Pain* 2008; **140**: 401–4.

17. Liebeskind DS, Kidwell CS, Sayre JW and Saver JL. Evidence of publication bias in reporting acute stroke clinical trials. *Neurology* 2006; **67**: 973–9.

18. Mathews DJ, Sugarman J, Bok H, *et al.* Cell-based interventions for neurologic conditions: ethical challenges for early human trials. *Neurology* 2008; **71**: 288–93.

19. Duggan PS, Siegel AW, Blass DM, *et al.* Unintended changes in cognition, mood, and behavior arising from cell-based interventions for neurological conditions: ethical challenges. *Am J Bioeth* 2009; **9**: 31–6.

20. van der Worp HB, de Haan P, Morrema E, *et al.* Methodological quality of animal studies on neuroprotection in focal cerebral ischaemia. *J Neurol* 2005; **252**: 1108–14.

21. Gibson CL, Gray LJ, Bath PM, *et al.* Progesterone for the treatment of experimental brain injury; a systematic review. *Brain* 2008; **131**: 318–28.

22. O'Collins VE, Macleod MR, Donnan GA, *et al.* 1,026 experimental treatments in acute stroke. *Ann Neurol* 2006; **59**: 467–77.

23. Banwell V, Sena ES and Macleod MR. Systematic review and stratified meta-analysis of the efficacy of interleukin-1 receptor antagonist in animal models of stroke. *J Stroke Cerebrovasc Dis* 2009; **18**: 269–76.

24. Benatar M. Lost in translation: treatment trials in the SOD1 mouse and in human ALS. *Neurobiol Dis* 2007; **26**: 1–13.

25. Crossley NA, Sena E, Goehler J, *et al.* Empirical evidence of bias in the design of experimental stroke studies: a metaepidemiologic approach. *Stroke* 2008; **39**: 929–34.

26. Sena ES, van der Worp HB, Bath PM, *et al.* Publication bias in reports of animal stroke studies leads to major overstatement of efficacy. *PLos Biol* 2010; **8**: e1000344.

27. Marks WJ, Jr., Ostrem JL, Verhagen L, *et al.* Safety and tolerability of intraputaminal delivery of CERE-120 (adeno-associated virus serotype 2-neurturin) to patients with idiopathic Parkinson's disease: an open-label, phase I trial. *Lancet Neurol* 2008; **7**: 400–8.

28. Kimmelman J. *Gene Transfer and the Ethics of First-in-human Research: Lost in translation.* Cambridge: Cambridge University Press, 2010.

29. Kimmelman J, London AJ, Ravina B, *et al.* Launching invasive, first-in-human trials against Parkinson's disease: ethical considerations. *Mov Disord* 2009; **24**: 1893–901.

30. Kimmelman J. Stable ethics: enrolling non-treatment-refractory volunteers in novel gene transfer trials. *Mol Ther* 2007; **15**: 1904–6.

31. Frank SA, Wilson R, Holloway RG, *et al.* Ethics of sham surgery: perspective of patients. *Mov Disord* 2008; **23**: 63–8.

32. de la Fuente-Fernandez R, Schulzer M and Stoessl AJ. The placebo effect in neurological disorders. *Lancet Neurol* 2002; **1**: 85–91.

33. Lublin FD and Reingold SC. Placebo-controlled clinical trials in multiple sclerosis: ethical considerations. National Multiple Sclerosis Society (USA) Task Force on Placebo-Controlled Clinical Trials in MS. *Ann Neurol* 2001; **49**: 677–81.

34. Miller A. Ethical issues in MS clinical trials. *Mult Scler* 2005; **11**: 97–8.

35. National Multiple Sclerosis Society. Ethics of Placebos in MS Clinical Trials Reassessed in New Publication. 2008. http://www.nationalmssociety.org/news/news-detail/index.aspx?nid=202 (Accessed November 2, 2010.)

36. National Placebo Working Committee. National Placebo Initiative (NPI). Health Canada. 2005. http://www.hc-sc.gc.ca/dhp-mps/prodpharma/activit/proj/npinotice_inpavis-eng.php (Accessed November 2, 2010.)

37. Kaptchuk TJ, Goldman P, Stone DA, *et al.* Do medical devices have enhanced placebo effects? *J Clin Epidemiol* 2000; **53**: 786–92.

38. Watts RL, Freeman TB, Hauser RA, *et al.* A double-blind, randomised, controlled, multicenter clinical trial of the safety and efficacy of stereotaxic intrastriatal implantation of fetal porcine ventral mesencephalic tissue (Neurocelli-PD) vs. imitation surgery in patients with Parkinson's disease (PD). *Parkinsonism and Related Disord* 2001; 7(S87).

39. Lidstone SC and Stoessl AJ. Understanding the placebo effect: contributions from neuroimaging. *Mol Imaging Biol* 2007; **9**: 176–85.

40. de la Fuente-Fernandez R, Ruth TJ, Sossi V, *et al.* Expectation and dopamine release: mechanism of the placebo effect in Parkinson's disease. *Science* 2001; **293**: 1164–6.

41. Lidstone SC, Schulzer M, Dinelle K, *et al.* Effects of expectation on placebo-induced dopamine release in Parkinson disease. *Arch Gen Psychiatry* 2010; **67**: 857–65.

42. Weijer C. I need a placebo like I need a hole in the head. *J Law Med Ethics* 2002; **30**: 69–72.

43. Lang AE, Gill S, Patel NK, *et al.* Randomized controlled trial of intraputamenal glial cell line-derived neurotrophic factor infusion in Parkinson disease. *Ann Neurol* 2006; **59**: 459–66.

44. Bjorklund A, Dunnett SB, Brundin P, *et al.* Neural transplantation for the treatment of Parkinson's disease. *Lancet Neurol* 2003; **2**: 437–45.

45. Macklin R. The ethical problems with sham surgery in clinical research. *N Engl J Med* 1999; **341**: 992–6.

46. London AJ and Kadane JB. Placebos that harm: sham surgery controls in clinical trials. *Stat Methods Med Res* 2002; **11**: 413–27.

47. Horng SH and Miller FG. Placebo-controlled procedural trials for neurological conditions. *Neurotherapeutics* 2007; **4**: 531–6.

48. Cohen PD, Herman L, Jedlinski S, *et al.* Ethical issues in clinical neuroscience research: a patient's perspective. *Neurotherapeutics* 2007; **4**: 537–44.

49. Goulart BH, Clark JW, Pien HH, *et al.* Trends in the use and role of biomarkers in phase I oncology trials. *Clin Cancer Res* 2007; **13**: 6719–26.

50. Ryberg H, Askmark H and Persson LI. A double-blind randomized clinical trial in amyotrophic lateral sclerosis using lamotrigine: effects on CSF glutamate, aspartate, branched-chain amino acid levels and clinical parameters. *Acta Neurol Scand* 2003; **108**: 1–8.

51. Agulnik M, Oza AM, Pond GR, *et al.* Impact and perceptions of mandatory tumor biopsies for correlative studies in clinical trials of novel anticancer agents. *J Clin Oncol* 2006; **24**: 4801–7.

52. Katzman GL, Dagher AP and Patronas NJ. Incidental findings on brain magnetic resonance imaging from 1000 asymptomatic volunteers. *JAMA* 1999; **282**: 36–9.

53. Illes J, Kirschen MP, Edwards E, *et al.* Ethics. Incidental findings in brain imaging research. *Science* 2006; **311**: 783–4.

54. Wolf SM, Lawrenz FP, Nelson CA, *et al.* Managing incidental findings in human subjects research: analysis and recommendations. *J Law Med Ethics* 2008; **36**: 219–48.

55. Illes J, Kirschen MP, Edwards E, *et al.* Practical approaches to incidental findings in brain imaging research. *Neurology* 2008; **70**: 384–90.

56. London AJ and Kimmelman J. Justice in translation: from bench to bedside in the developing world. *Lancet* 2008; **372**: 82–5.

57. Adab N, Tudur SC, Vinten J, *et al.* Common antiepileptic drugs in pregnancy in women with epilepsy. *Cochrane Database Syst Rev* 2004; **3**: CD004848.

58. Avorn J. *Powerful Medicines: The Benefits, Risks, and Costs of Prescription Drugs* – Chapter 7. New York, Vintage Books, 2005.

59. Leppik IE, Brodie MJ, Saetre ER, *et al.* Outcomes research: clinical trials in the elderly. *Epilepsy Res* 2006; **68** Suppl 1: S71–6.

60. Winerip M. Fighting for Jacob. *The New York Times* 1998.

61. The hard way to a Bill of Rights. *Lancet Neurol* 2005; **4**: 787.

62. Patient choice in clinical trials. *Lancet* 2005; **365**(9476): 1984.

63. Chen PW. Bending the Rules of Clinical Trials. *The New York Times* 2009.

64. Wilson JM. Medicine. A history lesson for stem cells. *Science* 2009; **324**: 727–8.

65. Lingler JH, Parker LS, DeKosky ST, *et al.* Caregivers as subjects of clinical drug trials: a review of human subjects protection practices in published studies of Alzheimer's disease pharmacotherapies. *IRB* 2006; **28**: 11–8.

66. Kimmelman J. Medical research, risk, and bystanders. *IRB* 2005; **27**: 1–6.

67. Kimmelman J. Missing the forest: further thoughts on the ethics of bystander risk in medical research. *Camb Q Healthc Ethics* 2007; **16**: 483–90.

68. Baker M. Tumours spark stem-cell review. *Nature* 2009; **457**: 941.

69. Lau D, Ogbogu U, Taylor B, *et al.* Stem cell clinics online: the direct-to-consumer portrayal of stem cell medicine. *Cell Stem Cell* 2008; **3**: 591–4.

The informed consent process: Compliance and beyond

Scott Y. H. Kim

Introduction

This chapter provides an evidence-based and practical overview of informed consent for neurological clinical trials, in four parts. The first part places the doctrine of informed consent within an overall framework of clinical research ethics, along with a brief history of informed consent. The second part discusses the three key elements of informed consent: how and what information to disclose; ensuring voluntary consent; and how to assess the decision-making capacity of potential subjects with cognitive impairment. The third part discusses issues to consider when considering enrollment of subjects based on surrogate consent. The conclusion critically examines the widely discussed concept of therapeutic misconception and suggests how to enhance the quality of subjects' decision-making about research participation.

The purpose of informed consent

The place of informed consent in research ethics

What makes clinical research ethical? Perhaps the first thing that comes to mind is informed consent. This is not surprising since autonomy, the ethical basis for informed consent, has become the dominant concept in Western bioethics [1]. But informed consent is only one among several requirements of ethical clinical research. If one were to review the various ethics codes, commission reports, declarations, and scholarly literature from around the world on clinical research ethics and reduced them to a set of common principles, one will likely find the seven principles identified by Emanuel *et al.*: social or scientific value, scientific validity, fair subject selection, favorable risk-benefit ratio, independent review, informed consent, and

respect for potential and enrolled subjects [1]. These requirements for ethical clinical research are in roughly sequential order in the process of evaluating the ethics of a research protocol.

There are five requirements that precede the question of informed consent. In other words, a clinical research protocol must satisfy five other requirements before it is deemed ethically permissible to even offer research participation to potential subjects. Thus, informed consent cannot make ethical the involvement of a person in a clinical trial that is of dubious scientific or social value, or that uses shoddy methods, or that targets a sample only for convenience, or that has not minimized the risks, or that has not undergone independent review. Although some of these elements are commonly thought of only as scientific criteria for evaluating research protocols, they are actually important ethical criteria that precede the question of informed consent.

So what role does informed consent play in research ethics? In general, rather than making a research *protocol* ethical, informed consent makes the *involvement of specific subjects* in ethically approved research ethical. It is a duty owed to specific individuals that shows respect for their right to self-determination.

History of informed consent for research

The purpose of research is fundamentally different from that of treatment. When a surgeon recommends an operation to her patient, the patient can reasonably assume that the surgeon's primary purpose in recommending the procedure is to improve his health and welfare. When a researcher offers a research protocol to a patient, on the other hand, the primary purpose of that research protocol is not the specific subject's health and welfare. The primary goal is the generation of scientific knowledge. This primary research goal implies a *potential* for some degree of sacrifice – of health,

Clinical Trials in Neurology, ed. Bernard Ravina, Jeffrey Cummings, Michael P. McDermott, and R. Michael Poole. Published by Cambridge University Press. © Cambridge University Press 2012.

welfare, or comfort – on the part of the subject for the sake of generating scientific knowledge. The amount of such trade-off will vary depending on the clinical trial.

At one extreme might be research involving placebos when effective treatments exist. Some have even argued that as long as the research subject does not suffer permanent serious injury or death, the trade-off may be permissible [2] whereas others have proposed a lower limit on risk in such situations [3]. On the other hand, for some research protocols, especially when they involve diseases for which no effective treatments exist and the proposed intervention is not too risky or burdensome, the amount of trade-off may be less. In either case, the main goal of clinical trials is, by treating the subject as a means (with his or her permission), to generate knowledge that can be applied to persons with the same medical condition; the primary goal is not to treat the specific individuals enrolling in the study.

The doctrine of informed consent in the treatment context was developed largely through case law in 1950s to 1970s [4]. But given the important distinction between research and treatment, the necessity of informed consent for research was recognized much earlier (even if it was not called informed consent at that time). For example, as early as 1907, Sir William Osler was asked to testify to the British Royal Commission on Vivisection regarding the ethics of Major Walter Reed's experiment on yellow fever [5]. When Osler was asked by the Commission whether 'to experiment upon man with possible ill results was immoral,' he answered, 'It is always immoral, without a definite, specific statement from the individual himself, with a full knowledge of the circumstances' [Osler quoted in [5] p. 131]. In fact, the essential difference between treatment and research was formally recognized even earlier [6].

The practice of informed consent for research

In order for a person to provide valid, informed consent, three conditions must be met. The person must be provided adequate *information*. He or she must possess *decision-making capacity*. And the decision must be made *voluntarily*, without coercion or undue influence.

Information to be disclosed for research consent

For most clinical research (and for most clinical trials in neurology), written informed consent will be required. The US Federal regulations are explicit about what needs to be disclosed to potential subjects; these elements are summarized in Table 17.1.

Because the disclosure elements are so explicitly spelled out, an investigator will find that his or her local research ethics review board (an institutional review board, or IRB, in the US) will have considerable say over what goes into an informed consent document. In fact, IRBs usually have a detailed template that the investigator will be expected to use.

Although the IRB's job is to ensure that the informed consent forms are 'understandable,' the tendency of IRB requirements regarding informed consent forms often go in the other direction, albeit unintentionally. Research shows that informed consent documents are written at a high level of reading difficulty. In fact, IRBs use language in their informed consent templates that are far above the levels they require their investigators to use (typically 8th grade level) in informed consent forms, by an average of almost three grade levels (average text level was 10.6th grade) [7].

What should the investigator do? IRBs vary considerably in their oversight practices and policies [8,9]. The researcher may not be able to do much in some cases. For instance, one of the most bureaucratic and difficult to understand passages in most clinical research informed consent forms is the section on 'Privacy and Confidentiality' because it is often written in lawyerly language in complying with the Federal HIPAA (Health Insurance Portability and Accountability Act) Privacy Rule. In spite of these bureaucratic constraints there are a few things that a researcher can do to improve the quality of disclosure.

The very nature of research involves uncertainties and probabilities. How to best communicate probabilities of risk and potential benefits is a common and complex issue [10]. First, should probabilities be expressed using words such as 'possible,' 'rare,' 'unlikely' or by numerical expressions? Studies have shown that it is generally better to use numerical expressions in the form of natural frequencies (i.e., '5 out of 100') rather than relying solely on verbal expressions of probability [10]. Also, although 'possible' and 'probable' seem to indicate quite different likelihood of an event occurring, many factors affect perceptions of such probability expressions; for example, mere valence (i.e., 'possible' has positive valence) of a verbal expression can create perceptions of probability that are much greater than what one might intend [11]. Second, being sensitive to how the probability statements are

Table 17.1 Legally required disclosure elements for informed consent for research (Title 45 Code of Federal Regulations 46.116a&b)

Always required:

(1) A statement that the study is research, its purpose and procedures

(2) Any reasonably foreseeable risks or discomforts

(3) Any benefits that may be reasonably expected

(4) Any alternative treatments that might be advantageous to the subject

(5) Degree of confidentiality expected

(6) Compensation, if any, and whether and nature of treatment available if injury occurs

(7) Contact information for further questions

(8) Statement that participation is voluntary

Required when appropriate:

(1) A statement regarding currently unforeseeable risks

(2) When the investigator may terminate the subject's participation

(3) Any additional costs to the subject that may result from participation in research

(4) Consequences of withdrawal from study and procedures for orderly withdrawal

(5) A statement that significant new findings during the study which may relate to continued participation by the subject will be provided

(6) Approximate number of subjects in the study

framed is important. Thus, when discussing potential benefits and risks, it may be important to present both the likelihood of a good outcome and the likelihood of bad outcome, especially if the outcome in question is central to the risk-benefit analysis that could affect a person's willingness to participate. Thus, instead of saying 'serious bleeding is rare,' it may be better to say, 'it is expected that if 100 persons were given this medication, on average 3 persons will experience severe bleeding and 97 persons will not.'

If the protocol is long and complex, it may be useful to prepare a short one page summary document (which will need to be approved by the IRB) of the long informed consent form. IRBs will not allow such forms to replace the longer form, but such a summary may be a useful tool to reinforce the key points and to provide an easy-to-grasp overview of the clinical trial.

In representing the risks and burdens of a study protocol, being clear and straightforward will serve the project well in the long run. Drop-outs are expensive and compromise the quality of science. An important ingredient in subjects' motivation to participate is the trust and confidence they feel in the researchers and their institutions [12]. Candor and transparency go a long way in earning such trust and confidence.

As the burdens or risks involved in a research study increases, greater the effort should be in ensuring that subjects' understanding is optimal. A variety of methods have been attempted, including multimedia interventions, enhanced consent forms, extended discussion formats, and test/feedback procedures [13]. A review of 42 such studies showed that, perhaps not surprisingly, the most effective means of improving understanding is extended, one-on-one discussions with the subjects [13].

Voluntary consent

The Federal regulations require that informed consent will be sought 'only under circumstances that provide the prospective subject or the representative sufficient opportunity to consider whether or not to participate and that minimize the possibility of coercion or undue influence' (45CFR46.116). Of the three elements of informed consent, this one is the least well conceptualized and studied [14].

Although evidence is scarce, it is highly unlikely that research subjects participate from coercion or undue influence. A recent study of 88 subjects enrolled in clinical trials for a variety of conditions found 'little evidence' of constraints on voluntariness [15]. Participation in clinical trials requires a good deal of cooperation based on trust. It is unlikely that a subject who feels coerced or feels external pressure would volunteer to participate, and even less likely that such a subject would continue to cooperate. Thus, discussions in bioethics regarding threats to voluntary decision-making have focused on other ways in which a subject may make a less than optimal decision – either by being misled by the information provided or misunderstanding the nature of research participation due to internal pressures (such as a desperate desire to benefit therapeutically). Systematic studies of informed consent forms do not reveal that subjects are given inaccurate information [16]. However, concerns that very sick individuals desperate for relief may conflate research with treatment (the so-called 'therapeutic misconception') remain [17]. These concerns are discussed in the final part of this chapter.

Decision-making capacity and cognitive impairment in neurological disorders

Many neurological conditions involve impaired cognitive function. Conditions such as Alzheimer's disease (AD) have a devastating impact on their victims. We cannot currently alter the course of the disease and the best hope for advances in treating persons with such illnesses rests on research. However, the assault on the brain that impairs the overall cognitive and decision-making abilities creates the ethical problem of needing to conduct research with those who are often not capable of providing their own informed consent.

The dementing illnesses have a major impact on consent capacity, even when the disease is in the early stages. In a study of 60 patients with mild cognitive impairment (MCI) with a mean mini-mental state examination (MMSE) score of 28.4, 27% to 53% were deemed to have capacity for treatment consent that was 'marginal or below,' depending on the standard of capacity used. In this study, 'marginal or below' was defined psychometrically as persons falling 1.5 standard deviations below the control group mean [8]. In a study that examined 40 persons with MCI regarding research consent capacity for a typical phase 3 drug clinical trial, expert judges categorized subjects using audio-taped capacity interviews. They found that 40% of MCI subjects were incapable of providing informed consent, despite a MMSE mean score of 28.3 (SD1.1) [19]. In a study of persons with AD (mean MMSE 22.9) using the same capacity instrument (MacArthur Capacity Assessment Tool-Clinical Research), 66% of the mild to mild-moderate AD patients failed a clinician panel-validated threshold on at least one of four

standards of decision-making ability [20]. Clearly, the capacity to consent to research or treatment is impaired very early in conditions such as AD.

Other neurodegenerative disorders with cognitive impairment will of course be associated with impaired decision-making abilities. For example, depending on the legal standard used, 25% to 80% of Parkinson's disease patients with 'mild' level of cognitive impairment were found to be marginally incapable or incapable of providing consent for treatment [21].

Assessment of capacity

The practice of capacity assessment is still an evolving field, especially when done to assess capacity for research consent. In contrast to the other two elements of informed consent (disclosure and voluntariness), the Federal regulations are silent in terms of criteria for assessing capacity. Over the past several years, some states in the US have passed specific laws regulating research with adults lacking capacity and some of these discuss the criteria for capacity. A recent New Jersey statute defines 'unable to consent' as:

> '…unable to voluntarily reason, understand, and appreciate the nature and consequences of proposed health research interventions… and to reach an informed decision' [22].

The principles of capacity assessment in the treatment context generally apply to the research context as well [23]. All adults are presumed to have decision-making capacity (DMC), although that presumption can be challenged, as in cases where the subject is known to have a cognitive disorder that often impairs a person's DMC.

The terms 'capacity,' 'decision-making capacity,' and 'competence' can be used interchangeably to indicate a clinical determination approximating what a court would decide; the latter can be specified as *adjudicated* competence or capacity, to avoid any confusion [23].

The assessment of decision-making capacity is measured according to four standards or abilities: evidencing a choice, understanding, appreciation, and reasoning [24]. Although the exact terms may be different, most statutes and policy documents mention (or can reasonably be interpreted to overlap with) these four abilities [23]. Evidencing a choice is a minimal standard, merely the ability to state a preference that is stable enough to be implemented. Understanding is the ability to comprehend intellectually the facts of the decision-making situation. Appreciation is the ability to apply those facts to one's own situation, and involves an ability to form appropriate beliefs. For instance, a person with AD may acknowledge that the researchers are telling him that he has dementia (thus exhibiting understanding of what the researchers are saying), and yet fail to believe that he actually has dementia (thus failing to appreciate the fact). The ability to reason refers to general procedural ability to process information without obvious processing defects; it is not a standard about the 'reasonableness' the subject's decision.

DMC is distinct from a diagnosis. It is a functional concept. Even if one has AD, the old fashioned, vague label of 'unsound mind' cannot be used to justify categorizing someone as lacking capacity. A person lacks capacity if he or she is unable to carry out the requisite abilities underlying decision-making, not simply because he or she has a diagnosis.

DMC is context sensitive. A capacity assessment is largely an exercise in balancing the duty to respect the person's autonomy interests with the duty to protect his welfare interests. Thus, in assessing whether a person lacks capacity, the potential welfare implications for the subject must be taken into account: the greater the potential for harm and lower the potential for benefit, the higher the level of abilities needed to be deemed competent. This is a long-standing principle that is widely accepted in policy documents [25, 26] and in practice [27].

Recommendations regarding capacity assessment

The decision as to whether a specific plan for capacity assessment is required in a clinical trial generally rests with the local IRB. However, there are no uniform standards for formulating such plans. Such plans need to be flexible and adapted to the particular context. The investigator should, at minimum, be familiar with the laws and regulations of one's own jurisdiction (and one's own institution's interpretation of those laws and regulations). The investigator should also be familiar with the elements of the modern practice of capacity assessment, along with the available empirical data on capacity for the population of interest, if available. Because the level of knowledge regarding these matters may vary considerably among IRBs, the investigator may need to educate his or her IRB.

The rigor or intensiveness of capacity evaluation should vary depending on the subject population and the risk-benefit profile of the protocol. At one extreme may be an informal judgment of capacity made by a research assistant. This may be appropriate, for example, for a minimal risk observational or interview study involving AD patients, with no sensitive information. Sometimes brief forms or questionnaires might be used to guide the assessment and to document the fact that subjects have understood the essential elements of informed consent, or for use as an initial screen to determine whether further, more intensive assessment is needed [28].

At the other extreme, the capacity evaluation procedures may need to be a systematic, structured evaluation by an experienced, independent mental health professional (or perhaps even a panel of such experts) who renders his judgment using a detailed and validated capacity assessment tool. This may be an appropriate standard when enrolling potentially impaired persons who provide their own informed consent for a high-risk study, such as first in human neurosurgical experiments.

Surrogate consent for research

Although the need for informed consent in research has long been recognized, controversy about how best to regulate research involving those who cannot consent for themselves remains, not only in the US [29] but also internationally [30]. Because the situation varies according to jurisdiction, it is impossible to give a uniform guidance on how to involve decisionally incapacitated subjects in neurological research. The investigator will need to work closely with his or her IRB. An excellent, detailed guidance on how to work with one's IRB on these issues has been published by the Alzheimer's Association [31]. Some of the key questions that will need to be addressed by the investigator and the IRB are as follows.

In practice, close family members tend to serve as de facto surrogates. We have found that persons at risk for AD, family caregivers, and the general public are all broadly in favor of de facto family consent [32–34]. But policy is not so clear. The US Federal research regulations require that for an incompetent adult, a legally authorized representative (LAR) provide permission for the incapacitated subject to participate in research (45 CFR 46.102c). However, the regulations defer to the states on who can serve as LAR. Although California, Virginia, and New Jersey have recently enacted laws that answer this question, most states have not addressed the issue clearly, if at all [22, 35–37].

The Federal regulations do not provide explicit guidance. Published documents by various groups do not agree [29–31]. For example, the recent law passed in California does not limit the research by specifying risk-benefit categories, leaving the judgment to local IRBs, whereas laws in Virginia and New Jersey do spell out the types of research allowed in terms of risks and benefits, such as excluding psychosurgery, and limiting risk on 'non-therapeutic' research. Most attempts to articulate a policy on this topic tend to focus on whether research holding no prospect for direct benefit to the subjects can involve risks that are greater than 'minor increase over minimal risk' [31].

When a person is able to provide affirmative agreement to participate, even if not capable of informed consent, it is generally agreed that such *assent* is essential. Dissent by an incompetent adult should generally be respected as well. Excellent discussion and recommendations regarding this issue can be found elsewhere [38]. Another widely discussed principle is that persons with incapacity may not be enrolled in research unless that research focuses on the subjects' medical condition [30]. Also, some advocate that research should not be performed with incompetent persons if it can be performed with competent persons (although this can be more complicated than it seems: see next part).

Ethical analysis: Should only competent subjects be enrolled in certain types of research?

When involving cognitively impaired subjects in clinical trials, the 'right thing to do' will require a deliberative process of thinking through various options, in working with independent ethics review bodies. It may be useful therefore to work through a realistic example that an investigator may encounter, as an exercise in ethical analysis.

Are there certain types of research that are so risky that only competent subjects – even if they have a disorder such as AD – should be allowed to enroll? Recently the Recombinant DNA Advisory Committee (RAC) of the National Institutes of Health recommended to researchers proposing to conduct a phase 2 sham control gene transfer study for AD that: (a) only competent subjects be enrolled and (b) requiring permission from a caregiver be prohibited because it would 'undermine the autonomy' of the subject [39].

The main consideration in favor of this 'competent only' requirement is the advantage of autonomous decision-making by the AD patient who can provide his or her own consent. Many people feel that if a competent person decides to take on a high-risk option, then it is more permissible than allowing an incapacitated person to take on that risk based on a surrogate's permission. This follows the logic of autonomy, at least theoretically.

A 'competent only' policy has obvious limitations as well. Since the threshold for capacity should be sensitive to the risk-benefit context, when a study's risk-benefit ratio is seen as quite high – i.e., those cases likely to elicit a competent only policy – very few AD patients will be competent to consent. Involving those few, perhaps atypical, AD patients may limit the generalizability of the clinical trial's findings. It will also make recruitment more difficult and expensive. But the point of a competent only policy may just be that sometimes the quality of science and the extra costs are the price to pay to uphold an important ethical principle. This trade-off is probably the most obvious focus when trying to balance the pros and cons of a policy of enrolling only competent subjects.

However, it may be useful to examine what such a policy might look like at the level of implementation, as a way of thinking through the merits of a competent only policy. Ethicists, often non-clinicians who advocate a competent only policy may not realize that a capacity determination is not a straightforward assessment. In fact, although capacity researchers have developed methods for measuring the abilities relevant to DMC in a dimensional sense, there is very little guidance on how to make a *categorical* determination of capacity, i.e., there is no 'gold standard' we can use to determine whether a cognitively impaired person is in fact competent [40]. Because the capacity for research consent is a relatively new domain of assessment, there can be widely differing opinions about where this line should be drawn, even among clinicians who routinely perform capacity assessments in other settings [27].

Is it possible then that a competent only policy places too much emphasis on a difficult to implement distinction? A person with well diagnosed AD who is deemed 'competent' remains a highly vulnerable subject because he is still cognitively impaired. On the other hand, there is considerable evidence that even if a person with mild to moderate AD is deemed 'incompetent,' he may still retain important, ethically relevant abilities, such as the ability to convey a preference, the ability to work cooperatively with a loved one, or the ability to delegate authority to a trusted surrogate [41].

In studies of persons with AD, it has been repeatedly shown that despite the obvious and significant loss in the ability to provide *independent* informed consent, such persons still tend to make medical treatment and research participation choices that are similar to age-matched controls and choices that are, in the main, quite reasonable [42, 43].

Is it better policy to require the 'competent' but vulnerable subjects to stand alone (i.e., prohibit a joint permission from a close relation) based on a difficult assessment; or, to require a broader approach by respecting their remaining abilities (by maximizing their involvement in decision-making) and yet providing additional safeguards, such as the informed permission of a family member?

Another consideration is that even if a person with AD is 'capable' of consenting to a highly risky study, it is quite likely that he or she will lose that capacity during the trial and will need a surrogate's permission to maintain that person's enrollment in the study [26]. Thus, even if a policy of competent only enrollment is used, the de facto practice will have to involve a person who agrees to serve as a surrogate. From a legal point of view, a surrogate's permission at the beginning of the study, if the subject is deemed competent, may not be necessary. But is there a reason to *prohibit* a surrogate's informed permission, especially since a de facto agreement from that surrogate is needed anyway? Also, since no one has a legal right to participate in a research study, it would seem reasonable for researchers to exercise the option of requiring informed decisions from both the subject and the prospective surrogate, if the researcher believes this will enhance the protection of a vulnerable research subject.

The point is not that a competent only policy is necessarily right or wrong. The answer will surely vary for different clinical trials. The investigator should carefully think through such a policy in working with his ethics review committee, and make sure that the theoretical rationale of upholding subject autonomy is not outweighed by other real-world ethical considerations.

Conclusion: Helping potential subjects make good decisions

Concern over therapeutic misconception

Some of the most devastating human illnesses are neurological disorders, with only marginally effective symptomatic treatment available. It is understandable that there is an increasing focus on novel and often aggressive interventions to treat these disorders, including brain stimulation, gene transfer, and cell transplants, among others [44–47].

The much needed effort to find new interventions is accompanied by a long-standing concern that persons with serious, incurable disorders may be so desperate for improvement that they are particularly vulnerable to what is called the therapeutic misconception (TM), which was first described over 25 years ago by Appelbaum and colleagues [48] as the tendency of research subjects to conflate research with treatment, thereby generating mistaken beliefs about the purpose and nature of research procedures, including the potential for benefits and harms [17].

Although the concept of TM seems intuitive, the term is used in the literature 'to denote a number of related, but not always identical concepts' [49]. For instance, in one study the investigators defined TM as the sum of three types of phenomena: subjects' therapeutic motivation for participation, their perception of therapeutic benefit, and their failure to understand the purpose of research [50]. It is likely that most persons with serious, often devastating, conditions with inadequate treatment options will volunteer for clinical trials because they are hoping for therapeutic benefit, even for early phase studies [12, 50]. But to assume that merely having such a motivation is a form of a misconception seems inaccurate. Motivation and understanding may influence one another, but they are not the same thing. Subjects motivated by personal benefit may in fact understand that the purpose of the clinical trial is scientific, for the benefit of society [50]. They may, for example, see themselves as using the clinical trial as an opportunity to receive benefit, in a kind of a gamble [12].

However, it is also reasonable to worry that when patients feel desperate about obtaining therapeutic benefit and volunteer for a clinical trial on that basis, they may not be in an optimal position to coolly absorb and weigh all of the relevant elements of a clinical trial. That is, although it is wrong to *equate* therapeutic motivation with a misunderstanding, it is reasonable to be on guard against the natural human tendency to interpret facts in line with one's motivations. As one subject put it in one of our studies, 'I really don't remember thinking about what [the researchers] were trying to accomplish as much as how it was going to affect me… I wasn't sure at the beginning, to tell you the truth, even though I went through the study. Then I realized that what they were trying to do was to see if there was any harm done. That was really the basis of the study' [12]. A subject who fails to see the experimental purpose of a clinical trial may in turn fail to understand and appreciate the details of the clinical trial.

Preventing therapeutic misconception

Informed consent for research has become institutionalized. This can encourage a 'compliance' mindset in which informed consent is seen as merely a vehicle for transferring information. People are seen as information receptacles that need to filled with the right kind of information [51]. The focus becomes the informed consent document which becomes longer and longer as more and more information is deemed necessary to 'transfer' to the subject.

But suppose informed consent is seen as more than compliance with regulations. What if it were seen as a conversation designed to promote good decision-making by potential subjects and investigators? The concern over TM is valuable. It serves as a reminder that the informed consent conversation should take into account where the patients are starting from, rather than seeing them as empty information receptacles.

The therapeutic motivation common in research subjects should therefore be an essential element in framing the informed consent conversation. Such a conversation at some point should involve an explicit question to the potential subject: 'Mr. Jones, can you tell me what your main reasons are for wishing to participate in this clinical trial?' Such a question is not required by the Federal regulations, and no IRB requires that an investigator ask it.

But the question will often bring out on the table a subject's therapeutic motivation. This will provide the investigator with an essential point of contrast between the scientific purpose of the clinical trial and the subject's underlying motivation: 'Although we hope that it might help you, our main concern is to see whether or not the experimental therapy is safe and effective. We are doing an experiment to answer that scientific question. That is why we will follow procedures that we would never use if our main goal were to benefit you.'

The investigator can then go on to explain those elements of research design such as randomization, use of placebos (such as use of sham surgery), limits on use of other medications, etc. that are done for the sake of answering the scientific question. In this way, informed consent can go beyond just disclosure of information. Instead, informed consent can become a means of

helping potential subjects make decisions, by providing a framework for an interactive conversation that places the concerns of the subject and the aims of the clinical trial in context.

Acknowledgments

Supported in part by a Greenwall faculty scholars Award in Bioethics.

References

1. Emanuel EJ, Wendler D and Grady C. What makes clinical research ethical? *JAMA* 2000; **283**: 2701–11.

2. Temple R and Ellenberg SS. Placebo-controlled trials and active-control trials in the evaluation of new treatments. *Ann Int Med* 2000; **133**: 455–63.

3. Emanuel EJ and Miller FG. The ethics of placebo-controlled trials – a middle ground. *New Engl J Med* 2001; **345**: 915–19.

4. Faden RR and Beauchamp TL. *A History and Theory of Informed Consent*. New York: Oxford University Press, 1986.

5. Jonsen AR. *The Birth of Bioethics*. New York: Oxford University Press, 1998.

6. Vollmann J and Winau R. The Prussian regulation of 1900: early ethical standards for human experimentation in Germany. *IRB* 1996; **18**: 9–11.

7. Paasche-Orlow M, Taylor HA and Brancati FL. Readability standards for informed consent forms as compared with actual readability. *New Engl J Med* 2003; **348**: 721–26.

8. McWilliams R, Hoover-Fong J, Hamosh A, *et al.* Problematic variation in local institutional review of a multicenter genetic epidemiology study. *JAMA* 2003; **290**: 360–66.

9. Dziak K, Anderson R, Sevick MA, *et al.* Variations among Institutional Review Board reviews in a multisite health services research study. *Health Serv Res* 2005; **40**: 279–90.

10. Lipkus IM. Numeric, verbal, and visual formats of conveying health risks: Suggested best practices and future recommendations. *Med Decis Making* 2007; **27**: 696–713.

11. Teigen KH and Brun W. Verbal probabilities: A question of frame? *J Behav Decision Making* 2003; **16**: 53–72.

12. Kim SYH, Schrock L, Wilson RM, *et al.* An approach to evaluating the therapeutic misconception. *IRB: Ethics & Hum Res* 2009; **31**: 7–14.

13. Flory J and Emanuel E. Interventions to improve research participants' understanding in informed

consent for research: A systematic review. *JAMA* 2004; **292**: 1593–1601.

14. Appelbaum PS, Lidz CW and Klitzman R. Voluntariness of consent to research: a conceptual model. *Hastings Cent Rep* 2009; **39**: 30–39.

15. Appelbaum PS, Lidz CW and Klitzman R. Voluntariness of consent to research: a preliminary empirical investigation. *IRB* 2009; **31**: 10–14.

16. Horng S, Emanuel EJ, Wilfond B, *et al*. Descriptions of benefits and risks in consent forms for phase I oncology trials. *New Engl J Med* 2002; **347**: 2134–140.

17. Lidz CW and Appelbaum PS. The therapeutic misconception: Problems and solutions. *Med Care* 2002; **40** (Suppl V): V55–63.

18. Okonkwo O, Griffith HR, Belue K, *et al*. Medical decision-making capacity in patients with mild cognitive impairment. *Neurology* 2007; **69**: 1528–35.

19. Jefferson AL, Lambe S, Moser DJ, *et al*. Decisional capacity for research participation in individuals with mild cognitive impairment. *J Am Geriatr Soc* 2008; **56**: 1236–43.

20. Kim SYH, Caine ED, Currier GW, *et al*. Assessing the competence of persons with Alzheimer's disease in providing informed consent for participation in research. *Am J Psychiatr* 2001; **158**: 712–17.

21. Dymek MP, Atchison P, Harrell L, *et al*. Competency to consent to medical treatment in cognitively impaired patients with Parkinson's disease. *Neurology* 2001; **56**: 17–24.

22. New Jersey, Access to Medical Research Act, Title 26, 14.1–14.5. In: 2008; 14.11–14.15.

23. Kim SYH. *Evaluation of Capacity to Consent to Treatment and Research*. New York: Oxford University Press, 2010.

24. Appelbaum PS. Assessment of patients' competence to consent to treatment. *New Engl J Med* 2007; **357**: 1834–40.

25. President's Commission for the Study of Ethical Problems in M, Biomedical, Behavioral R. Making health care decisions: the ethical and legal implications of informed consent in the patient-practitioner relationship, 1982. Report No. One.

26. National Bioethics Advisory C. Research Involving Persons with Mental Disorders That May Affect Decisionmaking Capacity. Rockville, MD, NBAC, 1998.

27. Kim SYH, Caine ED, Swan JG, *et al*. Do clinicians follow a risk-sensitive model of capacity determination? An experimental video survey. *Psychosomatics* 2006; **47**: 325–29.

28. Palmer BW, Dunn LB, Appelbaum PS, *et al*. Assessment of capacity to consent to research among older persons with schizophrenia, Alzheimer disease, or diabetes

mellitus: Comparison of a 3-item questionnaire with a comprehensive standardized capacity instrument. *Arch Gen Psychiatr* 2005; **62**: 726–33.

29. Kim SYH, Appelbaum PS, Jeste DV, *et al*. Proxy and surrogate consent in geriatric neuropsychiatric research: Update and recommendations. *Am J Psychiatr* 2004; **161**: 797–806.

30. Wendler D and Prasad K. Core safeguards for clinical research with adults who are unable to consent. *Ann Int Med* 2001; **135**: 514–23.

31. Alzheimer's A. Research consent for cognitively impaired adults: Recommendations for Institutional Review Boards and investigators. *Alzheimer's Dis Assoc Disord* 2004; **18**: 171–175.

32. Kim SYH, Kim HM, McCallum C, *et al*. What do people at risk for Alzheimer's disease think about surrogate consent for research? *Neurology* 2005; **65**: 1395–1401.

33. Kim S, Wall I, Stanczyk A, *et al*. Assessing the public's views in research ethics controversies: deliberative democracy and bioethics as natural allies. *J Emp Res Hum Res Ethics* 2009; **4**: 3–16.

34. Kim SYH, Kim HM, Langa KM, *et al*. Surrogate consent for dementia research: A National Survey of Older Americans. *Neurology* 2009; **72**: 149–55.

35. California Health and Safety Code, Amendment to Section 24178, 2002.

36. Code of Virginia, Title 32.1, Section 162.16–162–18. 2002; Section 162.116–162.119.

37. Saks ER, Dunn LB, Wimer J, *et al*. Proxy Consent to Research: Legal Landscape. *Yale J Health Law Policy Ethics* 2008; **8**: 37–78.

38. Black BS, Rabins PV, Sugarman J, Karlawish JH. Seeking assent and respecting dissent in dementia research. *Am J Geriatr Psychiatr* 2010; **18:** 77–85.

39. Minutes of the Recombinant DNA Advisory Committee. 2008. http://oba.od.nih.gov/oba/RAC/meetings/Sept2008/RAC_Minutes_09-08.pdf. (Accessed January 27, 2010.)

40. Kim SYH. When does decisional impairment become decisional incompetence? Ethical and methodological issues in capacity research in schizophrenia. *Schizophr Bull* 2006; **32**: 92–7.

41. Kim SYH and Appelbaum PS. The capacity to appoint a proxy and the possibility of concurrent proxy directives. *Behav Sci Law* 2006; **24**: 469–78.

42. Kim SYH, Cox C and Caine ED. Impaired decision-making ability and willingness to participate in research in persons with Alzheimer's disease. *Am J Psychiatr* 2002; **159**: 797–802.

43. Marson DC, Cody HA, Ingram KK, *et al*. Neuropsychological predictors of competency in

Alzheimer's disease using a rational reasons legal standard [comment]. *Arch Neurol* 1995; **52**: 955–59.

44. Lozano AM, Dostrovsky J, Chen R, *et al.* Deep brain stimulation for Parkinson's disease: disrupting the disruption. *Lancet Neurol* 2002; **1**: 225–31.

45. Kaplitt MG, Feigin A, Tang C, *et al.* Safety and tolerability of gene therapy with an adeno-associated virus (AAV) borne GAD gene for Parkinson's disease: an open label, phase I trial. *Lancet* 2007; **369**: 2097–105.

46. Freed CR, Greene PE, Breeze RE, *et al.* Transplantation of embryonic dopamine neurons for severe Parkinson's disease. *New Engl J Med* 2001; **344**: 710–19.

47. Hochberg LR, Serruya MD, Friehs GM, *et al.* Neuronal ensemble control of prosthetic devices by a human with tetraplegia. *Nature* 2006; **442**: 164–71.

48. Appelbaum PS, Roth LH and Lidz C. The therapeutic misconception: informed consent in psychiatric research. *Int J Law Psychiatry* 1982; **5**: 319–29.

49. Appelbaum PS, Lidz CW and Grisso T. Therapeutic misconception in clinical research: frequency and risk factors. *IRB Ethics & Human Research* 2004; **26**: 1–8.

50. Henderson GE, Easter MM, Zimmer C, *et al.* Therapeutic misconception in early phase gene transfer trials. *Soc Sci Med* 2006; **62**: 239–53.

51. Manson N and O'Neill O. *Rethinking Informed Consent in Bioethics*. New York: Cambridge University Press, 2007.

18
Evidentiary standards for neurological drugs and biologics approval

Russell Katz

Introduction

The evidentiary standards for the approval of drugs to treat human disease are set forth in the relevant sections of the Food, Drug, and Cosmetic Act (the Act) [1]. This statute, enacted by Congress in 1938, and amended in important ways numerous times since, describes the evidence a sponsor must submit, and that the FDA (the Agency) must find acceptable, in order for a drug to be approved for marketing in the US. The law set out broad standards for both the demonstration of effectiveness and safety, and implementing regulations written by the Agency further define, more specifically, how the statutory standards can be met. Both the Act and the regulations are sufficiently flexible to accommodate a wide variety of clinical situations; that is, they anticipate, and allow for, different standards for drug approval for the myriad conditions and diseases that afflict patients. The Public Health Service Act is the statute under which biological products ('…any virus, therapeutic serum, toxin, antitoxin, or analogous product…') are regulated; this statute requires, as a standard of effectiveness, that these products be shown to be 'potent'. For all intents and purposes, the standards for the demonstration of effectiveness are identical for drugs and biologics [2]. This chapter will focus primarily on some of the more important and current issues related to the demonstration of effectiveness of drugs and biologics.

General effectiveness

The basic legal requirement for a demonstration of effectiveness is codified in the Act at Section 505(d), and is described as follows:

'…substantial evidence that the drug will have the effect it purports or is represented to have under the conditions

of use prescribed, recommended, or suggested in the proposed labeling thereof…'

Until 1997, the Act defined 'substantial evidence' as follows:

'…evidence consisting of adequate and well-controlled investigations, including clinical investigations, by experts qualified by scientific training and experience to evaluate the effectiveness of the drug involved, on the basis of which it could fairly and responsibly be concluded by such experts that the drug will have the effect it purports or is represented to have under the conditions of use prescribed, recommended, or suggested in the labeling or proposed labeling thereof [1].'

The requirement that substantial evidence of effectiveness derive from clinical investigations was intended to embody the accepted scientific standard for independent replication or corroboration. That is, a 'positive' finding in a single study (perhaps even performed by a single investigator) was not considered to be adequate to support a conclusion that a drug was effective; such a finding had to be independently (e.g., by other investigators studying other patients) confirmed.

However, in 1997, Congress amended the Act by passing the Food and Drug Administration Modernization Act (FDAMA). Among other important changes, a new definition of substantial evidence of effectiveness was added to the law. The relevant language is given below:

'If the Secretary determines, based on relevant science, that data from one adequate and well-controlled clinical investigation and confirmatory evidence (obtained prior to or after such investigation are sufficient to establish effectiveness, the Secretary may consider such data and evidence to constitute substantial evidence…[3]'

The law now contains both definitions of substantial evidence, and either can be applied in any given case.

Clinical Trials in Neurology, ed. Bernard Ravina, Jeffrey Cummings, Michael P. McDermott, and R. Michael Poole. Published by Cambridge University Press. © Cambridge University Press 2012.

Although replication is most commonly required, the law provides no guidance as to when the alternative definition of substantial evidence was to be applied, nor does the law provide a definition of confirmatory evidence. However, the Agency has described some of the elements of a single trial that might permit it to constitute, with confirmatory evidence, substantial evidence of effectiveness. Some of these elements include:

1) a small p-value (demonstrating that the findings are very unlikely to have occurred by chance)
2) multiple outcomes showing statistically significant differences from the control
3) multiple study centers showing positive findings
4) multiple sub-groups (e.g., both mildly and severely impaired patients) equally benefitted by drug
5) multiple dose groups showing benefit

Although not all of these elements need to be positive in such a setting, the more robust the findings, the more likely that the results of a single study can be considered to constitute substantial evidence of effectiveness [4].

Surrogate markers as primary outcome measures

Another critical change to the law introduced with FDAMA was a provision regarding the use of surrogate markers as primary outcome measures.

Ordinarily, drugs are approved on the basis of a showing of an effect on a measure that is of clear clinical benefit to patients. In essentially all cases, drugs to treat neurological disease are approved on the basis of clinical trials that examine the drug's effects on a face valid measurement with clinical meaning (e.g., scales that measure symptoms, event [seizures], time to events of interest, etc.).

As part of FDAMA, however, Congress granted the FDA the authority to approve a drug on the basis of an effect on what can be called an 'unvalidated' surrogate marker. As described below, under its Fast Track provisions, the Agency may approve a drug:

> '...upon a determination that the product has an effect on ... a surrogate endpoint that is reasonably likely to predict clinical benefit [1].'

A surrogate marker is (typically) a laboratory test (biochemical test, imaging test, etc.) that, by itself, bears no direct relationship to how a patient feels or functions. For example, although a patient's blood pressure may be high, he or she does not ordinarily experience any clinical symptom reflective of this measurement, nor exhibit any clinical manifestations of an improvement in that measurement.

The Agency has for many years approved treatments on the basis of studies that examine a treatment's effects on surrogate markers, without any assessment of the patient's clinical symptoms (common examples include anti-hypertensives, cholesterol lowering drugs, treatments for glaucoma). The justification for relying on these measurements in these cases is that evidence exists demonstrating that changes in these surrogates are reflected (usually in the relatively distant future) in changes in clinically important outcomes (for example, a decrease in heart attacks and strokes for anti-hypertensives and cholesterol-lowering agents, and preservation of normal vision for treatments for glaucoma). Because there is evidence establishing the relationship between a treatment's effects on these surrogates and clinically important outcomes, these surrogates are considered 'validated'.

As a general matter, reliance on a drug's effect on a surrogate marker for approval is applied in those cases in which the clinical outcome of interest is likely to be demonstrable only over many years. That is, in these cases, studies capable of examining the treatment's effects directly on the clinical outcome(s) of interest may need to be impractically long.

FDAMA permits the Agency to approve treatments on the basis of their effects on what may be called 'unvalidated' surrogates (this standard has been in the regulations since 1992). Unvalidated surrogates are those for which the relationship between the treatment's effects on the surrogate and the clinical outcome(s) of interest has not been established. The law does require, as described above, that there be a 'reasonably likely' relationship between the effect on the surrogate and the clinical outcome of interest; the basis for such a conclusion can vary, but is ultimately a judgment.

Because the reasonably likely standard introduces a degree of uncertainty about the treatment's utility that does not exist with the usual basis for drug approval (after all, the effect on the surrogate may not predict the hoped-for clinical benefit), the law stipulates that this standard for approval be applied only in those cases where the disease being treated is serious or life-threatening and where the treatments already available are inadequate. In addition, the law requires that the surrogate be validated after the drug is approved.

Although the potential to approve drugs on the basis of their effects on unvalidated surrogate markers is attractive for many reasons, such approvals raise serious questions.

Most important, as alluded to above, because the effect on the surrogate need only be reasonably likely (and not established by evidence) to predict the clinical benefit, it could turn out that the treatment, in fact, does not predict the hoped-for clinical benefit. Indeed, numerous examples in the literature describe studies in which the proposed treatment did affect the surrogate in the desired way but had either no effect, or a deleterious effect on the ultimate clinical outcome. The relationship between the surrogate and the clinical outcomes in the untreated state may not continue to exist under treatment conditions.

There can be many reasons for the potential dissociation between the effects of a drug on an (unvalidated) surrogate and the clinical outcome with which the surrogate is correlated in the untreated state. In general, however, they are probably related to the fact that drugs can have both desirable and undesirable effects, many of which are unknown and unpredictable. Based on our understanding of the mechanism of action of a drug, we might predict that its effects on both the surrogate and clinical outcomes will be beneficial. In reality, it may 'fix' the surrogate and have other unpredicted actions that make the patient's clinical symptoms worse. Alternatively, there may be many underlying pathophysiological pathways that lead to clinical symptoms in a particular disease. Although a drug may have effects on a pathway that result in a desirable change on a surrogate outcome measure, it may have no effect or harmful effects on other pathways, resulting in an overall effect on the patient that is either null or harmful [5].

For these reasons, we would be most confident that a drug's effect on the surrogate will translate into a clinical benefit when we have a complete understanding of all of the drug's actions, as well as a complete understanding of all of the physiologic events underlying the production of symptoms. Of course, we never have such a complete understanding of either the treatment or the disease; in this respect, the conclusion that a drug's effect on an unvalidated surrogate marker will predict the clinical outcome of interest is always uncertain.

Pediatric studies

In an effort to promote the development of drugs to treat pediatric patients, several statutory mechanisms have been adopted.

The Pediatric Research Equity Act (PREA) was passed by Congress in 2003. This legislation requires sponsors to develop treatments for pediatric patients (defined as patients 16 years of age and younger) for those indications approved in adults [6].

Of course, the indication for which the drug is approved in adults must exist in at least some subset of pediatric patients in order for the requirements for pediatric studies to apply. For those subsets of pediatric patients in which the disease in adults does not exist, the Agency will grant a waiver of the requirements.

The specific kind of pediatric data required will depend on the specific clinical setting. If it can be demonstrated that: 1) the condition for which the drug is approved in adults is essentially the same as in pediatric patients; 2) there is evidence that pediatric patients will respond similarly to the drug as do adults; 3) there is evidence that pediatric patients will respond to the same doses (or plasma exposures) as adults, the only specific pediatric requirement may be for pharmacokinetic studies to determine an appropriate dosing regimen in pediatric patients that will produce relevant plasma exposures. On the other hand, if there is uncertainty about the similarity of the disease or the exposure-response relationship in pediatric and adult patients, a single controlled trial in pediatric patients will usually be required.

Independent of the specific requirements imposed for pediatric effectiveness data, there will almost always be a requirement for safety data in pediatric patients. Although some adult safety data may be relevant to the pediatric population, the Agency will almost always be interested in defining the effects of the treatment on the developing child, including an assessment on growth (height and weight), cognitive and neuropsychological development, sexual maturation, and other issues. Furthermore, additional special studies may be required for drugs known to have effects that may be particularly problematic on the developing human (e.g., pediatric patients may require specific bone density assessments when treated with drugs that affect bone metabolism).

In addition to the PREA requirements for pediatric studies, the Agency has another statutory mechanism for obtaining data in pediatric patients.

The Best Pharmaceuticals for Children Act (BPCA) was passed by Congress in 2002. The provisions of this act, unlike PREA, are voluntary. Specifically, BPCA provides that if sponsors perform and submit by a specified time, studies in pediatric patients requested by the Agency, any existing marketing exclusivity for a drug will be extended by 6 months (that is, generic versions of the drug will not be permitted for this additional 6 months). This exclusivity is extended whether or not the studies performed demonstrate that the treatment is effective or safe in pediatric patients. Under BPCA, the Agency can ask for studies not only in those indications already approved in adults but also for indications where the Agency considers that the treatment is likely to be used in pediatric patients. By contrast, the PREA requires pediatric studies only in the same indication for which the drug is approved in adults). Typically, studies required in pediatric written requests (PWRs) include extensive dose finding and pharmacokinetic studies, controlled trials, and safety data [7].

Because the sponsor may accrue a large financial benefit by conducting the studies requested by the Agency regardless of the outcome of the studies, and because the goal is to design and conduct studies optimally designed to yield useful information in the pediatric population, great energy is expended to ensure, to the extent possible, that the controlled trials conducted by the sponsors are designed to maximize the potential of the studies to detect a treatment effect, if there is one. This imperative may result in the imposition of specific requirements that may not always be part of studies performed in adults.

For example, although it is always important for adequate dose finding to be performed, it is particularly important in studies done to satisfy BPCA. If a sponsor proposes to study a single dose in a pediatric study that has been shown to be effective in adults, and that dose is not shown to be effective in pediatric patients, such a study is not likely to be considered adequate to satisfy the demands of BPCA, because pediatric patients may have a different dose-response than adults. Indeed if, a priori, we knew that pediatric patients responded similarly to a given dose as adults, a controlled trial in pediatric patients would be unnecessary. For this reason, PWRs typically require studies that explore the full tolerated dose range in pediatric patients to ensure, to the extent possible, that an effect will be demonstrated if it exists. Similarly, sample sizes for pediatric patients are typically calculated on estimates of effect size and data variability obtained in adults. Of course, these measures may be different in the pediatric population, so studies conducted to satisfy BPCA may need to incorporate interim analyses to assess whether these parameters are as predicted; if they are not, the sample size or other study parameters may need to be amended.

Orphan diseases

Rare diseases raise numerous questions related to the evidentiary standards for drug approval. The Agency defines orphan diseases as those with a prevalence of less than 200 000 in the US [8]. Although there are numerous benefits associated with the designation of a treatment as an 'orphan drug', including grants, tax advantages, and a waiver of the requirement to perform studies in pediatric patients, neither the law, nor the regulations describe any different standard of evidence (either for safety or effectiveness) required for the approval of treatments for orphan or non-orphan diseases. For example, the determination of effectiveness for an orphan indication must meet one of the two definitions of substantial evidence discussed above. However, of course, the specific data necessary to support approval of an orphan treatment will depend upon the specific clinical setting. For example, the requirements (for the demonstration of both safety and effectiveness) for approval of a drug intended to treat an orphan disease with a prevalence of 3000 people are likely to be substantially different from those imposed on a treatment intended to treat an orphan disease with a prevalence of 150 000 people.

Types of acceptable study designs

Although the Act does not define 'adequate and well-controlled investigations', the implementing regulations describe five different types of clinical trials that can, depending upon the clinical setting, be considered to contribute to a finding of substantial evidence of effectiveness. These following five studies are described at 21 Code of Federal Regulations (CFR) 314.126:

1) Placebo concurrent control-patients are assigned (typically randomly) to treatment with the investigational drug or an inactive placebo.
2) Dose-comparison concurrent control-patients are assigned (typically randomly) to one of several doses of the investigational drug; in this design, there may also be a placebo group.
3) No treatment concurrent control-patients are assigned (typically randomly) to the investigational treatment or to standard care, but no placebo.
4) Active treatment concurrent control-patients are assigned (typically randomly) to the investigational drug or to an active drug already approved for that indication. This design may also incorporate several fixed doses of either treatment as well as placebo.

5) Historical control-patients are given the investigational drug but there is no concurrent control group; the responses of the patients are compared to responses in a cohort of patients with the same condition not included in the study.

Although the five types of control groups described above as providing substantial evidence of effectiveness may all be appropriate under certain circumstances, in the development of treatments for patients with neurological illness, the use of historical controls is rarely acceptable. It is rarely, if ever, the case that a concurrent control cannot be included in a study of a neurological treatment.

Historical controls are the weakest type of control, primarily because there is usually considerable uncertainty that the patients being given the investigational drugs are similar in all relevant aspects to the patients constituting the historical control. The great advantage to utilizing a concurrent control group to which patients have been randomized is that randomization can be counted on (in most cases) to create treatment groups that are similar in the attributes (both known and unknown) that might affect response to treatment. If attributes that can affect patients' responses to the applied treatment are mal-distributed among groups, this is likely to result in a bias (that is, one group will be more likely to respond than another, unrelated to the treatment itself) that may be extraordinarily difficult to detect. If a difference between treatments is detected in such a study, it will be difficult, if not impossible, to determine if the difference is related to the treatment or the differences in responsiveness of the groups themselves. The use of non-concurrent historical controls will invariably raise questions of interpretability that may be impossible to answer. If there were conditions for which detailed information was available about the natural history of the untreated condition (for example, obtained from a large cohort of patients followed prospectively), and we were reasonably certain that the patients constituting this cohort were essentially identical to the ones being treated with the investigational drug (including elements of the standard of care of the historical control and the study population), and the effect produced by the treatment was extremely large, so that it could not reasonably be attributed to the fact that patients knew they were on active treatment, it might be possible to interpret a difference between the responses of the two cohorts as being due to the treatment. Unfortunately, we do not typically have this information for most of the conditions for which sponsors are currently developing treatments.

A critical aspect in the interpretation of the results of almost all clinical trials of neurological treatments is the requirement that a difference in outcomes be shown between the investigational treatment and the control in order for the results to be interpretable. The design that is usually most efficient in this regard employs a concurrent placebo control (such a design may also include multiple fixed doses and/or an active control), though this is almost never required. Of course, a trial that does not distinguish between the effects of an applied treatment and a placebo group cannot be interpreted as demonstrating an effect of the drug.

By contrast, trials employing an active control are often designed to demonstrate equivalence of two treatments with the intention of drawing the conclusion that the new treatment is effective. In most cases, a trial that fails to distinguish an effect between an investigational treatment and an active control is uninterpretable.

Such an outcome has two possible interpretations: either both drugs were effective, or both drugs were ineffective. The first interpretation seems the most logical; after all, a new drug was shown to be 'equivalent' to a drug known to be effective.

The flaw in this argument is that it is often impossible to know (with any reasonable degree of certainty) that the active control was effective *in this particular study*. Not every drug previously determined to be active (on the basis of adequate and well-controlled trials) is effective at all times, in all populations. Using this design, the only way to conclude that the investigational drug was effective is to show that the active treatment was also effective in this particular study; this can only be shown by demonstrating that patients *not* treated with the active control would have had a worse outcome. In this sense, an active control trial that fails to show a difference between treatments can be considered a type of historical controlled trial, the weakest, most difficult to interpret trial design, as discussed above [9–11].

One circumstance (perhaps the only one) in which an active control trial that does not distinguish treatments can appropriately be interpreted as establishing the effectiveness of the new treatment is the case in which there is a very large dataset of controlled trials that has uniformly demonstrated the effectiveness of the active control in patients essentially the same as those enrolled in the active controlled study itself. Typically, we would expect that the previous trials would have uniformly demonstrated superiority of the active control to a control (usually placebo) in many well-designed and conducted trials. Even one trial in which the active control was not superior to placebo would raise questions about whether or not the active control could reasonably have been known to have been effective in the trial in which it was included as a control. If there were a large such number of trials of the active control, all of them positive, we might be confident that it was effective in the trial in which it was compared to the investigational drug. Unfortunately, such a large, robust, clinical trial database in which a proposed active control has been uniformly shown to be superior to placebo (or other control) does not exist for most, if any, of the drugs sponsors have proposed as active controls in studies of neurological disease. For this reason, a trial of a neurological treatment that does not distinguish the effects of that treatment and an active control is typically considered to be uninterpretable.

Of course, if an investigational drug is shown to be superior to an active control, this can be interpreted as being a 'positive' study. In this case, we may not know if the active control was effective or not, but if it was not, then the new treatment has been shown to be superior to what, in effect, was a placebo (at least in this trial), which is the usual source of evidence of effectiveness. The only caveat about interpreting a difference between an investigational treatment and an active control is that, in order to interpret this difference as demonstrating a beneficial effect of the new treatment, we must assume that the active control did not make patients worse than they would have been without the treatment. This is usually a reasonable assumption, but there may be cases in which such an assumption is wrong. For example, there are certain anti-epilepsy drugs (AEDs) that are considered to exacerbate certain specific seizure types. If one of these AEDs were used as an active control in a study of an investigational treatment for that seizure type, any apparent superiority of the new treatment may be spurious.

Similarly, there are studies in which all patients receive the investigational treatment for a specified period of time, after which they are randomized to continue on the treatment or receive placebo (so-called randomized withdrawal designs). In these studies, the outcome measure is typically either the time to, or the proportion of patients, reaching a specified failure event. Although these are ordinarily acceptable designs (and are frequently used to establish long-term

effectiveness), in some of these cases, patients randomized to placebo may suffer withdrawal phenomena immediately after randomization, during which their condition may be worse than if they had never received treatment at all. In this case also, any difference seen between the patients continuing on drug and those experiencing withdrawal on placebo might inappropriately be attributed to a beneficial effect of the drug [12]. Additionally, withdrawal symptoms attributable to the investigational agent might unblind investigators to treatment assignments and create bias in a particular study. In some cases, withdrawal symptoms may be mitigated by slowly withdrawing treatment over time in patients randomized to placebo. Nonetheless, any difference between the new treatment and a control can be interpreted to support a beneficial effect of the new treatment.

Although a difference between the new treatment and almost any control can be interpreted to demonstrate an effect of the new treatment, as noted earlier, the most efficient and most common control group is a placebo group. Almost all trials of new agents to treat neurological disease employ a placebo group, even though there may be cases in which all patients are on other background treatments as well. In these studies, so-called add-on studies, patients are randomized to have the new drug, or the placebo, added on to their background medications; these studies can demonstrate that the new treatment is effective when added to other treatments, but not to establish that the new treatment is effective by itself.

Although an argument has been made that a group in which patients receive only placebo is unethical when alternative treatments are available for the condition under investigation, the international community, including the FDA, has not routinely adopted this position. To be sure, if the condition under study is serious or life-threatening, and the available treatments have been shown to prevent significant morbidity or mortality, these treatments cannot ethically be withheld. However, in many cases, the available treatments provide only symptomatic benefits, and withholding them for the relatively short durations necessary to establish the effectiveness of a new treatment does not expose the patient to any important risk. In these cases, it is perfectly acceptable from an ethical point of view to randomize patients to placebo. Indeed, if patients were required to receive the best available care in all cases in which treatments were available, no new treatments could ever be developed, because it would be ethically unacceptable to withhold the available treatments from patients, which means that they could not receive any new treatment that had not yet been established to be effective. The previous point notwithstanding, if the only studies that could be done were those that employed active controls, it is likely that many of these would not be interpretable, for the reasons discussed earlier. The conduct of clinical trials that are known to be uninterpretable is itself seriously problematic from an ethical point of view.

Disease modification and prevention

To date, the treatments available to treat progressive neurological disease are, almost without exception, considered to provide symptomatic benefit to patients; that is, there is no evidence that the available treatments slow the progression of the underlying disease process. However, at this time, numerous treatments are being developed that are believed to slow the progression of the underlying disease. It is worth considering the elements of clinical trial designs that could support such a claim.

In the typical case, patients are randomized to receive investigational drug or a control (usually placebo). Any difference in favor of drug is considered to demonstrate an effect of the drug, but such a design cannot distinguish between a symptomatic effect of the drug, and an effect on the underlying progression of the disease. For this reason, numerous clinical trial designs have been proposed as being capable of detecting a disease-modifying effect of a treatment.

It is commonly proposed that a trial (or outcome) that shows an increasing difference between study treatments over time defines a disease-modifying effect. In this view, symptomatic effects (which are usually seen early after treatment initiation and are typically considered to wane over time) could not possibly increase over time because the disease itself is progressing. Therefore, it is argued, such an outcome must reflect an effect of the treatment on the underlying disease process. Although this response could reflect a disease-modifying effect, it is possible that a symptomatic effect could, in fact, increase over time as the disease process progresses. The possibility that such an outcome may not represent a disease-modifying effect has made this scenario unacceptable (at this time) as establishing a disease-modifying effect of any treatment.

More commonly, many sponsors have proposed that surrogate markers be used in the service of establishing a treatment's effect on slowing disease progression. Specifically, it is postulated that a treatment's effect on a given surrogate reflects an effect on the disease itself. For example, a treatment may decrease the appearance of brain atrophy as imaged on MRI in patients with Alzheimer's disease, and this would be taken as evidence that the drug had an effect on the underlying disease. Another example would be a treatment that decreased the amount of amyloid in the brains of patients with AD, as seen on PET scanning. It is clear both atrophy and amyloid deposition increase with the progression of AD, and the assumption, therefore, is that a treatment that interrupts this process is considered to, almost by definition, slow the progress of the disease.

However, as stated earlier, the approval of a treatment (in this case, for a claim for disease modification) based on an effect on an 'unvalidated' surrogate is problematic. At this time, the Agency has determined that a treatment that has been demonstrated to have an effect on such a surrogate would not, by itself, be adequate to support a disease-modifying effect. However, a treatment shown to have an effect on a clinical outcome as well as on a proposed surrogate, might, under certain circumstances (including a wide consensus among the community of experts about the relationship of the surrogate to the progression of the disease) be considered to support a disease-modification claim. More appropriately, the Agency has endorsed a study design which is considered adequate to demonstrate a disease-modifying effect.

In this design, patients are randomized to either drug or placebo, as in the standard study design, and the expectation is that a difference will emerge between the treatments at an appropriate time (this is identical to the typical design and outcome that support a standard claim). At this point, patients originally assigned to drug are switched over to placebo, and patients originally treated with placebo continue to receive placebo. In this second phase, if patients originally assigned to drug (and now receiving placebo), approach the ratings of the patients continuing on placebo, the effect seen in the first phase is considered to reflect a symptomatic treatment (that is, when the treatment is withdrawn, they respond as if they had been on placebo all along). If, however, the patients originally assigned to drug do not approach (or reach) the original placebo patients when they are switched to placebo, the implication is that their original treatment with drug fundamentally altered their disease (otherwise, they would have 'caught up' to the original placebo patients). A similar design, except that in the second phase patients originally assigned to placebo are switched to drug, and those originally assigned to drug remain on drug, has also been proposed. These so-called randomized withdrawal and randomized start designs, respectively, have the great advantage of essentially 'forcing' a conclusion that the treatment has modified the disease, as opposed to relying on numerous assumptions about drug effects and pathophysiological events leading to disease that other approaches to disease modification require for interpretation. However, the randomized withdrawal (and start) designs are complicated and pose numerous methodological problems (for example, how long should the second phase be to accurately determine whether or not patients are 'approaching' each other; what are the statistical criteria to determine if patients are approaching each other; how should dropouts be handled in these long-term studies, etc.). Nonetheless, these designs have the great advantage of requiring few assumptions in order for a disease modification claim to be supported.

Another related issue of considerable interest is the determination of an effect of treatment on preventing neurological disease.

The design of a trial designed to prevent disease raises numerous questions, including the fundamental question of what constitutes a disease. In most degenerative diseases of the nervous system, the pathological hallmarks of the disease can predate the onset of clinical symptoms (and therefore diagnosis) by decades. Does a treatment that prevents the onset of symptoms (but that is applied after the onset of the pathology) truly prevent the disease?

An important point to make in this context is that delaying the time to diagnosis or the onset of symptoms is not the same as prevention. Delaying the time to diagnosis or symptoms, although perfectly acceptable as an outcome supporting drug approval, is entirely consistent with a symptomatic effect, and therefore cannot be considered to establish a preventive effect.

Similarly, long trial duration in asymptomatic patients, cannot, by itself, be considered to establish a preventive effect. For most diseases, the period of risk continues for the patient's life. For this reason, a study of even several years duration, in which drug-treated patients do not develop symptoms, cannot definitively establish that patients will not become symptomatic later. In some cases, if the period of risk of developing symptoms is known and finite, a trial duration of

appropriate length could, in theory, establish an effect on prevention, but these circumstances are rare, if they exist at all.

Regardless, many sponsors are contemplating developing treatments to be applied to patients with signs of pathology (either imaging or biochemical) but without clinical symptoms, in the hope of preventing those symptoms from occurring. Beside the obvious advantages to public health of doing so, recent experience with various treatments suggests that treating patients with purported disease-modifying agents once clinical symptoms have occurred may be futile, because the damage to necessary structures makes these treatments ineffective. For this reason, it might be necessary to study pre-symptomatic patients simply in order to establish an effect of the treatment. As noted above, in most cases, these trials would not be capable of establishing that the treatment prevented the disease, but could reliably be interpreted as delaying the time to the onset of symptoms (that is, they could detect a meaningful effect of the drug).

In most cases, the hope would be to treat patients many years before the expected onset of symptoms. In this setting, a trial of any reasonable duration would not be expected to show an effect on clinical symptoms. Therefore, a surrogate marker would most likely be acceptable as a primary outcome measure. However, as previously discussed, considerable information about the effect of the drug on the surrogate and the expected clinical outcome would need to be available in order for the Agency to conclude that the effect seen on the surrogate would be 'reasonably likely' to predict the desired effect on the clinical outcome. For example, in the case of AD, studies in patients with very early AD (i.e., mildly symptomatic patients) might establish a relationship between the treatment and the surrogate and clinical symptoms. Such data might then provide confidence that an effect on the surrogate alone (in the pre-symptomatic patients) would predict the delay to the onset of clinical symptoms that we would require in order to grant a claim.

Comparative effectiveness and safety

Another area of increasing interest is the area of comparative effectiveness and/or safety. For various reasons, there is considerable interest in the design of clinical trials that will demonstrate either the superior effectiveness of one treatment compared to another, or, alternatively, the superior safety profile. These comparisons are important, but trials designed to demonstrate the superiority of one treatment compared to another are potentially problematic.

In particular, the critical consideration in these comparisons is that any trial designed to demonstrate superiority should incorporate elements to ensure that the comparison is a fair one. For example, in trials designed to demonstrate that one drug is more effective than another, it is critical that appropriate doses of each treatment are compared. The choice, for instance, of a maximally tolerated high dose of the new treatment compared to a low dose of the control will result in an unfair comparison, and will not be adequate to conclude that the new treatment is superior to the old. Further, if the old treatment must be titrated, but is not titrated in the trial in which it is used as a control, any finding of superiority of the new treatment may be biased and uninterpretable. Another consideration would involve the appropriate choice of outcome measures. One drug may be superior to another on a particular measure of effectiveness, but the opposite may be true for a different measure of effectiveness. The over-arching principle to be applied in such studies is that the control treatment must be administered under conditions in which it will be maximally effective and which examine all relevant measures of effectiveness; if those conditions are not obtained in the comparative trial, any statement about the superior effectiveness of the new treatment will be questionable.

Similarly, if a claim of superior tolerability is to be granted, the study on which such a claim is to be granted must be a fair one. In this case, a critical consideration in the design of such trials is that the treatments be compared on doses that are equi-effective. If a finding of increased tolerability of one drug occurs in the setting of a dose of that drug that is less effective than the control, that finding may be misleading. This requirement can be problematic, because a showing of 'equi-effectiveness' may be difficult, given that it can only be formally demonstrated through a finding of non-inferiority, a difficult outcome to achieve. Again, as in the case of an attempt to establish superior effectiveness, the ideal study would compare a range of doses of both drugs.

In the case of a trial designed to establish the superior safety profile of one drug compared to another, it is also critical that the trials examine a full range of adverse events and employ methods sensitive enough to adequately assess them. If Drug A is not associated with an adverse event seen with Drug B, but Drug A causes an adverse event not seen with Drug B (or

increases the severity or frequency of this latter event), it may be inappropriate to permit a claim of superior tolerability for Drug A.

Of course, it may be possible for a trial to enroll patients who cannot tolerate Drug A (either because of a specific adverse reaction of due to a general lack of tolerability), and compare the tolerability of Drug A with Drug B. In such a trial, patients would be randomized to one or the other drug, and the comparative tolerability could be examined. Even if Drug B caused a 'new' adverse event in these patients, they may still prefer Drug B to Drug A.

References

1. Federal Food, Drug, and Cosmetic Act (FD&C Act). United States Code (U.S.C.) Title 21, Chapter 9.

2. Myers AM, *et al.* An overview of the drug approval process: An FDA perspective. In: Hartzema AG, Tilson HH, Chan KA. *Pharmacoepidemiology and Therapeutic Risk Management.* Harvey Whitney Books Company. 2008; 67–94.

3. Food and Drug Modernization Act (FDAMA) of 1997. Public Law 105–115. November 21, 1997.

4. Guidance document: Providing Clinical Evidence of Effectiveness for Human Drug and Biological Products. 1998. http://www.fda.gov/Drugs/GuidanceComplianceRegulatoryInformation/Guidances/ucm065012.htm

5. Fleming T and DeMets D. Surrogate end points in clinical trials: Are we being misled? *Ann Intern Med* 1996; **125**: 605–613.

6. Pediatric Research Equity Act (PREA) of 2003. Public Law 108–155. December 3, 2003.

7. Best Pharmaceuticals for Children Act (BPCA). Public Law 107–109. January 4, 2002.

8. Orphan Drug Act. Public Law 97–414. January 4, 1983.

9. Leber PD. Hazards of inference: the active control investigation. *Epilepsia* 1989; (30) Suppl 1:S57–63; discussion S64–8.

10. Temple R and Ellenberg SS. Placebo-controlled trials and active control trials in the evaluation of new treatments. Part 1: ethical and scientific issues. *Ann Intern Med* 2000; **133**: 455–63.

11. Temple R and Ellenberg SS. Placebo-controlled trials and active control trials in the evaluation of new treatments. Part 2: practical issues and specific cases. *Ann Intern Med* 2000; **133**: 464–70.

12. Leber PD and Davis CS. Threats to the validity of clinical trials employing enrichment strategies for sample selection. *Control Clin Trials* 1988; **19**: 178–87.

Chapter 19

Premarket review of neurological devices

Eric A. Mann and Peter G. Como

Introduction

The US neurological device market is one of the fastest growing segments in the country's medical device industry. The global neurological device market is predicted to exceed $5 billion by 2016 [1]. Factors expected to spur this growth include changing patient demographics, increasing physician adoption of innovative technologies, patient demand, and the availability of reimbursement for device-related procedures. In particular, neurological disorders such as epilepsy, chronic migraine headache, stroke, and neurodegenerative disorders (e.g., Alzheimer's disease, Parkinson's disease) affect large patient groups, many of which are rapidly increasing in size with the overall aging of the country's population.

Neurostimulation devices [e.g. deep brain stimulators (DBS), spinal cord stimulators, peripheral nerve stimulators, and vagus nerve stimulators] are the fastest growing category within the neurological device market [1]. Currently, FDA-approved indications for neurostimulation devices include the treatment of debilitating conditions such as treatment-resistant depression, epilepsy, gastroparesis, urinary incontinence, chronic pain, Parkinson's disease, essential tremor, dystonia, and obsessive compulsive disorder. Additionally, research is underway to expand the indications for use of neurostimulation devices to other important conditions such as obesity, stroke, Alzheimer's disease, hypertension, migraine, and neuropsychiatric disorders (e.g. Tourette syndrome and addictive disorders). Neurostimulation devices may, in fact, be cost-effective alternatives to traditional pharmacologic therapy for some disorders [2].

Neurointerventional devices constitute another rapidly growing segment of the neurological device market [3]. These devices include catheter-based systems designed to retrieve clots in patients experiencing acute ischemic stroke as well as a variety of coils, stents, flow diverters, and injectable agents designed to embolize and/or occlude intracranial aneurysms and arteriovenous malformations. These 'minimally invasive' technologies offer an alternative to open surgical procedures, and may have comparatively lower complication rates and shorter hospital stays.

Overall, the US neurological device market currently appears to be in a similar situation to that of the cardiovascular device market of the 1990s. That is, the substantial unmet need for effective treatments of neurological disorders, coupled with a large and expanding patient population, is expected to spur growth in the neurological device field in coming years.

The role of the FDA

The mission of the Center for Devices and Radiological Health (CDRH) within the FDA is to promote and protect the health of the American public by assuring the safety and effectiveness of medical devices and the safety of radiological products marketed in the US. The enormous scope of this mission is exemplified by the tremendous diversity and number of products regulated as devices including tongue depressors, wheelchairs, tanning beds, in vitro and radiological diagnostic devices, cardiac pacemakers, prosthetic joints, and DBSs. Overall, there are approximately 1700 different generic types of devices identified in the regulations [4]. In 2006 alone, expenditures on medical devices in the US were estimated at $131.6 billion [5].

FDA's legal authority to regulate medical devices derives from the Medical Device Amendments of 1976 to the Federal Food, Drug, and Cosmetic Act (FD&C Act). As defined under the Act [6], a medical device is:

Clinical Trials in Neurology, ed. Bernard Ravina, Jeffrey Cummings, Michael P. McDermott, and R. Michael Poole. Published by Cambridge University Press. © Cambridge University Press 2012.

Table 19.1 Risk-based classification of medical devices

Class	Risk	Regulatory requirements	Neurological device examples
Class I	Low	General controls	Manual surgical instruments, neurological pinwheel, tuning fork, neurosurgical chair
Class II	Moderate	General controls and special controls	EEG cortical and cutaneous electrodes, neurological endoscope, evoked response stimulators
Class III	High	General controls and premarket approval	DBS, VNS[a], cortical stimulators, dural sealants, polymerizing neurovascular embolization agents

[a] DBS: deep brain stimulator; VNS: vagus nerve stimulators.

An instrument, apparatus, implement, machine, contrivance, implant, in vitro reagent, or other similar or related article, including a component part, or accessory which is:

- recognized in the official National Formulary, or the US Pharmacopoeia, or any supplement to them,
- intended for use in the diagnosis of disease or other conditions, or in the cure, mitigation, treatment, or prevention of disease, in man or other animals, or
- intended to affect the structure or any function of the body of man or other animals, and which does not achieve any of it's primary intended purposes through chemical action within or on the body of man or other animals and which is not dependent upon being metabolized for the achievement of any of its primary intended purposes.

If the primary intended use of the product is achieved through chemical action or by being metabolized by the body, the product is usually regulated as a drug or biological product. The regulatory framework for devices differs from that for drugs and biologics in that a risk-based classification system determines the level of regulatory oversight for a specific device type. This regulatory approach is consistent with both the wide spectrum of risk levels posed by devices as well as the frequent, incremental modifications made to devices to enhance safety and effectiveness with rapid technological advancement. Requiring at least two adequate and well-controlled clinical investigations, the usual evidentiary standard per the drug regulations, would be inappropriate for many devices (e.g. tongue depressors, bedpans) and impractical and unnecessary for other devices (e.g. minor modifications or design enhancements to currently approved devices). However, evidentiary standards for devices, drugs, and biologics all share the common goal of ensuring both the safety and effectiveness of these products in the US.

Regulatory classification of devices

As described above, the Medical Device Amendments of 1976 established a risk-based classification system for medical devices [6]. The goal of this system is to tailor the degree of regulatory oversight to the risks posed by a particular device type. Each generic type of device is assigned to one of three regulatory classes, each with distinct regulatory requirements (see Table 19.1). A list of classification regulations for various types of diagnostic, surgical, and therapeutic neurological devices, and their regulatory classification is found in the Code of Federal Regulations (CFR) under 21 CFR 882[7]. The following sections will provide an overview of the regulatory requirements for each of these classes.

Class I devices

Class I devices are low risk devices for which FDA has determined that general controls alone will provide a reasonable assurance of safety and effectiveness. General controls are the baseline regulatory requirements of the FD&C Act that apply to all three classes of medical devices. These controls include:

- Adulteration and Misbranding provisions (Sections 501 and 502 of the FD&C Act)

In general, a device will be considered *adulterated* (and in violation of the FD&C Act) if it is unsanitary, contains a poisonous substance or unsafe color additive, differs from its claimed purity or quality, or fails to meet a required performance standard. The main provisions regarding *misbranding* require that the labeling not be false or misleading, that the device packaging bear a label containing certain information (e.g. name and address of manufacturer, device's established name, quantity of contents), and that the device bear adequate directions for use including appropriate warnings for over-the-counter devices.

- Good manufacturing practices

The device manufacturer must conform to the Quality System Regulation (21 CFR 820) which contains general requirements in the areas of: organization and personnel; design practices and procedures; buildings and environmental control; design of labeling and packaging; controls for components, processes, packaging and labeling; finished device evaluation; distribution and installation; device and manufacturing records; complaint processing; and QA system audits.

- Registration and listing

All manufacturers are required to register their establishments with FDA and submit a list of all devices they manufacture. This information is maintained in databases within FDA.

- Repair, replacement or refund provisions

The FD&C Act authorizes the Agency, after offering an opportunity for an informal hearing, to order manufacturers, importers, or distributors to repair, replace, or refund the purchase price of devices that present an unreasonable risk to health.

- Records and reports on devices

Section 519 of the FD&C Act authorizes FDA to promulgate regulations requiring manufacturers, importers, or distributors to maintain records and reports to assure that devices are not misbranded or adulterated.

- Restricted devices

Under Section 520 (e) of the Act, FDA may restrict the sale, distribution, or use of a device if necessary to provide a reasonable assurance of safety and effectiveness. For example, if adequate directions for use for a device can not be written that will assure safe use of a device by the lay public, the device can be restricted through prescription use. Other restrictions may pertain to labeling or other requirements. For example, hearing aid devices are not restricted through prescription use, but are restricted by regulation regarding specific labeling requirements (e.g. user brochure, technical data to be provided) and the requirement for a medical evaluation by a licensed physician within 6 months of the hearing aid being dispensed.

- Banned devices

If a device presents such deception or risk of illness or injury, which cannot be corrected by a change in labeling, then FDA may publish a proposed regulation to ban the device. To date, only one device (prosthetic hair fibers) has been banned by FDA regulation.

- Premarket notification

Section 510(k) of the FD&C Act requires a manufacturer who intends to market a new medical device to submit a premarket notification [also known as a '510(k)'] to the Agency. This 510(k) premarket application is described in further detail in 'Types of FDA Premarket Applications' below.

Of note, as a result of the 1997 Food and Drug Administration Modernization Act (FDAMA), almost all Class I devices are now exempt from the premarket notification requirement. However, there are limitations to this exemption, as outlined in 21 CFR 882.9 for neurological devices.

Thus, manufacturers are required to comply with the general controls outlined above in order to legally market a Class I medical device. Examples of Class I neurological devices include various simple diagnostic devices (e.g. tuning fork, neurological pinwheel, percussion hammer) and various manual surgical instruments.

Class II devices

Class II devices are moderate risk devices for which FDA has determined that special controls, in addition to the general controls (as outlined above), are necessary to provide a reasonable assurance of safety and effectiveness. The special controls which apply to a certain device type depend on the specific safety and effectiveness issues associated with it, and may include special labeling requirements, mandatory performance standards and post-market surveillance requirements (e.g. patient registry or device-tracking requirements that facilitate device recalls or patient notifications if necessary). For example, the special control for neurovascular embolization devices such as embolization coils (which are Class II devices) is a special controls guidance document created by FDA [8] which outlines specific risks to health posed by these devices (e.g. blood vessel perforation, unintended thrombosis, adverse tissue reaction, infection, hematoma formation) and recommended measures to mitigate these risks (e.g. pre-clinical testing, animal testing, clinical testing, labeling). Thus, any manufacturer intending to market a new neurovascular embolization coil device will need to adequately address the issues outlined in this guidance document and will need to obtain FDA marketing clearance through the premarket notification [510(k) process which is described below. Unlike Class I devices, most Class II devices still require clearance through the 510(k) process prior to marketing.

Class III devices

Class III is the most stringent regulatory classification for devices. Class III devices are those for which insufficient information exists to assure safety and effectiveness solely through general or special controls. Typically, such devices support or sustain human life, are of substantial importance in preventing impairment of human health, or present a potential, unreasonable risk of illness or injury.

In addition to the General Controls that also apply to Class I and Class II devices, premarket approval (PMA) is the required process of scientific review to ensure the safety and effectiveness of Class III devices (see further description of the PMA process in the following account). Examples of Class III devices which require PMA include DBSs, cortical stimulators, and vagus nerve stimulators.

Types of FDA premarket applications

Premarket notification

A premarket notification or 510(k) is the type of the premarket application required by FDA for most Class II devices and some class I devices [9]. The 510(k) must demonstrate that the device to be marketed is at least as safe and effective, that is, 'substantially equivalent', to a legally marketed device (or devices) that is not subject to PMA. A legally marketed device, as described in 21 CFR 807.92(a)(3), is a device that was either:

1. Legally marketed prior to the Medical Device Amendments of 1976 (pre-amendments device), for which a PMA is not required, or
2. A device which has been reclassified from Class III to Class II or I, or
3. A device which has been found substantially equivalent through the 510(k) process.

This legally marketed device to which equivalence is drawn is commonly known as the 'predicate' device. Although devices most recently cleared under 510(k) are often selected as the predicate to which substantial equivalence is claimed, any legally marketed as defined above may be used as a predicate.

A device is substantially equivalent if, in comparison to a predicate, it:

- has the same intended use as the predicate; *and* has the same technological characteristics as the predicate; or has the same intended use as the predicate; *and* has different technological characteristics and the information submitted to FDA:
  - does not raise new types of safety and effectiveness questions; *and*
  - demonstrates that the device is at least as safe and effective as the legally marketed device.

A claim of substantial equivalence does not mean that the new and predicate devices must be identical. Substantial equivalence is established with respect to intended use, design, energy used or delivered, materials, chemical composition, manufacturing process, performance, safety, effectiveness, labeling, biocompatibility, standards, and other characteristics, as applicable. If there are differences in these areas between the new device and the predicate which could impact safety and/or effectiveness, the applicant must provide performance data (e.g. bench, animal, and/or clinical data) in the 510(k) to show that the new device is at least as safe and effective as the cited predicate. Until the submitter receives an order from FDA declaring a device to be substantially equivalent, the submitter may not proceed to market the device. This determination, which is referred to as a 'clearance' for marketing (as opposed to 'approval' for marketing under the PMA process as described below), is usually made within 90 days of FDA review time and is made based on the information submitted by the applicant.

Over the past decade (1999–2009), FDA has cleared approximately 1800 neurological devices. A significant portion of these 510(k) cleared devices include devices which assess brain function (e.g. EEG monitors, EEG electrodes, depth of anesthesia monitoring systems, intracranial pressure monitors), diagnostic devices such as hearing screeners, biofeedback systems, transcutaneous electrical nerve stimulator (TENS) devices, and various neurological and neurosurgical instruments. An online searchable database of FDA-cleared devices is available at: http://www.accessdata.fda.gov/scripts/cdrh/cfdocs/cfPMN/pmn.cfm

As noted above, most Class I devices (and some Class II devices) are now exempted by regulation from the 510(k) requirements. However, these exemptions are subject to limitations under the regulations (i.e., if a new device that falls under these 'exempted' device types has either a new indication for use or new technology which could impact its safety or effectiveness compared to other legally marketed predicate devices within that device type, then the manufacturer would be required to obtain 510(k) clearance prior to marketing the new device).

Premarket approval

The PMA process [4] is the most stringent type of device marketing application and is required by FDA for Class III devices. The applicant must receive FDA approval of its PMA application prior to marketing the device. PMA approval is based on a determination by FDA that the PMA contains sufficient valid scientific evidence to assure that the device is safe and effective for its intended use(s). An approved PMA is, in effect, a private license granting the applicant permission to market the device.

Information contained in a PMA submission typically includes the following: an in-depth device description and indications for use, a description of alternative practices and procedures for the proposed indications for use, a marketing history of the device outside of the US if applicable, detailed manufacturing information, reference to any performance standard or voluntary standard used in the development and testing of the device, results of non-clinical laboratory studies, results of clinical investigations involving human subjects, and copies of all proposed labeling for the device.

The regulations provide 180 days for FDA to review the PMA and make a decision. However, the overall review time may be longer because of deficiencies or questions raised by FDA that need to be addressed by the applicant. An online searchable database of PMA-approved devices is available at: http://www.accessdata.fda.gov/scripts/cdrh/cfdocs/cfPMA/pma.cfm

Among the most prominent neurological devices approved under the PMA process are the DBS devices which have been PMA-approved for Parkinson's disease and essential tremor. The first of these neurostimulators was approved by FDA in 1997 (Medtronic Activa Tremor Control System™). This device system (DBS lead electrodes, lead extensions, implantable pulse generator, memory module, console programmer, burr hole ring and cap, magnet, test stimulator, lead frame kits and accessories) was initially approved for the following indication: 'unilateral thalamic stimulation for the suppression of tremor in the upper extremity in patients who are diagnosed with essential tremor or parkinsonian tremor not adequately controlled by medications and where the tremor

constitutes a significant functional disability.' Since the original approval, the sponsor has submitted approximately 82 supplemental applications to the original PMA to date which have been approved for a variety of changes to the device hardware (e.g., rechargeable battery) and indications for use (e.g., bilateral implantation, management of the advanced symptoms of Parkinson's disease).

Humanitarian device exemption

A humanitarian use device (HUD) is a device that is intended to benefit patients by treating or diagnosing a disease or condition that affects or is manifested in fewer than 4000 individuals in the US per year. A device manufacturer's research and development costs could exceed its market returns for diseases or conditions affecting small patient populations. The HUD provision of the regulations (21 CFR 814 Subpart H) provides an incentive for the development of devices for use in the treatment or diagnosis of diseases affecting these populations.

To obtain marketing approval for an HUD, a humanitarian device exemption (HDE) application is submitted to FDA. An HDE is similar in both form and content to a PMA application, but is exempt from the effectiveness requirement of a PMA. That is, an HDE application is not required to demonstrate that the device is effective for its intended purpose. The application, however, must contain sufficient information for FDA to determine that the device does not pose an unreasonable or significant risk of illness or injury, and that the *probable benefit to health* outweighs the risk of injury or illness from its use, taking into account the probable risks and benefits of currently available devices or alternative forms of treatment. Additionally, the applicant must demonstrate that no comparable devices (other than another HDE device) are available to treat or diagnose the disease or condition, and that they could not otherwise bring the device to market.

An approved HDE authorizes marketing of the HUD. However, an HUD may only be used in facilities that have established a local institutional review board (IRB) to supervise clinical use of HDE-approved devices. The labeling for an HUD must state that the device is a humanitarian use device and that, although the device is authorized for marketing by Federal Law, the effectiveness of the device for the specific indication has not been demonstrated.

Over the past 13 years, FDA has approved nearly 50 HDEs. Several of these have included neurological device technology including neurostimulator devices indicated for restoring or promoting bladder function, gastric emptying, and diaphragmatic function; for aiding in the management of chronic, intractable primary dystonia; and for the treatment of patients with obsessive-compulsive disorder who are resistant to medical therapy. Several other HDEs have been approved for neurovascular indications (stroke, wide-necked intracranial aneurysms) in HUD populations.

A listing of HDE approvals can be found at the FDA website at: http://www.fda.gov/MedicalDevices/ProductsandMedicalProcedures/DeviceApprovalsandClearances/HDEApprovals/ucm161827.htm

Investigational device exemptions

The investigational device exemptions (IDE) regulation (21 CFR 812) pertains to devices that have not been approved or cleared for marketing or that are being tested for indications not previously approved or cleared. The IDE allows the investigational device to be used in a clinical study in order to collect safety and effectiveness data required to support a PMA or, less frequently, a 510(k) or HDE premarket submission. An IDE application to FDA is required for any *significant risk device*, as defined below.

Significant risk device

A significant risk device presents a potential for serious risk to the health, safety, or welfare of a subject. Significant risk devices may include implants, devices that support or sustain human life, and devices that are substantially important in diagnosing, curing, mitigating or treating disease, or in preventing impairment to human health. Examples of neurological devices currently considered as significant risk devices include implanted intracerebral/subcortical stimulators, implanted spinal cord and peripheral nerve stimulators, neurovascular embolization devices, hydrocephalus shunts, and electroconvulsive therapy devices.

FDA guidance on distinguishing between significant risk and non-significant risks studies is available in the document 'Significant Risk and Nonsignificant Risk Medical Device Studies' [10]. FDA is the final arbiter in deciding whether a device study poses significant risk (SR) or non-significant risk (NSR). It should be noted, however, that FDA generally only sees those studies that sponsors submit to the agency or those studies for which an IRB or clinical investigator asks for FDA's opinion. If FDA disagrees with an IRB's NSR determination, the sponsor may not begin their study until FDA approves an IDE. If a sponsor submits an IDE to FDA because the sponsor presumed it to be an SR study, and FDA determines that the device study is a NSR, FDA will inform the sponsor in writing. The study may then be reviewed by the IRB as an NSR study.

Non-significant risk device

Non-significant risk devices are devices that do not pose a significant risk to subjects in a research study. Examples of NSR neurological devices include EEG, functional non-invasive electrical neuromuscular stimulators, and TENS devices for treatment of pain (except chest pain/angina).

A NSR device study requires only IRB approval prior to initiation of a clinical study. Sponsors of studies involving NSR devices are not required to submit an IDE application to FDA for approval.

IDE application process

An IDE application to FDA must include information on relevant preclinical studies and any available clinical data. The sponsor (or sponsor/investigator in the case of an individual or group of individuals not associated with a device manufacturer) must also submit an investigational research plan that describes the research design and analytic methods to be used. This plan should define the study design, study objectives or hypotheses, device description, subject inclusion/exclusion criteria, procedures, data monitoring plan, statistical analysis plan, including sample size estimates and power calculations to detect a significant effect, specification of primary and secondary outcome measures, risks/risk monitoring plan, number of investigators/sites, and whether or not a data safety monitoring committee is planned. Extensive online information is available to assist industry and investigators in the planning, design and conduct of IDE studies at: http://www.fda.gov/MedicalDevices/DeviceRegulationandGuidance/HowtoMarketYourDevice/InvestigationalDeviceExemptionIDE/ucm162453.htm

An IDE study cannot proceed until the IDE is approved by FDA and an IRB. FDA and investigators or sponsors may engage in extensive discussions about the characteristics and objectives of research studies to support any future claims of safety and effectiveness.

These discussions often occur through the pre-IDE process (see next section).

Upon receipt of an IDE application, sponsors are notified in writing of the date that FDA received the original application and an IDE number assigned for tracking purposes. An IDE application is considered approved 30 days after it has been received by FDA, unless FDA otherwise informs the sponsor within 30 calendar days from the date of receipt that the IDE is approved, approved with conditions, or disapproved. In cases of disapproval, a sponsor has the opportunity to either respond to the deficiencies or to request a regulatory hearing.

Once an IDE application is approved, the following requirements must be met in order to conduct the investigation in compliance with the IDE regulation:

- Labeling – The device must be labeled in accordance with the labeling provisions of the IDE regulation (21 CFR 812.5) and must bear the statement 'CAUTION – Investigational Device. Limited by Federal (or United States) law to investigational use.'
- Distribution – Investigational devices can only be distributed to qualified investigators [21 CFR 812.43(b].
- Informed Consent – Each subject must be provided with and sign an informed consent form before being enrolled in the study. 21 CFR 50, Protection of Human Subjects, contains the requirements for obtaining informed consent.
- Monitoring – All investigations must be properly monitored to protect the human subjects and assure compliance with approved protocols (21 CFR 812.46).
- Prohibitions – Commercialization, promotion, and misrepresentation of an investigational device and prolongation of the study are prohibited (21 CFR 812.7).
- Records and Reports – Sponsors and investigators are required to maintain specified records and make reports to investigators, IRBs, and FDA (21 CFR 812.140 and 21 CFR 812.150).

IDE exempt investigations

All clinical investigations of devices must have an approved IDE or otherwise be exempt from the IDE regulation. Studies exempt from the IDE regulation [21 CFR 812.2(c] include those involving:

1. A legally marketed device when used in accordance with its labeling
2. A diagnostic device if it complies with the labeling requirements in 21 CFR 809.10(c) and if the testing:
    a. is non-invasive;
    b. does not require an invasive sampling procedure that presents significant risk;
    c. does not by design or intention introduce energy into a subject; and
    d. is not used as a diagnostic procedure without confirmation by another medically established diagnostic product or procedure.

3. Consumer preference testing, testing of a modification, or testing of a combination of devices if the device(s) are legally marketed device(s) [that is, the devices have an approved PMA, cleared Premarket Notification 510(k), or are exempt from 510(k] *and* if the testing is not for the purpose of determining safety or effectiveness and does not put subjects at risk.
4. A device intended solely for veterinary use.
5. A device shipped solely for research with laboratory animals and contains the labeling 'CAUTION – Device for investigational use in laboratory animals or other tests that do not involve human subjects.'

Depending upon the nature of the investigation, those studies which are exempt from the requirements of the IDE regulation may or may not be exempt from the requirements for IRB review.

Pre-IDE process

The pre-IDE process provides a means for gaining FDA comments and feedback on proposed preclinical or clinical studies intended to support a marketing application. This includes studies for both SR and NSR devices or post-market studies which do not require an IDE submission, but which will generate data to support an eventual marketing submission. This process is especially beneficial for medical device manufacturers or sponsors/investigators who have not had previous contact with the FDA, and whose device utilizes new technologies or involves new uses of existing technologies. Early interaction with the agency may help to increase the sponsor's understanding of FDA requirements, regulations, and guidance documents, and will

Table 19.2 FDA Medical Device Advisory Panels

Anesthesiology and Respiratory Therapy Devices Panel	Hematology and Pathology Devices Panel
Circulatory System Devices Panel	Immunology Devices Panel
Clinical Chemistry and Clinical Toxicology Devices Panel	Microbiology Devices Panel
Dispute Resolution Panel	Molecular and Clinical Genetics Panel
Ear, Nose and Throat Devices Panel	Neurological Devices Panel
Gastroenterology and Urology Devices Panel	Obstetrics and Gynecology Devices Panel
General and Plastic Surgery Devices Panel	Ophthalmic Devices Panel
Dental Products Panel	Orthopaedic and Rehabilitation Devices Panel
General Hospital and Personal Use Devices Panel	Radiological Devices Panel

allow FDA personnel to familiarize themselves with the new technologies. Increased interaction between FDA and sponsors and investigators may also help to speed the regulatory process and minimize delays in the development of clinically useful devices. The communication with FDA may take the form of a 'pre-IDE submission' and/or a 'pre-IDE meeting'. Pre-IDE submissions often focus on troublesome parts of a planned IDE application (e.g., clinical protocol design, preclinical testing proposal, pre-clinical test results, and protocols for foreign studies when the studies will be used to support future marketing applications to be submitted to FDA). Upon completion of the review of the pre-IDE submission, the reviewing division within CDRH will issue comments and responses to questions posed by the sponsor within the submission in a timely manner, usually within 60 days of receipt. Pre-IDE meetings may take the form of telephone conference calls, video conferences, or face-to-face meetings and typically focus on specific questions or issues raised during the review of the pre-IDE submission.

Role of FDA advisory panels

The Medical Devices Advisory Committee consists of 18 panels (see Table 19.2). With the exception of the Medical Devices Dispute Resolution Panel, these panels advise the Agency about issues related to the safety and effectiveness of medical devices. The Medical Devices Dispute Resolution Panel provides advice to the Commissioner on complex or contested scientific issues between the FDA and medical device sponsors, applicants, or manufacturers. CDRH has established advisory committees to provide independent, professional expertise and technical assistance on the development, safety and effectiveness, and regulation of medical devices and electronic products that produce radiation. Each committee consists of experts with recognized expertise and judgment in a specific field. Members have the training and experience necessary to evaluate information objectively and to interpret its significance. While these members are not regular employees of FDA, they are paid as 'special government employees' for the days they participate as members of a panel and assist FDA in its public health mission. The committees are advisory – they provide their comments and recommendations regarding issues and questions posed by FDA – but final decisions are made by the Agency. Panel input is often requested for 'first of kind' devices or applications which pose challenging safety and/or effectiveness issues.

The majority of neurological device issues requiring panel input are brought before the Neurological Devices Advisory Panel. However, depending on the proposed indication for use of the device under consideration, other advisory panels may be involved. For example, neurostimulation devices to promote gastric or bladder emptying would likely be presented to the Gastroenterology and Urology Devices Panel which would have the most appropriate clinical and scientific expertise to evaluate the safety and effectiveness issues associated with such devices. Alternatively, experts from other advisory panels within FDA may be used to augment necessary areas of expertise for the Neurological Devices Advisory Panel for specific device issues.

Summary

FDA uses a tiered, risk-based classification of medical devices, including neurological devices, in determining the regulatory requirements for the premarket review process. General regulatory requirements (i.e., general controls) apply to all classes of devices and are, by themselves, sufficient to assure the safe and effective use of low risk (Class I) devices. Additional 'special controls' such as post-market surveillance, conformance to standards and guidance documents, supplement these general controls for moderate risk (Class II) devices. Finally, the PMA process is used to ensure the safety and effectiveness of high risk (Class III) devices. In addition to reviewing premarket applications for these devices [510(k)s, PMAs, HDEs], the FDA is responsible for the regulatory oversight of clinical studies for significant risk investigational devices. The agency actively collaborates with industry and investigators in developing rigorous clinical studies that will provide adequate safety and effectiveness data to support FDA clearance or approval of devices that will benefit the American public. The data generated by such studies may be presented to a CDRH Advisory Panel of external clinical and scientific experts for recommendation and comment for devices with novel technologies, indications for use, or for applications which pose specific challenging safety and effectiveness issues. During the premarket review of neurological and other device types, the FDA strives to fulfill its dual mission of both promoting and protecting the public health by assuring the safety and effectiveness of medical devices.

References

1. PRLog Free Press Release. Prospects of the Neurology Devices Market to 2016. 2010. http://www.prlog. org/10544597-prospects-of-the-neurology-devices-market-to-2016.html

2. Weaver FM, Follett K, Stern M, *et al.* Bilateral deep brain stimulation vs best medical therapy for patients with advanced Parkinson disease: A randomized controlled trial. *JAMA* 2009; **301**: 63–73.

3. Pena C, Li K, Felten R, *et al.* An example of US Food and Drug Administration device regulation: Medical devices indicated for use in acute ischemic stroke. *Stroke* 2007; **38**: 1988–1992.

4. Premarket Approval Manual. HHS Publication FDA 97–4214, January 1998; 1–2.

5. Donahoe G and King G. Estimates of Medical Device Spending in the United States. 2009. http://www.advamed.org/NR/rdonlyres/6ADAAA5B-BA37–469E-817B-3D61DEC4E7C8/0/King2009FINALREPORT52909.pdf

6. Federal Food, Drug, and Cosmetic Act (as amended March, 2005). U.S. Government Printing Office. Washington, D.C. 2005. http://www.fda.gov/RegulatoryInformation/Legislation/FederalFoodDrugandCosmeticActFDCAct/default.htm

7. Code of Federal Regulations. U.S. Government Printing Office. Washington, D.C. http://www.accessdata.fda.gov/scripts/cdrh/cfdocs/cfcfr/cfrsearch.cfm

8. Center for Devices and Radiological Health FDA. Guidance for industry and FDA staff – Class II special controls guidance document: vascular and neurovascular embolization devices. Silver Spring, MD. http://www.fda.gov/MedicalDevices/DeviceRegulationandGuidance/GuidanceDocuments/ucm072013.htm

9. Center for Devices and Radiological Health FDA. Guidance on the CDRH premarket notification review program. 510(k) Memorandum #K86–3. Silver Spring, MD. http://www.fda.gov/MedicalDevices/DeviceRegulationandGuidance/GuidanceDocuments/ucm081383.htm

10. Information Sheet Guidance for IRBs, Clinical Investigators, and Sponsors: Significant and nonsignificant risk medical devices. http://www.fda.gov/downloads/RegulatoryInformation/Guidances/ucm126418.pdf

Chapter

20

Parkinson's disease

Karl Kieburtz and Jordan Elm

Introduction

In the early nineteenth century James Parkinson described the cardinal motor features of Parkinson's disease (PD), which remain the hallmark of early diagnosis to this time. His initial observations emphasized the slowness of movement (bradykinesia), rhythmic shaking of the limbs at rest (resting tremor), resistance of the limbs to passive movement (rigidity), and stooped posture with impaired balance (postural change and instability). Later in the nineteenth century these clinical features were confirmed by other neurologists and codified by Charcot. Although the initial description did not include impairment in cognitive functioning, some concerns were raised about this, and other aspects of mood and personality, as a greater understanding of the disease developed. Furthermore, it was recognized as an illness that is chronic and progressive, with no clear treatments that could modify the course.

The underlying neuropathology of this disorder only came to light in the early twentieth century, with the identification of cell loss and atrophy of brain stem and mid-brain nuclei of neurons. Loss was particularly notable in the pigmented pars compacta of the substantia nigra of the mid-brain. However, other pigmented nuclei of the brain stem, such as the locus coeruleus and the dorsal motor nucleus of the vagus, also had evidence of neuronal loss. An understanding of the underlying neurochemical defects in PD did not emerge until the second half of the twentieth century. Several investigators, including Oleh Hornykiewicz, Arvid Carlsson, and others, identified the striatal deficiency of dopamine that was a corollary of the loss of neurons in the substantia nigra pars compacta. This identification of a dopaminergic deficit led to the proposal, and subsequent testing, of replacement of the deficient dopamine via oral supplementation of levodopa, a metabolic precursor of dopamine. Although initial investigation was of uncertain benefit, eventually levodopa emerged as a dramatically effective treatment in reversing most of the motor features of PD, particularly rigidity and bradykinesia.

The ultimate cause of PD remains uncertain, although there are genetic forms of illness (both autosomal recessive and dominant) with clinical and some pathological features similar to otherwise 'idiopathic' PD. Still, the vast majority of PD does not have a clear genetic cause, although many investigators believe there is an important interplay between genes and the environment in its pathogenesis. Current hypotheses regarding the mechanism of neurodegeneration include abnormalities in protein folding and trafficking, bioenergetic defects, free radical injury and induction of cell death programs, perhaps with an interaction among all. Potential therapies targeting these mechanisms are under active investigation.

Goals of intervention

With the advent of effective treatment of the classic motor features of PD, a better understanding of the complexity of the clinical features of PD emerged in the last few decades of the twentieth century. Complex motor features such as freezing of gait, falling and motor fluctuations, including wearing off of the response to levodopa and involuntary movements called dyskinesias (often in response to levodopa dosing), were identified. These motor features, particularly freezing and falling, were relatively resistant to the beneficial effects of levodopa, in comparison to rigidity and bradykinesia. In addition, despite the effective treatment of the classic motor features of

Clinical Trials in Neurology, ed. Bernard Ravina, Jeffrey Cummings, Michael P. McDermott, and R. Michael Poole. Published by Cambridge University Press. © Cambridge University Press 2012.

PD, additional non-motor features emerged, perhaps reflecting the more extensive neuropathology of PD that involves more than dopaminergic nerve cells. Chief among these non-motor features is impairment in cognition, which may be subtly present even at the earliest diagnosis, but in a proportion of patients will advance to functionally limiting cognitive impairment and dementia. Mood is also impaired in PD most often manifested by depression, but the depression often has atypical anxious features, and the response to standard anti-depressive medications is uncertain. Autonomic function is also impaired in PD with fluctuation in control of blood pressure, gastrointestinal function and urinary bladder emptying. There is often disruption in sleep, sometimes preceding the diagnosis of PD, with various problems including REM behavior sleep disorder, restless legs symptoms, and vivid dreaming. Night-time vivid dreaming sometimes extends into daytime hallucinations, usually of a visual nature, that seem to be precipitated or exacerbated by dopaminergic medications. Although not well studied, many PD patients have complaints of pain, that may represent inadequately treated motor symptoms, but pain is often not responsive to standard dopaminergic medications.

In summary, although the classic and initial features of PD are primarily motoric, a range of symptoms involving cognition, mood, autonomic function, and sleep are also part of the constellation of PD signs and symptoms. While some of the motor features may respond very well to levodopa and other dopaminergic treatment, many of the non-motor features are either non-responsive or are exacerbated by dopaminergic therapies, and currently lack definitive effective treatments. All of the signs and symptoms of PD are progressive in nature and ultimately culminate in significant disability for a majority of people with PD, despite the use of dopaminergic therapies. While mood and sleep disruption may be early features of PD, significant cognitive impairment, autonomic dysfunction, and hallucinations tend to be later features of the illness.

Clinical trials in PD have focused in two major areas: treatments designed to alleviate signs and symptoms in the short run, and treatments designed to modify the long-term progression of the illness. As might be expected, the trial designs and outcome measures for studies addressing these two very different aims are also different. We will review both categories of trials separately.

Study populations

Because of the progressive nature of the disease, randomized trials tightly define the target population depending on the goal of the intervention. In general, clinical trials in PD enroll patients all within the same course of their disease. Frequently, clinical trials enroll one of three groups of patients: 1) early, untreated PD patients; 2) patients who are just initiating dopaminergic therapy; or 3) advanced patients who are experiencing motor fluctuations.

Measurement tools and biomarkers

In clinical trials of short-term improvement with early PD patients the most common primary outcome measure is the Unified Parkinson's Disease Rating Scale (UPDRS) [1]. This rating scale was developed by expert consensus rather than through a traditional clinicometric process. The UPDRS is divided into three main sections: mentation, activities of daily living, and motor. Recently the UPDRS has been updated and modified as the Movement Disorder Society-UPDRS (MDS-UPDRS) [2], in an attempt to create better clinicometric properties. The classic UPDRS focuses on the traditional motor features (rigidity, bradykinesia, tremor), which were most responsive to levodopa. Hence, as an outcome measure it is most sensitive to improvement in the core or classic PD motoric features. It is not particularly good at assessing other aspects of PD including mood and cognition.

In clinical trials of advanced patients, aimed at reducing 'off' time, the most common primary outcome measures are patient-completed diaries, usually on a half hour basis, where the subject indicates whether they are 'on' (medication controlling symptoms), 'off' (medication not controlling symptoms), or asleep. These diaries are typically collected for 2–3 days before a baseline visit and before subsequent and final visits to assess whether the amount of time spent in the 'on' condition has been extended. Additionally, UPDRS scores may be obtained in both the 'on' and 'off' states to determine if the medication has lessened the severity of symptoms in the 'off' condition. Most trials are not attempting to improve the best 'on' state.

Clinical trials to address short term improvement in signs and symptoms

As already mentioned, early in the course of PD the classic motor signs predominate the clinical picture.

Table 20.1 Recent randomized, multi-center clinical trials in early PD

Trial	Design	Total sample size	Primary efficacy outcome	Duration
STEP-UP, 1997 [5]	Double-blind, placebo-controlled, parallel-group, multi-arm	264	Change in Total UPDRS	10 wks
Shannon, Bennett, Friedman study of pramipexole, 1997, [6]	Double-blind, placebo-controlled, parallel-group	335	Change in ADL and Motor UPDRS	Up to 32 wks
The 056 study of ropinirole, 1998 [7]	Double-blind, parallel-group	268	Percentage improvement in motor UPDRS	Interim analysis at 26 wks
TEMPO, 2002 [8]	Double-blind, placebo-controlled, parallel-group, multi-arm	404	Change in Total UPDRS	26 wks
PATCH, 2003 [4]	Double-blind, placebo-controlled, parallel-group, multi-arm	242	Change in Motor+ADL UPDRS	14 wks

Table 20.2 Recent randomized, multi-center clinical trials of PD motor fluctuations

Trial	Design	Total sample size	Primary efficacy outcome	Duration
SEESAW, 1997 [12]	Double-blind, placebo-controlled, parallel-group	205	Change in percentage of 'on' time	24 wks
Lieberman, Ranhosky, Korts (1997) study of pramipexole [13]	Double-blind, placebo-controlled, parallel-group	360	Change in ADL UPDRS (average of 'on' and 'off' ratings), change in motor UPDRS	32 wks
Lieberman et al (1998) study of ropinerole [14]	Double-blind, placebo-controlled, parallel-group	149	Number of patients with 20% or greater decrease in L-dopa dose and 20% or greater reduction in percent time spent 'off'	26 wks
Waters et al (2004) study of Zydis Selegiline [15]	Double-blind, placebo-controlled, parallel-group	140	Change in percentage of total daily 'off' time	12 wks
PRESTO, 2005 [11]	Double-blind, placebo-controlled, parallel-group, multi-arm	472	Change in total daily 'off' time	26 wks
Rascol, Brooks, Melamed, LARGO, 2005 [17]	Double-blind, placebo-controlled, parallel-group	687	Change in total daily 'off' time	18 wks

Clinical trials at this stage are largely aimed at improving motor function. Traditionally in clinical practice, levodopa, a potent treatment for the motor signs and symptoms of PD, is delayed until there is significant motor disability. The rationale behind this practice was a concern that levodopa could either hasten the progression of illness, or that the duration of its beneficial effect may be limited and should be preserved until such time as disability warrants therapy. Both of these concerns have subsequently been questioned, but the tradition of delaying dopaminergic therapy in patients with an early diagnosis of PD persists. In this setting, patients who have been identified with idiopathic PD are recruited to test novel interventions which may have anti-parkinsonian effects as monotherapy. Most clinical trial designs have been relatively straightforward and simplistic in this stage of therapeutic development. Usually studies are double-blind, placebo-controlled,

include measurement of ambulatory capability and ability to function in the home or work environment. Although the Schwab and England ADL scale was initially developed with this in mind, its clinicometric properties are not well studied, and it tends to focus on motor function. Validated overall measures of disability in PD based on motor and non-motor features are being developed. In response to this lack of single measurement of disability or overall PD severity, analytic strategies such as global statistical tests have been proposed. In such an approach, rather than selecting a single primary outcome measure, multiple outcome measures assessing relevant domains are used. They are then analyzed in a single synthetic way using a global statistical test that takes into account an individual's performance on a series of measures [45]. This seems like a reasonable and fairly efficient approach until a single, more global measurement of functioning in PD can be established.

We have largely used the clinical manifestations of PD as a measurement of the underlying progression of the illness. This approach is fraught with difficulties since there are so many treatments to modify the expression of the clinical features which we don't believe have any impact on the underlying disease (although this may be a mistake). Ideally we would have some way of assessing the extent and progression of the disease process, whether that is a measure of neuronal atrophy and death, a loss of important physiological compensatory mechanisms, impairment of glial function or structure, or all of the above. Unfortunately such a biomarker of disease progression is lacking. Attempts at developing imaging biomarkers including those that measure the dopamine transporter, the metabolic capacity of dopaminergic neurons, vesicular transporter mechanisms, or pre-synaptic receptor binding have not emerged as effective outcome tools in the setting of clinical trials of PD progression. Measurements of the deposition of alpha synuclein protein, or of inflammation, are other approaches to measuring disease progression in PD, but are largely experimental at this time. There have been analogous attempts to measure changes in body fluid (blood, CSF, urine) markers including alpha-synuclein, indices of cell death, and indices of oxidative stress. While some of these appear promising, none have emerged as an effective biomarker in the context of PD trials. While it will be a very long road for any of these biomarkers to be accepted as surrogate endpoints in the context of disease progression studies, using them as supportive

and complimentary evidence in the context of studies relying on clinical measures could give us a better framework to understand the clinical effects we observe in trials.

Trial design

Confirmatory (phase 3) clinical trials in PD typically require long-term follow-up (months or years for trials of disease modification) and relatively large sample sizes for definitive evidence of efficacy. As such, it is sensible to perform pilot testing of potential agents. Ideally, phase 2 testing will be conducted quickly in a small sample of patients, so as not to delay the drug development process. Phase 2 tests of potential disease modifying agents in PD have relied on short-term improvement (observed over 1 year or less) in order to complete a phase 2 study within a reasonable time frame. This prompts the question of whether such short-term improvement is purely symptomatic or truly reflecting disease modification. An examination of 1 and 3 month time points compared to 12 months can help alleviate this concern. Moreover, as alluded to before, in order to be able to detect short-term change, phase 2 testing is frequently done in an early, untreated PD sample, making the generalizability of results to treated patients more difficult [46].

Phase 2 or pilot testing of several potential disease modifying agents has been done using a futility design [47]. This design is frequently used in cancer clinical trials to quickly rule out clearly ineffective treatments. Rather than testing for efficacy, each treatment arm is compared to a futility threshold (a predefined maximum worsening to warrant further study of the drug). If the drug is worse than this threshold, then the drug would be discarded as futile. Failure to reject the null hypothesis would imply that further study of the drug should be undertaken in a phase 3 setting. Cancer futility designs are typically single-armed studies in which there is no placebo group, thereby reducing the overall study sample size. However, given the variability of the placebo rate in PD and changes in practice over time, it is advisable to include a concurrent placebo control group and test the futility hypothesis as a two-group comparison. Phase 2 dose-ranging trials (where the maximum tolerated dose is already known) can be performed as a test of linear trend (of the doses) [48]. Two-stage selection/futility designs have been proposed to select among more than one dose arm in the phase 2 setting and are in use in other areas of neurology

[49–50]. Because of the long-term follow-up required for pilot trials in PD, pilot designs that incorporate early stopping rules are not as efficient from a sample size perspective as in disease areas where follow-up time is short. This is because most patients have been enrolled by the time the first cohort completes follow-up or recruitment must be halted after enrollment of the first cohort. All of these designs require a smaller sample size (with the same power) compared to a study designed to test the null hypothesis of equal efficacy in a two-group comparison (treatment vs. placebo). For a pilot study, a smaller sample size can be achieved by setting the false positive rate (alpha) at 0.1 or 0.25 (rather than the conventional 0.05); this is justified since the drug will be tested again in a confirmatory trial [51]. Phase 2 trials also address safety, tolerability, and feasibility issues.

Multiple trial designs have been proposed and used in studies to assess disease modification in PD. The original DATATOP [52] used a 2×2 factorial design and randomized subjects to deprenyl, tocopherol, the combination, or placebo. A factorial design permits for an evaluation of the interaction of the two drugs. Under the assumption that there is no significant drug interaction, the sample size is more efficient than testing both drugs alone. The groups were followed over time regarding the development of sufficient disability to warrant dopaminergic therapy. Similar double-blind placebo controlled, parallel-group studies have been conducted using agents including Co-enzyme Q_{10}, CEP-1347 [53] and TCH-346 [54]. These studies either used change in UPDRS as an outcome measure or time until development of disability warranting dopaminergic therapy. The deprenyl and Co-enzyme Q_{10} studies suggested a beneficial effect of the intervention studied. However, the apparent change in the long-term course of illness may have been a manifestation of short-term improvement in PD signs and symptoms (shifting the progression curve to the left) that confounded the ability to detect a change in the long-term course of PD. Post-hoc disease progression modeling studies [55] suggest that there is both a short-term symptomatic improvement and long-term disease modification in the deprenyl studies, but such post-hoc analyses need to be interpreted cautiously. In an attempt to address this issue of short-term symptomatic vs. disease modification effects, two-period designs have been proposed.

Two-period designs are those in which, after an initial period of randomization to active and placebo, both groups then experience a second period where they are on the same treatment status [56]. In a delayed start design the two groups are initially randomized to active and placebo, and in the second period the placebo group begins on active medication while the active group continues on the original assignment. At the end of the second period, any difference that exists between the two groups is hard to explain as short-term symptomatic improvement alone since both groups are on the medication in the final period. An alternate approach is to randomize subjects to active and placebo and then withdraw the active in the second period, the so called withdrawal design. The advantage of this design is that in the second period neither group is on active medications and if any difference persists it is more likely to represent a more 'structural,' or disease-modifying effect, than a symptomatic effect. On the other hand, study designs which require both groups to be on extended periods of placebo intervention are problematic, and determining the adequate length of the withdrawal period is difficult. A recent example of a delayed start design with rasagiline has been published [57], which suggests that the 1 mg dosage is of benefit regarding disease modification, but the 2 mg failed. The reasons for the differences in these two responses will likely be the source of speculation for some time, and helps to point out some of the methodological difficulties and uncertainties regarding two-period design clinical trials.

Several statistical analyses of hypotheses of disease modification are possible with two-period designs. The FDA is currently considering the methodological merit of various approaches [58]. In the delayed start design, three analyses of the primary outcome (e.g., total UPDRS change) are of interest: 1) within period 1, the rate of change in the active group is less than (slower than) the placebo group; 2) the early-start group has a lower change from baseline compared to the delayed-start group (patients who received the drug early have a better final outcome than those starting drug later; 3) the rate of change within period 2 in the early-start group is the same as the rate of the delayed-start group as demonstrated by a test of non-inferiority.

Other trial designs have not focused on trying to differentiate short-term symptomatic improvement from long-term disease modification regarding the clinical features of PD, but instead have focused on determining if there is a long-term change in disability. Long-term disability trials do not necessarily try to imply the mechanism of reduction in disability (i.e., they do not necessarily try to differentiate symptomatic from disease-modifying effects) but focus on the ultimate outcome of subjects randomized to different treatment strategies. In the long-term trial planned by the NET-PD group over 1700 subjects were randomized to receive either placebo or creatine 10 g per day and will be followed for a minimum of 5 years. During the time of randomized treatment, the subjects may receive any other PD treatments available including surgery. The primary outcome is a set of outcome measures designed to assess disability. The Symbol Digit Test is used to assess cognition, the Rankin Scale to assess overall functional capability, the Schwab and England Scale to assess PD function, ambulatory capability is assessed by selected UPDRS scores, and the PDQ-39, a PD specific health related quality-of-life instrument. These outcomes will be analyzed using a global statistical test comparing those receiving creatine with those receiving placebo to determine the overall disability at the end of a minimum of 5 years of treatment. If a single overall disability scale were to emerge in the meantime, it could be proposed as an alternative primary outcome measure.

Lastly, large pragmatic trials of different treatment strategies, or comparative effectiveness trials have been proposed. The PD-MED and PD-SURG [19] trials in the UK are examples of these. Subjects are randomized to different treatment strategies without the use of a placebo control arm. Follow-up assessment is relatively brief and infrequent, and the primary outcome measure is the PDQ-39, a health-related quality-of-life instrument. Entry criteria are few and the trial can be conducted by both neurologists and gerontologists. The advantage of large pragmatic trials is that their external validity or generalizability is likely higher than more explanatory trials. This means that the results of them are likely more directly applicable to the management of community-based patients with PD. The mechanism of impact of interventions in such trials will not be clear, but that may not be needed in order to choose a treatment strategy which will be most beneficial in the long run. Comparative effectiveness trials largely fall into this type of clinical trial approach.

Standards for efficacy and special safety concerns

Several particular safety concerns have emerged in the context of PD clinical trials. In the early studies with dopamine agonists a phenomenon originally called 'sleep attacks' was identified. Individuals who denied prior sleepiness reported falling asleep suddenly, for example while driving. In follow-up of this phenomenon it appears that in fact subjects were drowsy but were unaware of this due to the chronic nature of the drowsiness associated with the treatments. Dopaminergic therapies in general can cause a mild degree of sedation which can lead to excessive daytime sleepiness and to episodes of falling asleep. Hence measuring the extent of excessive daytime sleepiness, also present in unmedicated PD, is important in the context of clinical trials. The Epworth Sleepiness Scale has emerged as a reliable standard tool to measure [59] symptoms of daytime sleepiness in individuals with PD. A cutoff point of 10 is usually suggested as threshold for excessive sleepiness.

Early in the development of levodopa there was a concern that it could induce or promote melanomas or the proliferation of pigmented skin cells. While several epidemiological studies have not confirmed an increased risk for melanomas with dopaminergic medications, it is clear that PD populations are at about a 2–3-fold risk of melanomas compared to the population without PD. This is distinctive as the risk of other cancers in PD is normal or slightly lower. In the context of clinical trials, increased surveillance for melanomas and other skin cancers is warranted.

While the phenomena of impulse control disorders, especially pathological gambling and inappropriate sexual behavior, have been reported for decades in the context of PD, a recent resurgence in interest of this came from the apparent increase in these behaviors with the co-administration of dopamine agonists and levodopa. Impulse control disorder assessment tools (including the modified Minnesota Impulse Disorders Interview (mMIDI) [60–61] and the Questionnaire for Impulsive-Compulsive Behaviors in Parkinson's Disease (QUIP) [62], may be useful in the context of clinical trials to assess baseline and subsequent change in these behaviors. This kind of adverse event raises the issue of low frequency events that are of high importance but that are difficult to measure in the context of clinical trials. These instruments are based on self-reporting and many of these behaviors are considered inappropriate or potentially shameful; hence patients and families are less likely to be willing to report them. Active investigation for such events is necessary.

Lastly, although suicide is an unusual event in PD there is continued interest in observing for the occurrence of suicidal behaviors or suicide. The Beck Depression Inventory (BDI-II) is a widely used screening measure of depression, and it includes a question on suicidal thoughts [63]. The Columbia Suicide and Severity Rating Scale has been developed by the FDA in collaboration with academic investigators. It has been used in trials of PD with relative ease.

Challenges/controversies

One of the biggest controversies in trials of disease modification of PD is the appropriate patient population. While many of the studies have focused on early untreated PD, it remains uncertain as to whether there is truly a population of patients who are early and appropriately not treated any longer. Some investigators feel that early initiation of dopaminergic therapy is warranted for the best long-term outcome, whereas others still believe that delaying initiation of dopaminergic therapy until significant motor disability has emerged is the best course. No clear standard has emerged for the design of trials to assess slowing disease progression, although the FDA and other investigators are working on models of disease progression as one approach. This methodological uncertainty is not present for trials of symptom improvement. In the setting of this controversy it has been increasingly difficult to identify and recruit subjects in this 'early untreated' state to clinical trials. This also raises the question of equitable access to and knowledge about clinical trials for patients and families with PD. Many organizations have attempted to increase the awareness of clinical trials so that those who are interested can participate, but dissemination of information about clinical trials remains suboptimal, in particular among patients of racial or ethnic minority groups [64].

The use of sham controls in high-risk or intensity intervention studies remains controversial. The rigor of placebo or sham controlled trials has been useful in identifying ineffective therapies thought to be effective in unblinded studies. Fetal nigral tissue transplantation was essentially halted until aspects of it can be optimized. It is likely that gene therapy and stem cell treatments will be subjected to similarly rigorous trial designs. Seeking information about attitudes and beliefs of subjects and their families, as well as researchers, on the appropriateness of such sham control studies is important [65–66].

Studies of disease modification in PD will be long term by definition. In all long-term trials some subjects will stop participation before the intended completion. Hence, there will always be missing data from clinical trials. Alternatively, subjects may participate in clinical trials but elect to no longer take the study medication.

They will contribute data but it will not be data derived from the treated state. There exists significant controversy about how to deal with truly missing data. Methodologically sound clinical trials will perform an intent-to-treat analysis, whereby all patients who are randomized are included in the primary analysis. Patients for whom data are not available will have their missing data imputed (or assigned, in some accepted way). Historically, PD patients participating in clinical trials are adherent to study medications and dropout rates are low. However, because of the progressive nature of the disease it is difficult for many PD patients to remain untreated or remain on a stable dose of dopaminergic therapy for the duration of trial follow-up. The presence of missing data poses a challenge to the conduct of two-period designs (delayed start or withdrawal designs) which may be increasingly used in disease modification trials. Using a delayed start design (rather than a withdrawal design) may circumvent the likelihood that patients are more likely to discontinue under withdrawal. In early trials that are measuring time for need for levodopa or UPDRS scores, subjects that require additional therapy will not be able to contribute data beyond that point. Hence, they also contribute to the missing data pool. How to handle such missing data and impute data to replace it is an area of active investigation. Frequently this is done by simply carrying forward the patient's score at the last visit in which the patient initiated dopaminergic therapy or required additional therapy. Better approaches to impute these types of missing data are statistically complex and, as yet, remain an area of continued theoretical research. While some PD clinical trials have discontinued follow-up of patients once they are no longer able to follow the study protocol, there is an emerging consensus that subjects who are in a trial but discontinue the study drug should continue with all protocol assessments. The data generated are not on active intervention, but are data which reflect the status of the subject in any case. Data in study subjects, off study medication is likely to be much more informative than any imputed data that replace missing data.

References

1. Fahn S and Elton RL, Members of the UPDRS Development Committee. The Unified Parkinson's Disease Rating Scale. In: Fahn S, Marsden CD, Calne DB and Goldstein M, editors. *Recent Developments in Parkinson's disease*, Vol 2. Florham Park, NJ, Macmillan Health Care Information. 1987; 153–164: 293–304.

2. Goetz CG, Tilley BC, Shaftman SR, *et al.* Movement Disorders Society-sponsored revision of the Unified Parkinson's Disease Rating Scale (MDS-UPDRS): scale presentation and clinimetric testing results. *Mov Disord* 2008; **23**: 2129–70.

3. Parkinson Study Group. Safety and efficacy of pramipexole in early Parkinson disease. A randomized dose-ranging study. *JAMA* 1997; **278**: 125–30.

4. Parkinson Study Group. A controlled trial of rotigotine monotherapy in early Parkinson's disease. *Arch Neurol* 2003; **60**: 1721–8.

5. Parkinson Study Group. Safety and efficacy of pramipexole in early Parkinson disease. A randomized dose-ranging study. *JAMA* 1997; **278**: 125–30.

6. Shannon KM, Bennett JP, Jr and Friedman JH. Efficacy of pramipexole, a novel dopamine agonist, as monotherapy in mild to moderate Parkinson's disease. The Pramipexole Study Group. *Neurology* 1997; **49**: 724–8.

7. Rascol O, Brooks DJ, Brunt ER, *et al.* Ropinirole in the treatment of early Parkinson's disease: a 6-month interim report of a 5-year levodopa-controlled study. 056 Study Group. *Mov Disord* 1998; **13**: 39–45.

8. Parkinson Study Group. A controlled trial of rasagiline in early Parkinson disease: the TEMPO study. *Arch Neurol* 2002; **59**: 1937–43.

10. Parkinson Study Group. A controlled, randomized, delayed-start study of rasagiline in early Parkinson disease. *Arch Neurol* 2004; **61**: 561–6.

11. Parkinson Study Group. A randomized placebo-controlled trial of rasagiline in levodopa-treated patients with Parkinson disease and motor fluctuations. The PRESTO Study. *Arch Neurol* 2005; **62**: 241–8.

12. Parkinson Study Group. Entacapone improves motor fluctuations in levodopa-treated Parkinson's disease patients. *Ann Neurol* 1997; **42**: 747–55.

13. Lieberman A, Ranhosky A and Korts D. Clinical evaluation of pramipexole in advanced Parkinson's disease: results of a double-blind, placebo-controlled, parallel-group study. *Neurology* 1997; **49**: 162–8.

14. Lieberman A, Olanow CW, Sethi K, *et al.* A multicenter trial of Ropinirole as adjunct treatment for Parkinson's disease. Ropinirole Study Group. *Neurology* 1998; **51**: 1057–62.

15. Waters CH, Sethi KD, Hauser Ra, *et al.* Zydis Selegiline reduces off time in Parkinson's disease patients with motor fluctuations: a 3-month, randomized, placebo-controlled study. *Mov Disord* 2004; **19**: 426–32.

17. Rascol O, Brooks DJ, Melamed E, *et al.* Rasagiline as an adjunct to levodopa in patients with Parkinson's disease and motor fluctuations (LARGO, Lasting effect in Adjunct therapy with Rasagiline Given Once daily, study): a randomized, double-blind, parallel-group trial. *Lancet* 2005; **365**: 947–54.

18. Weaver FM, Follett K, Stern M, *et al.* Bilateral deep brain stimulation vs. best medical therapy for patients with advanced Parkinson disease: A randomized controlled trial. *JAMA* 2009; **301**: 63–73.

19. Williams A, Gill S, Varma T, *et al.* Deep brain stimulation plus best medical therapy versus best medical therapy alone for advanced Parkinson's disease (PD SURG trial): a randomized, open-label trial. *Lancet Neurol* 2010; **9**: 581–91.

20. Follett KA, Weeaver FM, Stern M, *et al.* Pallidal versus subthalamic deep-brain stimulation for Parkinson's disease. *NEJM* 2010; **362**: 2077–91.

21. Freed CR, Breeze RE, Rosenberg NL, *et al.* Survival of implanted fetal dopamine cells and neurologic improvement 12 to 46 months after transplantation for Parkinson's disease. *N Engl J Med* 1992; **327**: 1549–55.

22. Hauser RA, Freeman TB, Snow BJ, *et al.* Long-term evaluation of bilateral fetal nigral transplantation in Parkinson's disease. *Arch Neurol* 1999; **56**: 179–87.

23. Schumacher JM, Ellias SA, Palmer EP, *et al.* Transplantation of embryonic porcine mesencephalic tissue in patients with PD. *Neurology* 2000; **54**:1042–50.

24. Patel NK, Bunnage M, Plaha P, *et al.* Intraputamenal infusion of glial cell line-derived neurotrophic factor in PD: a two-year outcome study. *Ann Neurol* 2005; **57**: 298–302.

25. Slevin JT, Gash DM, Smith CD, *et al.* Unilateral intraputaminal glial cell-line derived neurotrophic factor in patients with Parkinson's disease: response to 1 year of treatment and 1 year of withdrawal. *J Neurosurg* 2007; **106**: 614–20.

26. Stover NP, Bakay RAE, Subramanian T, *et al.* Intrastriatal implantation of human retinal pigment epithelial cells attached to microcarriers in advanced Parkinson's disease. *Arch Neurol* 2005; **62**: 1833–7.

27. Marks WJ, Ostrem JL, Verhagen L, *et al.* Safety and tolerability of intraputaminal delivery of CERE-120 (Adeno-associated virus serotype 2-neurturin) to patients with idiopathic Parkinson's disease: an open-label, phase I trial. *Lancet Neurol* 2008; **7**: 400–8.

28. Freed CR, Greene PE, Breeze RE, *et al.* Transplantation of embryonic dopamine neurons for severe Parkinson's disease. *N Engl J Med* 2001; **344**: 710–19.

29. Olanow CW, Goetz CG, Kordower JH, *et al.* A double-blind controlled trial of bilateral fetal nigral transplantation in Parkinson's disease. *Ann Neurol* 2003; **54**: 403–14.

30. Lang AE, Gill S, Patel NK, *et al.* Randomized controlled trial of intraputaminal glial cell line-derived neurotrophic factor infusion in Parkinson's disease. *Ann Neurol* 2006; **59**: 459–66.

31. Koller WC, Hutton JT, Tolosa E, Capilldeo R, and the Carbidopa/Levodopa Study Group. Immediate-release

and controlled-release carbidopa/levodopa in PD. A 5-year randomized multicenter study. *Neurology* 1999; **53**: 1012–19.

32. Dupont E, Andersen A, Boas J, *et al*. Sustained-release Madopar HBS compared with standard Madopar in the long-term treatment of de novo parkinsonian patients. *Acta Neurol Scan* 1996; **93**: 14–20.

33. Rinne UK, Bracco F, Chouza C, *et al*. Early treatment of Parkinson's disease with Cabergoline delays on the onset of motor complications. Results of a double-blind levodopa controlled trial. *Drugs* 1988; **55** (Suppl): 23–9.

34. Parkinson Study Group. Pramipexole vs. levodopa as initial treatment for Parkinson disease. A randomized controlled trial. *JAMA* 2000; **284**: 1931–8.

35. Rascol O, Brooks DJ, Korczyn AD, *et al*. A five-year study of the incidence of dyskinesias in patients with early Parkinson's disease who were treated with Ropinirole or levodopa. *N Engl J Med* 2000; **342**: 1484–91.

36. Oertel WH, Wolters E, Sampaio C, *et al*. Pergolide versus levodopa monotherapy in early Parkinson's disease patients: the PELMOPET study. *Mov Disord* 2006; **21**: 343–353.

37. Allain H, Destee A, Petit H, *et al*. Five-year follow-up of early lisuride and levodopa monotherapy in de novo Parkinson's disease. The French Lisuride Study Group. *Eur Neurol* 2000; **44**: 22–30.

38. Rinne UK. Lisuride, a dopamine agonist in the treatment of early Parkinson's disease. *Neurology* 1989; **39**: 336–9.

39. Nakanishi T, Iawata M, Goto I, *et al*. Nation-wide collaborative study on the long-term effects of Bromocriptine in the treatment of parkinsonian patients. Final report. *Euro Neurol* 1992; **32**(Suppl 1): 9–22.

40. Olanow CW, Hauser RA, Jankovic J, *et al*. A randomized, double-blind, placebo-controlled, delayed start study to assess rasagiline as a disease modifying therapy in Parkinson's disease (the ADAGIO study): rationale, design, and baseline characteristics. *Mov Disord* 2008; **23**: 2194–201.

41. The NINDS NET-PD Investigators. A randomized clinical trial of coenzyme Q10 and GPI-1485 in early Parkinson's disease. *Neurology* 2007; **68**: 20–8.

42. Goetz CG, Stebbins GT, Wolff D, *et al*. Testing objective measures of motor impairment in early Parkinson's disease: Feasibility study of an at-home testing device. *Mov Disord* 2009; **24**: 551–6.

43. Parkinson Study Group. DATATOP: A multicenter controlled clinical trial in early Parkinson's disease. *Arch Neurol* 1989; **46**: 1052–60.

45. Huang P, Goetz CG, Woolson RF, *et al*. Using global statistical tests in long-term Parkinson's disease clinical trials. *Mov Disord* 2009; **24**: 1732–39.

46. Elm JJ, Goetz CG, Tilley B, *et al*. A responsive outcome for Parkinson's disease neuroprotection futility studies. *Ann Neurol* 2005; **57**: 197–203.

47. Tilley BC, Palesch YY, Kieburtz K, *et al*. Optimizing the ongoing search for new treatments for Parkinson disease: Using futility designs. *Neurology* 2006; **66**: 628–33.

48. Shults CW, Oakes D, Kieburtz K, *et al*. Effects of Coenzyme Q10 in early Parkinson Disease. Evidence of slowing the functional decline. *Arch Neurol* 2002; **59**: 1541–50.

49. Levy G, Kaufmann P, Buchsbaum R, *et al*. A two-stage design for a phase II clinical trial of coenzyme Q10 in ALS. *Neurology* 2006; **66**: 660–3.

50. Cheung YK, Gordon PH and Levin B. Selecting promising ALS therapies in clinical trials. *Neurology* 2006; **67**: 1748–51.

51. Schoenfeld D. Statistical considerations for pilot studies. *Int J Radiat Oncol Biol Phys* 1980; **6**: 371–4.

52. Parkinson Study Group. Effects of tocopherol and deprenyl on the progression of disability in early Parkinson's disease. *N Engl J Med* 1993; **328**: 176–83.

53. Parkinson Study Group PRECEPT Investigators. Mixed lineage kinase inhibitor CEP-1347 fails to delay disability in early Parkinson disease. *Neurology* 2007; **69**: 1480–90.

54. Olanow W, Schapira AHV, LeWitt PA, *et al*. TCH346 as a neuroprotective drug in Parkinson's disease: a double-blind, randomized, controlled trial. *Lancet Neurol* 2006; **5**: 1013–20.

55. Holford NHG, Chan PL, Nutt JG, *et al*. Disease progression and pharmacodynamics in Parkinson disease – Evidence for functional protection with levodopa and other treatments. *J Pharmacokinet Pharmacodyn* 2006; **33**: 281–311.

56. McDermott MP, Hall WJ, Oakes D, *et al*. Design and analysis of two-period studies of potentially disease-modifying treatments. *Control Clin Trials* 2002; **23**: 635–49.

57. Olanow CW, Rascol O, Hauser R, *et al*. A double-blind, delayed-start trial of Rasagiline in Parkinson's disease. *N Engl J Med* 2009; **361**: 1268–78.

58. Bhattaram VA, Siddiqui O, Kapcala LP, *et al*. Endpoints and analyses to discern disease-modifying drug effects in early Parkinson's disease. *AAPS J* 2009; **11**: 456–64.

59. Johns MW. A new method for measuring daytime sleepiness: the Epworth sleepiness scale. *Sleep* 1991; **14**: 540–45.

60. Christenson GA, Faber RJ, and deZwaan M. Compulsive buying: descriptive characteristics and psychiatric comorbidity. *J Clin Psychiatry* 1994; **55**: 5–11.

61. Weintraub D, Siderowf AD, Potenza MN, *et al*. Association of dopamine agonist use with impulse

control disorders in Parkinson disease. *Arch Neurol* 2006; **63**: 969–73.

62. Weintraub D, Stewart S, Shea JA, *et al.* Validation of the Questionnaire for Impulsive-Compulsive Behaviors in Parkinson's Disease (QUIP). *Mov Disord* 2009; **24**: 1461–67.

63. Beck AT, Steer RA, and Brown GK. *Manual for Beck Depression Inventory II*. San Antonio, TX, Psychological Corporation, 1996.

64. Schneider MG, Swearingen CJ, Shulman LM, *et al.* Minority enrollment in Parkinson's disease clinical trials. *Parkinsonism Relat Disord* 2009; **15**: 258–62.

65. Kim SYH, Frank S, Holloway R, *et al.* Science and ethics of sham surgery. A survey of Parkinson disease clinical researchers. *Arch Neurol* 2005; **62**: 1357–60.

66. Kim SYH, Holloway RG, Frank S, *et al.* Volunteering for early phase gene transfer research in Parkinson disease. *Neurol* 2006; **66**: 1010–15.

Chapter

21

Alzheimer's disease

Joshua D. Grill and Jeffrey Cummings

Biological basis for therapies

This chapter will provide an overview of the fundamentals of clinical trials in Alzheimer's disease (AD). A basic understanding of disease biology and clinical presentation is necessary to interpret matters regarding AD trials and we begin with an overview of the disease. We review the goals of AD trials, the basic tools used in their conduct, current and future trial designs, limitations and challenges to trial conduct, and controversies that exist in the field of AD clinical research. The field of AD trials is a rapidly evolving one. We attempt to address recent changes in trial conduct and to consider future changes that will be needed.

Introduction to Alzheimer's disease

Alzheimer's disease is a progressive neurodegenerative disorder characterized over 100 years ago but still lacking adequate therapies. To date, the US FDA has approved five drugs for the treatment of AD. Most studies suggest that these agents provide only symptomatic improvement in AD and pursuit of treatments capable of altering the natural history of AD is rigorous. Therefore, clinical trials of new therapies in AD in the coming years will continue to be a mainstay of AD research.

Recent decades have brought significant increases in the understanding of AD pathogenesis. Much of the focus in AD research continues to revolve around the two hallmarks of disease pathology first described by Alzheimer himself, the neuritic plaque and the neurofibrillary tangle (NFT). These two brain lesions, and the proteins that are most readily used to identify them in immunocytochemical study, have become the focus of research in both disease etiology and treatment development. Neuritic plaques are largely composed of the fibrillogenic 42-amino acid length form of the

beta amyloid protein ($A\beta_{42}$). Neurofibrillary tangles are composed primarily of hyperphosphorylated aggregations of the microtubule-associated protein tau. The molecular events that lead to the formation of these two brain lesions provide ample opportunity for therapeutic intervention. Most attempts at developing disease-modifying drugs to this point have focused on the $A\beta$ cascade (Figure 21.1). Proteolytic processing of the large membrane-bound amyloid precursor protein results in the formation of both seemingly benign and synapto- and neurotoxic proteins of varying sizes. $A\beta_{42}$ is the result of sequential cleavage by beta and gamma secretase enzymes. The presence of $A\beta_{42}$ is characteristic of AD. Its presence in neuritic plaques, combined with demonstration that mutations to the genes for amyloid precursor protein or the catalytic subunits of gamma secretase result in an autosomal dominant, inherited early onset form of AD, suggest that it is this post-translational product that is critical to the disease pathogenesis.

Formation of $A\beta$ plaques results from a series of stages of aggregation. It is not clear which or how many of these stages are neuro- or synaptotoxic. Soluble low number combinations of monomeric $A\beta$ may be most toxic. The number of $A\beta$ monomers aggregated into soluble combinations collectively termed *oligomers* ranges from 2 to 12. Soluble oligomers appear to be more toxic than monomeric $A\beta$ or the insoluble fibrillar aggregates of $A\beta$ found in diffuse or neuritic plaques [1]. Synaptic function is altered in neuronal processes in proximity to $A\beta$ plaque deposition [2].

Tau is an endogenous microtubule-associated protein critical to axonal transport and neuronal health and function. The hyperphosphorylation of tau can occur through activity of a variety of kinases, but glycogen synthase kinase 3β appears to be a primary mechanism for tau hyperphosphorylation. Once

Clinical Trials in Neurology, ed. Bernard Ravina, Jeffrey Cummings, Michael P. McDermott, and R. Michael Poole. Published by Cambridge University Press. © Cambridge University Press 2012.

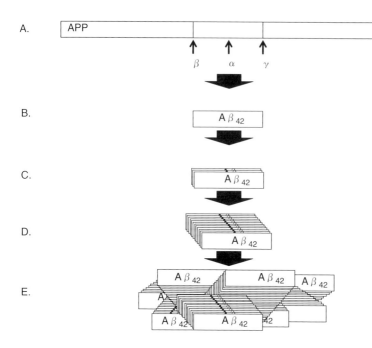

A.

B.

C.

D.

E.

Figure 21.1. The Aβ cascade. A. The amyloid precursor protein is a large peptide that undergoes proteolytic process at characterized sites, including β-, α-, and γ-sites. B. Serial cleavage at the β- and γ-sites liberates the 42-amino acid-length peptide fragment Aβ$_{42}$. C. Low *n* combinations of monomeric Aβ combine into high-molecular weight soluble oligomers that represent synapto- and neurotoxic elements. D. Aggregation of Aβ continues into fibrillar forms such as protofibrils and fibrils. E. Fibrillar Aβ forms diffuse and neuritic Aβ plaques.

hyperphosphorylated, tau condenses, dissociates from microtubules, and aggregates, impairing axonal transport and giving the characteristic appearance of a NFT. Formation of NFTs proceeds topographically and has been used to stage disease severity upon pathological examination. While there is overlap among Aβ and NFT regional pathology, pathological burden in early disease differs between the two hallmark signs in the AD brain. Aβ plaque deposition is first observed in the posterior cingulate cortex and other cortical areas, while NFT formation occurs initially in the entorhinal cortex and hippocampus of the medial temporal lobe.

Aβ plaques and NFTs are accompanied by a variety of other cellular and molecular changes within the AD brain. Inflammatory responses are evident and include increased recruitment of microglia, which are associated with Aβ plaques. As neurons are lost, characteristic depletions of neurotransmitters occur. One such neurotransmitter decrease was discovered early in modern AD research and resulted in the development of the mainstay of current therapies, cholinesterase inhibitors.

Alzheimer's disease pathology begins a decade or more prior to dementia onset: 20–40% of elderly individuals with normal cognition qualify for post-mortem diagnostic criteria for AD [3]. While this may contradict current pathological theories of AD, it seems probable that such individuals were destined for cognitive impairment and, eventually, full blown dementia.

Thus, Alzheimer's *disease* is present prior to the onset of Alzheimer's *dementia*. Efforts are underway to better understand the earliest stages of biological and clinical AD. Attempts to better characterize the earliest stages of AD resulted in construction of the clinical syndrome mild cognitive impairment (MCI), which is defined as subtle cognitive impairment that distinguishes one from an age-matched cohort but does not impair activities of daily living (ADL). The cognitive impairment is most commonly defined as performance on standardized cognitive tasks that is 1.5 or 2.0 standard deviations below the mean for an age-cohort, adjusted for education. Individuals with MCI are at significantly increased risk for all types of dementia. Individuals who suffer from amnestic MCI (characterized by the presence of memory impairment specifically, either alone or concomitantly with impairments to other cognitive domains) are at significantly increased risk for AD dementia specifically. A concerted effort is underway, including the National Institute on Aging- and industry-sponsored collaborative Alzheimer's Disease Neuroimaging Initiative, to better characterize the biological markers that predict future dementia among MCI and non-impaired persons. Biological signatures associated with AD predict future AD dementia among MCI cohorts. These include characteristic atrophy of brain volume assessed by MRI, brain hypometabolism as measured by fluorodeoxyglucose (FDG) PET amyloid burden as measured by amyloid-specific ligands with PET imaging, and changes in CSF protein levels. Individuals who meet MCI criteria and also demonstrate a biological signature of AD have been defined as *prodromal* AD [4]. Alternatively, individuals who carry the biological signature of AD but for whom no demonstrable cognitive impairment is present may be defined as *preclinical* AD.

A wide array of therapeutic interventions for AD are being developed. These include therapies that aim to halt the underlying biology of AD, as well as therapies that aim to improve cognitive function despite the pathological burden of disease. As is the case for many therapeutic realms, clinical trials represent the rate-limiting step to the testing of new therapies for AD. Trials of AD therapies, however, bring unique challenges related to study design and enrollment. Further, it is likely that only through clinical testing of targeted therapies, perhaps in the prodromal and preclinical phases of disease, will many of the debates related to AD pathology be resolved.

Goals of intervention in AD

Alzheimer's disease is characterized by episodic memory impairments (initially manifest as impairments to short-term episodic memory); language changes such as anomia and fluent aphasia; visuospatial impairments; and executive function compromise. Behavioral impairments such as apathy, depression, and agitation also are common. The course of AD is unrelenting; life expectancy after diagnosis is 8–12 years and quality of life will decline through this period.

Definitive diagnosis of AD is reached only upon post-mortem examination or brain biopsy, demonstrating the presence of fibrillar amyloid. The clinical diagnosis of probable AD is based on symptom presentation, is sensitive and specific when performed by a specialist, and is often supported by biological testing. Screening tools for AD exist and can assist in identification of individuals with cognitive impairment. Neuropsychological assessment is often used to further delineate the type and extent of cognitive abnormality present. Biological measures also can aid in diagnosis, especially differentiating AD from reversible forms of cognitive impairment or other dementias.

Among the biological changes that can be used in the diagnosis of AD, brain atrophy in the hippocampus and entorhinal cortex is well described in the earliest stages. Similarly, bilateral hypometabolism in the temporal lobe, parietal cortex, and posterior cingulate cortex are consistently observed in AD with FDG PET. Recently, disease-specific ligands for use with PET, such as the amlyloid-specific Pittsburgh compound B (PIB), florbetaben, and AV-45 have become available for use in AD research and appear to have good specificity and sensitivity for AD identification. Analysis of CSF proteins can be used in diagnostic assessment, although consistency in cutoff points and protein level measures across laboratories is still lacking. Decreased levels (<190 pg/mL) of CSF Aβ are expected in AD, hypothetically due to the accumulation of Aβ into plaques in the brain. Concomitant increases in CSF tau and hyperphosphorylated tau occur and are good predictors of AD diagnosis (Figure 21.2).

Currently available treatments include the cholinesterase inhibitors donepezil, galantamine, and rivastigmine, and the glutamate receptor antagonist memantine. None have been demonstrated to possess disease-modifying properties. Symptomatic therapies improve patient performance on cognitive tasks, global measures, ADL, and behavior. Alternatively,

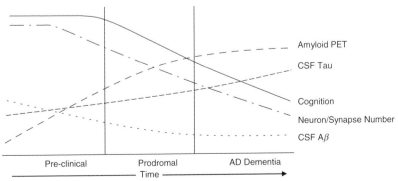

Figure 21.2. Markers of AD progression. AD progresses from an asymptomatic pre-clinical stage, to a period of mild cognitive impairment during which criteria for AD are not met (prodromal AD), and eventually to AD dementia. Biological signs of AD, including reduced CSF Aβ, increased CSF Tau, positive signal on amyloid PET imaging, and brain atrophy (neuron loss) are present in preclinical AD and increase in magnitude with disease progression. CSF Aβ and amyloid PET imaging progress at approximate equal rates, in opposite directions, as amyloid is accumulating in the brain and accordingly decreasing in level in the CSF. Declines in cognition are delayed, relative to the onset of biological changes, and better correlate neuron and synapse number.

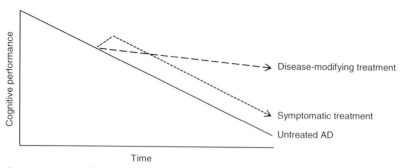

Figure 21.3. Distinction of symptomatic from disease-modifying therapies. The solid line represents a hypothetical model of disease progression (with the caveat that disease progression in AD is not linear). Initiation of symptomatic therapy results in immediate increase in performance, but an unaltered decline in function over time (slope). Disease-modifying therapies, alternatively, may or may not provide symptomatic improvement upon initiation, but alter the course of disease progression (slope) over time, resulting in preservation in cognitive function over time and delay to milestones related to overall cognitive function.

disease-modifying therapies offer a different type of benefit, though the specific definition of that benefit is actively debated.

Disease-modifying therapies may not provide an immediate recovery of memory function. Over time, however, the rate of decline in memory would be slowed, relative to the untreated patient (Figure 21.3). One proposed definition for disease modification requires that the underlying biology must be altered. Alternatively, a patient-centered perspective provides a definition whereby clinical milestones must be delayed, such as the ability to perform ADL or nursing home placement. Purely cellular or molecular milestones may not confer clinical benefit. Similarly, symptomatic therapies may improve clinical outcomes without truly altering disease biology. Therefore, we use a definition that combines these two requirements: disease-modifying therapies must both alter the underlying biology of AD that results in cell death and, as a product of that biological effect, produce a measurable impact on clinical disease progression [5]. Given the long course, the apparent preclinical period of potential intervention, and the late-life age-of-onset of AD, the medical and economic ramifications of developing disease-modifying drugs are substantial and research related to development of these therapies is intense. A drug that can delay the onset of AD dementia by 5 years could decrease disease prevalence by 50%. A drug that delays AD dementia by 10 years will alleviate the public health crisis of AD [6].

Alzheimer's disease clinical trial measurement tools

Clinical trials of the first approved treatments for AD have largely guided subsequent trials, though the targets, mechanisms of action, and intended indications

of investigational treatments have evolved. To receive marketing approval from the FDA, a new AD drug must demonstrate efficacy on co-primary outcomes, including a cognitive measure and a functional or global measure in two well conducted trials [7]. Randomized trials of cholinesterase inhibitors were parallel group 3- and 6-month studies. Subjects were blindly assigned to therapy or placebo and cognitive performance was assessed with the AD Assessment Scale which included the cognitive subscale (ADAS-cog) and the non-cognitive (ADAS-noncog) portion. Since these initial trials, the ADAS-cog has remained the cognitive scale used in most trials conducted in mild to moderate AD (Table 21.1). The ADAS-cog is a 70-point scale that assesses performance in memory, orientation, comprehension of language and commands, naming, word finding, and ideational and constructional praxis. An 80-point version of the ADAS-cog that includes a delayed recall task is also available. Attention, working memory, and executive function are largely overlooked by the ADAS-cog; an expanded ADAS-cog 13 with cancellation and maze tasks is available [8]. Standard cholinergic therapy provides a benefit of approximately 2 points on the ADAS-cog after 6 months.

Evaluation of placebo groups in large trials suggests that the ADAS-cog scores decline roughly 4 to 6 points per year in AD [9, 10]. In the single largest AD trial to date, mean ADAS-cog scores in the placebo group declined 4.28 and 7.08 points at 12 and 18 months, respectively [11]. Other studies have demonstrated annual rates of decline as high as 11.4 points [12]. These discrepancies result from the fact that disease progression measured with the ADAS-cog is not linear and populations in different trials differ in their rate of decline. Ito and colleagues performed a meta-analysis of ADAS-cog decline in acetylcholinesterase clinical trials. They found that baseline mini-mental

Table 21.1 Co-primary outcomes used in phase 3 clinical trials in AD

Phase 3 trial [Reference]	Disease stage	Cognitive primary outcome	Global or functional primary outcome
Tacrine[42]	Mild-to-Moderate	ADAS-cog	CIBI
Donepezil[43]	Mild-to-Moderate	ADAS-cog	CIBIC-Plus
Rivastigmine[44]	Mild-to-Moderate	ADAS-cog	CIBIC-Plus
Galantamine[45, 46]	Mild-to-Moderate	ADAS-cog	CIBIC-Plus
Rivastigmine [transdermal][47]	Mild-to-Moderate	ADAS-cog	ADCS-CGIC
Donepezil[48]	Severe	SIB	ADCS-ADL
Donepezil[16]	Severe	SIB	CIBIC-Plus
Memantine[23]	Moderate-to-Severe	SIB	ADCS-ADL
Tarenflurbil[11]	Mild-to-Moderate	ADAS-cog	ADCS-ADL
Tramiprosate[34]	Mild-to-Moderate	ADAS-cog	CRD-SB
Bapineuzumab[34]	Mild-to-Moderate	ADAS-cog	DAD
Dimebon [drug naïve][34]	Mild-to-Moderate	ADAS-cog	CIBIC-Plus
Dimebon [donepezil add on][34]	Mild-to-Moderate	ADAS-cog	ADCS-ADL
Dimebon [memantine add on][34]	Moderate-to-Severe	SIB	ADCS-ADL
Solanezumab[34]	Mild-to-Moderate	ADAS-cog	ADCS-ADL
LY450139[34]	Mild-to-Moderate	ADAS-cog	ADCS-ADL

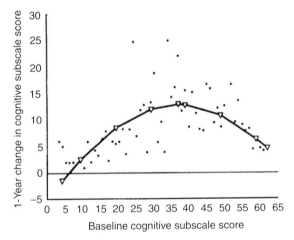

Figure 21.4. One-year changes in ADAS-cog score. Taken from Stern *et al.* [13] this figure demonstrates changes in performance in the ADAS-cog based on baseline entry score on the same outcome measure. The figure clearly illustrates that the greatest annual change in ADAS-cog performance occurs in moderate disease, with minimal changes in very mild and very severe disease. Reprinted with permission from the *American Journal of Psychiatry*, Copyright 1994, American Psychiatric Association.

state examination (MMSE) scores above 27 (or ADAS-cog below 10) were associated with an annual decline of 2.97 ADAS-cog points/year, but baseline MMSE below 12 (ADAS-cog above 40) was associated with an annual decline of 7.52 ADAS-cog points [10]. Similarly, Doraiswamy and colleagues noted an 84% greater decline in the ADAS-cog after 6 months among participants with baseline MMSE 12–18, relative to those with baseline MMSE 19–23. Stern and colleagues examined 1-year change in ADAS-cog among participants with a range of baseline ADAS-cog scores. They noted that in very mild and more severe AD, annual decline is reduced, relative to moderate disease [13] (Figure 21.4). Neither age nor ApoE genetic status appears to impact the rate of decline on ADAS-cog [14].

Because of the performance characteristics of the ADAS-cog, particularly in the earliest stages of disease, Harrison and colleagues developed the Neuropsychological Test Battery (NTB), specifically for use in clinical trials [15]. The NTB uses nine validated components to examine cognitive function in the domains of visual and verbal memory, and executive function. The NTB appears to demonstrate linear decline for both mild and moderate dementia. The NTB has been used in only a few trials and its performance across trials is not yet well understood.

All cholinesterase inhibitors are approved for mild-to-moderate AD and two medications (memantine and donepezil) have been approved by the FDA for severe dementia. Approval in the severe disease stage

all associated with a lack placebo group decline on the ADAS-cog. Schneider and Sano recently assessed placebo group decline in eleven 18-month trials for which data were available [40]. They noted a wide range of mean placebo decline on the ADAS-cog in these studies from 4.34 to 9.10 points, despite largely similar inclusion criteria. Mean placebo group decline at 18 months for the examined trials was 6.5 points and roughly 25% of patients declined by 1 point or less.

Trials of disease-modifying therapies are generally at least 18 months in length to allow for sufficient placebo group decline. It remains unclear if this is sufficient time to demonstrate disease-modifying efficacy. Recent large 18-month trials of tramiprosate and tarenflurbil failed to demonstrate significant differences from placebo.

Most 18-month trials are powered to detect a difference of 2 points in mean ADAS-cog scores at study conclusion. Depending on the expected slowing of rate of decline, however, this suggests that the rate of decline observed in these studies might or might not be sufficient for a positive trial. A drug that slows rate of decline by 50% would require 18 months to demonstrate efficacy if the placebo group was declining by 3 points annually. A drug that slowed decline by 25% would require a 3-year trial to demonstrate efficacy under the same parameters. Such effectiveness, however, might represent a significant improvement in the quality of care and is still worthy of marketing. Uncertainties related to effect sizes of potential disease modifying therapies and variance in placebo group decline make planning of well-powered but cost-effective large-scale trials difficult.

Finally, it is clear that AD biology begins prior to clinical phenomenology and this window of time may represent the ideal point of intervention. Trials enrolling individuals who fit criteria for preclinical or prodromal AD may have the greatest likelihood of success, since the pathological burden of disease is minimal. Further, cognitive rescue is greatest in this disease phase. Conducting trials in such populations is difficult, however. Individuals must be identified, informed of their condition, and recruited to long-term participation. Fulfillment of entry criteria, by definition, includes presence of a biomarker of disease. Currently, the biological marker with the greatest predictive sensitivity for AD dementia is CSF analysis via lumbar puncture (LP). Convincing individuals who may think that they are cognitively normal to undergo LP so that they can then learn that they have a disease and/or are likely to soon develop AD dementia is a difficult and ethically challenging arena.

Methodological limitations/ controversies

The rapid and substantial increase in research focus, drug development, and trial conduct in AD has not been without challenges. Concerns exist over the lack of regulatory guidance for the next age of AD drug development, i.e., therapies that slow disease progression rather than or in addition to causing symptomatic benefit. It is unclear what information will be included in the prescribing information of the first agent that demonstrates such efficacy. It is also unclear what requirements will be necessary to make such a claim.

New diagnostic criteria for AD have been proposed but have not been endorsed by regulatory bodies [4]. It is a consensus among investigators that implementation of such criteria would improve trials and increase likelihood of success. Such criteria include clinical and biomarker evidence of AD. Alternatively, the use of biomarkers as key secondary outcome measures has become common, but no biological measure of disease has been accepted as a surrogate marker for disease progression or drug efficacy.

Because of the lack of surrogate markers, current trials rely upon clinical assessment tools as primary outcome measures. The minimal clinically significant benefit of therapy for disease-modifying agents is controversial. A European group of experts concluded that a 2-point difference from placebo on the ADAS-cog at 18 months was a 'minimal clinically important change' [41]. Others, however, regard global and/or functional measures as being of greater importance. For these tools as well, however, the minimal difference and time course for establishing such a difference remain debated and lacking regulatory guidance.

The recent failures in large-scale phase 3 trials has led to questions regarding which agents should be taken forward into large scale clinical development. Data from phase 2 are often limited to non-significant results on measures of efficacy and whether such clinical data represent sufficient rationale for moving to phase 3 is debated. Support of such decisions with biomarker data and POP studies should be used more readily.

Finally, it remains unclear if the dominant theory in AD is correct and if the majority of disease modifying therapies aim at the appropriate target. The amyloid hypothesis remains well-supported by basic and clinical research. Alternate hypotheses exist, however, and the need to pursue other lines of therapeutic research is compelling. Therapies that aim at other pathological characteristics of AD are in development, but lag behind those that aim at Aβ. Inhibitors of the kinases that phosphorylate tau and phosphatases that attempt to reverse this phosphorylation are in development. Agents that aim to protect neurons from death, independent of the cause of that death, including mitochondrial stabilizers and neurotrophic factors, are also in development. Agents that aim at the intrinsic mechanisms of aging, the single greatest risk factor for AD, such as resveretrol and other antioxidants are now being tested clinically.

In summary, AD trials represent an area of urgent need, tremendous enthusiasm, and great promise. An unprecedented number of trials are currently under way at all levels of development. A wide array of mechanisms of action and therapeutic targets are being pursued. Despite this diversity, trial designs and tools are largely unchanged in the modern era of AD research. It is possible that similar evolution in the way that trials are conducted will be needed before effective disease modifying therapies can be demonstrated as clinically effective, approved for large-scale marketing, and utilized to avoid an extraordinary health care burden.

References

1. Shankar GM, Li S, Mehta TH, *et al*. Amyloid-beta protein dimers isolated directly from Alzheimer's brains impair synaptic plasticity and memory. *Nat Med* 2008; **14**: 837–42.

2. Meyer-Luehmann M, Spires-Jones TL, Prada C, *et al*. Rapid appearance and local toxicity of amyloid-beta plaques in a mouse model of Alzheimer's disease. *Nature* 2008; **451**: 720–24.

3. Price JL, McKeel DW, Jr., Buckles VD, *et al*. Neuropathology of nondemented aging: presumptive evidence for preclinical Alzheimer disease. *Neurobiol Aging* 2009; **30**: 1026–36.

4. Dubois B, Feldman HH, Jacova C, *et al*. Research criteria for the diagnosis of Alzheimer's disease: revising the NINCDS-ADRDA criteria. *Lancet Neurol* 2007; **6**: 734–46.

5. Cummings JL. Defining and labeling disease-modifying treatments for Alzheimer's disease. *Alzheimers Dement* 2009; **5**: 406–18.

6. Brookmeyer R, Gray S, and Kawas C. Projections of Alzheimer's disease in the United States and the public health impact of delaying disease onset. *Am J Public Health* 1998; **88**: 1337–42.

7. Leber P. Observations and suggestions on antidementia drug development. *Alzheimer Dis Assoc Disord* 1996; **10** Suppl 1: 31–5.

8. Mohs RC, Knopman D, Petersen RC, *et al*. Development of cognitive instruments for use in clinical trials of antidementia drugs: additions to the Alzheimer's Disease Assessment Scale that broaden its scope. The Alzheimer's Disease Cooperative Study. *Alzheimer Dis Assoc Disord* 1997; **11** Suppl 2: S13–21.

9. Holford NH and Peace KE. Results and validation of a population pharmacodynamic model for cognitive effects in Alzheimer patients treated with tacrine. *Proc Natl Acad Sci U S A* 1992; **89**: 11471–5.

10. Ito K, Ahadieh S, Corrigan B, *et al*. Disease progression meta-analysis model in Alzheimer's disease. *Alzheimers Dement* 2010; **6**: 39–53.

11. Green RC, Schneider LS, Amato DA, *et al*. Effect of tarenflurbil on cognitive decline and activities of daily living in patients with mild Alzheimer disease: a randomized controlled trial. *JAMA* 2009; **302**: 2557–64.

12. Suh GH, Ju YS, Yeon BK, and Shah A. A longitudinal study of Alzheimer's disease: rates of cognitive and functional decline. *Int J Geriatr Psychiatry* 2004; **19**: 817–24.

13. Stern RG, Mohs RC, Davidson M, *et al*. A longitudinal study of Alzheimer's disease: measurement, rate, and predictors of cognitive deterioration. *Am J Psychiatry* 1994; **151**: 390–96.

14. Kleiman T, Zdanys K, Black B, *et al*. Apolipoprotein E epsilon4 allele is unrelated to cognitive or functional decline in Alzheimer's disease: retrospective and prospective analysis. *Dement Geriatr Cogn Disord* 2006; **22**: 73–82.

15. Harrison J, Minassian SL, Jenkins L, *et al*. A neuropsychological test battery for use in Alzheimer disease clinical trials. *Arch Neurol* 2007; **64**: 1323–9.

16. Black SE, Doody R, Li H, *et al*. Donepezil preserves cognition and global function in patients with severe Alzheimer disease. *Neurology* 2007; **69**: 459–69.

17. Feldman H, Sauter A, Donald A, *et al*. The disability assessment for dementia scale: a 12-month study of functional ability in mild to moderate severity Alzheimer disease. *Alzheimer Dis Assoc Disord* 2001; **15**: 89–95.

18. Schneider LS, Raman R, Schmitt FA, *et al*. Characteristics and performance of a modified version of the ADCS-CGIC CIBIC+ for mild cognitive impairment clinical trials. *Alzheimer Dis Assoc Disord* 2009; **23**: 260–7.

19. Morris JC. The Clinical Dementia Rating (CDR): current version and scoring rules. *Neurology* 1993; **43**: 2412–4.

20. Lyketsos CG, Lopez O, Jones B, *et al.* Prevalence of neuropsychiatric symptoms in dementia and mild cognitive impairment: results from the cardiovascular health study. *JAMA* 2002; **288**: 1475–83.

21. Cummings JL, Mega M, Gray K, *et al.* The Neuropsychiatric Inventory: comprehensive assessment of psychopathology in dementia. *Neurology* 1994; **44**: 2308–14.

22. Doody RS, Gavrilova SI, Sano M, *et al.* Effect of dimebon on cognition, activities of daily living, behaviour, and global function in patients with mild-to-moderate Alzheimer's disease: a randomised, double-blind, placebo-controlled study. *Lancet* 2008; **372**: 207–15.

23. Tariot PN, Farlow MR, Grossberg GT, *et al.* Memantine treatment in patients with moderate to severe Alzheimer disease already receiving donepezil: a randomized controlled trial. *JAMA* 2004; **291**: 317–24.

24. Winblad B, Gauthier S, Scinto L, *et al.* Safety and efficacy of galantamine in subjects with mild cognitive impairment. *Neurology* 2008; **70**: 2024–35.

25. Wimo A, Winblad B, Shah SN, *et al.* Impact of donepezil treatment for Alzheimer's disease on caregiver time. *Curr Med Res Opin* 2004; **20**: 1221–5.

26. Wimo A, Winblad B, Stoffler A, *et al.* Resource utilisation and cost analysis of memantine in patients with moderate to severe Alzheimer's disease. *Pharmacoeconomics* 2003; **21**: 327–40.

27. Logsdon RG, Gibbons LE, McCurry SM, and Teri L. Assessing quality of life in older adults with cognitive impairment. *Psychosom Med* 2002; **64**: 510–19.

28. Shin IS, Carter M, Masterman D, *et al.* Neuropsychiatric symptoms and quality of life in Alzheimer disease. *Am J Geriatr Psychiatry* 2005; **13**: 469–74.

29. Salloway S, Sperling R, Gilman S, *et al.* A phase 2 multiple ascending dose trial of bapineuzumab in mild to moderate Alzheimer disease. *Neurology* 2009; **73**: 2061–70.

30. Bateman RJ, Siemers ER, Mawuenyega KG, *et al.* A gamma-secretase inhibitor decreases amyloid-beta production in the central nervous system. *Ann Neurol* 2009; **66**: 48–54.

31. Doody RS, Ferris SH, Salloway S, *et al.* Donepezil treatment of patients with MCI: a 48-week randomized, placebo-controlled trial. *Neurology* 2009; **72**: 1555–61.

32. Salloway S, Ferris S, Kluger A, *et al.* Efficacy of donepezil in mild cognitive impairment: a randomized placebo-controlled trial. *Neurology* 2004; **63**: 651–7.

33. Cummings JL, Doody R, and Clark C. Disease-modifying therapies for Alzheimer disease: challenges to early intervention. *Neurology* 2007; **69**: 1622–34.

34. www.clinicaltrials.gov.

35. Mohs RC, Doody RS, Morris JC, *et al.* A 1-year, placebo-controlled preservation of function survival study of donepezil in AD patients. *Neurology* 2001; **57**: 481–8.

36. Sano M, Ernesto C, Thomas RG, *et al.* A controlled trial of selegiline, alpha-tocopherol, or both as treatment for Alzheimer's disease. The Alzheimer's Disease Cooperative Study. *N Engl J Med* 1997; **336**: 1216–22.

37. Gomez-Isla T, Blesa R, Boada M, *et al.* A randomized, double-blind, placebo controlled-trial of triflusal in mild cognitive impairment: the TRIMCI study. *Alzheimer Dis Assoc Disord* 2008; **22**: 21–29.

38. de Jong D, Jansen R, Hoefnagels W, *et al.* No effect of one-year treatment with indomethacin on Alzheimer's disease progression: a randomized controlled trial. *PLoS One* 2008; **3**: e1475.

39. Gold M. Study design factors and patient demographics and their effect on the decline of placebo-treated subjects in randomized clinical trials in Alzheimer's disease. *J Clin Psychiatry* 2007; **68**: 430–8.

40. Schneider LS and Sano M. Current Alzheimer's disease clinical trials: methods and placebo outcomes. *Alzheimers Dement* 2009; **5**: 388–97.

41. Vellas B, Andrieu S, Sampaio C, and Wilcock G. Disease-modifying trials in Alzheimer's disease: a European task force consensus. *Lancet Neurol* 2007; **6**: 56–62.

42. Knapp MJ, Knopman DS, Solomon PR, *et al.* A 30-week randomized controlled trial of high-dose tacrine in patients with Alzheimer's disease. The Tacrine Study Group. *JAMA* 1994; **271**: 985–91.

43. Rogers SL, Doody RS, Mohs RC, Friedhoff LT. Donepezil improves cognition and global function in Alzheimer disease: a 15-week, double-blind, placebo-controlled study. Donepezil Study Group. *Arch Intern Med* 1998; **158**: 1021–1031.

44. Rosler M, Anand R, Cicin-Sain A, *et al.* Efficacy and safety of rivastigmine in patients with Alzheimer's disease: international randomised controlled trial. *BMJ* 1999; **318**: 633–8.

45. Tariot PN, Solomon PR, Morris JC, *et al.* A 5-month, randomized, placebo-controlled trial of galantamine in AD. The Galantamine USA-10 Study Group. *Neurology* 2000; **54**: 2269–76.

46. Raskind MA, Peskind ER, Wessel T, Yuan W. Galantamine in AD: A 6-month randomized, placebo-controlled trial with a 6-month extension. The Galantamine USA-1 Study Group. *Neurology* 2000; **54**: 2261–8.

47. Winblad B, Cummings J, Andreasen N, *et al.* A six-month double-blind, randomized, placebo-controlled study of a transdermal patch in Alzheimer's disease –

rivastigmine patch versus capsule. *Int J Geriatr Psychiatry* 2007; **22**: 456–67.

48. Winblad B, Kilander L, Eriksson S, *et al*. Donepezil in patients with severe Alzheimer's disease: double-blind, parallel-group, placebo-controlled study. *Lancet* 2006; **367**: 1057–65.

49. Shumaker SA, Legault C, Rapp SR, *et al*. Estrogen plus progestin and the incidence of dementia and mild cognitive impairment in postmenopausal women: the Women's Health Initiative Memory Study: a randomized controlled trial. *JAMA* 2003; **289**: 2651–62.

50. Shumaker SA, Legault C, Kuller L, *et al*. Conjugated equine estrogens and incidence of probable dementia and mild cognitive impairment in postmenopausal women: Women's Health Initiative Memory Study. *JAMA* 2004; **291**: 2947–58.

51. Sano M, Jacobs D, Andrews H, *et al*. A multi-center, randomized, double blind placebo-controlled trial of estrogens to prevent Alzheimer's disease and loss of memory in women: design and baseline characteristics. *Clin Trials* 2008; **5**: 523–33.

52. Meinert CL, McCaffrey LD, Breitner JC. Alzheimer's Disease Anti-inflammatory Prevention Trial: design, methods, and baseline results. *Alzheimers Dement* 2009; **5**: 93–104.

53. DeKosky ST, Williamson JD, Fitzpatrick AL, *et al*. Ginkgo biloba for prevention of dementia: a randomized controlled trial. *JAMA* 2008; **300**: 2253–62.

54. Vellas B, Andrieu S, Ousset PJ, *et al*. The GuidAge study: methodological issues. A 5-year double-blind randomized trial of the efficacy of EGb 761 for prevention of Alzheimer disease in patients over 70 with a memory complaint. *Neurology* 2006; **67**: S6–11.

55. Thal LJ, Ferris SH, Kirby L, *et al*. A randomized, double-blind, study of rofecoxib in patients with mild cognitive impairment. *Neuropsychopharmacology* 2005; **30**: 1204–15.

56. Feldman HH, Ferris S, Winblad B, *et al*. Effect of rivastigmine on delay to diagnosis of Alzheimer's disease from mild cognitive impairment: the InDDEx study. *Lancet Neurol* 2007; **6**: 501–12.

57. Petersen RC, Thomas RG, Grundman M, *et al*. Vitamin E and donepezil for the treatment of mild cognitive impairment. *N Engl J Med* 2005; **352**: 2379–88.

58. Petersen RC, Smith GE, Waring SC, *et al*. Mild cognitive impairment: clinical characterization and outcome. *Arch Neurol* 1999; **56**: 303–8.

59. Faison WE, Schultz SK, Aerssens J, *et al*. Potential ethnic modifiers in the assessment and treatment of Alzheimer's disease: challenges for the future. *Int Psychogeriatr* 2007; **19**: 539–558.

Acute ischemic stroke

Devin L. Brown, Karen C. Johnston, and Yuko Y. Palesch

Overview

In this chapter, we will discuss clinical trials in acute ischemic stroke. Stroke is one of the leading causes of death in the US and the leading cause of adult disability. Unfortunately, there is currently only one FDA-approved treatment for this devastating and common disease. Ischemic stroke prevention and rehabilitation strategies share little in common with acute therapies so we will focus on acute therapies.

Biological basis

Recanalization

Cerebral infarction is the result of severe enough ischemia for a sufficient time to result in cell death. The progression toward infarction includes protein synthesis failure, anaerobic metabolism, release of neurotransmitters, energy failure, and ultimately, when the threshold of <0.15 cc/gm/min of blood flow is reached, anoxic depolarization [1]. If hypoperfusion can be remedied quickly, penumbral tissues which were not yet critically hypoperfused can be saved. This is the physiological basis of recanalization therapy with lytics and mechanical agents. Ultrasound and physiological studies have shown that recanalization with intravenous recombinant tissue plasminogen activator (IVrt-PA) is associated with tissue salvage and better clinical outcomes [2, 3]. Clinical trials have shown that IV rt-PA is associated with better outcomes compared with control groups [4, 5]. Similarly, successful endovascular clot removal, retrieval, and lysis have been associated with better clinical outcomes than persistent arterial occlusion [6–8]. However, no mechanical system has yet been tested in clinical efficacy studies.

Neuroprotection

An alternative or complementary strategy to recanalization is neuroprotection aimed at interruption of the ischemic cascade for tissue preservation. Numerous aspects such as energy supply failure, membrane depolarization, excitatory amino acid release, intracellular calcium accumulation, free radical elaboration, and cellular edema can be targeted [1]. Despite successes in animal models, no neuroprotective agent has yet been successful in humans. The multitude of failed neuroprotective clinical trials led to the development of the Stroke Therapy Academic Industry Roundtable (STAIR) recommendations [9]. These recommendations describe guidelines for preclinical development of potential neuroprotective agents in the hopes that more rigorous preclinical preparation and drug selection will ultimately yield a successful neuroprotective agent.

Time window

Because ischemia causes time dependent tissue injury, time is critical in initiation of acute stroke therapies. If efficacious therapies can be initiated early enough, the ischemic penumbra can be salvaged, tissue damage can be limited, and clinical outcomes can be improved. Even the most efficacious therapy will fail however if the stroke is completed and no viable tissue remains to be rescued at the time of drug administration. Time is our best marker of salvageable tissue currently, although clearly individuals respond differently to duration of ischemia likely dependent on collateral flow, age, and many other factors. Functional imaging, originally with PET, but now more commonly with CT perfusion and MR perfusion imaging can be used to study the ischemic penumbra. When mismatch of infarct and perfusion deficit is identified, salvageable penumbra

Clinical Trials in Neurology, ed. Bernard Ravina, Jeffrey Cummings, Michael P. McDermott, and R. Michael Poole. Published by Cambridge University Press. © Cambridge University Press 2012.

may exist. Studies have shown that thrombolytic therapy is more efficacious in those with existing penumbra [10], but no efficacy study has yet proven that functional imaging can be used to extend the time window for thrombolytic administration [11]. The NINDS rt-PA Stroke Study [5] showed that IV rt-PA is efficacious when used in the first 3 hours of stroke symptom onset, and ECASS III [4] extended this to 4.5 hours. PROACT II [8] showed that endovascular prourokinase when initiated within 6 hours of proximal middle cerebral artery occlusion, and infused over 2 hours, also improves clinical outcomes. Other single arm studies [6] have initiated endovascular recanalization therapy out to 8 hours, but no randomized, controlled efficacy study has proven any clinical benefit to any recanalization therapy initiated after 6 hours. Increased risk of intracranial hemorrhage and less benefit was found in PROACT II compared with the NINDS rt-PA Stroke Study, but this may be due to the more severely affected patients in the endovascular treatment trial.

Goals of intervention

Reduction of death and disability

The main purpose of acute stroke therapy is to reduce death and disability. The only currently FDA-approved therapy for acute ischemic stroke, IV rt-PA, has been proven to reduce disability but does not have an affect on mortality [5]. One would assume that a significant and early reduction in post-stroke deficits should reduce potentially fatal stroke-related complications such as aspiration pneumonia and pulmonary emboli, common causes of death post stroke. Nevertheless, functional recovery is a highly meaningful outcome measure.

Reduction of brain injury volume through penumbral salvage (primary injury)

As discussed above, at the initiation of ischemia, there is a core of infarction surrounded by viable but impaired tissue. Expeditious reperfusion can save the impaired tissue and return it to normal function. Failure to save this tissue results in permanent structural changes and ultimately necrosis of neuronal cells. Volume of infarction does relate to ultimate outcome, but the relationship is non-linear, and depends on location, age, and other factors. Furthermore, there is some evidence that the effects of infarcted tissue, even if it does not directly result in disability, accumulate and may contribute to cognitive dysfunction and poor brain 'reserve.'

Therefore, preservation of brain tissue is also a goal. In addition to limiting the primary injury cause by ischemia through penumbral salvage, interruption of the ischemic cascade through neuroprotection may decrease secondary injury. Ultimately, the tissue goal is similar: to limit the amount of infarcted brain.

Properties and measurement tools

Biomarkers/biological outcome

Biomarkers may provide an efficient means of determining biological effects of new agents and are useful outcomes in middle development because they predict a clinical endpoint. Surrogate markers, biomarkers that capture the full major effects of a treatment [12, 13], are used to substitute for clinical outcome measures, but have not been accepted in late development acute stroke trials.

Recanalization/reperfusion

Recanalization, the re-establishment of arterial patency can be assessed by angiography and indirectly by transcranial Doppler ultrasound [14], and graded. Results may be confusing due to inconsistencies in the application of recanalization rating scales, and therefore, it has been recommended that all trials reporting angiographic outcomes include information on target vessel patency, distal filling, and capillary phase perfusion [15]. Recanalization relates but is not identical to antegrade reperfusion, which is volume of flow through the previously occluded vessel, and collateral perfusion which represents the volume of flow through collaterals to the ischemic region. Even when recanalization is successful, the region may remain ischemic due to distal emboli. Furthermore, flow may be established too late for some or all of the ischemic tissue to be preserved. Therefore, recanalization can be an important marker of treatment effects, but alone is not sufficient to determine whether a treatment is going to be effective. In middle development studies, early recanalization should be assessed in addition to assessment of late infarct volume [15]. PROACT I provides an example of a middle phase study that used recanalization as the primary endpoint [16]. Subjects with M1 or M2 occlusions had prourokinase or placebo infused directly into the proximal portion of the thrombus, initiated within 6 hours of stroke symptom onset. Both groups received heparin. The primary efficacy outcome was recanalization of the M1 or M2 2 hours after the initiation of the treatment. There was also a primary safety outcome: symptomatic intracerebral hemorrhage within 24 hour of treatment.

Imaging outcomes

Infarction size on CT or MRI can be used as an outcome measure in middle phase studies. Final difference between treatment groups can be compared, or alternatively, differences between baseline infarction size and final size can be compared when baseline measures are feasible. However, location of infarction and clinical deficits are also important factors in ultimate outcome in addition to lesion size.

Safety outcome measures

Symptomatic intracranial hemorrhage

Symptomatic intracranial hemorrhage (sICH) is a highly feared complication of acute stroke recanalization therapies because it carries with it a high risk of poor outcome including death. It has been defined differently in different trials but is often characterized by any hemorrhage on CT scan within the first 24–48 hours after stroke symptom onset accompanied by a meaningful deterioration in neurological status sometimes defined by a worsening on the NIHSS by 4 or more points [17]. CT evidence of hemorrhage has been graded by the European Cooperative Acute Stroke Studies (ECASS) investigators into four categories: hemorrhagic infarction-1 (HI-1) with small petechial hemorrhage, hemorrhagic infarction-2 (HI-2) with confluent petechial hemorrhage, parenchymal hematoma-1 (PH-1) where the hematoma consumes less than 30% of the infarcted area with a mild space-occupying effect, and parenchymal hematoma-2 (PH-2) where the hematoma takes up greater than 30% of the infarcted area and exerts a significant space-occupying effect. Most definitions of sICH do not include a requirement for parenchymal hematoma, but risk of neurological deterioration is more likely with larger amounts of hemorrhage.

Asymptomatic ICH

It has been argued that while parenchymal hematomas are due to a thrombolytic effect, that hemorrhagic transformation is related to other factors and is an irrelevant epiphenomenon [18]. Hemorrhagic transformation is often not typically accompanied by symptomatic worsening. However, there is some recent evidence that HI-2 is associated with poor clinical outcomes and that the outcome is proportional to the extent of hemorrhage [19]. It is uncertain whether asymptomatic ICH is a meaningful safety outcome because of its lack of clear clinical significance. However, asymptomatic hemorrhage is more common in lytic treated subjects and may be a marker for lytic activity [17].

Neurological worsening

Neurological deterioration may be due to a variety of causes such as sICH, seizure, intracranial hypertension, recurrent stroke, and medical illnesses that include pneumonia and urinary tract infections. Neurological worsening is often specified as a deterioration in NIHSS of 4 points or more, and usually triggers a mandatory head CT to investigate the possibility of sICH. Neurological worsening is typically a safety outcome which is not necessarily reported in the primary trial publication; it is often due to the underlying disease and not the study treatment. Because there can be temporary fluctuations early after stroke, the duration of worsening that constitutes neurological worsening is often specified.

Serious adverse events

Although, in accordance with Good Clinical Practice guidelines, all serious adverse events (SAEs) should be collected in a clinical trial, many SAEs in the 3 months after stroke are related to the underlying stroke rather than the study treatment. However there are drug- and device-related SAEs in addition to sICH. For instance, thrombolytic treatment can cause angioedema and associated respiratory compromise, although this is uncommon. Use of recanalization devices can cause arterial dissection, vascular perforation, and embolization into a previously unaffected vessel; while angiography itself carries a risk of retroperitoneal hemorrhage and contrast-related complications. Intubation is required for many recanalization procedures which also can result in complications.

Death

Death is a clinical outcome that is recorded in stroke studies as an SAE but is also often a part of a pre-specified outcome measure, such as in the modified Rankin Scale. On many rating scales, death is ascribed the worst outcome score (e.g., modified Rankin Scale), while with other scales there is no provision for death (e.g., Barthel Index).

Clinical efficacy outcome measures – definitive endpoint

Traditional scales

The selection of an endpoint for a clinical trial depends on the intervention's mechanism of action and expected effect. Ideally an endpoint should be reliable, reproducible, sensitive, easy to measure, and clinically

Table 22.1 Common stroke outcome measures

	Measurement	Scoring
Neurological impairment		
NIH Stroke Scale[18]	Neurological examination based on 13 clinical items	Ordinal scale ranging from 0 (best) to 2 or 3 or 4 (worst) for each of 13 items
Disability measures		
Modified Rankin Scale[12]	Functional assessment ranging from no symptoms to death	Ordinal scale ranging from 0 (no symptoms) to 6 (death)
Barthel Index[13]	Activities of daily living based on 10 questions on feeding, bathing, grooming, dressing, toilet use, transfers, mobility, stairs, bowel, and bladder continence.	Total score from 10 items ranging from 0 to 100 (best)
Quality of life		
Stroke Impact Scale[26]	59 questions covering 9 domains: (strength, hand function, activities of daily living, mobility, communication, emotion, memory and thinking, and social participation).	Each domain ranging from 0–100 (best)
Stroke Specific Quality of Life[25]	49 questions covering 12 domains (energy, family roles, language, mobility, mood, personality, self-care, social roles, thinking, upper extremity function, vision, and work/productivity).	Overall score is the average of all domains

meaningful (for later stage trials). The use of more sensitive outcome measures should in general help reduce sample size requirements. For middle phase studies, the endpoint should relate to the mechanism of action of the treatment, even if it is not the most clinically relevant outcome, given the goal of identifying a biological effect with the fewest patients necessary.

A variety of measures can be used to assess recovery post stroke, and there is no consensus about which measure or what cutoffs to use (Table 22.1). The most common efficacy endpoint measures in acute stroke therapy trials are the modified Rankin Scale and the NIHSS [20], most often performed at 3 months post stroke. To improve standardization, certified personnel should be used to administer the NIHSS, and a structured interview should be used for the modified Rankin Scale. The modified Rankin Scale while simple and reliable, is insensitive and only has 7 categories [21]. The Barthel Index is valid and reliable but is insensitive to small changes and is limited by a ceiling effect [21]. Those attaining the highest (i.e., best) score can nonetheless have significant disabilities [22]. Because placebo-treated patients tend to achieve a 'favorable outcome' more frequently for disability than for neurological impairment measures, larger sample sizes may be required when using a disability index, such as the modified Rankin Scale. Required sample sizes may be lower when using the modified Rankin Scale than the Barthel Index given that the modified Rankin Scale is more sensitive to change [23, 24]. Two more comprehensive and stroke-specific outcome measures were more recently developed: the Stroke-Specific Quality of Life (SS-QOL) [25] and the Stroke Impact Scale (SIS) [26]. Both expand the spectrum of limitations in activities, physical abilities, and participation. These stroke-specific measures are increasing in use in clinical trials as secondary outcomes.

Non-traditional scales

As mentioned, quality of life is an important measurement that represents a comprehensive patient-oriented outcome measure. When measured, it is typically relegated to a secondary outcome. Cognitive outcomes are also gaining recognition as important post-stroke measures. No single measure of cognitive function post stroke is accepted, and measurements are complicated by aphasia.

Global statistics

Global statistics incorporate results of more than one measure simultaneously and therefore may increase the chance of identifying a treatment effect especially within a heterogeneous study population [22]. Study power using a global measure is at least equal to and often greater than using a single measure, assuming a common treatment effect among the measures. For these reasons, it was used to test the primary hypothesis of part II of the NINDS rt-PA Stroke Study. The global statistic incorporated the results of four pre-specified outcome measures: the NIHSS, Barthel Index, modified Rankin Scale, and the Glasgow Outcome Scale [5]. Patients who were deceased at the time of the outcome assessment at 90 days were ascribed the lowest score in each scale. The global statistics test was significant, as were the tests of the individual outcome measures. Because the results of a global statistic may be difficult to interpret clinically, the FDA may require justification for its use in an acute stroke trial, where a single outcome measure may be sufficient to capture the effect of the treatment.

Early vs. late clinical outcomes

Three months is the most common clinical endpoint in late phase acute stroke trials [21]. Much of the recovery from acute stroke is thought to have occurred by this time, and thus greater differences between the treatment groups may be seen. However, this later endpoint may introduce additional variability compared with earlier time points, from factors unrelated to the treatment allocation. For instance, differences in recurrent stroke or rehabilitation programs may contribute to late outcome differences that are unrelated to the study treatment. Earlier endpoints, such as 24 hours or 7 days, may be feasible depending on the mechanism of action of the treatment. Furthermore, the use of early outcomes in adaptive designs (see below) could result in increased selection efficiency, and a shortend duration in comparision with non-adaptive trials. Middle development studies often use earlier outcomes as primary endpoints. For instance, the IVrt-PA bridging study – a middle phase randomized, controlled trial of IVrt-PA compared with placebo – used a reduction in NIHSS by 4 or more points or NIHSS of zero at 24 hours as the primary outcome measure [27]. NIHSS at 24 hours has been shown to predict the modified Rankin Scale at 3 months [28].

Treatment of outcome analytically – dichotomous, ordinal, continuous, sliding dichotomy

Dichotomous treatment of ordinal outcome scales is common in acute stroke trials. For example, the modified Rankin scale is often dichotomized into 0–1 vs. 2–6, for trials where very good outcomes are anticipated [5, 29] or into 0–2 vs 3–6 where reduction

in poor outcome is of interest [8, 29]. This approach is advantageous because it is analytically simple, and creates results that are clinically meaningful and interpretable and easily described to patients. The most significant disadvantage, however, is loss of information, where small but potentially meaningful improvements can be missed. Occasionally, ordinal outcomes are trichotomized, such as in the GAIN Americas trial [30]. In this study, the Barthel Index was trichochomized into 95–100, 60–90, and 0–55 or dead. The extended Mantel-Haenszel test was used to test whether the distribution of scores was different between the treatment groups.

Shift analysis, also known as analysis of distributions or proportional odds model analysis, assesses differences in the distribution of treatment groups across the full range of an outcome scale [31, 32]. It can account for realistic treatment goals and does not require that the most severe patients demonstrate a dramatic, and perhaps unrealistic, improvement in order for the treatment to be called a success. As an example, the Stroke–Acute Ischemic NXY Treatment II (SAINT II) trial compared distribution of modified Rankin Scale scores at 90 days between those treated with a putative neuroprotectant agent, NXY-059, and placebo [33]. Because the SAINT II investigators anticipated the benefits of a neuroprotective agent to affect all levels of severity moderately, they opted to use shift analysis rather than analysis of the dichotomized modified Rankin Scale where only subjects with minimal or no disability would be counted as a 'success.' Distributions of scores were compared with a generalized Cochran-Mantel-Haenszel test [33] adjusting for three baseline covariates. This test does not assume proportionality of odds ratio (i.e., does not assume that the odds ratio would be the same regardless of the choice of cutpoint for dichotomization on the ordinal scale). In this study, there was no difference between the groups, but had there been, explanation of the magnitude of treatment benefit to a patient or his/her family may have been somewhat challenging.

The use of a single measure of success applied to a heterogeneous study population may obscure benefit. Therefore, some investigators have proposed different criteria for favorable outcome depending on baseline severity. For example, in the Abciximab in Emergency Stroke Treatment Trial–II (AbESTT-II)[29], this type of sliding dichotomy, or responder analysis, was used. A successful outcome, a so called 'responder,' was defined as follows: if the baseline NIHSS was 4–7, the goal was a modified Rankin Scale=0; if the baseline NIHSS was 8–14, the goal was a modified Rankin Scale=0–1; if the baseline NIHSS was 15–22, the goal modified Rankin Scale was 0–2. This is one reasonable and analytically simple way of accounting for expected differences in benefit based on initial severity. The results can also be reasonably communicated to patients by referring to percentage in each treatment group with a favorable outcome.

Studies using individual level patient data from randomized controlled stroke trials demonstrated that tests that maintain the ordinal level of data are typically more efficient than treating functional outcome measures dichotomously [34]. In fact, on average, while maintaining the same statistical power, trials analyzed using an ordinal approach could have been 28% smaller than those measured using a binary approach. However, the analytic approach planned for a trial should be pre-specified based on a variety of factors, including the anticipated treatment effect. Simulation studies have suggested that depending on the pattern of treatment benefit, shift analysis or dichotomous analyses can be more efficient [31]. Shift analysis is likely to be more efficient for treatments that result in uniform mild benefit across outcome levels. However, since the distribution of the outcome data are unknown when designing a trial, the sample size and analysis plan should consider the effect of violation of primary analysis model assumptions, if any, on the statistical power and inferences at the conclusion of the study.

Clinical trial design used in development

Early and middle development

Dose finding

Early and middle development studies of new compounds for acute stroke require pharmacologic data such as determination of the effective plasma level, delineation of the minimum dose that achieves 95% of the maximum effect (i.e., the ED_{95}), optimal dose, time window, and duration of therapy, and contribute to safety data. Early middle phase studies are also needed to determine safety and to gain information on efficacy. For these, broad eligibility criteria are sensible, so that danger to those with comorbidities and the elderly can be determined. Later middle phase studies may benefit from a narrowing of eligibility so that biological effects

can be more easily detected. Traditional dose-finding studies, open-label dose escalation studies where a small group of patients are treated with successively higher doses of drug pending the lack of sufficient adverse events, or treated with lower doses if adverse events occur, have been used successfully. This approach was used to develop IV rt-PA. In the first IV rt-PA pilot study [35], 74 patients were treated within 7 dose tiers ranging from 0.35 mg/kg and ending with 1.08 mg/kg within 90 minutes of stroke symptom onset. Members of the safety and monitoring committee and the investigators made consensus decisions about the number of subjects treated per dose and dose advancement. The absence of a single intracranial hematoma in at least six consecutively treated patients in a dosing tier prompted a dose advancement after review. Higher numbers of subjects were required for the highest dose tiers. Two major bleeding complications in six patients at a particular dose resulted in a dose tier reduction. No intracranial hematomas occurred in any of the 58 subjects treated with ≤0.85 mg/kg; although, dose tier did not relate to infarction volume. In the second IV rt-PA pilot study [36], where subjects were treated within 91–180 minutes, 20 patients were tested in 3 dose tiers: 0.6 mg/kg, 0.85 mg/kg, and 0.95 mg/kg. One fatal intracranial hemorrhage occurred in each of the highest dose tiers.

One middle development study, the *Albumin in Acute Stroke* (ALIAS) trial used its dose escalation results to assess for an efficacy signal by grouping their dose tiers. ALIAS was an open-label, dose-escalation study that tested the safety of moderate to high doses of 25% human albumin in acute ischemic stroke. Six doses were administered; the lowest three were thought to be subtherapeutic based on preclinical studies. The investigators therefore grouped the outcome of the lowest three tiers and the highest three. They also compared the highest three dose tiers with data from the NINDS rt-PA Stroke Study [37].

Adaptive designs (see Chapter 9) are an efficient way of learning the dose-response relationship in real time, but have been applied infrequently in acute stroke trials. One example is the Acute Stroke Therapy by Inhibition of Neutrophils (ASTIN) study [38] which tested a neutrophil inhibitory factor in 15 doses ranging from 10–120 mg and placebo using a Bayesian adaptive dose-response finding study. This approach was designed for early termination for efficacy or futility using a clinically relevant outcome measured at 90 days post stroke. A sequential stopping rule was applied where the effect compared with placebo of the ED_{95} was iteratively calculated and if it reached a preset threshold, would trigger study termination for futility or efficacy. The study was terminated for futility after 966 subjects had been treated.

Single treatment arm studies

When new endovascular mechanical treatments are introduced, no dose-finding studies are necessary. Single treatment arm studies are often performed where patients who meet certain selection criteria are all offered the new treatment. An example of this is mechanical clot removal for larger artery occlusions with the Merci device in the Mechanical Embolus Removal in Cerebral Ischemia (MERCI) trials [6]. The primary outcome was recanalization of the target vessel, while important safety outcomes, such as sICH and device-related complications, and clinical outcomes were also reported they could not be compared to a contemporaneous control group. Outcomes were compared between those who had recanalization and those who did not. On the basis of mere single arm study results, the Merci retriever system received FDA approval to 'restore blood flow in the neurovasculature by removing thrombus in patients experiencing ischemic stroke' [39], highlighting differences in approval between drugs and devices.

Historical controls

Rather than acquiring contemporaneous controls, some single-arm studies use historical controls. These controls can be gathered through case series, or more practically by using the placebo arm of previously conducted randomized studies. For instance, the outcomes of the placebo arm and treatment arm of the NINDS rt-PA Stroke Study were compared with outcomes of those treated with combined IV and intra-arterial (IA) rt-PA in the Interventional Management of Stroke (IMS) study in the primary outcome publication [40]. The placebo group of PROACT-II was used as the comparison for the MERCI trials given that both groups were large artery occlusions and treated in a similar time window [41]. These types of comparisons can provide some useful information; however, because they are not randomized, there are likely to be inherent differences between the two groups that contribute to differential outcomes. Because the controls are not contemporaneously ascertained, secular trends may also contribute to bias. Therefore, this type of study is inappropriate for a late phase study to ascertain

definitively the treatment effect. However, a middle phase study using historical control data can provide preliminary information about the treatment effect more efficiently since it requires about one-fourth of the sample size of a concurrently controlled study with the same study parameters.

Futility

The purpose of middle development futility studies is to discard treatments with a small likelihood of success, and to maintain promising treatments to test in late phase studies (see Chapter 8). These protocols are typically conducted as single-arm studies in which all subjects receive the treatment under question. Outcomes used for comparison are obtained from placebo groups of other trials conducted in similar study populations, case-series, or from clinical consensus/ judgment of the expected outcome in the untreated patient population. The smallest effect size considered clinically meaningful is determined to provide the threshold that the treatment must pass. To illustrate the utility of performing middle development futility analyses, investigators performed simulated futility analyses applied to data from a convenience sample of a mixture of positive and negative previously published late phase acute stroke trials [42]. In this analysis, futility was established based on the simulations for three treatments, all of which had negative late phase results, using only a small fraction of the sample size that was required for the late phase studies. Three studies did not show futility; one of these had a positive result in the late phase study. Thus, with a fraction of the sample size required for an efficacy study, a single arm futility study can help discard treatments with a low likelihood of success.

Late phase

Parallel group randomized controlled trial

Use of placebos vs. active control (IVrt-PA)

When the NINDS rt-PA Stroke Study was performed, there were no approved acute therapies with which IVrt-PA could be compared. Differences between a new intervention and placebo are generally greater than between a new intervention and a proven treatment. Now that IVrt-PA is FDA-approved, and has been shown to be an efficacious treatment in clinical trials, alternative lytics must be tested against IVrt-PA rather than a placebo within the 3 hour window, and due to ECASS III [17], within the 3–4.5 hour window as well. However, patients with very severe strokes, or other particular patient groups that would have been excluded from ECASS III trial enrollment, can be enrolled in a placebo-controlled acute stroke therapy trial within the 3–4.5 hour window. Studies that test new devices and drugs within the 4.5 hour window in subjects who may have been treated with IV rt-PA should block stratify based on IVrt-PA treatment.

Randomization allocation ratio

In acute stroke trials, subjects are generally randomized to treatment groups in a 1:1 fashion, where trial power is optimized. However, it may entice patients to enroll if the chance of receiving a placebo is reduced below 50%. For instance, in PROACT II, subjects were allocated in a 2:1 fashion to active treatment and control groups [8]. Uneven group allocation may also allow additional experience to be obtained with a treatment or within a patient subset. However, if the allocation ratio is or exceeds 3 (i.e. the proportion on the treatment exceeds 0.75) statistical test power is significantly reduced for the same total sample size.

Subject selection

Eligibility criteria can be broad, or more focused in an attempt to find subjects who will have more similar responses. Widened eligibility criteria improve generalizability, and increase the available sample population. However, it introduces heterogeneity and may include subjects with a low likelihood of response to the treatment. In early and mid-development studies, limiting the sample to those who are most likely to benefit or establishing those most likely to benefit is helpful in proving proof of concept. Similar eligibility criteria are then applied to the initial late phase studies. Once there is evidence of success, further trials can be designed to expand the population. For example, limiting the time window to 3 hours in the NINDS rt-PA Stroke Study [5] and then following this with other late phase studies of a more expanded window proved successful. However, there are circumstances where eligibility criteria are liberalized for the later phase studies.

Baseline severity is an important consideration. It is well known from the NINDS rt-PA trial that patients with a very high NIHSS have less dramatic recoveries. Patients with a low NIHSS on the whole tend to do quite well and are often normal or near normal at 3 months. Therefore, the greatest benefit may be seen when enrollment focuses on those with moderate

deficits, such as an NIHSS between 7 and 20. Inclusion of the severity extremes will increase the variability of response and will require a larger sample size. To help account for expected differences in outcomes based on initial severity, some trials have stratified by baseline NIHSS. For instance, the Glycine Antagonist in Neuroprotection (GAIN) Americas trial stratified by age (≤75 vs. >75 years) and NIHSS (2–5, 6–13, or ≥14), creating six strata [30]. Accounting for baseline severity at the time of analysis is another strategy for accounting for this heterogeneity (see above 'Treatment of outcome analytically – dichotomous, ordinal, continuous, sliding dichotomy'). In smaller trials, where the benefits of stratification are greatest, only a few stratification variables should be selected to minimize the numbers of strata. It has been recommended that the number of strata be less than the total number of subjects divided by four times the block size [43].

Imaging can also be used for patient selection. The ECASS investigators elected to exclude subjects from thrombolytic trials based on early evidence of ischemia in greater than a third of the MCA territory [4]; however, an analysis in the NINDS rt-PA Stroke Study data did not support a treatment by early ischemic change interaction [44]. Some multimodal imaging studies have shown that lack of evidence of penumbra suggests against a thrombolytic response [10]. Eliminating subjects who are unlikely to respond helps reduce study sample size.

Masking

Maintaining proper treatment masking is essential to reduce assessment bias in randomized trials. When treatment allocation masking is not possible, the clinical outcomes assessor should be masked. This can be accomplished by using two different treating and rating investigators or other study team members. Boluses and infusions of study drug and placebos can be prepared to look identical, out of the sight of investigators by an investigational pharmacist. Masking can become more complex when combinations of agents are tested. For instance, in the Combined approach to Lysis utilizing Eptifibatide And Recombinant tissue-type plasminogen activator (CLEAR) stroke study, standard dose IV rt-PA was tested against a lower dose of IV rt-PA plus eptifibatide using a double-dummy approach [45]. All patients received either 10% of the standard dose or 15% of the lower dose bolus in 10 ml. Patients then received the remainder of the standard dose of IV rt-PA in two sequential infusions over 30 minutes each, or the remainder of the low dose IVrt-PA over 30 minutes followed by 30 minutes of placebo. The patients who received low dose IV rt-PA were given a 2 hour infusion of eptifibatide, and those who received standard dose IV rt-PA were given a 2 hour infusion of placebo. Volumes given to both groups at all phases were identical, and all infusions were clear.

Effect size

For sample size calculations, a minimum clinically important difference (MCID) or the effect size must be specified. Because the sample size increases with the inverse square of the MCID, detecting small differences requires a very large sample size. In general, the effect size used is the smallest clinically relevant effect. Selecting an effect size from that observed in middle phase studies can be misleading. Middle phase studies tend to have smaller sample size and hence a smaller number of clinical sites, and more homogeneous samples, and often, this leads to an observed treatment effect that is larger than what could be observed in larger late-phase studies with greater variability in patient characteristics as well as in clinical management at a larger number of sites. Therefore, the effect size sought should be derived from a clinical perspective and the observed treatment effect from the middle phase studies used to determine whether the MCID selected for the late phase study can be reasonably achieved. As an example, the ECASS II investigators pre-specified a 10% difference in favorable outcome between the groups. Prior data do often inform the expected treatment difference selected in late phase studies. Examples include the benefit of PROACT I on PROACT II [8], and the influence of prior pooled data from other late phase studies on the extended time window for ECASS III [4]. Estimates of the probability of favorable outcome in the placebo group can be obtained from prior natural history studies.

Study design

Superiority

Most trials are analyzed to compare outcomes between two groups with respect to superiority in an intent-to-treat fashion. This is frequently performed by comparing the proportion of favorable outcome between the two randomized treatment groups, sometimes adjusted for baseline factors such as NIHSS score [8, 30]. Rather than a comparison between a primary outcome measured only at the final visit, comparison adjusting for the baseline value of the outcome generally increases

power by decreasing the standard error of the treatment effect.

Non-inferiority

In the post IVrt-PA era, a new treatment can be tested to see if it is superior to IV rt-PA, or whether it is as good as (i.e., not inferior to) IV rt-PA. In acute stroke therapies, identifying something that works equivalently to, or not worse than, IV rt-PA would not represent an important impact on patient care, unless the treatment were clearly safer than IV rt-PA. Hence, the usefulness of non-inferiority studies is currently minimal in acute stroke therapy trials [see Chapter 13]. Furthermore, depending on the threshold used to determine non-inferiority, the sample size for these studies is often quite large. Therefore, to test a new thrombolytic agent thought to be similarly effective but with a lower sICH risk, it may be more efficient to incorporate sICH into the primary outcome measure such as devising a scheme in which the outcome score would be penalized for an sICH. Finally, the FDA has stringent criteria for non-inferiority studies where superiority of the active control must be well established from placebo-controlled late phase studies.

Adaptive designs

Using group sequential analysis designs, interim analyses that control for overall type I as well as type II errors can be applied so that trials can be stopped early for efficacy and/or futility. GAIN Americas performed two interim analyses in addition to the final analysis using a group sequential design to limit type I error [30]. The NINDS rt-PA Stroke Study described interim analyses after each three sICH subjects so that the trial could be stopped early if IVrt-PA were found to be harmful.

Conditional power can be calculated to determine whether trial continuation is futile. PROACT II for instance, had a preplanned futility analysis conducted after the first 42% of patients had completed their 3 month follow up.

Although not performed frequently, sample size can be recalculated during the trial if parameters unrelated to efficacy comparison (i.e., nuisance parameters) from the current trial data suggest that the information on which the original sample size calculations were based were different. For instance, if the proportion of favorable outcome in the placebo group is closer to 50% from either direction, the sample size is likely to be inadequate, if the original assumption for the placebo group success rate was much less than or much greater than 50%. Also, if the variance of the estimate of a continuous outcome measure was underestimated prior to study initiation, it may be prudent to re-estimate the sample size, preferably in a blinded manner using aggregate data, to ensure adequate statistical power for the final analysis. A plan for sample size re-estimation at some point in the trial should be pre-specified prior to beginning the trial.

An efficient method for adjusting sample size while preserving alpha is adaptive randomization. A recent example of this was planned for the recently published, but early terminated, TNK trial [46]. This was planned as a single overarching study including a seamless transition between a middle and late phase. The first piece of the study was designed to select one of three doses of tenecteplase to use for comparison with IV rt-PA through an adaptive design based on a 24 hour outcome measure. This outcome incorporated favorable outcome and sICH using the following scoring system: sICH (0), major neurological improvement (2), neither sICH nor major improvement (1). When the one of the three dose arms fell behind the best dose group by 6 points, the dose was discarded. One dose of tenecteplase was eliminated using a sequential selection procedure based on only 14 triplets' (each assigned to the three different doses) 24 hour data.

Standards for efficacy and special safety issues

Adjusted primary analysis

Even with balanced randomization, heterogeneity is known to result in bias towards the null in clinical trial analyses of dichotomous variables or survival data [47]. Adjustment for important baseline characteristics that are associated with outcome thus results in increased efficiency. For example, a reanalysis of the NINDS rt-PA Stroke Study data showed that adjustment for age, NIHSS, stroke subtype, prior disability, diabetes, and history of stroke resulted in a more extreme odds ratio (i.e., greater treatment effect) than bivariate analysis [48]. This would have resulted in a 13% smaller required sample size. Accordingly, pre-specification of a risk-adjusted analysis should be considered in stroke trials that use a binary (or survival) outcome.

Interaction with IV rt-PA

Because patients who are eligible for IV rt-PA therapy should not be denied this approved treatment in favor of enrollment in a non-thrombolytic trial, studies that include IV rt-PA eligible patients now have to account for the effects of the IV rt-PA treatment. As an example, in the SAINT II study, randomization was stratified on intent to administer IV rt-PA, in addition to country, baseline NIHSS, and side of infarction [33]. This stratification is appropriate because IV rt-PA is associated with the primary outcome. Similarly the analysis was stratified by use of IV rt-PA, NIHSS, and side of infarct. To answer the question as to whether the effect of the study drug differed based on IV rt-PA administration, an interaction was investigated, but not identified.

Implementation issues

Recruitment and consent

Recruitment of acute stroke subjects is challenging. Patients with acute stroke often are unable to consent for themselves, 70% in the NINDS rt-PA Stroke Study [49], requiring family members to act as surrogate decision makers for research. The superimposed challenge is that decisions must be made very quickly and in the setting of a stressful event – an acute medical illness. Some small studies have suggested that acute stroke study consent does not always fulfill the objectives of consent and that patients often have significant misconceptions about the trial design, purpose, and certainty of benefit [50, 51]. Laws and other regulations that govern the use of surrogate consent vary at the country, state, and institutional levels. Further complications include the lack of a federal statutory provision specifying the qualifications of a legally authorized representative, and the inconsistencies in state and Institutional Review Board (IRB) rules on this subject. However, the use of surrogate consent is essential to acute stroke research for two reasons. First, a requirement for self-consent would eliminate the majority of otherwise eligible subjects, thereby substantially increasing study recruitment duration. And second, there are significant differences between patients who can and cannot consent for themselves with respect to age, stroke severity, infarction volume, side of infarction, and ultimate recovery [49, 52]. Studies have not shown an interaction between ability to consent for oneself and IV rt-PA response, however [49].

When surrogate consent is necessary and the legally authorized representative is not physically present, opportunities for obtaining informed consent are limited. Some IRBs allow the use of telephonic consent if the consent form can be viewed by the surrogate and a signed copy can be returned. This is possible if the surrogate has easy access to a fax machine. In a novel permutation of this process, the Field Administration of Stroke Therapy-Magnesium (FAST-MAG) investigators have pilot tested and are using a consent process that begins during ambulance transport to the hospital [53]. Other investigators have focused on aerial flight rather than ambulance transport. Patients at rural or other non-urban hospital emergency departments are often transferred by helicopter to tertiary care stroke centers after initial evaluation. The ability to capture patients for acute stroke trials during transport would increase early trial enrollment and extend trial opportunities to those who live in non-urban areas who would otherwise arrive too late. The feasibility of obtaining consent from patients or their surrogates during helicopter transport has been demonstrated [54].

Obstacles to recruitment

Recruitment in acute stroke trials is a challenge for many reasons. There is usually a very limited time window in which patients can be enrolled, leaving few patients eligible. This is combined with a very time-limited consent process, an actively sick patient, and often a drug that can cause major adverse events, making the process even more challenging. In drug trials, the study agent is often not available outside of the clinical trial; however, with endovascular treatments, the procedure is often available outside of the research setting because of the different standard for FDA device approvals compared with drugs. For instance, while clinical trials of the Merci retriever are currently ongoing, its use as part of routine clinical care is common. If faced with the option of a randomized trial of recanalization with the Merci retriever or Merci retriever use outside of research, families will often choose the 'sure thing' despite the lack of known risk/benefit ratio. Interventionalists may also be tempted to use devices and receive standard reimbursement versus enroll in research with lower reimbursement. These issues negatively affect recruitment into trials and diminish trial generalizability. Centers that are enrolling in catheter-based therapy trials need to consider whether they will offer routine clinical use of these unproven treatments to patients who are otherwise eligible for study enrollment. A commitment to avoid this would improve trial recruitment and expedite the advancement of stroke therapies. Similarly, the

financial disincentives for centers to participate in device-related acute stroke trials needs to be addressed, otherwise the ability to develop any proven endovascular therapies will be jeopardized.

Randomization in multi-center trials under the time constraints

The time pressures of acute stroke study enrollment are fierce and include the consent process, review of eligibility criteria, randomization, and study treatment preparation. Local randomization procedures are typically simpler and easier to implement than central randomization, but may result in imbalances in the overall treatment assignment as well as in baseline characteristics in the total study population across sites. A new method, step-forward randomization [55], has been proposed as a hybrid approach. The first subject of a multi-center trial has a treatment assigned before trial enrollment. After enrollment of each successive subject, a single randomization assignment is made for only the next subject at that site based on the baseline characteristics and treatment assignments of all prior subjects across all sites. This dynamic randomization technique keeps randomization one step ahead of subject enrollment. After each enrollment, the study team enters the enrollment information about the subject just enrolled into the study website, so that the assignment for the next eligible patient can be made prior to the patient's presentation. The approach allows for incorporation of blinding. The step-forward randomization expedites the treatment assignment process. This randomization scheme has been proposed and applied to acute stroke trials coordinated by the Medical University of South Carolina [55]. Their experience with ALIAS and IMS III suggests the success of the procedure for maintaining covariate balance. However, they caution that step-forward randomization should probably be limited to studies with no more than two strata.

Methodological limitations/ controversies

Conducting trials in the face of evolving treatments

The technology of mechanical thrombectomy is evolving faster than the technologies can be tested adequately in clinical trials. This creates a complexity where an improved device becomes available while the prior device is being tested. For instance, when recruitment for the Multi MERCI single arm study began in January 2004, only the first generation retriever devices, X5 and X6 were available [6]. Only during the study, in August of 2004 did the L5 second generation retriever gain FDA clearance. To address this issue, the investigators performed a non-inferiority analysis testing whether the newer device was not inferior to the older device.

Clinical trials in the setting of variation in the definitions of terms

The NIH-NINDS has initiated a process of creating and defining Common Data Elements (CDEs) for stroke trials [56]. The common utilization of terms is expected to reduce variability and maximize comparability amongst trials. The first draft of the CDEs is now available (www.commondataelements.ninds.nih.gov/Stroke.aspx). It is anticipated that different trials will utilize different elements and that the definitions of elements may evolve to some degree.

Race/ethnicity and gender breakdown of trial participants

Some trials in stroke prevention may naturally enroll a non-representative race/ethnic distribution of subjects by virtue of the disease it targets, such as sickle cell disease or intracranial atherosclerosis. Based on the epidemiology of stroke, the most common minority groups should be overrepresented in US acute stroke trials given their higher risk of stroke compared with non-Hispanic whites. However, this does not appear to be the case, especially for Hispanics, who are now the largest minority group in the US. As an example, the NINDS rt-PA Stroke Study enrolled only 5–8% Hispanics in each treatment group despite their prevalence in the 2000 US census of 12.5% [57]. Further complicating the assessment of this issue is the lack of reporting of race/ethnicity in many publications [6, 11, 45] and international trials where the background population representation of these groups differs. To a lesser degree, women also seem to be underrepresented in trials [5, 8], which may be due to their tendency to have strokes later in life, and thus may be differentially excluded by an age limit. The lack of representation of race and ethnic minority groups may limit the generalizability of these clinical trials.

Emergency exception to informed consent

In the US, a provision for emergency exceptions from informed consent has existed since 1996. This provision can be applied to acute stroke therapeutic research if a number of qualifications are met [58]. These include: the condition is life-threatening; available treatments are unsatisfactory or unproven; obtaining informed consent is not feasible and the research cannot be practicably performed without the waiver; direct benefit to the participant is possible; if the potential therapeutic window permits, contact was attempted with the legally authorized representative; there is an IRB-approved protocol and consent. Additional provisions must also be in place including at a minimum: community consultation; public disclosure of the trial and consent process (and later, the results); an independent data monitoring committee; documentation that any family member was called in attempt to allow him/her to object; after enrollment, the patient, legally authorized representative, or any family member must be sought out to discuss the research to provide the opportunity for research participation to be discontinued. Most acute stroke research easily fits within these confines. However, there are some controversial areas. An approved therapy is available, IV rt-PA, but some have argued that it is unsatisfactory due to hemorrhage risk, moderate benefit, and a short therapeutic window [59]. Furthermore, although consent is possible in some stroke patients or with their legally authorized representatives, exclusion of groups unable to consent, such as those with aphasia, would bias study results. Many acute stroke trials have been carried out to date without invoking the exception to informed consent requirement for emergency research. Because informed consent is so intrinsic to clinical research ethics, if this exception is to be applied, it should be done so with great care and extensive consideration.

Conclusion

Stroke is a very common and often devastating disease with important public health impact. Unfortunately, despite a multitude of completed clinical trials, only one currently FDA-approved treatment is available. Rigorous clinical trial design is needed to progress new therapies through early, middle, and late development in order to identify efficiently a new treatment for acute ischemic stroke.

Reference

1. Hossmann KA. Viability thresholds and the penumbra of focal ischemia. *Ann Neurol* 1994; **36**: 557–65.

2. Heiss WD, Grond M, Thiel A, *et al.* Tissue at risk of infarction rescued by early reperfusion: A positron emission tomography study in systemic recombinant tissue plasminogen activator thrombolysis of acute stroke. *J Cereb Blood Flow Metab* 1998; **18**: 1298–1307.

3. Molina CA, Montaner J, Abilleira S, *et al.* Time course of tissue plasminogen activator-induced recanalization in acute cardioembolic stroke: a case-control study. *Stroke* 2001; **32**: 2821–7.

4. Hacke W, Kaste M, Bluhmki E, *et al.* Thrombolysis with alteplase 3 to 4.5 hours after acute ischemic stroke. *N Engl J Med* 2008; **359**: 1317–29.

5. The National Institute of Neurological Disorders and Stroke rt-PA Stroke Study Group. Tissue plasminogen activator for acute ischemic stroke. The National Institute of Neurological Disorders and Stroke rt-PA Stroke Study Group. *N Engl J Med* 1995; **333**: 1581–7.

6. Smith WS, Sung G, Saver J, *et al.* Mechanical thrombectomy for acute ischemic stroke: final results of the Multi MERCI trial. *Stroke* 2008; **39**: 1205–12.

7. Bose A, Henkes H, Alfke K, *et al.* The Penumbra System: a mechanical device for the treatment of acute stroke due to thromboembolism. *AJNR, American Journal of Neuroradiology* 2008; **29**: 1409–13.

8. Furlan A, Higashida R, Wechsler L, *et al.* Intra-arterial prourokinase for acute ischemic stroke. The PROACT II study: a randomized controlled trial. Prolyse in Acute Cerebral Thromboembolism. *JAMA* 1999; **282**: 2003–11.

9. Recommendations for Standards Regarding Preclinical Neuroprotective and Restorative Drug Development. *Stroke* 1999; **30**: 2752–8.

10. Albers GW, Thijs VN, Wechsler L, *et al.* Magnetic resonance imaging profiles predict clinical response to early reperfusion: the diffusion and perfusion imaging evaluation for understanding stroke evolution (DEFUSE) study. *Ann Neurol* 2006; **60**: 508–17.

11. Hacke W, Furlan AJ, Al-Rawi Y, *et al.* Intravenous desmoteplase in patients with acute ischaemic stroke selected by MRI perfusion-diffusion weighted imaging or perfusion CT (DIAS-2): a prospective, randomised, double-blind, placebo-controlled study. *Lancet Neurol* 2009; **8**: 141–50.

12. Prentice RL. Surrogate endpoints in clinical trials: definition and operational criteria. *Stat Med* 1989; **8**: 431–40.

13. De Gruttola VG, Clax P, DeMets DL, *et al.* Considerations in the evaluation of surrogate endpoints in clinical trials: Summary of a National Institutes of Health Workshop. *Control Clin Trials* 2001; **22**: 485–502.

14. Alexandrov AV, Molina CA, Grotta JC, *et al.* Ultrasound-enhanced systemic thrombolysis for acute ischemic stroke. *N Engl J Med* 2004; **351**: 2170–8.

15. Saver JL, Albers GW, Dunn B, *et al.* Stroke therapy academic industry roundtable (STAIR) recommendations for extended window acute stroke therapy trials. *Stroke* 2009; **40**: 2594–600.

16. del Zoppo GJ, Higashida RT, Furlan AJ, *et al.* PROACT: A phase ii randomized trial of recombinant pro-urokinase by direct arterial delivery in acute middle cerebral artery stroke. *Stroke* 1998; **29**: 4–11.

17. Hacke W, Kaste M, Fieschi C, *et al.* Intravenous thrombolysis with recombinant tissue plasminogen activator for acute hemispheric stroke. The European Cooperative Acute Stroke Study (ECASS). *JAMA* 1995; **274**: 1017–25.

18. Thomalla G, Sobesky J, Kohrmann M, *et al.* Two tales: Hemorrhagic transformation but not parenchymal hemorrhage after thrombolysis is related to severity and duration of ischemia: MRI study of acute stroke patients treated with intravenous tissue plasminogen activator within 6 hours. *Stroke* 2007; **38**: 313–8.

19. Dzialowski I, Pexman JHW, Barber PA, *et al.* Asymptomatic hemorrhage after thrombolysis may not be benign: Prognosis by hemorrhage type in the Canadian alteplase for stroke effectiveness study registry. *Stroke* 2007; **38**: 75–9.

20. Fisher M, Hanley DF, Howard G, *et al.* Recommendations from the STAIR V meeting on acute stroke trials, technology and outcomes. *Stroke* 2007; **38**: 245–8.

21. Duncan PW, Jorgensen HS, Wade DT. Outcome measures in acute stroke trials: A systematic review and some recommendations to improve practice. *Stroke* 2000; **31**: 1429–38.

22. Fisher M, for the Stroke Therapy Academic Industry Roundtable IV. Enhancing the development and approval of acute stroke therapies: Stroke Therapy Academic Industry Roundtable. *Stroke* 2005; **36**: 1808–13.

23. Weimar C, Kurth T, Kraywinkel K, *et al.* Assessment of functioning and disability after ischemic stroke. *Stroke* 2002; **33**: 2053–9.

24. Young FB, Lees KR, Weir CJ. Strengthening acute stroke trials through optimal use of disability end points. *Stroke* 2003; **34**: 2676–80.

25. Williams LS, Weinberger M, Harris LE, *et al.* Development of a stroke-specific quality of life scale. *Stroke* 1999; **30**: 1362–9.

26. Duncan PW, Bode RK, Min Lai S, *et al.* Rasch analysis of a new stroke-specific outcome scale: the stroke impact scale. *Arch Phys Med Rehabil* 2003; **84**: 950–63.

27. Haley EC, Brott TG, Sheppard GL, *et al*. Pilot randomized trial of tissue plasminogen activator in acute ischemic stroke. The TPA Bridging Study Group. *Stroke* 1993; **24**: 1000–4.

28. Brown DL, Johnston KC, Wagner DP, *et al*. Predicting major neurological improvement with intravenous recombinant tissue plasminogen activator treatment of stroke. *Stroke* 2004; **35**: 147–50.

29. Adams HP, Jr., Effron MB, Torner J, *et al*. Emergency administration of Abciximab for treatment of patients with acute ischemic stroke: Results of an international phase III trial: Abciximab in Emergency Treatment of Stroke Trial (AbESTT-II). *Stroke* 2008; **39**: 87–99.

30. Sacco RL, DeRosa JT, Haley EC Jr, *et al*. Glycine antagonist in neuroprotection for patients with acute stroke: GAIN Americas: a randomized controlled trial. *JAMA* 2001; **285**: 1719–28.

31. Saver JL, Gornbein J. Treatment effects for which shift or binary analyses are advantageous in acute stroke trials. *Neurology* 2009; **72**: 1310–15.

32. Saver JL. Novel end point analytic techniques and interpreting shifts across the entire range of outcome scales in acute stroke trials. *Stroke* 2007; **38**: 3055–62.

33. Shuaib A, Lees KR, Lyden P, *et al*. NXY-059 for the treatment of acute ischemic stroke. *N Engl J Med* 2007; **357**: 562–71.

34. Optimising Analysis of Stroke Trials Collaboration. Calculation of sample size for stroke trials assessing functional outcome: comparison of binary and ordinal approaches. *Int J Stroke* 2008; **3**: 78–84.

35. Brott TG, Haley EC Jr, Levy DE, *et al*. Urgent therapy for stroke. Part I. Pilot study of tissue plasminogen activator administered within 90 minutes. *Stroke* 1992; **23**: 632–40.

36. Haley EC, Levy DE, Brott TG, *et al*. Urgent therapy for stroke. Part II. Pilot study of tissue plasminogen activator administered 91–180 minutes from onset. *Stroke* 1992; **23**: 641–5.

37. Palesch YY, Hill MD, Ryckborst KJ, *et al*. The ALIAS pilot trial: A dose-escalation and safety study of albumin therapy for acute ischemic stroke – II: Neurologic outcome and efficacy analysis. *Stroke* 2006; **37**: 2107–4.

38. Krams M, Lees KR, Hacke W, *et al*. Acute stroke therapy by inhibition of neutrophils (ASTIN): An adaptive dose-response study of UK-279,276 in acute ischemic stroke. *Stroke* 2003; **34**: 2543–8.

39. 501(k) summary. http://www.accessdata.fda.gov/cdrh_docs/pdf3/k033736.pdf.

40. The IMS II Trial Investigators. The interventional management of stroke (IMS) II Study. *Stroke* 2007; **38**: 2127–35.

41. Josephson SA, Saver JL, Smith WS, *et al*. Comparison of mechanical embolectomy and intraarterial thrombolysis in acute ischemic stroke within the MCA: MERCI and Multi MERCI compared to PROACT II. *Neurocrit Care* 2009; **10**: 43–9.

42. Palesch YY, Tilley BC, Sackett DL, *et al*. Applying a Phase II futility study design to therapeutic stroke trials. *Stroke* 2005; **36**: 2410–4.

43. Kernan WN, Viscoli CM, Makuch RW, *et al*. Stratified randomization for clinical trials. *J Clin Epidemiol* 1999; **52**: 19–26.

44. Patel SC, Levine SR, Tilley BC, *et al*. Lack of clinical significance of early ischemic changes on computed tomography in acute stroke. *JAMA* 2001; **286**: 2830–8.

45. Pancioli AM, Broderick J, Brott T, *et al*. The combined approach to lysis utilizing eptifibatide and rt-PA in acute ischemic stroke: The CLEAR Stroke Trial. *Stroke* 2008; **39**: 3268–76.

46. Haley EC, Thompson JLP, Grotta JC, *et al*. Phase IIB/III trial of Tenecteplase in acute ischemic stroke: Results of a prematurely terminated randomized clinical trial. *Stroke* 2009; **41**: 707–711.

47. Gail MH, Wieand S, and Piantadosi S. Biased estimates of treatment effect in randomized experiments with nonlinear regressions and omitted covariates. *Biometrika* 1984; **71**: 431–44.

48. Johnston KC, Connors AF, Jr., Wagner DP, *et al*. Risk adjustment effect on stroke clinical trials. *Stroke* 2004; **3**: e43–e45.

49. Flaherty ML, Karlawish J, Khoury JC, *et al*. How important is surrogate consent for stroke research? *Neurology* 2008; **71**: 1566–71.

50. Kasner SE, Del Giudice A, Rosenberg S, *et al*. Who will participate in acute stroke trials? *Neurology* 2009; **72**: 1682–8.

51. Mangset M, Førde R, Nessa J, *et al*. I don't like that, it's tricking people too much…: acute informed consent to participation in a trial of thrombolysis for stroke. *J Med Ethics* 2008; **34**: 751–6.

52. Dani KA, McCormick MT, and Muir KW. Brain lesion volume and capacity for consent in stroke trials: potential regulatory barriers to the use of surrogate markers. *Stroke* 2008; **39**: 2336–40.

53. Saver JL, Kidwell C, Eckstein M, *et al*. Physician-investigator phone elicitation of consent in the field: a novel method to obtain explicit informed consent for prehospital clinical research. *Prehosp Emerg Care* 2006; **10**: 182–5.

54. Leira EC, Ahmed A, Lamb DL, *et al*. Extending acute trials to remote populations: a pilot study during interhospital helicopter transfer. *Stroke* 2009; **40**: 895–901.

55. Zhao W. Step-forward randomization in multi-site emergency treatment clinical trials. *Acad Emerg Med* 2009; **17**: 659–65.

56. Saver JL, Warach S, Janis S, *et al.* Standardizing the structure of stroke clinical and epidemiologic research data: The NINDS Stroke Common Data Element (CDE) Project. *Stroke* 2012; in press.

57. United States Census 2000. The Hispanic population: Census 2000 brief. http://www.census.gov (Accessed June 1, 2004.)

58. 21 CFR §50.24.

59. Bateman BT, Meyers PM, Schumacher HC, *et al.* Conducting stroke research with an exception from the requirement for informed consent. *Stroke* 2003; **34**: 1317–23.

Multiple sclerosis

Richard A. Rudick, Elizabeth Fisher, and Gary R. Cutter

Biological basis for therapies

Pathogenesis of MS on which experimental therapies are based

Multiple sclerosis (MS) is classified as an organ-specific autoimmune disease. Genome-wide association studies have linked HLA and immune system genes to the disease, leaving little doubt that immunological factors contribute to disease pathogenesis [1]. In the early stages of MS, scattered foci of inflammation occur in the central nervous system, the target of the inflammatory response. When these inflammatory foci involve motor, sensory, or visual pathways, clinical relapses occur. With resolution of inflammation, patients recover and enter a clinical remission. Relapses occur during the relapsing-remitting stage of MS (RRMS) at a variable rate, both across and within patients. Studies using MRI have revealed frequent new lesions, defined as gadolinium-enhancing lesions or as new T2-hyperintense lesions. The frequency of new lesions seen on MRI exceeds that of clinical relapses by approximately 10 to 1. For MS treatment, all currently approved disease-modifying drugs target inflammation and are generally indicated for reduction of relapse frequency.

In MS patients, relapses become less frequent over the initial 10–20 years of the disease, and are replaced by slowly advancing neurological disability. This stage is referred to as secondary progressive MS (SPMS). Mechanisms underlying the transition from RRMS to SPMS are not entirely understood, but there appears to be a transition from a mostly inflammatory pathology to one that is neurodegenerative and no longer dependent on inflammation. Although neurodegeneration is presumed to underlie progressive neurological disability in SPMS, axonal transection occurs at sites of CNS inflammation [2] and causes neurodegeneration during the early disease stages. There are no approved disease-modifying drugs that directly target neurodegeneration in MS.

A subtype of MS, primary progressive MS (PPMS), occurs in approximately 15% of patients and is characterized by continuous progression of neurological disability in the absence of relapses from disease onset forward. Mechanisms underlying PPMS are presumed to be similar to those underlying SPMS. Therapies targeting inflammation have been tested in PPMS but have not been beneficial.

The role of animal models in developing MS treatments

No naturally occurring animal model of MS exists. However, for nearly a century, experimental autoimmune encephalomyelitis (EAE) models have provided great insight into the mechanism of immune-initiated inflammation within the CNS. EAE can be induced in a variety of animal species and strains by immunization with CNS constituents or passive transfer of T cells or antibodies from immunized animals, resulting in immunologically mediated inflammatory injury to the CNS. Gold and colleagues extensively reviewed the value and limitations of EAE models in MS research [3]. They point out the tremendous heterogeneity in clinical manifestations and pathology, depending on the animal species or strain and the immunogen. After decades of study of rat and guinea pig models of EAE, mouse models were developed, and recently, various transgenic or knock-out mouse models have been used.

These models have yielded important information about immune-mediated CNS tissue injury, but the

Clinical Trials in Neurology, ed. Bernard Ravina, Jeffrey Cummings, Michael P. McDermott, and R. Michael Poole. Published by Cambridge University Press. © Cambridge University Press 2012.

value of EAE in screening therapeutic agents has been limited. First, no single EAE model reliably mimics all aspects of MS. Secondly, in many models inflammation predominates while demyelination is sparse. Further, no generally accepted models exhibit the marked neurodegeneration observed in later stages of MS although more recent models may be useful to investigate the axonopathy seen in SPMS [4]. The most significant limitation of the EAE model is that the outcomes of therapeutic strategies tested in EAE do not reliably predict results in humans. Positive therapeutic studies in the EAE model have not always translated into effective treatments in patients with MS, and conversely some beneficial therapies (e.g., interferon therapy) were not preceded by strong efficacy results in animal models. The EAE models appear to be most useful and significant for studies of immune pathogenesis. Consequently, they have not achieved a prominent role in the screening of therapies for MS to date.

Derfuss and colleagues [5] demonstrated that the axoglial protein contactin 2 and its rat homologue TAG-1 may be important autoantigens in the gray matter pathology that has recently been identified in MS. Adoptive transfer of TAG-1-reactive T cells resulted in inflammation predominately in spinal cord and cortex gray matter; when myelin-oligodendrocyte glycoprotein-specific antibodies were coadministered, focal cortical perivascular demyelination also developed. Contactin 2-induced EAE may represent a new model to analyze mechanisms of and interventions for MS gray matter pathology [6, 7].

'Neuroprotective' vs. 'anti-inflammatory' therapy

All current therapies for MS target neuroinflammation, with the aim of reducing the frequency of gadolinium-enhancing or new T2 lesions (which are markers of inflammation) and the frequency of relapse, and thus slowing disease progression. Because axons are transected at sites of acute inflammation [2], anti-inflammatory therapy may be neuroprotective by preventing axonal injury and transection. A number of studies [8] have demonstrated that the rate of brain tissue loss, as measured by MRI volumetric studies, slows after effective anti-inflammatory therapy, adding evidence to support the concept that anti-inflammatory therapy may be neuroprotective in the early stages of MS. Anti-inflammatory therapy, however, has not been effective in the later stages of MS,

presumably because inflammation is not essential to the ongoing neurodegeneration in the later stages. A range of potential treatments directed at neurodegeneration may be neuroprotective. Some strategies aim to increase axon stability or alter processes that damage axons. Others include remyelination strategies that promote differentiation of oligodendrocyte precursors into myelin-producing cells or the use of mesenchymal or bone marrow-derived stem cells [9]. To date, no trial of neuroprotective therapy in MS has been positive. However, evaluating the efficacy of potential neuroprotective agents is complex because there are no validated methodologies to demonstrate neuroprotection (see below).

Newer hypotheses concerning multiple sclerosis etiology

New hypotheses have emerged regarding the role of ultraviolet light and vitamin D [10–12], vascular comorbidity in driving disability progression [13], and venous obstruction [14]. These hypotheses each lead directly to therapeutic strategies – e.g., vitamin D supplementation, prevention and treatment of vascular comorbidities, or treatment of venous obstruction. As with any intervention, studies will require large sample sizes and rigorous designs, and results will depend on the validity of the underlying hypothesis.

Goals of intervention

Modifying the disease process vs. relieving symptoms

The goals of disease-modifying therapy in MS – reducing relapse frequency or reducing disability progression – may or may not improve quality of life in the short term. An entirely separate approach targets MS symptoms; symptom therapies may significantly benefit patients by reducing morbidity or improving quality of life. Symptom-based therapies for MS are often used off-label, e.g., use of antidepressants or analgesics is common. Additionally, drug development recently has focused on symptom management. Studies of 4-amino pyridine (dalfampridine-SR) have targeted walking speed in patients with MS; studies of dextromethorphan together with quinidine (AVP 923) have targeted pseudobulbar affect; duloxetine and dronabinol have targeted neuropathic pain; solifenacin succinate, bladder symptoms; and modafinil, fatigue. Table 23.1

Table 23.1 Drugs currently under development for symptomatic treatment of multiple sclerosis

Drug	ClinTrials.gov identifier	Symptoms targeted	Current status	Sponsor
4-amino pyridine (dalfampridine-SR)	NCT00053417	Walking speed (timed 25-foot walk)	Approved	Accorda Therapeutics
dextromethorphan + quinidine Neudexta	NCT00573443	Pseudobulbar affect	Approved	Avanir Pharmaceuticals
duloxetine	NCT00755807 NCT00457730	Neuropathic pain	Completed Recruiting	Eli Lilly
dronabinol	NCT00959218	Neuropathic pain	Ongoing	Bionorica Research GmbH
solifenacin succinate	NCT00629642	Bladder symptoms	Completed	Astellas Pharma Inc
modafinil	NCT00220506	Fatigue	Recruiting	Sheba Medical Center
	NCT00142402	Memory, fatigue, anxiety and depression	Ongoing	Kessler Foundation
modafinil + interferon β-1a*	NCT00210301	Cognition and fatigue (secondary outcomes)	Recruiting	Institute for Clinical Research
armodafinil	NCT00981084	Cognitive function and cognitive fatigue	Enrolling, by invitation	University of Missouri, Kansas City

* To test the safety of the combination.

lists drugs currently being developed for symptomatic treatment – the clinical development pipeline for MS symptom relief is robust.

Lessons learned from the development of interferon β to reduce relapses

Development of interferon β for MS [15] was a watershed event because interferon β-1b was the first disease-modifying drug approved by regulatory agencies to treat MS. Thus, its approval ushered in the current therapeutic era in MS. Importantly, approval was supported by a prominent reduction in new T2 hyperintense brain lesions. This firmly established MRI lesions as an important secondary outcome measure for MS clinical trials. Approval of interferon β-1b was quickly followed by approval of intramuscular interferon β-1a and subcutaneous interferon β-1a. Whereas interferon β-1b was approved based on its effect on relapse rate, intramuscular interferon β-1a was approved based on its effect of delaying the time to confirmed worsening on the Kurtzke Expanded Disability Status Scale (EDSS). Disability progression was defined as an increase in the EDSS level, confirmed at the next 6-month scheduled visit. This has led to a still-unresolved debate concerning the methodology used to measure disability progression in RRMS. Despite the controversy about the meaning of confirmed EDSS worsening in RRMS, virtually all subsequent clinical trials of disease-modifying drugs in MS, including those leading to approval of subcutaneous interferon β-1a, used measures of confirmed EDSS worsening.

Study populations

Classification of MS subtypes

In 1996, Lublin and Reingold published the results of an international survey that established standard terminology and categories for the different MS subtypes: RRMS, SPMS, PPMS, and progressive-relapsing MS (PRMS) [16]. This classification has profoundly influenced development of MS therapies because the clinical category has been used as a study entry criterion for nearly all trials of disease-modifying therapy. More recently, clinically isolated syndrome (CIS) has been added as a new category. This refers to the occurrence of a typical clinical syndrome suggesting inflammatory demyelination. When CIS is accompanied by multiple lesions on brain MRI, the likelihood of new MRI lesions or clinical relapses is extremely high [17], but patients with CIS do not meet current international panel criteria for a diagnosis of definite MS [18]. All MS clinical trials enrolling CIS patients have required multiple T2 hyperintense brain lesions as an inclusion criterion [19–21]. This represents a form of 'informative enrollment' (see below). Recently, a consensus panel called for a more precise definition of CIS [22]. In 2009, incidental MRI abnormalities that suggested MS was described and termed as the 'radiologically isolated syndrome' [23]. No studies to date have entered patients with radiologically isolated syndrome into randomized clinical trials.

The benefits of early treatment

In patients with CIS, interferon β has been shown to reduce conversion to RRMS by 50% [19]. In RRMS, interferon β therapy reduces the frequency of relapses by 33% [24–26]. Studies of interferon β therapy in patients with SPMS or PPMS have been negative. These findings suggest the possibility that anti-inflammatory therapy is most effective at earlier disease stages. Additionally, pathology studies demonstrated transected axons in the inflammatory lesions of patients in early RRMS. Inhibiting inflammation at an early stage, therefore, would seem a good strategy. A crossover study comparing early and delayed subcutaneous interferon β-1a therapy showed that those patients initially treated with placebo for 2 years and then switched to interferon β-1a, were worse at 4 years compared with patients who received interferon β-1a treatment for all 4 years, supporting the contention that early treatment is better than delayed treatment [27]. These observations led to the concept that early treatment is preferable to delayed treatment, and the MS clinical trial field has moved in that direction, testing interventions in CIS patients and testing aggressive immunomodulatory treatment very early in the disease.

Special issues concerning primary progressive MS and pediatric MS

To date, no treatments have shown significant benefits in patients with PPMS (Table 23.2 [28–34]), although most published studies are relatively small. A notable exception was the PROMiSe trial, in which 943 patients were randomly assigned to receive glatiramer acetate or placebo for 3 years. The two arms did not significantly differ on the primary outcome of delay in disability progression. Patients in the treatment arm had a significant decrease in the number of gadolinium-enhancing lesions and smaller increases in T2 lesion volume although this difference was not significant. The lower-than-expected disability progression rate as

well as study drug discontinuation may have contributed to the negative findings [29]. Presumably, results in PPMS trials have been negative because inflammation drives the pathologic process to a lesser degree in PPMS compared with RRMS and because mechanisms driving neurodegeneration were not specifically targeted. As no approved therapies exist for PPMS, placebo-controlled trials are ethical and needed, and this is an area of extremely high unmet need. Childhood MS [35] has been emphasized recently, but randomized controlled trials in the pediatric MS populations are just beginning.

Informative enrollment in MS clinical trials

The most common approaches to trial enrollment are: 1) selection of patients with a history of relapses in the year or two prior to trial entry; 2) selection of patients with 'disability progression,' usually defined as worsening by a specified amount on the EDSS scale; or 3) patients with one or more gadolinium-enhancing lesions on cranial MRI during a run-in or at study entry. As with other inclusion and exclusion criteria, informative enrollment strategies will restrict generalizability of the results. In addition to limiting generalizability, informative enrollment strategies raise other considerations. First, entrance criteria may significantly influence trial results. As noted above, studies of a given drug show a greater effect on relapse frequency in CIS populations compared with RRMS populations, which in turn show greater efficacy than studies in SPMS populations. Thus, restricting trial entry to patients in earlier stages of MS may result in higher observed efficacy. Selecting patients who demonstrated increased EDSS scores may bias trial results in the direction of lower efficacy, since patients remain at various EDSS steps for periods that approach or exceed the duration of clinical trials. Thus, entering patients who recently moved to a higher EDSS level may ensure fewer EDSS events rather than enriching the cohort for added events. Finally, enrolling patients with more progressive disease may enrich the trial for patients more refractory to treatment. Thus, the main advantage of informative enrollment based on disease activity – increased events during the trial – must be balanced against the likely effect of the informative enrollment strategy on the outcome.

Another consideration is that standardized, validated methods to identify patients based on disease activity before randomization are not available. One common approach is to require pre-study relapses for

Table 23.2 Summary of randomized placebo-controlled clinical trials for PPMS

Study	Placebo (n)	Treatment (n)	Drug(s)	Outcome measures	Outcome
Hawker et al. [28]	147	292	rituximab 2 1000-mg infusions/24 weeks for 96 weeks	• Time to sustained disease progression on EDSS • Changes on MRI	Groups did not significantly differ in time to progression. Patients receiving treatment had a significantly smaller increase in T2 lesion volume. Subgroup analyses suggested that treatment may delay disease progression in younger patients, particularly those with inflammatory (gadolinium-enhancing) lesions.
Wolinsky et al. [29]	316	627	glatiramer acetate 20 mg SC/day for 36 months	• Time to sustained disease progression on EDSS • Changes on MRI	Groups did not significantly differ in time to progression. MRI lesion burden was significantly less in the treatment group. Treatment may have slowed progression in males with rapid progression. Because the trial was stopped early and the event rate was low, the trial may have been underpowered to detect a treatment effect.
Montalban [30]	37	36	IFN β-1b 8 MIU SC every other day for 2 years	• Time to sustained disease progression on EDSS • Change in MSFC • QOL measures • Changes on MRI	No significant differences were found in disability progression as assessed by EDSS. However, significant differences favoring interferon β-1b treatment were seen in the MSFC score, T2 and T1 lesion volumes, suggesting that IFN β-1b may have a beneficial effect in PPMS.
Leary et al. [31]	20	30	IFN beta-1a, IM 30 μg or 60 μg 1x/wk for 24 months	• Time to sustained disease progression on EDSS • Changes on MRI • 10-meter walk, 9-hole peg test	No difference in EDSS. T2 lesion load less in 30 μg treatment group but brain volume loss greater with 60 μg
Rammohan et al. [32]	72	72	modafinil, oral Crossover design with titration up from 200 mg to 400 mg	• FSS score • MFIS score • VAS-F score • EDSS score	Fatigue significantly improved with 200 mg treatment on all measures
Rice et al. [33]	54	105	cladribine, SC, 0.07 mg/kg/day for 5 consecutive days every 4 weeks for 2 or 6 cycles (total dose, 0.7 mg/kg or 2.1 mg/kg, respectively), followed by placebo, for a total of 8 cycles (12 months)	• Mean change in EDSS • Scripps Neurologic Rating Scale • MRI changes	Treatment did not significantly affect the absolute change or time to progression in EDSS or SNRS scores. Both doses significantly reduced the presence, number, and volume of gadolinium-enhanced T1 brain lesions, and cladribine 2.1 mg/kg decreased the T2 lesion load accumulation.
Filippi et al. [34]	48	14	cladribine, SC, 0.07 mg/kg/day for 5 consecutive days every 4 weeks for 2 or 6 cycles (total dose, 0.7 mg/kg or 2.1 mg/kg, respectively), followed by placebo, for a total of 8 cycles (12 months)	• Change in brain volume	Brain volumes decreased in all patients as a group and in placebo-treated patients when analyzed alone. Neither cladribine dose had any effect on brain volume loss over time. In the placebo group, changes in brain volume did not correlate with changes in other MRI measures.

EDSS = Kurtzke Extended Disability Status Scale; MSFC = Multiple Sclerosis Functional Composite; QOL = quality of life; SC = subcutaneous; IM = imtramuscular; MIU = million international units; FSS = Fatigue Severity Scale; MFIS = Modified Fatigue Impact Scale; VAS-F = Visual Analogue Scale for Fatigue; ESS = Epworth Sleepiness Scale.

trial eligibility, but defining pre-study relapse rate is subjective. Thus, clearly defining the population studied may be difficult.

Lastly, methods to enroll patients based on biological factors, while appealing, are in their infancy in MS. For example, the HLA-DRB1*15 allele is more common in MS patients, and is associated with more rapid MS disease progression. An informative enrollment strategy would be to enroll only HLA-DRB1*15-positive patients. However, the responsiveness of this patient subgroup to a particular therapy cannot be known in advance, so a more appealing strategy would be to conduct pre-planned subgroup analyses in patients positive for HLA-DRB1*15 before using this marker for informative enrollment.

Properties of measurement tools

Clinical measures: relapses, physical function, neuropsychological performance

The most common outcome measure for RRMS trials is the relapse number or rate. This was the primary outcome measure in two of the three pivotal trials of interferon for RRMS [26, 36], the glatiramer acetate trial [24], and the placebo-controlled natalizumab trial [37]. Relapses are relatively simple to count, and by definition have a clinical impact on the patient. However, the relationship between relapses and eventual disability is weak [38]; relapses are sometimes subjective and open to bias, over- or under-reporting, and treatment unmasking; and generally accepted methods for quantifying the severity of each relapse, or for quantifying recovery are not developed.

The EDSS is an ordinal scale from 0 to 10 that captures the level of disability according to 19 steps [39]. Between 0.0 (normal neurological examination) and 3.5 (moderate disability in more than one functional system) the score is determined by combinations from seven separate functional system scales (e.g., visual, motor, cerebellar, sensory, bowel, bladder, etc.). From 4.0 to 6.0, the scale measures limitations in distance walking. Level 6.0 indicates the need for unilateral assistance to walk, 6.5 bilateral assistance, and ≥ 7.0 measures severity in non-ambulatory patients. There is considerable debate whether the EDSS measures disability accurately at the low end, and whether the middle and high ranges are optimally sensitive for clinical trials. Despite criticism, the EDSS has been the standard measure of neurological disability in nearly all MS clinical trials.

Since the mid-1990s, the EDSS has been used to determine confirmed worsening from the baseline score determined at study entry. Kaplan-Meier analysis of survival curves plotting the time to onset of confirmed disability worsening in each treatment arm have been used to estimate hazard ratios for disability progression with active treatment. Worsening of the EDSS score has been confirmed at a 3-month study visit in most trials; a minority of trials have required 6-month confirmation. The EDSS may revert to baseline more commonly if the 3-month definition is used [40]. Also, the relevance of confirmed EDSS worsening in the early stages of MS is uncertain, although a recent report demonstrated a correlation between 6-month confirmed EDSS worsening and clinical outcome 8 years later [41].

Because of perceived limitations of the EDSS, a National Multiple Sclerosis Society task force recommended the MS Functional Composite (MSFC), a three-part composite consisting of timed measures of ambulation, upper extremity function, and cognition [42]. The MSFC has been extensively tested and validated but has yet to achieve its intended purpose – to replace the EDSS as a primary clinical measure of MS-related disability. A substantial part of the problem lies in interpreting the clinical relevance of the results. As originally recommended, the three MSFC measures are transformed to a single Z score, defined as the average of the Z scores from the ambulation, upper extremity, and cognitive tests. The optimal population used to normalize the clinical trial test scores has been a subject of debate, since the choice of reference population influences the weighting of the different components within the MSFC [43]. Recently, a group analyzed MSFC data collected during the AFFIRM trial and proposed using the MSFC to identify a disability progression event, analogous to how the EDSS is used [44]. Disability progression as demonstrated by the MSFC score correlated with traditional measures of disease activity and progression, and the MSFC score as a measure of progression showed treatment effects similar to EDSS. It is expected that adding a visual assessment measure to the MSFC and possibly substituting a cognitive measure with less learning effect than the Paced Auditory Serial Addition Test (PASAT) will improve the MSFC performance characteristics and allow the MSFC to replace the EDSS as a more useful measure of disability.

Neuropsychological impairment, particularly in processing speed, complex attention, and verbal learning, has been identified in approximately 50% of MS cases in population-based studies [45]. The effects of treatment on neuropsychological test performance have been reported, although the popularity of neuropsychological testing in MS clinical trials has declined because of time and cost considerations. Six randomized clinical trials have been published that investigate disease-modifying medications and also assess neuropsychological outcome [46], with mixed results. Neuropsychological testing is most appropriate for a study that specifically targets neurocognitive deficits in MS. Efforts are under way to develop and validate brief neuropsychological test batteries that are more practical for MS clinical trials [47].

Patient-reported quality-of-life measures [48]

Many health-related quality-of-life (HR-QOL) scales have been used in MS trials. Generic HR-QOL measures include the Symptom Impact Profile and the Medical Outcomes Study 36-Item Short-Form Survey (SF-36). Hybrid measures are the MS Quality of Life Index and MSQOL-54; MS-specific instruments include the Functional Assessment of MS and MS Impact Scale-29. No consensus exists concerning the optimal patient self-report HR-QOL instrument for MS clinical trials. At least eight clinical trials have reported the effects of interferon or glatiramer acetate treatment on quality of life in MS. The AFFIRM study revealed a strong association between the physical component score of the SF-36 and both the EDSS score and relapse rate and number, and showed significant treatment effects [49]. Patient-reported HR-QOL measures are appealing in that they capture the overall burden of MS, but they are somewhat insensitive in that clinical changes can occur while HR-QOL remains the same. In addition, many HR-QOL measures are non-specific and are therefore most appropriate as secondary outcome measures.

Conventional MRI measures

Measures using MRI, such as the number of contrast-enhancing lesions and T2 hyperintensity volumes, are routinely used in MS clinical trials. Lesions that enhance on T1-weighted images acquired after injection with a paramagnetic contrast agent (typically, gadolinium-DTPA) indicate blood-brain barrier disruption and inflammatory activity. Frequent MRI studies have shown that gadolinium-enhancing lesions

occur much more often than clinical relapses. However, enhancement only lasts for 1 to 4 weeks, so enhancing lesions will be missed when periods between serial MRIs are longer. During and following enhancement, most lesions appear hyperintense on T2-weighted MRIs. Once formed, T2 hyperintense lesions may persist indefinitely. Because serial MRIs are costly and impractical for most studies, clinical trials typically include counts of both gadolinium-enhancing lesions and new or enlarging T2 hyperintensities as measures of inflammatory activity. The number of combined unique active lesions is a single measure that has been proposed for use in clinical trials to avoid double counting of enhancing lesions and new T2 lesions [50]. All currently approved MS disease-modifying therapies have been shown to reduce enhancing lesions.

The total volume of T2 hyperintense lesions is considered an estimate of overall MS disease burden. Reductions in the accrual of T2 lesion volume have been reported in the active treatment arms compared to placebo for most MS trials. The significance of these volume reductions has been questioned because the accrual of T2 lesion volume only weakly correlates with disability progression over the short term [51]. Furthermore, post-mortem studies have shown that only about half of T2 hyperintense lesions correspond to focally demyelinated MS lesions [52]. Pathologically, T2 lesions range from transient edema to severe tissue destruction, complicating interpretation. Despite these issues, T2 lesion volume correlates modestly with future brain atrophy [53], and it remains an important measure in trials for confirming that treatment arms are well-matched at baseline.

Lesions that appear persistently hypointense on unenhanced T1-weighted images (T1 black holes) have been shown to correspond to regions with axonal loss [54]. However, black hole total volume correlates strongly with T2 lesion volume, and has not been particularly useful as a clinical trial outcome measure. Recently, the percentage of enhancing lesions that evolve into chronic T1 black holes has been proposed as a marker of neuroprotection [55].

Brain atrophy is a conventional MRI measure that is considered to be a marker of severe tissue destruction. Measurement of changes in normalized brain volume [56] and direct measurement of changes in brain edges from pairs of registered MRIs [57] have been applied in MS clinical trials to estimate whole brain atrophy. Like T2 lesion volume, normalized brain volume can be considered a marker of overall disease burden, but it has some advantages over lesion measurements. Importantly, it reflects the net effect of the destructive processes due to MS. Brain atrophy correlates more strongly with disability than any other conventional MRI measurement and predicts subsequent disability [58]. However, some important issues relate to the interpretation of atrophy measurements from clinical trials. In the initial period after starting most anti-inflammatory therapies, there is typically an accelerated reduction in brain volume, termed pseudoatrophy [8], which presumably is due to the resolution of inflammatory edema rather than actual tissue loss. Therefore, sometimes treatment effects on atrophy can only be observed after the first of treatment. Also, although changes in brain volume are much higher in MS patients than in healthy controls, the changes are still very small, on the order of 0.5% to 1% per year. Therefore, highly reproducible methods and studies of adequate duration are required.

Generally, MRI measures have the advantage of being more objective and more sensitive than clinical measures. However, because no MRI measures meet the stringent definition of a surrogate marker of MS, MRI is not accepted by regulatory agencies as a primary outcome for phase 3 trials, although gadolinium-enhancing lesions are commonly used as the primary outcome in phase 2 trials. Sormani and colleagues conducted a pooled analysis of 23 clinical trials that tested the effect of interventions on relapse rate and included MRI lesion measures [59]. The effect of the intervention on MRI lesions accounted for 81% of the variance in the treatment effect on relapses, thus showing a strong association between reduction in MRI lesions and reduction in relapses. Consistency in MRI acquisition is a significant issue in clinical trials. Volumetric measures are highly sensitive to changes in scanner hardware of software and changes in sequence parameters, whereas count measures, e.g., enhancing lesions, are relatively robust. Scanner upgrades can be disastrous for clinical trials, and care must be taken to prospectively plan for unavoidable changes in MRI hardware and software over the study period.

Pharmacodynamic markers

Many different assays have been used in pharmacodynamic studies to measure or monitor biological effects of specific therapies. For instance, B-cell numbers are monitored in rituximab trials because rituximab depletes B cells. For interferon trials, interferon-stimulated gene products may be monitored. Pharmacodynamic markers are useful in early studies to determine the dose or dosing interval, monitor patients for tachyphylaxis, and compare the magnitude of biological effects across doses or agents. With the exception of antibodies to biological agents, few studies have shown correlations between the effect of therapy on a pharmacologic marker and clinical response to therapy.

New approaches to measuring MS

Measures based on MRI have been continually evolving with new image acquisition methods and higher magnet strengths. Several non-conventional MRI techniques are under development for use in MS clinical trials [60]. These include magnetization transfer imaging, T1 and T2 relaxation time measurements, magnetic resonance spectroscopy, diffusion tensor imaging, functional MRI, ultra-high field strength imaging, and molecular imaging. These measures provide greater sensitivity and specificity, allowing quantitative assessment of pathophysiological mechanisms in MS. Challenges remain related to validation, optimization, and standardization that would permit newer measures to be used in multi-center trials.

Interest in optical coherence tomography (OCT), a newer technique that quantifies the retinal nerve fiber layer (RNFL), was stimulated by findings that MS patients have reduced low-contrast letter acuity [61]. These studies demonstrated that the RNFL is thinner in patients than controls, even in those without a history of optic neuritis [62], raising the possibility that OCT could be used to assess treatment effects on the thickness of the RNFL. As of yet, no study has demonstrated that treatment affects the fiber layer.

Clinical trial designs and analytical methods used in development

Conventional designs: Preclinical through phase 3 studies

Conventional designs for phase 1 through phase 3 trials are well known and established. The primary objectives of phase 1 clinical trials are to identify an effective dose and assess toxicity. In phase 2 trials, the objectives are to insure that the drug provides some degree of effectiveness and insure safety without excess toxicity in the disease population. It is critical that phase 3 trials demonstrate clinical effectiveness, but they also provide information about side effects and tolerability of treatments, as well as their impact on quality of life.

Delayed start

Placebo treatment arms are ethically questionable, and increasingly so as more effective drugs are approved. However, active arm comparator designs (e.g., head-to-head trials) require more patients than placebo-controlled trials with the same endpoints. The BEYOND Trial, which compared two doses of interferon β-1b with glatiramir acetate, randomized 2244 patients [63]. Such large sample sizes are driving the need for alternative trial designs that can be accomplished without an active comparator arm. For example, patients can be randomized to double-blinded early- or delayed-start treatment, with subjects in the delayed-start arm receiving placebo until the treatment phase is initiated for that arm. This design was used in the BENEFIT Trial, which randomized 487 patients to interferon beta-1b or placebo for up to 2 years and then initiated therapy. Here the question was timing of treatment and whether earlier intervention was beneficial [21]. The FDA (http://www.fda.gov/RegulatoryInformation/Guidances/ucm125802.htm) endorses such an approach and examines two outcomes: replicating the treatment effect in the patients initially receiving placebo and the sustained parallel differences between the treatment arms after placebo patients are switched to treatment. If a gap persists and treatment effects are replicated, it seems reasonable to conclude that the drug slows disease progression.

Standards for efficacy and special safety issues

Active arm comparison and combination trials

Ethical concerns surrounding placebo-controlled trials in RRMS involve the availability of effective disease-modifying drugs that reduced the severity of MS. One approach has been to conduct placebo-controlled trials in regions of the world where disease-modifying drugs are unavailable, but this does not satisfactorily address the ethical concerns. Another approach has been to offer placebo-controlled trials to patients who decline the use of available drugs [64], but this introduces selection biases. Consequently, MS trialists have moved in recent

years to active arm comparison trials and to trials of drugs in combination. Active arm comparisons and trials of combination therapy entail several considerations. The first involves sample size: as event rates are reduced by active therapy in the comparison arms, the number of cases necessary to achieve adequate power increases dramatically. In the example of the BEYOND trial, we saw an almost four-fold increase in sample size to 2244 compared to the placebo-controlled BENEFIT trial with 487 patients. Second, adverse events may escalate significantly with multiple drug therapy. Another issue is that the FDA often requires at least three arms in combination trials – the combination and each of the component drugs alone or in combination with a placebo. These three groups are necessary to provide evidence of a statistically significant superiority of the combination, say drugs A+B over A alone, and B alone. The rationale is that if A+B is not better than both drug A alone and drug B alone, there is no reason to expose the patient to both drugs. The Avonex Combination Trial tested the addition of methotrexate, methylprednisolone, or both to intramuscular interferon β-1a in patients with RRMS who had disease activity despite intramuscular interferon β-1a. Although combination therapy showed beneficial trends compared to monotherapy, they were not statistically, and probably not clinically, significant [65].

Adverse events

Opportunistic infections

Two cases of progressive multifocal leukoencephalopathy (PML) in patients participating in the SENTINEL trial [66] were sufficient to stop the study. Importantly the number of events, two, is insufficient statistically to call for stopping a trial. Such decisions are based on clinical judgment and the severity of the consequences of the events. In this situation, upon notification of the PML cases in February 2005, the FDA suspended use of natalizumab pending a detailed safety review of all patients exposed to the drug. Only after a complete analysis of the estimated risk for PML and other opportunistic infections was the drug reintroduced to the market in June 2006. Subsequent to the reintroduction, worldwide attention has focused on the risk of PML, on risk stratification methods, and on risk minimization and treatment of PML. The natalizumab experience has called into question the methods used in post-marketing surveillance for unusual severe adverse events such as opportunistic infections and has had tremendous implications for the use of potent immunomodulatory, immunosuppressive, and cytotoxic drugs for MS. Opportunistic infections have also been reported with current drugs in development, including but not limited to fingolimod [67, 68] and cladribine [69].

Cancer

Mitoxantrone (Novantrone) was approved for relapsing and progressive MS. It was rapidly adopted due to the lack of approved treatments for progressive MS. Shortly thereafter it became clear that mitoxantrone was linked to acute leukemia [70], which has significantly limited its use. Cladribine, which is used to treat leukemia, has been associated with second cancers in that setting, and MS clinical trials have thus far demonstrated some increase in cancer in cladribine recipients relative to placebo recipients [69].

Other significant adverse events

Fingolimod has been associated with atrioventricular block, bradycardia, mildly increased blood pressure, and occasionally, macular edema [71]. These 'off target' effects of fingolimod appear to be mild enough to allow use of the drug. At times, off-target effects have been significant enough to stop development of potential MS drugs. In the mid-1990s, linomide (Roquinimex) was in phase 3 clinical studies for RRMS and SPMS. Approximately 1200 participants were enrolled. Development was stopped when eight patients experienced myocardial infarction and two died. It was later determined that linomide caused pericarditis. Subsequently, a chemical derivative of linomide, laquinimod, was developed. It does not appear to be cardiotoxic and is in phase 3 testing at present.

Implementation issues – challenges in the conduct of the trial

Recruitment challenges

Two decades ago when trials in MS were starting, patient recruitment was not a problem. Today, phase 2 and phase 3 MS trials have recruited patients overseas where regulatory processes are less onerous, trial costs are lower, and patients have fewer therapeutic options. Trial recruitment difficulties may also stem from increased media coverage of clinical trials, where negative media coverage trials may damage the public's trust in biomedical research. On the other hand, media reports can create a clamor for treatments that remain unproven. A recent example is the fervor surrounding chronic cerebrospinal venous insufficiency as a possible cause of MS, leading to the demand for endovascular intervention, despite the lack of trial results demonstrating treatment benefits.

Few trials today recruit ahead of schedule, and most suffer from 30% to 40% slower recruitment than planned. Aban *et al.* discussed their experience in planning and launching a multinational study in myasthenia gravis [72]. They highlighted the additional steps required for international sites and provided estimates of the time required to bring US and non-US sites into full regulatory compliance before they could initiate recruitment. Delays for non-US centers were 13.4 ± 0.96 months as compared with US centers, of 9.67 months ($p = 0.02$). The delay for non-US sites was attributable to Federal Wide Assurance certification and State Department clearance.

Historically MS trials have enjoyed very high retention rates, usually exceeding 90% in 1- or 2-year studies. However, as the MS treatment options increase, more patients can be expected to exit trials when they experience disease activity or side effects.

Effect of multiple trials within MS centers

When multiple trials exist within an MS center, competition for patients can occur. In such circumstances, if researchers recruit potential study patients according to the trial in which they believe the patient will do best, the trial results may not be generalizable. In many industry-sponsored studies, when speed of recruitment is an important goal, randomization is often not done within each center. When selection biases occur, particularly under circumstances of competing trials, the treatment effects can be confounded by both center and the small patient numbers within a center. There are no statistical remedies for this confounding and its impact on generalizability.

MS severity 'drift'

The changing patterns of relapses over time with an apparent lessening, even in placebo groups, as well as somewhat reduced disability progression raises the question of changes in MS severity over time. If such drift is occurring, is it a result of changing incidence and newer forms of MS, or differing subgroups of patients detected with differing prognoses? Is earlier diagnosis changing the patterns observed from prior decades of observation, in the era before disease-modifying therapy? Or does therapy have a cumulative effect on clinician awareness and response to the disease? Drift is important, as it changes the risk-benefit equations that patients and clinicians need to consider when selecting treatments.

Country effects

The participation of multiple countries and centers in MS research includes many untested assumptions concerning bias and trial design. The origin of the patients, the medical care system, the investigative teams and their views, and approaches to clinical trials combine to challenge the assumptions made in trial design – that the effects of drugs are independent of country, center, etc. Ultimately, the confounding of such effects with treatment effects may affect the generalizability of the results if assumptions concerning these important covariates are false, but more importantly, effective therapies may be missed due to increased variability.

Challenges and controversies

What is the relationship of treatment to relapses, EDSS, and MRI parameters?

Figure 23.1 shows the course of destructive pathology in the central nervous system in MS. During the initial 10 to 20 years of symptoms, relapses result in periodic neurological problems, but patients tend to function relatively well and would not be considered to be disabled. As the pathology progresses and is superimposed on the aging process, a threshold is surpassed, beyond which progressive neurological disability ensues, and the patient enters the secondary progressive phase.

All approved therapies for MS at present have been directed at the RRMS and have targeted inflammation. The degree to which such treatments inhibit and halt

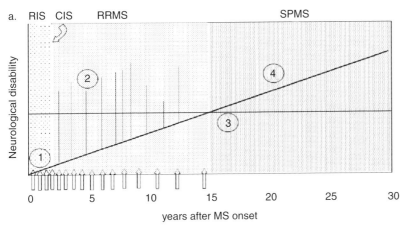

Figure 23.1a. The natural course of multiple sclerosis without disease-modifying drug therapy.

The figure shows the stages of MS (see text): RIS – radiologically isolated syndrome; CIS – clinically isolated syndrome; RRMS – relapsing remitting MS; SPMS – secondary progressive MS. (1) Many patients presenting with CIS already have multicentric MRI lesions, indicating preceding subclinical disease activity, designated as new MRI lesions (↑). At the time of CIS and at the time of relapses (2), transient neurological disability appears (vertical lines). Once a threshold of CNS pathology is surpassed (3), disability ceases to be transient, and ongoing disease pathology is manifest as progressively worse neurological disability. The presence of ongoing tissue injury (4) is suggested by MRI studies showing progressive brain atrophy starting early in the disease.

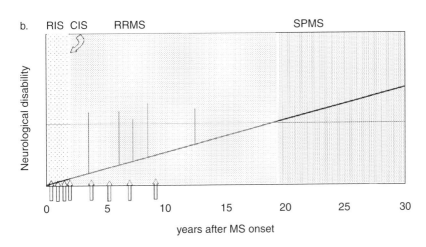

Figure 23.1b. The course of multiple sclerosis with disease-modifying drug therapy initiated at the time the patient presents with CIS.

All current approved disease-modifying drugs target brain inflammation and reducing new brain MRI lesions and relapses. The figure shows a hypothetical modified course of MS in the presence of disease-modifying drug therapy. New MRI lesions are reduced by about 70%, relapses by 50%, and the rate of progression of ongoing tissue injury by about 35%. Lowering the rate of ongoing tissue injury delays the onset of SPMS to about 20 years from symptom onset and lowers the eventual level of neurological disability.

the CNS pathology is of considerable debate. The traditional measures of relapses and MRI lesions are useful because they measure benefit to patients, but the long-term benefits of drug treatment on clinically significant disability and development of SPMS are still uncertain. Part of the problem relates to the unclear relationship between treatment effect on relapses or MRI lesions and later clinically significant impact on disability. The EDSS has been used in an attempt to define progressive disability in RRMS. Commonly, a defined amount of worsening from the score at study entry is required and must be confirmed at least 3 months later. Many have equated confirmed EDSS worsening as synonymous with progressive disability in RRMS patients, but this remains controversial and uncertain. The EDSS is somewhat imprecise at the low disability end of its range, and in a substantial proportion of patients, reports have documented recovery from confirmed EDSS worsening of 1 point after 3 months [40]. Long-term longitudinal studies are required to determine the relevance of relapses, lesions, and confirmed EDSS worsening as predictors of clinically significant disability and SPMS. Further, it is necessary to determine whether, and to what degree, improvements on these parameters translate into clinical benefits years later in the form of reduced disability. Many experts believe that decreases in relapses, confirmed EDSS worsening, and lesions represent intermediate outcome measures that predict a beneficial long-term effect, but this has not been firmly established.

Is 'disease free' a useful concept in MS trials?

The concept of 'disease free' (which derives from cancer trials) in MS is based on results from the natalizumab trials, which reported the proportion of patients with no indication of disease activity during treatment. Disease-free is defined as no new MRI lesions, no active MRI lesions during the trial, no relapses, and no worsening on the EDSS score. Although a useful concept, it is not certain that disease-free equates to pathology-free status. For example, much of the MS pathology has been localized to gray matter, and gray matter pathology is not detectable with conventional MRI techniques.

What is the role of brain atrophy studies in clinical trials?

Although brain atrophy has been measured in MS trials for almost two decades, the interpretation of

atrophy results has been controversial. Volumetric changes are pathologically non-specific. Some portion of the change reflects real tissue loss due to MS, but superimposed on the disease-related changes are possible physiological fluid shifts related to hydration status [8, 73], effects of gliosis or steroids [74], and possibly cytotoxic effects [75]. These confounding effects are difficult, if not impossible, to control. Despite these complex issues, MS patients lose greater brain volume over time than age-matched healthy controls, and atrophy correlates with and predicts disability [76], suggesting that atrophy measurements mainly reflect disease-related change. Currently available MS disease-modifying therapies have been shown to slow atrophy 30% to 50% in the second year of treatment [56, 77, 78]. This finding has been relatively consistent across trials, therapies, and measurement methodologies. However, more recently, a few MS trials have reported complete cessation or even reversal of brain atrophy [63, 79], the meaning of which is under investigation.

The lack of a validated, pathologically specific measure of neuroprotection has prompted further discussion on the utility of brain atrophy measurements. In 2008, a meeting was convened to develop a consensus on how to measure neuroprotection and repair in MS clinical trials [80]. The panel concluded that brain atrophy measurements are the most feasible, well-characterized, and useful marker of neuroprotection currently available. More specific measures of neuroprotection and repair are essential and are currently being sought.

What are we missing?

An important limitation to using MRI for evaluating disease burden in MS is that abnormalities revealed by conventional MRI are restricted to the white matter. Pathology studies have shown that, in addition to the classic white matter plaques, significant tissue damage occurs in the gray matter and in white matter regions outside areas of focal demyelination [81]. However, most MRI outcome measures in MS (including gadolinium-enhancing lesions, T2 lesions, and T1 black hole lesions) are insensitive to both gray matter pathology and diffuse white matter damage. With conventional MRI acquisitions, only atrophy measurements are sensitive to the effects of damage in the gray matter and normal-appearing white matter. Gray matter atrophy has been shown to be correlated with disability and is currently under investigation as a feasible outcome measure in trials [82]. Advanced MRI acquisition methods have been applied to detect MS pathology outside of white matter lesions, including magnetization transfer ratio and double inversion recovery [83, 84]. For technical reasons, these non-conventional imaging techniques are not yet ready for use in large multi-center trials.

Design limitations specific to MS

Alternative statistical designs for MS have been discussed extensively. Most are not new, but just have not been implemented in MS. Part of the reason for this is the interaction between regulatory authorities and pharmaceutical companies. Each in its own way is conservative, opting for tried and true. Additional regulatory forces, such as ethics boards, increase the inherent difficulty of more adventurous designs in MS. For example, adaptive designs require elaborate *a priori* decision-making and often changes to sample sizes, duration of treatment, etc., which require further discussions with IRBs and ethics boards. The practical aspects often outweigh the statistical design properties and even potential cost savings attributed to modifications of the design. A single change in protocol could cost $150 000 if there were 100 centers at $1500 per change.

References

1. International Multiple Sclerosis Genetics Consortium, Hafler DA, Compston A, et al. Risk alleles for multiple sclerosis identified by a genomewide study. *N Engl J Med* 2007; **357**: 851–62.

2. Trapp BD, Peterson J, Ransohoff RM, et al. Axonal transection in the lesions of multiple sclerosis. *N Engl J Med* 1998; **338**: 278–85.

3. Gold R, Linington C, and Lassmann H. Understanding pathogenesis and therapy of multiple sclerosis via animal models: 70 years of merits and culprits in experimental autoimmune encephalomyelitis research. *Brain* 2006; **129**: 1953–71.

4. Soulika AM, Lee E, McCauley E, et al. Initiation and progression of axonopathy in experimental autoimmune encephalomyelitis. *J Neurosci* 2009; **29**: 14965–79.

5. Derfuss T, Parikh K, Velhin S, et al. Contactin-2/TAG-1-directed autoimmunity is identified in multiple sclerosis patients and mediates gray matter pathology in animals. *Proc Natl Acad Sci USA* 2009; **106**: 8302–7.

6. Steinman L. The gray aspects of white matter disease in multiple sclerosis. *Proc Natl Acad Sci USA* 2009; **106**: 8083–4.

7. Rudick RA and Trapp BD. Gray-matter injury in multiple sclerosis. *N Engl J Med* 2009; **361**: 1505–6.

8. Zivadinov R, Reder AT, Filippi M, et al. Mechanisms of action of disease-modifying agents and brain volume changes in multiple sclerosis. *Neurology* 2008; **71**: 136–44.

9. Greenberg BM and Calabresi PA. Future research directions in multiple sclerosis therapies. *Semin Neurol* 2008; **28**: 121–7.

10. Ramagopalan SV, Maugeri NJ, Handunnetthi L, et al. Expression of the multiple sclerosis-associated MHC class II allele HLA-DRB1*1501 is regulated by vitamin D. *PLoS Genet* 2009; **5**: e1000369.

11. Ebers GC. Environmental factors and multiple sclerosis. *Lancet Neurol* 2008; **7**: 268–77.

12. Giovannoni G and Ebers G. Multiple sclerosis: The environment and causation. *Curr Opin Neurol* 2007; **20**: 261–8.

13. Marrie RA, Rudick R, Horwitz R, et al. Vascular comorbidity is associated with more rapid disability progression in multiple sclerosis. *Neurology* 30: 1041–7.

14. Zamboni P, Galeotti R, Menegatti E, et al. Chronic cerebrospinal venous insufficiency in patients with multiple sclerosis. *J Neurol Neurosurg Psychiatry* 2009; **80**: 392–9.

15. Bermel RA and Rudick RA. Interferon-beta treatment for multiple sclerosis. *Neurotherapeutics* 2007; **4**: 633–46.

16. Lublin FD and Reingold SC. Defining the clinical course of multiple sclerosis: Results of an international survey. *Neurology* 1996; **46**: 907–11.

17. Brex PA, Ciccarelli O, O'Riordan JI, et al. A longitudinal study of abnormalities on MRI and disability from multiple sclerosis. *N Engl J Med* 2002; **346**: 158–64.

18. McDonald WI, Compston A, Edan G, et al. Recommended diagnostic criteria for multiple sclerosis: Guidelines from the international panel on the diagnosis of multiple sclerosis. *Ann Neurol* 2001; **50**: 121–7.

19. Jacobs LD, Beck RW, Simon JH, et al. Intramuscular interferon beta-1a therapy initiated during a first demyelinating event in multiple sclerosis. CHAMPS study group. *N Engl J Med* 2000; **343**: 898–904.

20. Comi G, Martinelli V, Rodegher M, et al. Effect of glatiramer acetate on conversion to clinically definite multiple sclerosis in patients with clinically isolated syndrome (PreCISe study): A randomised, double-blind, placebo-controlled trial. *Lancet* 2009; **374**: 1503–11.

21. Kappos L, Polman CH, Freedman MS, et al. Treatment with interferon beta-1b delays conversion to clinically definite and McDonald MS in patients with clinically isolated syndromes. *Neurology* 2006; **67**: 1242–9.

22. Miller DH, Weinshenker BG, Filippi M, *et al.* Differential diagnosis of suspected multiple sclerosis: A consensus approach. *Mult Scler* 2008; **14**: 1157–74.

23. Moore F and Okuda DT. Incidental MRI anomalies suggestive of multiple sclerosis: The radiologically isolated syndrome. *Neurology* 2009; **73**: 1714.

24. Johnson KP, Brooks BR, Cohen JA, *et al.* Copolymer 1 reduces relapse rate and improves disability in relapsing-remitting multiple sclerosis: Results of a phase III multicenter, double-blind placebo-controlled trial. the copolymer 1 multiple sclerosis study group. *Neurology* 1995; **45**: 1268–76.

25. Jacobs LD, Cookfair DL, Rudick RA, *et al.* Intramuscular interferon beta-1a for disease progression in relapsing multiple sclerosis. The Multiple Sclerosis Collaborative Research Group (MSCRG). *Ann Neurol* 1996; **39**: 285–94.

26. PRISMS (Prevention of Relapses and Disability by Interferon beta-1a Subcutaneously in Multiple Sclerosis) study group. Randomized double-blind placebo-controlled study of interferon beta-1a in relapsing/remitting multiple sclerosis. *Lancet* 1998; **352**: 1498–504.

27. PRISMS Study Group and the University of British Columbia MS/MRI Analysis Group. PRISMS-4: Long-term efficacy of interferon-beta-1a in relapsing MS. *Neurology* 2001; **56**: 1628–36.

28. Hawker K, O'Connor P, Freedman MS, *et al.* Rituximab in patients with primary progressive multiple sclerosis: Results of a randomized double-blind placebo-controlled multicenter trial. *Ann Neurol* 2009; **66**: 460–71.

29. Wolinsky JS, Narayana PA, O'Connor P, *et al.* Glatiramer acetate in primary progressive multiple sclerosis: Results of a multinational, multicenter, double-blind, placebo-controlled trial. *Ann Neurol* 2007; **61**: 14–24.

30. Montalban X. Overview of European pilot study of interferon beta-1b in primary progressive multiple sclerosis. *Mult Scler* 2004; **10** (Suppl 1): S62; discussion 62–4.

31. Leary SM, Miller DH, Stevenson VL, *et al.* Interferon beta-1a in primary progressive MS: An exploratory, randomized, controlled trial. *Neurology* 2003; **60**: 44–51.

32. Rammohan KW, Rosenberg JH, Lynn DJ, *et al.* Efficacy and safety of modafinil (provigil) for the treatment of fatigue in multiple sclerosis: A two centre phase 2 study. *J Neurol Neurosurg Psychiatry* 2002; **72**: 179–83.

33. Rice GP, Filippi M and Comi G. Cladribine and progressive MS: Clinical and MRI outcomes of a multicenter controlled trial. Cladribine MRI Study Group. *Neurology* 2000; **54**: 1145–55.

34. Filippi M, Rovaris M, Iannucci G, *et al.* Whole brain volume changes in patients with progressive MS treated with cladribine. *Neurology* 2000; **55**: 1714–8.

35. Banwell B, Ghezzi A, Bar-Or A, *et al.* Multiple sclerosis in children: Clinical diagnosis, therapeutic strategies, and future directions. *Lancet Neurol* 2007; **6**: 887–902.

36. Interferon beta-1b is effective in relapsing-remitting multiple sclerosis. I. clinical results of a multicenter, randomized, double-blind, placebo-controlled trial. The IFNB Multiple Sclerosis Study Group. *Neurology* 1993; **43**: 655–61.

37. Rudick RA, Stuart WH, Calabresi PA, *et al.* Natalizumab plus interferon beta-1a for relapsing multiple sclerosis. *N Engl J Med* 2006; **354**: 911–23.

38. Kremenchutzky M, Rice GP, Baskerville J, *et al.* The natural history of multiple sclerosis: A geographically based study 9: Observations on the progressive phase of the disease. *Brain* 2006; **129**: 584–94.

39. Kurtzke JF. Rating neurologic impairment in multiple sclerosis: An expanded disability status scale (EDSS). *Neurology* 1983; **33**: 1444–52.

40. Ebers GC, Heigenhauser L, Daumer M, *et al.* Disability as an outcome in MS clinical trials. *Neurology* 2008; **71**: 624–31.

41. Rudick RA, Lee J, Cutter GR, *et al.* Significance of disability progression in a clinical trial in relapsing-remitting multiple sclerosis: Eight-year follow-up. *Arch Neurol* 2010; **67**: 1329–35.

42. Rudick R, Antel J, Confavreux C, *et al.* Recommendations from the national multiple sclerosis society clinical outcomes assessment task force. *Ann Neurol* 1997; **42**: 379–82.

43. Fox RJ, Lee JC, and Rudick RA. Optimal reference population for the multiple sclerosis functional composite. *Mult Scler* 2007; **13**: 909–14.

44. Rudick RA, Polman CH, Cohen JA, *et al.* Assessing disability progression with the multiple sclerosis functional composite. *Mult Scler* 2009; **15**: 984–97.

45. Rao SM, Leo GJ, Bernardin L, *et al.* Cognitive dysfunction in multiple sclerosis. I. Frequency, patterns, and prediction. *Neurology* 1991; **41**: 685–91.

46. Cohen JA, Rudick RA, editors. *Multiple Sclerosis Therapeutics*. 3rd ed. London, UK, Informa Health care. 2007.

47. Benedict RH, Cookfair D, Gavett R, *et al.* Validity of the minimal assessment of cognitive function in multiple sclerosis (MACFIMS). *J Int Neuropsychol Soc* 2006; **12**: 549–58.

48. Rudick RA and Miller DM. Health-related quality of life in multiple sclerosis: Current evidence, measurement and effects of disease severity and treatment. *CNS Drugs* 2008; **22**: 827–39.

49. Rudick RA, Miller D, Hass S, *et al.* Health-related quality of life in multiple sclerosis: Effects of natalizumab. *Ann Neurol* 2007; **62**: 335–46.

50. Li DK and Paty DW. Magnetic resonance imaging results of the PRISMS trial: A randomized, double-blind, placebo-controlled study of interferon-beta1a in relapsing-remitting multiple sclerosis. *Ann Neurol* 1999; **46**: 197–206.

51. Barkhof F. MRI in multiple sclerosis: Correlation with expanded disability status scale (EDSS). *Mult Scler* 1999; **5**: 283–6.

52. Fisher E, Rudick RA, Cutter G, *et al.* Relationship between brain atrophy and disability: An 8-year follow-up study of multiple sclerosis patients. *Mult Scler* 2000; **6**: 373–7.

53. Rudick RA, Lee JC, Simon J, *et al.* Significance of T2 lesions in multiple sclerosis: A 13-year longitudinal study. *Ann Neurol* 2006; **60**: 236–42.

54. van Walderveen MA, Kamphorst W, Scheltens P, *et al.* Histopathologic correlate of hypointense lesions on T1-weighted spin-echo MRI in multiple sclerosis. *Neurology* 1998; **50**: 1282–8.

55. van den Elskamp IJ, Lembcke J, *et al.* Persistent T1 hypointensity as an MRI marker for treatment efficacy in multiple sclerosis. *Mult Scler* 2008; **14**: 764–9.

56. Rudick RA, Fisher E, Lee JC, *et al.* Use of the brain parenchymal fraction to measure whole brain atrophy in relapsing-remitting MS. Multiple Sclerosis Collaborative Research Group. *Neurology* 1999; **53**: 1698–704.

57. Smith SM, Zhang Y, Jenkinson M, *et al.* Accurate, robust, and automated longitudinal and cross-sectional brain change analysis. *Neuroimage* 2002; **17**: 479–89.

58. Fisher E, Rudick RA, Simon JH, *et al.* Eight-year follow-up study of brain atrophy in patients with MS. *Neurology* 2002; **59**: 1412–20.

59. Sormani MP, Bonzano L, Roccatagliata L, *et al.* Magnetic resonance imaging as a potential surrogate for relapses in multiple sclerosis: A meta-analytic approach. *Ann Neurol* 2009; **65**: 268–75.

60. Filippi M. Multiple sclerosis, part II: Nonconventional MRI techniques. Preface. *Neuroimaging Clin N Am* 2009; **19**: xiii–xiv.

61. Balcer LJ, Baier ML, Pelak VS, *et al.* New low-contrast vision charts: Reliability and test characteristics in patients with multiple sclerosis. *Mult Scler* 2000; **6**: 163–71.

62. Fisher JB, Jacobs DA, Markowitz CE, *et al.* Relation of visual function to retinal nerve fiber layer thickness in multiple sclerosis. *Ophthalmology* 2006; **113**: 324–32.

63. O'Connor P, Filippi M, Arnason B, *et al.* 250 microg or 500 microg interferon beta-1b versus 20 mg glatiramer acetate in relapsing-remitting multiple sclerosis: A prospective, randomised, multicentre study. *Lancet Neurol* 2009; **8**: 889–97.

64. Polman CH, Reingold SC, Barkhof F, *et al.* Ethics of placebo-controlled clinical trials in multiple sclerosis: A reassessment. *Neurology* 2008; **70**: 1134–40.

65. Cohen JA, Imrey PB, Calabresi PA, *et al.* Results of the avonex combination trial (ACT) in relapsing-remitting MS. *Neurology* 2009; **72**: 535–41.

66. Langer-Gould A, Atlas SW, Green AJ, *et al.* Progressive multifocal leukoencephalopathy in a patient treated with natalizumab. *N Engl J Med* 2005; **353**: 375–81.

67. Cohen JA, Barkhof F, Comi G, *et al.* Oral fingolimod or intramuscular interferon for relapsing multiple sclerosis. *N Engl J Med* 2010; **362**: 402–15.

68. Kappos L, Radue EW, O'Connor P, *et al.* A placebo-controlled trial of oral fingolimod in relapsing multiple sclerosis. *N Engl J Med* 2010; **362**: 387–401.

69. Giovannoni G, Comi G, Cook S, *et al.* A placebo-controlled trial of oral cladribine for relapsing multiple sclerosis. *N Engl J Med* 2010; **362**: 416–26.

70. Martinelli V. *J Neurol Sci* 2009; **30**: S167–70.

71. Kappos L, Antel J, Comi G, *et al.* Oral fingolimod (FTY720) for relapsing multiple sclerosis. *N Engl J Med* 2006; **355**: 1124–40.

72. Aban IB, Wolfe GI, Cutter GR, *et al.* The MGTX experience: Challenges in planning and executing an international, multicenter clinical trial. *J Neuroimmunol* 2008; **201–202**: 80–4.

73. Duning T, Kloska S, Steinstrater O, *et al.* Dehydration confounds the assessment of brain atrophy. *Neurology* 2005; **64**: 548–50.

74. Fox RJ, Fisher E, Tkach J, *et al.* Brain atrophy and magnetization transfer ratio following methylprednisolone in multiple sclerosis: Short-term changes and long-term implications. *Mult Scler* 2005; **11**: 140–5.

75. Chen JT, Collins DL, Atkins HL, *et al.* Brain atrophy after immunoablation and stem cell transplantation in multiple sclerosis. *Neurology* 2006; **66**: 1935–7.

76. Bermel RA and Bakshi R. The measurement and clinical relevance of brain atrophy in multiple sclerosis. *Lancet Neurol* 2006; **5**: 158–70.

77. Sormani MP, Rovaris M, Valsasina P, *et al.* Measurement error of two different techniques for brain atrophy assessment in multiple sclerosis. *Neurology* 2004; **62**: 1432–4.

78. Miller DH, Soon D, Fernando KT, *et al.* MRI outcomes in a placebo-controlled trial of natalizumab in relapsing MS. *Neurology* 2007; **68**: 1390–401.

79. Paolillo A, Coles AJ, Molyneux PD, *et al.* Quantitative MRI in patients with secondary progressive MS treated

with monoclonal antibody campath 1H. *Neurology* 1999; **53**: 751–7.

80. Barkhof F, Calabresi PA, Miller DH, *et al.* Imaging outcomes for neuroprotection and repair in multiple sclerosis trials. *Nat Rev Neurol* 2009; **5**: 256–66.

81. Ludwin SK. The pathogenesis of multiple sclerosis: Relating human pathology to experimental studies. *J Neuropathol Exp Neurol* 2006; **65**: 305–18.

82. Fisher E, Lee JC, Nakamura K, *et al.* Gray matter atrophy in multiple sclerosis: A longitudinal study. *Ann Neurol* 2008; **64**: 255–65.

83. Filippi M, Campi A, Dousset V, *et al.* A magnetization transfer imaging study of normal-appearing white matter in multiple sclerosis. *Neurology* 1995; **45**: 478–82.

84. Geurts JJ, Pouwels PJ, Uitdehaag BM, *et al.* Intracortical lesions in multiple sclerosis: Improved detection with 3D double inversion-recovery MR imaging. *Radiology* 2005; **236**: 254–60.

Chapter

24

Amyotrophic lateral sclerosis

Nazem Atassi, David Schoenfeld, and Merit Cudkowicz

Introduction

Amyotrophic lateral sclerosis (ALS) is a neurodegenerative disorder characterized by progressive muscle weakness that eventually affects respiratory muscles and causes death. There is a strong unmet need for development of treatments for people with ALS. In the past 10–15 years there has been an exponential growth in clinical trials in ALS [1]. Much has been learned from these studies about preclinical models and clinical trial design and conduct in ALS. The complexities of ALS still pose major challenges in translating progress in understanding disease mechanisms into effective novel therapies for people with ALS. The development of ALS therapeutics has followed a traditional discovery path with identification of potential targets from a variety of in vitro and in vivo preclinical models. The predictability of these preclinical tools for determination of efficacy in humans with ALS is not yet known. Once a candidate therapy has been identified, investigators are faced with additional challenges to identify compound bioavailability, dosing and pharmacodynamic properties and the optimal clinical trial design. Preclinical disease models, biomarkers, clinical trial design options, and challenges to the conduct of ALS clinical trials are discussed in this chapter.

Biological basis for interventions

People with ALS develop progressive muscle weakness, atrophy and spasticity, reflecting loss of lower motor neurons (LMNs) and upper motor neurons (UMNs) in the brain and spinal cord. No treatment prevents, halts or reverses the disease, although a small delay in mortality occurs with the drug riluzole [2]. While the majority of ALS cases are sporadic, about 10% of cases are familial and of these, 30% arise due to a hexanucleotide repeat expansion on chormosome 9 and 25% arise due to mutations in the gene encoding SOD1 [3, 4].

Therapeutic targets

The precise cause of selective motor neuron death in ALS is unknown. Many pathogenetic mechanisms have been proposed such as excitotoxicity, oxidative damage, mutant proteins, immune dysregulation, mitochondrial dysfunction, and growth factors (Table 24.1) [5, 6]. Advances in understanding the biology of motor neuron death in ALS has led to more than 32 compounds being tested in phase 2/3 clinical trials in ALS during the past 15 years (Table 24.1). The recent discovery of new ALS genes has expanded our understanding of the role of aberrant RNA metabolism in the pathogenesis of both familial and sporadic ALS.

Pre-clinical disease models

Valid disease models are critical to better understand disease pathogenesis and to the development of new treatments for ALS. A wide range of in vitro and in vivo models are available to both study disease biology and screen therapeutic compounds (Table 24.2). The G93A SOD1 mouse is used routinely as an in vivo model for ALS. Recently, skin fibroblasts from people with ALS were used to produce induced pluripotent stem cells (iPS) that are capable of differentiating into motor neurons and glia [7]. These recent advances in stem cell technology offer potential motor neuron models of sporadic ALS that can help understand disease pathogenesis and screen new drugs.

Challenges in translation from models to people

Most available cell and mouse models are based on the SOD1 mutation that is present in only about 2% of ALS patients. Currently, mice carrying 23 copies of the human G93A SOD1 transgene are considered the

---

Clinical Trials in Neurology, ed. Bernard Ravina, Jeffrey Cummings, Michael P. McDermott, and R. Michael Poole. Published by Cambridge University Press. © Cambridge University Press 2012.

Table 24.1 Examples of past ALS clinical trials and their proposed primary targets

Targeted pathway	ALS clinical trials
Excitotoxicity	Riluzole, gabapentin, topiramate, lamotrigine, dextromethorphan, celecoxib, talampanel Ceftriaxone*
Oxidative damage	Vitamin E, glutathione, N-acetylcysteine, selegiline,
Immunoregulation	Interferon β1a, ganglioside, cyclophosphamide, intravenous immunoglobulin, celecoxib, total lymphoid irradiation
Energy & mitochondria	Creatine monohydrate*, coenzyme Q10, branched chain amino acids, L-threonine, KNS-760704*, Olesoxime
Growth factors	Ciliary neurotrophic factor, brain-derived neurotrophic factor, thyrotropin releasing hormone [47], growth hormone, insulin-like growth factor [48], xaliproden, VEGF* (SB509 and sNN0029)
Apoptosis	Omigapil (TCH346), minocycline, pentoxifylline, tamoxifen*
Protein aggregation	Arimoclomol
Decrease SOD1 levels	ISIS-333611*, pyrimethamine
Stem cell replacement	Neural stem*

* Active trial.

Table 24.2 Common pre-clinical disease models

In vitro

1. Mature cells	• Organotypic spinal cord cultures from post-natal rats
	• NSC34 and HeLa cell lines expressing mutant SOD1
	• Glutamate excitotoxicity models
2. Embryonic cells	• Organotypic slice cultures from wild type/G93A embryonic spinal cords
	• Purified human motor neurons and astrocytes from human embryonic spinal cord anterior horns
	• Motor neurons from mice embryonic stem cells (ESCs)
	• Motor neurons from human ESCs and pluripotent cells
3. Neuroblastoma cell lines	

In vivo

1. Rodent models:	• Transgenic motor neuron disease rodent models: G93A SOD1, G85R SOD1, G37R SOD1 rodents, Dynamitin over-expression model
	• VEGF mouse model
	• PMN, Wobbler, HCSMA mouse models
2. Zebra fish models	

standard model for ALS therapeutic studies. While the G93A SOD1 is an invaluable tool to test proof of concept that the proposed therapy has the desired biological activity, this mouse model has several limitations [8]. Until there are more therapies that are effective in people, it is not possible to know whether the currently available preclinical models are valid screening tools.

Goals of interventions

Slow disease progression

Most therapeutic targets and preclinical disease models discussed in this chapter are focused on modifying disease progression. The primary goals of most clinical trials in ALS are to slow disease progression as measured either by function or survival. Functional scales include measures of strength, pulmonary function, and a questionnaire called the ALS functional rating scale-revised (ALSFRS-R) [9].

Treat ALS-related symptoms

In addition to muscle weakness, people with ALS suffer from many other ALS-related symptoms. Improving ALS symptomatic management is as important to ALS patients and their caregivers as disease modifying treatments. The improvement in survival in people with ALS seen in the past 10 years is likely secondary to improved multidisciplinary care and symptomatic treatments of dyspnea and dysphagia such as non-invasive ventilation and gastrostomy [10]. There have been very few studies to determine best approaches to manage most of the symptoms of ALS. This is an unmet need and one for which it is difficult to find funding.

Study population

Demographics

The incidence of ALS is approximately 2/100 000/year [11]. Fifty percent of people with ALS die within 3 years of onset of symptoms and 90% die within 5 years [12]. Variability in rate of disease progression and symptom progression is high among people with ALS. Age and gender are the only risk factors repeatedly documented in epidemiological studies [13].

Eligibility in ALS clinical trials

The goal of requiring specific eligibility criteria for subjects to enter ALS clinical trials is to achieve the balance between confidence of the diagnosis and early disease enrollment.

The wide variety of presenting symptoms in ALS makes absolute diagnosis difficult early in disease course and ALS diagnosis is often delayed for approximately 12 months after symptom onset [14]. The World Federation of Neurology Subcommittee on Motor Neuron Disease reached consensus on the criteria for the diagnosis of ALS in 1994 and these were revised in 2000 [15].

Clinical trials in ALS require a certain degree of certainty about the diagnosis based on the El Escorial diagnostic criteria. Clinical trials to assess efficacy of an intervention (phase 2 or 3) often enroll people early in the disease course. This would include people classified as possible, probable or definite by El Escorial criteria, who have a forced vital capacity above 60 or 70% of predicted normal and disease duration less than 2 or 3 years. The reasons for these criteria include wanting to treat people as early as possible in their disease course, minimizing patient to patient variability in rate of disease progression, and for studies whose primary outcome measure is function, ensuring that people can complete the study. Early phase safety and dosage finding studies (phase 1 or 2a) often include people with more advanced disease. There are trial-specific eligibility criteria that depend on the aims and the primary outcome measures of the trial. For example, trials of

drugs targeting SOD1 protein, such as ISIS-333116 and Arimoclomol, require genetic confirmation of SOD1 familial ALS.

Disease heterogeneity

Although ALS by definition involves both UMN and LMN dysfunction, some people have apparently only LMN (progressive muscular atrophy) or only UMN (primary lateral sclerosis) involvement which can be associated with prolonged survival [16]. Similarly, phenotypes that predominantly affect certain body areas (arm, leg, or bulbar) can be associated with different disease progression and survival. In addition, different SOD1 mutations are associated with different disease phenotypes and rates of progression. As ALS is characterized by marked phenotypic heterogeneity, variations in therapeutic response might be an important confounding factor in clinical trials which drives the need for larger sample size.

Statistical challenges because of disease heterogeneity

Most phase 2 or 3 efficacy clinical trials in ALS have not addressed phenotypic or genotypic heterogeneity. Currently there is one trial which is restricted to patients with familial ALS from genetic mutations in SOD1 mutations that are associated with a rapid rate of progression. The hope is that because the rate of disease progression is rapid and more homogeneous in this population of patients, determination of efficacy can be made with a smaller number of participants.

The question about whether to combine genotypes and phenotypes or to separate them is always problematic. In the 1960s cancer clinical trials for solid tumors often tested agents on many different tumor types. It was only after agents were targeted to specific tumors that progress began to be made. Currently cancer therapy is very specifically targeted to tumor pathology. As more is learned about the biology behind the different phenotypic forms of ALS, the field will learn whether this approach is feasible for ALS.

Measurement tools in ALS

One of the most essential steps in clinical trial design is choosing the outcome measure. The ideal outcome measure for an ALS clinical trial is sensitive to disease progression, clinically meaningful, and easy to administer even in advanced disease when patients are not able to come to clinic.

Clinical outcome measures

Survival

Survival is the gold standard primary endpoint for ALS trials. However, trials using survival as an outcome measure require prolonged durations (typically 18 months or more) and typically 400 people per arm. Survival is influenced by the individual's rate of disease progression, site of onset, nutrition status, use of riluzole, invasive and non-invasive ventilation, and gastrostomy. The occasional use of permanent assisted ventilation (PAV) by ALS patients confounds survival as a clinical trial endpoint since survival can be considerably extended by PAV [17]. At best this adds variation to a treatment comparison of mortality at worse there might be a treatment effect on the decision to start PAV. Sometimes the outcome measure is the time to death or the initiation of PAV. This also has difficulties as the decision about when to start PAV, in patients who want it, may be affected by treatment. There is currently no validated surrogate marker for survival. Several other outcome measures have been used in various ALS clinical trials (Table 24.3).

Vital capacity

Vital capacity (VC) is used in most ALS clinical trials as marker of respiratory muscle weakness. It is correlated with survival [18]. The major limitation of VC use is that patients with bulbar weakness cannot make a good seal around the mouth piece resulting in increased measurement variability. Time to a drop in VC has been used as a way to address this limitation (NCT00542412). One of the outcome measures in the current clinical trial of Arimoclomol in familial ALS is forced expiratory volume (FEV-6), a new measure that enables patients to reliably measure their respiratory status at home (NCT00706147).

Muscle strength

Measuring the decline in muscle strength using hand-held dynamometry, the Tufts quantitative neuromuscular examination (TQNE) or manual muscle testing, can be easily performed. It takes approximately 45 minutes to administer the TQNE, it requires expensive equipment and is not practical for home visits. In the clinical trial of topiramate in ALS, a significant difference in muscle strength was not associated with

excess mortality [19]. Manual muscle testing on the other hand, offers a faster and more portable method of muscle strength measurement that has comparable variability to the TQNE. The disadvantages of this technique are that grading is qualitative and it may be insensitive to small changes. A more promising technique uses a hand held dynamometer to test isometric strength of multiple muscles [20]. This technique is portable, fast, and has been validated against TQNE [21]. It been used in previous ALS clinical trials and is one of the outcome measures in the trial of ceftriaxone in ALS (NCT00349622). Muscle weakness is the major ALS symptom and it is important to include it in efficacy trials.

Motor unit number estimates [22]

Motor unit number estimates (MUNE) is an electrophysiological measure of lower motor neuron loss. It uses surface electromyography techniques to assess the progress of motor neuron loss and consequent re-enervation of denerved muscle fibers by surviving neurons. This measure can be reliably performed in a multi-center trial and yields results that show a consistent decline of MUNE overtime [23]. One of the advantages of MUNE is that it is one of the closest measures to disease pathology. It requires formal electrophysiology training and it takes approximately 30 minutes to compete. It might be a good outcome measure for a small phase 2, proof of concept, ALS clinical trial. Currently, there is an ongoing longitudinal study of MUNE as a potential outcome measure in ALS.

Patient-reported outcome measures

ALS Functional Rating Scale-Revised

The ALS Functional Rating Scale-Revised (ALSFRS-R) is widely used as a primary or secondary outcome measure in ALS clinical trials. It is an ordinal scale (0–4) used to determine patients' assessment of their capability and independence in 12 functional activities questions (total score of 48). It can be administered quickly (five minutes) in person or over the phone [24] and is also validated for administration from the caregiver [25]. Questions in ALSFRS-R cover four domains: gross motor, fine motor, swallowing, and breathing. The ALSFRS-R rate of decline was approximately 0.92 units per month with a standard error of 0.08 in the placebo arm of the trial of topiramate in ALS [19].

Table 24.3 Outcome measures used in past ALS clinical trials

Therapy	Primary outcome measure
Riluzole	Survival & ALSFRS
Gabapentin	MVIC
Topiramate	MVIC
Lamotrigine	Clinical scores (age of onset, bulbar and respiratory involvement, ambulation and functional disability) Functional decline (Norris, Plaitakis and Bulbar scales)
Dextromethorphan	Survival
Talampanel	ALSFRS-R
Ciliary neurotrophic factor	- Isometric muscle dynamometry - Combination of MVIC & VC
Insulin-like growth factor-1	Appel ALS score
Brain-derived neurotrophic factor	VC & Survival
Thyrotropin releasing hormone	- Tufts quantitative neuromuscular exam - Muscle strength
Xaliproden	Survival
Vitamin E	- Modified Norris limb scale - Survival
N-acetyl-L-cysteine	Survival
Selegeline	Appel ALS total score
Coenzyme Q10	MVIC
Creatine	- Survival - MVIC
Branched chain amino acids	- Muscle strength, maximal isometric muscle torque - Disability scales
Nimodipine	Isometric muscle strength
Verapamil	VC and limb megascores
TCH346	ALSFRS-R
Pentoxifylline	Survival
Minocycline	Safety/tolerability measures ALSFRS-R
Sodium phenylbutyrate	Safety and tolerability
Cyclophosphamide	Neurological function score
Bovine gangliosides	Neuromuscular function Various objective tests of muscle strength
Interferon beta (IFβ1a)	Non self supporting status (Medical Research Council Scale, Norris Scale, Bulbar scores)
Glutathione	Manual muscle testing
Oxandrolone	MVIC
Tamoxifen	Safety, MVIC
Lithium	Survival
Ceftriaxone	Survival
Arimoclomol in familial ALS	ALSFRS-R and survival
KNS-760704	ALSFRS-R and survival
ISIS-333611	Safety

ALSFRS-R: ALS functional rating scale-revised; MVIC: maximum voluntary isometric contraction; VC: vital capacity.

Appel rating scale

The Appel rating scale includes both subjective and objective assessments of bulbar, respiratory function, muscle strength, and upper and lower extremity function [26]. Appel scores range from 30 points (healthy) to 164 (maximum impairment).

ALS specific quality of life

Quality of life in ALS patients is not easily determined by standard scales, such as SF-36, that rely mainly on physical function as indicator of quality of life. The ALS specific quality of life (ALSSQOL) is a self-administered questionnaire that was developed, tested and validated to measure quality of life in ALS patients. It is usually used as a secondary outcome measure in ALS clinical trials [27]. The scale consists of 59 questions, each rated on a 1–10 scale, that ask about the severity of the symptoms of ALS, mood, affect, intimacy, and social issues.

Biomarkers

There are currently no reliable blood, cerebrospinal fluid or imaging biomarkers that track disease progression. The availability of biomarkers that were disease relevant and were related to disease progression could potentially greatly accelerate therapy in drug development. Establishing multi-center polling of a large number of blood, CSF and tissue samples is essential for biomarker discovery. In addition to the above mentioned disease-related biomarkers, there are biomarkers that are drug-specific. Measuring EAAT2 activity in olfactory nerve ending during the trial of ceftriaxone in ALS is one example of a drug-specific biomarker that tracks pharmacodynamic activity. Another example is measuring histone acetylation levels to determine the ideal dosage of sodium phenylbutyrate in a phase 2 study in ALS [28]. Neuroimaging has proved to be an invaluable biomarker for drug discovery in multiple sclerosis and Alzheimer's disease trials, and is a promising tool in ALS (reviewed in [29]).

Principles of statistics and outcome measures in ALS clinical trials

The statistical techniques used in ALS clinical trials depend on the outcome measure. The proportional hazard regression model is often used to analyze time to death or time to death or PAV; these trials need to be large because the mortality in a clinical trial population is about 15–20% per year. For instance to detect a 50% improvement would require approximately 600 patients followed for 2 years. The length of follow-up becomes a problem as patients tend to stop therapy early in ALS trials, which reduces the power of a trial that requires long follow-up.

Random effects models are used to analyze longitudinal measures such as vital capacity, ALSFRS-R, muscle strength, and MUNE. The most common primary efficacy measure is ALSFRS-R because it can be assessed by telephone if the patient is unable to travel to the clinic [24]. The random effects model specifies that each patient has a linear trajectory in the outcome measure. Their actual measurements will be normally distributed about this trajectory and the trajectories themselves will have normally distributed slopes and intercepts. The primary statistical hypothesis is that the mean slope of these trajectories is different in the active treatment group than it is in the placebo group. This model can be extended to situations where the trajectories are non-linear, where there are important covariates, and where the distributions are not normal.

Trials that use longitudinal outcomes tend to be smaller than trials focused on mortality, although they still are fairly large due to the variability in the rate of patient progression. For instance the standard deviation of the slope of ALSFRS-R is approximately 0.83 units/month. This implies that 11% of the patients will actually improve on placebo. The standard deviation around the trajectory is 2/units per month but the effect of this can be minimized by taking enough measurements.

The trial of lithium in ALS has used time to progression as an efficacy measure. Progression was defined as a 6 point drop in ALSFRS-R, death, or PAV. The advantage of this endpoint is that it shortened the trial for rapidly progressing patients on placebo and allowed them to switch to active treatment. The problem with this endpoint is that it is not as powerful as using the ALSFRS-R measurements themselves. One compromise is to use the design but to use a random effects model in the analysis.

Another proposal is to combine a longitudinal outcome with mortality using a rank-based approach which compares time to death when patients die and the last value of their longitudinal endpoint when they survive [30, 31].

Statistical challenges of ALS outcome measures

The largest challenge in clinical trials that use ALSFRS-R or other longitudinal outcomes measures is missing data.

Participants may drop out of the trial and not provide data on the outcome measure. Other patients die during the trial. It is not clear how to handle these missing data statistically. It appears that the usual random effects model is fairly robust to this missingness. Alternatives where the missingness process is explicitly modeled appear to give similar results. Methods that combine mortality and ALSFRS-R do not have this problem but have somewhat less power than random effects models unless there is a large effect on mortality that is independent of the relationship of mortality and ALSFRS-R.

Trial designs

ALS trial designs

Phase 1 trials in ALS

Phase 1 trials are designed to learn the pharmacokinetics, tolerable dosage ranges, and initial safety of single and multiple doses of the drug under investigation in humans. Approaches in ALS are similar to those used in other neurological and non-neurological disorders.

Phase 2 trial designs

Phase 2 trials in ALS usually enroll between 60 and 400 participants and trial duration is usually less than 12 months. The main purpose of phase 2 trials in ALS is to gather information about drug's biological activity (pharmacodynamics), dosage range and schedule, tolerability, side effects, and preliminary efficacy. This information will help guide the decision about whether to proceed to and how to best design a phase 3 trial [32].

Traditional phase 2 trials in ALS are not focused on evaluating efficacy. In addition to toxicity and safety information, it is useful to incorporate pharmacodynamic markers, predictive markers for therapeutic response (proof-of-concept), and explore a range of dosages.

Phase 2 or proof-of-concept designs are challenging in ALS because there is no short-term sensitive biomarker that can predict long-term therapeutic efficacy. Clinical trials that use available functional outcome measures such as ALSFRS-R, typically require approximately 200 subjects per arm and at least 9 months to have the statistical power to identify a treatment effect. To overcome these design challenges, other types of phase 2 designs are sometimes employed such as futility design, multi-arm selection design, and lead-in design [32, 33].

Futility design

The main purpose of futility design studies in ALS is to eliminate drugs that are not worthy of proceeding to phase 3 trials (discussed in Chapter 8). Two futility studies have been performed in ALS [34, 35] studying coenzyme Q10, and the combination of creatine and minocycline and creatine and celecoxib.

Multi-arm selection design

The purpose of selection designs is to use smaller sample sizes to select a superior treatment or dosage to move forward to a phase 3 trial (discussed in Chapter 8). This approach is particularly useful when there are several candidate treatments or dosages. For example, two doses of CoQ10 were compared and the winner was selected to be compared to placebo in a futility analysis [36] and in another trial, two drug combinations were compared [35].

Lead-in design

The lead-in design provides historical data about each patient prior to treatment onset hoping to reduce the variance of the outcome measure which will allow for smaller sample size. The main concerns of this design are the delay of treatment onset, enrollment difficulties, and non-linearity of the outcome measure. There are two approaches to analyzing these trials depending on whether you assume that the slope of the placebo group will not change after treatment is initiated. With this assumption the slope of the ALSFRS-R lead-in phase serves as a control for the treatment phase and augments the placebo sample size. This assumption has become suspect because in two recent ALS clinical trials (TCH346 and Minocycline), the slope of ALSFRS-R of the placebo arm changed after treatment had started [37, 38]. Without this assumption the slope of ALSFRS-R in the lead in phase is used as a prognostic covariate. With the latter analysis, the power advantage of a lead-in design is small because the lead-in phase is not as prognostic as one would expect. [32].

Phase 3 trial designs in ALS

Phase 3 trials are usually performed after successfully completing a phase 2 trial that provided some evidence of drug activity. A placebo arm is required in phase 3 trials and multiple dosages are sometimes desired. Phase 3 trials need to have adequate power to detect a clinical benefit if it is truly present. The primary outcome measure should be clinically meaningful and the goal of these studies is to conclusively demonstrate efficacy or lack of efficacy, in addition to long-term safety. Phase 3 trials in ALS need to be powered according to the primary outcome measure used in the trial. For example, approximately 200–250 subjects per arm followed for 9–12 months if ALSFRS-R is the primary outcome measure, and 400 subjects per arm followed for 18 months if survival is chosen to be the primary outcome measure. Traditionally phase 3 trials in ALS looked at survival as the primary endpoint; however, more recent phase 3 trials started using functional outcome measures such as ALSFRS-R as the primary endpoint in order to conduct smaller, shorter, and more efficient trials with fewer drop outs.

Adaptive designs

Adaptive design trials have been recently tried in ALS as a way to conserve on sample size, trial duration, and resources (see Chapter 9). The trials of CoQ10 and more recently the trial of ceftriaxone in ALS are examples of seamless adaptive trial designs using the first stage to determine the best dosage to be used in an efficacy later stage [34, 39]

Challenges in clinical trial design

Dosage selection

Picking the appropriate dosage and route of administration in humans is one of the most challenging aspects of drug development. Determining dosage response and maximum tolerated dosage can be costly but should be key components in phase 2/3 ALS trials. The phase 2/3 randomized trial of TCH347 [37] and the second study of riluzole [40] are examples of well-conducted ALS clinical trials that explored a broad range of dosages. Without determining the ideal therapeutic dosages, it is difficult to interpret the results of negative clinical trials which may result in erroneous rejection of drugs and scientific hypotheses because of a 'failed' trial.

Sample size

Sample size requirements vary based on the primary outcome measure and expected effect size. For example, 1200 participants are needed to demonstrate a 50% change in median survival during a 1 year follow up trial (90% power and alpha of 0.05), whereas only 200 participants are needed to show a 40% change in ALSFRS-R. However, large changes in ALSFRS-R may not mean similar large changes in survival. Many past ALS trials were insufficiently powered including trials of dexomethorphan ($n = 45$), vitamin E ($n = 104$), nimodipine ($n = 87$), verapamil ($n = 72$), and creatine, 5g ($n = 104$).

Drug interactions

It is very important to determine experimental drug interactions with riluzole and other commonly used symptomatic treatments. An experimental drug, such as minocycline, that can potentially increase riluzole levels may increase riluzole side effects and may also negatively affect ALSFRS-R scores [41]. Thus, drug interactions can cause apparent worsening of functional decline or mask positive effects of the experimental drug.

Standards for efficacy and special safety concerns

Efficacy in Phase 2/3 ALS trials (Riluzole is the new placebo)

Riluzole is the only FDA-approved treatment for ALS. In the US, only about 60% of people with ALS use riluzole because of its high cost relative to its minimal expected clinical benefit. Most ALS trials in the US enroll people regardless of their riluzole use and stratified enrollment based on riluzole use is usually implemented to balance treatment groups. Riluzole is more commonly used in Europe and Canada, subsequently; most ALS trials in Europe and Canada are considered 'add-on' trials.

Riluzole treatment during an ALS clinical trial potentially sets a higher bar for survival efficacy of the new experimental drugs. For example, a new investigational drug for ALS has to prolong median survival for at least 6 months which translates to a 30% decrease in ALSFRS-R rate of decline in a 12 month trial of more than 350 subjects.

Achieving balance between feasibility of high-cost large clinical trials in a rare disease like ALS is a major challenge.

Methods and standards of monitoring safety in ALS clinical trials

As ALS is a devastating disease the side effects of new treatments are usually acceptable as long as these treatments are effective. Therefore, the safety threshold in ALS clinical trials is relatively high and is comparable to cancer trials, and safety concerns in ALS trials are usually specific to the experimental treatment. High-risk phase 1 and all phase 2/ 3 ALS clinical trials typically have a Data Safety Monitoring Board (DSMB), that evaluates whether the clinical trial should continue as planned, requires modifications to the protocol, or should terminate early because of safety or toxicity concerns or convincing evidence of efficacy or futility. The recent trial of lithium (NCT00818389) is an example of an ALS trial that stopped early for futility.

Clinical trial conduct in ALS

Enrollment

The percentage of eligible people with ALS that enroll in trials is surprisingly small. In a recent poll of neurologists involved in ALS clinical research, average enrollment in ALS trials was 25% and highly variable between different sites. In a literature review of 36 completed clinical trials in ALS, the average enrollment rate was 2.2 participants/site/month [42]. Slow enrolling trials are more resource intensive and may end prematurely and without an answer due to insufficient power. Off-label use of study medication significantly delayed enrollment for topiramate, minocycline, and celecoxib clinical trials. Low enrollment rate is not unique to ALS trials but it has a bigger impact in ALS trials because it is an orphan disease. Recently, low enrollment has resulted in recent changes in trial design and eligibility criteria that allow early enrollment in more efficient trials.

Study retention

The dropout rate of past ALS clinical trials was high, particularly in trials of longer duration or with significant adverse events. With intent-to-treat (ITT) analyses, high dropout rates result in the dilution of the observed benefits of the new therapy. For longitudinal endpoints such as ALSFRS it can compromise the validity of the trial because of the assumption that patients who remain are no different from those who drop out. For example, in the 12- month trial of topiramate in ALS, 23% of the participants did not complete the trial because of subject's choice, disease progression, adverse events, and difficulty travelling [20]. Conducting shorter trials with fewer visits and offering home visits or travel compensation may ease the burden on the participants and improve study retention.

Diagnostic accuracy

Most ALS clinical trials require confirmed diagnosis and good respiratory function as part of the eligibility criteria. Amyotrophic lateral sclerosis is mainly a clinical diagnosis that follows the El Escorial criteria which is based on different degrees of certainty about

the diagnosis. The inclusion criteria of most ALS trials require the presence of both UMN and LMN dysfunction in multiple body segments to be confident about the diagnosis of ALS. This reduces the number of trial-eligible people and results in conducting trials on a subpopulation of people with advanced ALS that have probably missed their therapeutic window. Traditionally, people with 'possible ALS' according to the El Escorial criteria were excluded from enrollment in ALS trials, but more recently, people with 'possible ALS' are allowed to enroll in clinical trials. A prospective population study reported that 35% of the patients with ALS were considered trial ineligible at the time of diagnosis and 16% of patients die of ALS without being considered trial-eligible based on El Escorial criteria for 'possible ALS' [14]. Some of these patients have a very clear clinical presentation of early ALS but unfortunately they do not fulfill the strict diagnostic criteria to enter ALS clinical trials. Development of a sensitive and specific diagnostic biomarker for ALS can help early accurate diagnosis and enrollment in clinical trials, which allows earlier initiation of potential therapies.

Challenges and controversies

Changing natural history

An improvement in survival during the last decade has been demonstrated in different studies [43, 44]. In addition to FDA approval of riluzole treatment in ALS in the mid-1990s, symptom management of ALS has improved due to the introduction of multidisciplinary clinics [45], better hospital care, early use of non-invasive ventilation [46], and nutritional support with gastrostomy. Although survival has improved in the placebo arms of ALS trials, function measured by ALSFRS-R has not changed [10].

Multisystem disorder

Most ALS clinical trials target motor dysfunction and survival as outcome measures with minimal focus on other features of ALS such as cognitive dysfunction. The recognition of extra-motor involvement in ALS has changed the old definition of ALS as a pure motor neuron disease. Approximately half of people with ALS have frontal executive deficits. The lack of good disease models and outcome measures for cognitive dysfunction in ALS are the major challenges of conducting ALS trials targeting cognitive dysfunction.

What is missing? (symptomatic treatments)

Despite an increased number of candidate drugs and clinical trials in ALS, few trials target management of ALS-related symptoms. A survey of clinicians' practice in the symptomatic treatment of ALS revealed that consensus on treatments was rare among clinicians [47]. The Quality Standards Subcommittee of the American Academy of Neurology along with the ALS Practice Parameters Task Force issued an evidence-based review of the practice parameter in the care of people with ALS in 2009 [49]. Few evidence-based guidelines were produced for symptomatic treatments and further controlled trials were recommended.

Summary

Amyotrophic lateral sclerosis is an orphan neurodegenerative disorder that has one available treatment with modest impact on survival. In addition to the experience in clinical management and clinical trial design and conduct, an enormous amount of new and promising information about ALS genetics, pathophysiology, and biomarkers has become available. These are very exciting and hopeful times for ALS research and therapy discovery.

References:

1. Lanka V, Cudkowicz M. Therapy development for ALS: Lessons learned and path forward. *Amyotroph Lateral Scler* 2008; **9**: 131–40.

2. Bensimon G, Lacomblez L, and Meininger V. The ALSRSG. A Controlled Trial of Riluzole in Amyotrophic Lateral Sclerosis. *N Engl J Med* 1994; **330**: 585–91.

3. Rosen DR, Siddique T, Patterson D, *et al*. Mutations in Cu/Zn superoxide dismutase are associated with familial amyotrophic lateral sclerosis. *Nature* 1993; **362**: 59–62.

4. Renton AE, Majounie E, Waite A, *et al*. A hexanucleotide repeat expansion in C9ORF72 is the cause of chromosome 9p21-linked ALS-F70. *Neuron* 2011; **72**(2): 257–68.

5. Rothstein JD. Current hypotheses for the underlying biology of amyotrophic lateral sclerosis. *Ann Neurol* 2009; **65**(S1): S3–S9.

6. Cleveland DW and Rothstein JD. From Charcot to Lou Gehrig: Deciphering selective motor neuron death in ALS. *Nature Reviews Neuroscience* 2001; **2**(11): 806–19.

7. Dimos JT, Rodolfa KT, Niakan KK, *et al*. Induced pluripotent stem cells generated from patients with ALS can be differentiated into motor neurons. *Science* 2008; **321**: 1218–21.

8. Scott S, Kranz JE, Cole J, *et al*. Design, power, and interpretation of studies in the standard murine model of ALS. *Amyotroph Lateral Scler* 2008; **9**: 4–15.

9. Cedarbaum J, Stambler N, Malta E, *et al*. The ALSFRS-R: a revised ALS functional rating scale that incorporated assessments of respiratory function. *J Neurol Sci* 1999; **169**: 13–21.

10. Qureshi M, Schoenfeld DA, Paliwal Y, *et al*. The natural history of ALS is changing: Improved survival. *Amyotroph Lateral Scler* 2009; **10**: 324–31.

11. McGuire V, Longstreth Jr W, Koepsell T, *et al*. Incidence of amyotrophic lateral sclerosis in three counties in western Washington State. *Neurology* 1996; **47**: 571–3.

12. Kurtzke J and Kurland L. The epidemiology of neurologic disease. In: Joynt R, editor. *Clinical Neurology*. Philadelphia, J.B. Lippincot. 1989; 1–43.

13. Kurtzke JF. Risk factors in amyotrophic lateral sclerosis. *Adv Neurol* 1991; **56**: 245–70.

14. Traynor BJ, Codd MB, Corr B, *et al*. Clinical features of amyotrophic lateral sclerosis according to the El Escorial and Airlie House diagnostic criteria: A population-based study. *Arch Neurol* 2000; **57**: 1171–6.

15. Brooks B, Miller R, Swash M, *et al*. El Escorial revisited: revised criteria for the diagnosis of amyotrophic lateral sclerosis. *Amyotroph Lateral Scler Other Motor Neuron Disord* 2000; **15**: 293–9.

16. Gordon PH, Cheng B, Katz IB, *et al*. The natural history of primary lateral sclerosis. *Neurology* 2006; **66**: 647–53.

17. Conte A, Media F, Luigetti M, *et al*. Survival in ALS patients after tracheostomy. 20th Symposium on ALS/MND. Berlin. 2009.

18. Traynor BJ, Zhang H, Shefner JM, *et al*. Functional outcome measures as clinical trial endpoints in ALS. *Neurology* 2004; **63**: 1933–5.

19. Cudkowicz ME, Shefner JM, Schoenfeld DA, *et al*. A randomized, placebo-controlled trial of topiramate in amyotrophic lateral sclerosis. *Neurology* 2003; **61**: 456–64.

20. Goonetilleke A, Modarres-Sadeghi H and Guiloff R. Accuracy, reproducibility, and variability of hand-held dynamometry in motor neuron disease. *J Neurol Neurosurg Psych* 1994; **57**: 326–32.

21. Beck M, Giess R, Wurffel W, *et al*. Comparison of maximal voluntary isometric contraction and Drachman's hand-held dynamometry in evaluating patients with amyotrophic lateral sclerosis. *Muscle Nerve* 1999; **22**: 1265–70.

22. Raoul C, Estevez A, Nishimune H, *et al*. Motoneuron death triggered by a specific pathway downstream of Fas. potentiation by ALS-linked SOD1 mutations. *Neuron* 2002; **35**: 1067–83.

23. Shefner J, Rutkove SB, David W, *et al*. Modified incremental motor unit estimation in a longitudinal natural history study of subjects with ALS. 20th International Symposium on ALS/MND. Berlin. 2009.

24. Kaufmann P, Levy G, Montes J, *et al*. Excellent inter-rater, intra-rater, and telephone-administered reliability of the ALSFRS-R in a multicenter clinical trial. *Amyotrophic Lateral Sclerosis* 2007; **8**: 42–6.

25. Kasarskis EJ, Dempsey-Hall L, Thompson MM, *et al*. Rating the severity of ALS by caregivers over the telephone using the ALSFRS-R. *Amyotroph Lateral Scler Other Motor Neuron Disord* 2005; **6**: 50–4.

26. Appel V, Stewart S, Smith G, *et al*. A rating scale for amyotrophic lateral sclerosis: description and preliminary experience. *Ann Neurol* 1987; **22**: 328–33.

27. Simmons Z, Felgoise SH, Bremer BA, *et al*. The ALSSQOL: Balancing physical and nonphysical factors in assessing quality of life in ALS. *Neurology* 2006; **67**: 1659–64.

28. Cudkowicz ME, Andres PL, Macdonald SA, *et al*. Phase 2 study of sodium phenylbutyrate in ALS. *Amyotrophic Lateral Sclerosis* 2009; **10**: 99–106.

29. Turner MR, Kiernan MC, Leigh PN, *et al*. Biomarkers in amyotrophic lateral sclerosis. *Lancet Neurol* 2009; **8**: 94–109.

30. Finkelstein D and Schoenfeld D. Combining mortality and longitudinal measures in clinical trials. *Stat Med* 1999; **18**: 1341–54.

31. Cudkowicz M, Bozik ME, Ingersoll EW, *et al*. The effects of dexpramipexole (KNS-760704) in individuals with amyotrophic lateral sclerosis. *Nat Med* 2011; **17**(12): 1652–6.

32. Cudkowicz ME, Katz J, Moore DH, *et al*. Toward more efficient clinical trials for amyotrophic lateral sclerosis. *Amyotrophic Lateral Sclerosis* 2010; **11**: 259–65.

33. Schoenfeld DA and Cudkowicz M. Design of phase II ALS clinical trials. *Amyotrophic Lateral Sclerosis* 2008; **9**: 16–23.

34. Petra K, John LPT, Gilberto L, *et al*. Phase II trial of CoQ10 for ALS finds insufficient evidence to justify phase III. *Annals of Neurology* 2009; **66**: 235–44.

35. Gordon PH, Cheung Y-K, Levin B, *et al*. A novel, efficient, randomized selection trial comparing combinations of drug therapy for ALS. *Amyotrophic Lateral Sclerosis* 2008; **9**: 212–22.

36. Levy G, Kaufmann P, Buchsbaum R, *et al*. A two-stage design for a phase II clinical trial of coenzyme Q10 in ALS. *Neurology* 2006; **66**: 660–3.

37. Miller R, Bradley W, Cudkowicz M, *et al*. Phase II/III randomized trial of TCH346 in patients with ALS. *Neurology* 2007; **69**: 776–84.

38. Gordon PH, Moore DH, Miller RG, *et al*. Efficacy of minocycline in patients with amyotrophic lateral sclerosis: a phase III randomised trial. *Lancet Neurol* 2007; **6**: 1045–53.

39. Cudkowicz M, Greenblatt D, Shefner J, *et al*. Ceftriaxone in ALS: results of stages 1 and 2 of an adaptive design safety, pharmacokinetic and efficacy trial. 20th International Symposium on ALS/MND. Berlin. 2009.

40. Lacomblez L, Bensimon G, Leigh P, *et al*. Dose-ranging study of riluzole in amyotrophic lateral sclerosis. Amyotrophic Lateral Sclerosis/Riluzole Study Group II. *Lancet* 1996; **347**: 1425–31.

41. Aggarwal S and Cudkowicz M. ALS drug development: reflections from the past and a way forward. *Neurotherapeutics* 2008; **5**: 516–27.

42. Bedlack RS, Pastula D, Welsh E, *et al*. Scrutinizing enrollment in ALS clinical trials: Room for improvement? *Amyotroph Lateral Scler* 2008; **9**: 257–65.

43. Czaplinski A, Yen AA, Simpson EP, *et al*. Slower disease progression and prolonged survival in contemporary patients with amyotrophic lateral sclerosis: Is the natural history of amyotrophic lateral sclerosis changing? *Arch Neurol* 2006; **63**: 1139–43.

44. Testa D, Lovati R, Ferrarini M, *et al*. Survival of 793 patients with amyotrophic lateral sclerosis diagnosed over a 28-year period. *Amyotroph Lateral Scler Other Motor Neuron Disord* 2004; **5**: 208–12.

45. Traynor BJ, Alexander M, Corr B, *et al*. Effect of a multidisciplinary amyotrophic lateral sclerosis (ALS) clinic on ALS survival: a population based study, 1996–2000. *J Neurol Neurosurg Psychiatry* 2003; **74**: 1258–61.

46. Dattwyler RJ, Halperin JJ, Pass H, *et al*. Ceftriaxone as effective therapy in refractory lyme disease. *J Inf Dis* 1987; **155**: 1322–4.

47. Forshew DA and Bromberg MB. A survey of clinicians' practice in the symptomatic treatment of ALS. *Amyotroph Lateral Scler Other Motor Neuron Disord* 2003; **4**: 258–63.

48. Miller RG, Jackson CE, Kasarskis EJ, *et al*. Practice Parameter update: The care of the patient with amyotrophic lateral sclerosis: Drug, nutritional, and respiratory therapies (an evidence-based review): Report of the Quality Standards Subcommittee of the American Academy of Neurology. *Neurology* 2009; **73**: 1218–26.

49. Batshaw M, MacArthur R, and Tuchman M. Alternative pathway therapy for urea cycle disorders: twenty years later. *J Pediatr* 2001; **138**(Suppl 1): S46–55.

50. Leigh N, Groups atNAaEAI-S. The treatment of ALS with recombinant insulin-like growth factor (rhIGF-1): pooled analysis of two clinical trials. *Neurology* 1997; 1997(Suppl 1): A217–A8.

Epilepsy

John R. Pollard, Susan S. Ellenberg,
and Jacqueline A. French

Introduction

Epilepsy is a condition that is characterized by unprovoked recurrent seizures. It has also been called 'the epilepsies' since epilepsy is in fact comprised of a number of syndromes, and can be precipitated by a large variety of underlying causes. Seizures associated with epilepsy occur with unpredictable and variable timing and frequency. This variability is central to many of the issues surrounding epilepsy clinical trials, and as with all conditions that occur episodically, creates some complexity. Yet, antiepileptic drugs have been an active area of drug development, for several reasons.

The pathophysiology is understood; the preclinical models had good predictive value in treating human disease; and the clinical trials were relatively reliable because seizures were objective events that were easily analyzable. More recently the path to epilepsy drug approval has become somewhat more difficult. This chapter will illustrate the important issues to consider while shepherding a compound through epilepsy clinical trials.

There are several facets of epilepsy that deserve treatment but have not been the main objective of approval studies in the past. These include comorbidities such as depression or dementia, and more fundamental problems like status epilepticus or development of epilepsy (epileptogenesis.) This chapter will be limited to treatment of seizures.

Biological basis for interventions

It is generally accepted that a seizure results when excitation in one area of the brain exceeds inhibition. This imbalance results in synchronous depolarization of excitatory neurons (which far outnumber inhibitory ones) and ultimately this activity manifests as clinical seizures [1]. In practical application this theory has led to the development of several useful antiepileptic drugs [2]. However, this extremely useful theory is profoundly difficult to extend to the single cell level that makes extensive use of recent advances in genetics, functional genomics, proteomics, and signaling pathways. It is difficult to incorporate the variation in neuroanatomy, the differential effects of the drugs on excitatory versus inhibitory neurons, or the effects on astrocytes and glia. One result is that the mechanisms of action of many antiepileptic drugs are still under active investigation.

Complicating the understanding of the biological basis of epilepsy is the fact that there are a number of epilepsy syndromes that may represent fundamentally different types of dysfunction. Dysregulation of thalamocortical circuits probably underlies generalized onset seizures, which can either result from a primary genetic disorder (idiopathic generalized epilepsies such as juvenile myoclonic epilepsy and absence epilepsy) or conditions associated with diffuse brain disruption (symptomatic generalized epilepsies such as Lennox Gastaut syndrome, West syndrome). Partial onset seizures start focally or multifocally and then spread to involve adjacent or well-connected brain regions [1]. Usually this results from a focal anatomic brain disturbance (common etiologies include mesial temporal sclerosis, cortical dysplasia, stroke, and traumatic brain injury)[3].

Approximately one-third of patients with epilepsy are treatment resistant, and it is these patients for whom new drugs are often targeted. The mechanism of treatment resistance is poorly understood. Some theories include an inability of drugs to reach relevant targets due to overexpression of multidrug efflux transporters (such as P-glycoprotein), alteration of the targets in a way that makes common drugs ineffective, and/ or development of unique mechanisms of seizure genesis

Clinical Trials in Neurology, ed. Bernard Ravina, Jeffrey Cummings, Michael P. McDermott, and R. Michael Poole. Published by Cambridge University Press. © Cambridge University Press 2012.

in treatment resistant patients, that are not addressed by standard antiepileptic drugs. Thus, it is possible that drugs most appropriate for newly diagnosed patients may not be relevant for patients with treatment resistant epilepsy, who may need unique approaches [4].

The major known mechanisms of actions of antiepileptic drugs can be subdivided into those associated with alteration of voltage and receptor gated ion channels, (sodium, potassium, calcium), modulation of neurotransmitter release, and modulation of excitatory and inhibitory neurotransmitters [5]. Some antiepileptic drugs are developed as 'designer drugs', with a known mechanism as a target. This was the case for vigabatrin, which acts via irreversible inhibition of the GABA metabolizing enzyme GABA transaminase [6]. In contrast, a number of antiepileptic drugs are identified through high throughput screening (see below) or other means, and in these cases mechanisms may be unknown. Drugs identified this way will undergo testing to try to uncover important mechanisms of action. One or several may be discovered, and it is often difficult to confirm that any of these mechanisms discovered post hoc is the principle mechanism by which the drug exerts its efficacy. Occasionally, further investigation will uncover a completely novel mechanism. This was the case for levetiracetam, which ultimately was found to bind to synaptic vesicle protein 2A, and is thought to act through modifying the release of neurotransmitter, a previously unknown mechanism [7].

Understanding the putative mechanism of an antiepileptic drug may be important in determining the clinical population that will benefit from the drug. Some mechanisms of action have been associated with aggravation of some seizure types. Most notably, drugs that act either by fast sodium channel blockade (carbamazepine, phenytoin, oxcarbazepine) or GABA enhancement (vigabatrin, tiagabine) are known to exacerbate certain types of generalized seizures (absence, myoclonus) [8].

Preclinical assessment of antiepileptic drugs

One of the great boons to epilepsy drug development has been the availability of the NIH Anticonvulsant Screening Program, which provides preclinical screening at no cost to companies with potential antiepileptic compounds. It is estimated that over the last 35 years, nearly 32 000 investigational antiepileptic drugs have been evaluated by the program [9].

Screening focuses on high throughput models utilizing electrically or chemically induced seizures in normal animals, such as the maximum electroshock test and the pentylenetetrazol test, which in the past were believed to predict efficacy against tonic-clonic and absence seizures, respectively, and the 6 Hz model [10], which may better target drugs for treatment resistant epilepsy. More recently, these screens have been criticized as they do not truly model the human condition, even though they have been quite predictive of at least some efficacy in human clinical trials [11].

Newer models, such as pilocarpine, kainate, or electrically induced post-status epilepsy models, may be more useful for identifying compounds for treatment-resistant epilepsy, but are not useful for high-throughput screening of new chemical entities. Also gaining favor are genetic spike-wave models such as the WAG/RIJ rodent model [12], and the generalized absence epilepsy rat of Strasbourg which have a good record for predicting efficacy against generalized onset seizures associated with EEG spike-wave, and also can help predict the likelihood of seizure exacerbation [13].

Preclinical models are also used to evaluate pharmacokinetic parameters and toxicology. Of particular interest in antiepileptic drug development is testing in another non-rodent species to refine the model for estimating dosing in humans [14].

Study populations: Human

Populations for epilepsy clinical trials are usually subdivided based on epilepsy syndrome and patient age. It is difficult to enroll treatment sensitive patients into clinical trials once they are already on an established antiepileptic drug, and therefore the trials are also subdivided into those for newly diagnosed patients, and those who continue to have seizures despite therapy (treatment resistant).

The majority of epilepsy trials enroll patients with partial (focal) epilepsy, as defined in the International League Against Epilepsy seizure classification, which has recently been revised [15]. The previous classification is typically used for classifying seizures in antiepileptic drug trials, although this may change [16]. Two-thirds of all epilepsies are partial onset, and these can begin at any age. Seizures associated with partial epilepsies are classified depending on degree of spread, which translates to degree of clinical disruption. If a seizure involves a small amount of brain, and thus no alteration of awareness, it is referred to as a simple partial seizure. A seizure that involves more brain and results in alteration of awareness is called a complex partial seizure, and a seizure that spreads to involve the whole brain results in a secondary generalized tonic clonic seizure, often referred to as a 'convulsion'. Of these seizure types, the most common in clinical trials is the complex partial seizure, but each patient can have one, two or all of these seizure types. Partial onset types of seizures are by far the most common in drug resistant adult epilepsy patients, and therefore partial onset seizures form the basis of most pivotal trials to demonstrate efficacy and safety for initial drug registration [17]. The International League Against Epilepsy defines drug resistant epilepsy as: 'failure of adequate trials of two tolerated and appropriately chosen and used [antiepileptic drug] schedules (whether as monotherapies or in combination) to achieve sustained seizure freedom' [18].

The generalized onset epilepsy types typically begin in childhood or adolescence, and some will remit by adulthood. Seizure types for the more benign genetic (idiopathic) generalized epilepsies include absence, myoclonus and generalized tonic-clonic (often referred to as primarily generalized, to distinguish them from those that occur in the partial epilepsies, as described above). Which of these seizure types manifests, is determined by the specific syndrome. Clinical trials have been performed in patients with seizure types associated with juvenile myoclonic epilepsy, as well as in patients with generalized, tonic clonic seizures [19]. Occasionally, trials for absence seizures have been attempted, but these are difficult due to the fact that the majority of absence seizures are treatment sensitive [19].

The more devastating symptomatic generalized epilepsies are typically accompanied by multiple seizure types, including all of the types described for partial epilepsy, as well as 'atypical' absence, myoclonus, and tonic/atonic ('drop seizures'). Patients with the so-called Lennox-Gastaut Syndrome, which is characterized by multiple seizure types, developmental delay, and a characteristic slow-spike-wave EEG pattern, are usually selected for clinical trials of this epilepsy syndrome. This syndrome begins in childhood, but persists into adulthood [20].

Because of ethical considerations, it is considered unacceptable to leave an epilepsy patient untreated because standard of care therapy is effective in preventing serious injury. In addition, the relatively high efficacy of almost all the medications in treatment naïve patients often results in seizure freedom or rare seizures. These characteristics make new onset epilepsy patients a poor choice for initial registration studies, where the regulatory authorities typically insist on a placebo control. Thus, the default antiepileptic trial for drug approval in the US has become the add-on design enrolling drug resistant adult partial onset epilepsy subjects with a high enough seizure frequency to be able to demonstrate a drug effect.

Methods of delivery

The usual method of medication delivery in epilepsy is oral administration. Intravenous administration of these drugs in terms of approval studies has been restricted to use when oral medications are unable to be administered [21]. In practice intravenous administration is often used in emergency rooms to ensure that new onset epilepsy patients have achieved adequate serum concentrations before going home. Thus the availability of intravenous phenytoin has helped ensure its persistent status as one of the most prescribed antiepileptic drugs in the US. In addition, intravenous formulations are critical for treatment of patients with status epilepticus. However, clinical trials in this population are extremely difficult, so regulatory approval for this indication has not been sought.

Other methods of administration have been explored for acute and urgent use, where it is important to have an immediate drug exposure. Epileptic seizures have a tendency to cluster, and a new indication was created, namely 'acute repetitive seizures', when rectal diazepam underwent regulatory review [22]. In practice, rectal diazepam may also be used for status epilepticus prior to ambulance arrival, in children with very severe epilepsy. Intranasal therapy using midazolam is being tested for use in acute repetitive seizures and an intramuscular formulation of diazepam is under investigation for the same indication.

Measurement tools

The primary instrument for assessment of efficacy in epilepsy clinical trials is counting of seizure events over time. This is usually done by use of a seizure diary. The subjects work with the site investigator to define each seizure type the subject suffers and assign a letter designation for each. The subjects or their caregivers then record how many of each seizure type the subject had that day. If there were none, a box is checked to indicate this, and exclude a missing day of data.

There is some controversy over the use of the diary, and the diary restricts the type of patient that can enroll in the study. For example, a patient who is unaware of most of his seizures is ineligible. If patients cannot record their own seizures (either because they are not aware of them, or they have cognitive disturbance), they should have caregivers who can record this information for them. Living conditions should remain stable. If a subject is unaware that he is unaware of some seizures, moving in with a relative in the middle of the study could result in reporting of an artificial increase in seizure frequency. Inaccurate evaluation of each seizure type by the neurologist or imperfect administration by the subject may be a source of significant error in centers that are inexperienced in clinical trials. With studies increasingly involving less experienced centers from around the world, in some cases the diaries may be precise but not accurate. The diary is an imperfect tool, but the best available.

Seizures have a tendency to occur in clusters and flurries, which can occur over the course of minutes, hours, or even days. Seizure clusters represent a problem in epilepsy trials. If the patient cannot count the number of seizures that have occurred in a cluster, there may be issues in analysis. A patient who suffers seizures that cluster and uses frequent rescue medication (benzodiazepines for acute seizures, as described above), which is becoming more common, is also not ideal because if a patient randomized to placebo uses more rescue medication than a patient in the treatment group, there may be less separation between the groups. Finally, an effective new antiepileptic therapy can change a single seizure cluster into many countable seizures, and while this change would benefit patients, it could profoundly impact the measurement of the primary endpoints of a trial. However, frequency of use of rescue medications could be used as an outcome measure but this has not been widely done in the past.

At present, there is no EEG surrogate available that can replace or even enhance standard three month efficacy trials for partial onset seizures. Recording EEG intermittently to capture inter-ictal activity is not useful, as some antiepileptic drugs will be able to reduce seizure frequency, but will have no effect on inter-ictal activity, and some (carbamazepine is an example) are actually known to increase inter-ictal spikes [23]. Occasionally, when a drug is known to suppress inter-ictal spikes, spike counting can be used as a surrogate measure of drug effect [24]. There is no current means to record chronic EEG for long enough periods to be an effective surrogate marker for seizures. Video-EEG has been used in trials of patients with the Lennox-Gastaut syndrome to teach parents how to recognize seizures, but not as an outcome measure [25]. In a recent study, EEG has also been used as an accompaniment to seizure diaries comparing three treatments for absence seizures. In this case, children had a prolonged out-patient EEG with hyperventilation to confirm control of absence seizures, and to rule out unrecognized or unreported events [26].

Some studies have tried to capture the reduction in seizure severity that often occurs with the administration of an effective antiepileptic drug. In practice this type of analysis is difficult to quantitate and is not often used as a primary outcome variable [27].

There are many quality of life scales used in epilepsy studies. One of the most common is the Quality of Life in Epilepsy-31 (QOLIE-31)[28]. They are very helpful in certain circumstances but somewhat insensitive to the reduction in seizure frequency usually achieved by a new compound, likely reflecting the fact that in these trials, seizure freedom is rare, and thus the clinical impact of treatment may be small, rather than a defect in the instruments (see above 'Preclinical assessment of antiepileptic drugs') [29].

An extensive battery of neuropsychological assessment is seldom used in antiepileptic trials. The recent exception is the Stimulation of the Anterior Nucleus of the Thalamus for Epilepsy study of the deep brain stimulator in the anterior nucleus of the thalamus [30].

Treatment emergent adverse event frequency is usually assessed in comparison to placebo. This becomes more complicated, in the add-on trials used for registration of new antiepileptic drugs for partial onset seizures. In these trials, patients are typically receiving one to three background antiepileptic drugs, to which either a placebo or the new chemical entity are added. The baseline drugs the patient is on often have side effects which are similar to those of the study drug. The resulting pharmacodynamic impact for side effects can result in a high rate of adverse events or even result in subject drop out, potentially making the primary outcomes more difficult to reach [31]. Often, for this reason the side effect profile of new antiepileptic drugs is over estimated until monotherapy studies are performed later in development. Dropout rate and reason for dropout is another important outcome measure in all epilepsy therapeutic trials.

There are several different outcomes that have been employed in epilepsy clinical trials through use of the seizure diary. The seizure frequency is highly variable from patient to patient, and there is also variability from month to month within patient, which makes statistical assessment of outcome complex. For this reason, most chronic epilepsy trials employ a 6 to 12 week baseline to establish seizure frequency, followed by a treatment period. Most commonly, the primary outcome measure is assessment of seizure rate during the treatment period, compared to their baseline. This is usually assessed as median percent seizure reduction. Another common outcome measure is the 'responder rate.' This is a dichotomous assessment of the number of patients who achieve a certain percent of seizure reduction compared to baseline. Commonly, 50% seizure reduction is considered to be clinically meaningful, and thus patients who achieve this are designated as responders [32]. Patients with 75% response may also be reported. Seizure-free rates (100% seizure reduction) are also often reported, but the number of patients achieving this outcome tends to be small, and the reporting has been confounded by use of different definitions of seizure freedom. For example, in some studies, patients who dropped out early but have not had seizures prior to drop out are counted as seizure free. In other studies, patients would need to complete the entire treatment period to be counted [33]. Another complexity is that changes in seizure counts do not obey a normal distribution. This is because the seizure frequency can only be reduced by a maximum of 100%, but can increase by any amount. This is dealt with by normalization using various means, including logarithmic transformation. Bounded functions of seizure rates are often used as well. A common measure is the response ratio, which is the ratio of the difference between the treatment and baseline seizure rates to the sum of these two rates [34].

Monotherapy trials in patients newly diagnosed with epilepsy are usually performed as active control non-inferiority trials. Newly diagnosed patients have a much higher likelihood of seizure freedom, and comparison of the percent of patients that remain seizure free on each randomized therapy is usually used at the outcome measure. Recently, the Committee for Medicinal Products for Human Use (CHMP, European regulatory body) has provided relatively stringent criteria for assessment of seizure freedom in active control monotherapy trials. They suggest that seizure freedom should be compared for at least 6 months, and that the trial be continued for at least 1 year. They also suggest a relative -20% delta for the 95% CI, with 80% power.

Finally, an assessment can specify the overall effectiveness of the drug by assessing whether patients meet certain endpoints over a prespecified period of time. This outcome is used in withdrawal to monotherapy studies in patients with treatment resistant partial onset seizures. In this trial design, a number of exit criteria, which are indicators of worsening of seizures are pre-specified. The number of patients meeting the exit criteria over time is determined. This kind of assessment is also used in a 'time to n-th seizure design,' where patients exit the study after they have experienced a predetermined number of seizures. Time to exit has been used in studies of newly diagnosed subjects [35]. This outcome measure is considered to be a composite of efficacy and tolerability. This is said to provide information about drug 'effectiveness,' a better assessment of real-life impact, rather than efficacy. The outcome measure has been criticized by some, as drugs that are well tolerated but minimally efficacious can look equally as effective as drugs that are poorly tolerated but highly efficacious. For more information, refer to Section 2 of this book.

Clinical trial designs

Efficacy

Many drug trials are performed to achieve registration for specific indications by regulatory authorities. Ultimately these clinical trials are designed to demonstrate to the regulatory agencies that a drug is effective and safe. Often an early study is done to aid in dose finding. These are the first studies in epilepsy patients.

Due to the intermittent, unpredictable nature of the clinical manifestations of epilepsy and the various types of epilepsies secondary to variable etiologies, different pathophysiological mechanisms, as well as different clinical and electroencephalographic expressions, there are complexities in assessing efficacy of potentially new antiepileptic drugs in man in a rapid fashion.

One proof of concept study that had been gaining popularity is performed in patients with photosensitive epilepsy. These patients reliably have an epileptiform discharge known as a photoparoxysmal response on their EEG in response to specific frequencies of flashing light. The photoparoxysmal response can be used as a quantitative measure of photosensitivity and therefore epileptogenicity. To date, efficacy of a single

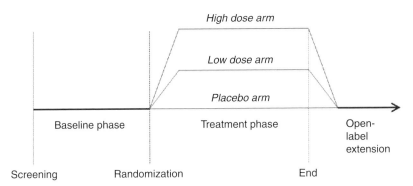

Typical phase 3 trial design for add-on therapy

Figure 25.1. Placebo controlled add-on design. All subjects stay on their prescreening antiepileptic drugs. Screening is followed by a baseline phase. Randomization occurs just before drug initiation. In this diagram there are two treatment arms and a placebo add-on. This is followed by an open-label extension in which the dose is determined by the investigator.

dose of drug in the photoparoxysmal response protocol has been a robust indicator of successful antiepileptic drugs (e.g., levetiracetam and lamotrigine). Combined with blood level monitoring, the model offers information about the time of onset and the duration of the antiepileptic action and side effects [36].

A dose-finding study is typically performed in early development, using different doses of the study drug to try to establish some trend towards efficacy in a dose-dependent manner. These studies are often not powered to detect significant efficacy or to establish definitive number of subjects experiencing adverse events.

There are alternative designs which have proven useful in the past both for initial demonstration of efficacy and for dose finding. One interesting alternative is a presurgical inpatient study. In this study subjects are enrolled while in an epilepsy monitoring unit. Typically, patients have been weaned off some or all of their background antiepileptic drugs in order to record seizures for surgical localization. Patients are then randomized to test drug or placebo, and finish involvement in the study when a prespecified number of seizures has occurred [37]. Although the design does provide a rapid assessment of drug efficacy in partial seizures, it is an expensive study, and is not considered by the regulatory agencies for drug approval. Ethical issues have also been raised in regards to maintaining patients on placebo alone for prolonged periods solely for the purpose of the trial, as post-ictal psychosis and other adverse events have occurred as a consequence [38].

Definitive proof of efficacy studies usually employ drug resistant partial onset seizure patients with at least three seizures per month. The subjects remain on their typical antiepileptic regimen, usually one to three antiepileptic drugs, in addition to the study drug. The outcomes are measured with a seizure diary.

The regulatory program leading to drug registration usually has approval for an indication as add-on therapy in treatment resistant partial onset seizures as the linchpin. Two adequate and well-controlled trials will need to demonstrate efficacy and safety. These regulatory studies usually enroll drug resistant partial onset seizure patients who are already on one to three antiepileptic drugs, not including a vagus nerve stimulator, and are having at least three or four countable partial seizures per month [39] (See Figure 25.1). After a 6–12 week baseline, patients are randomized to add-on placebo or one of several fixed doses of the test drug. Flexible dose trials are frowned upon by US regulatory agencies. There is typically a 1 to 4 week titration period, followed by a 12 week maintenance period (mandated by the regulatory authorities in Europe and the US to assure a long enough duration of therapy to assess drug affect). At the conclusion of the study, patients are usually offered a long-term maintenance phase. Patients who do not elect to continue on the drug are tapered off over a 1–3 week taper phase. The outcome of seizure reduction is measured with seizure diaries. Often the two definitive pivotal trials to demonstrate efficacy and safety for regulatory bodies are run nearly concurrently with one based in the US and Canada and one based in Europe to persuade the two most stringent regulatory agencies. At present, these large studies are run multinationally.

In addition to approval for partial onset seizures, many drugs are assessed for efficacy in one or more additional seizure types. One design utilizes patients with a very high seizure frequency, those with

Lennox-Gastaut. As noted above, the Lennox-Gastaut syndrome has onset in childhood, and is associated with a high seizure frequency. Some seizure types may be difficult to differentiate from behavioral problems, since the syndrome is associated with developmental delay which can at times be profound. Thus, the study measures both total seizures and frequency of one of the more clear cut seizure types (tonic and atonic seizures) and seizure severity. In other aspects, trial design is similar to that used for randomized placebo-controlled add-on study in partial onset seizures. Recently, the drug rufinamide was evaluated in Lennox-Gastaut syndrome [40].

Most epilepsy efficacy studies are followed by an open-label extension study. In this trial type, all subjects in the efficacy study who tolerated the medication are allowed a chance to try the study medication at a clinician estimated dose. This is used primarily to garner information on long-term use of the drug for safety and for approval [41].

Add-on trials may also be done in patients with idiopathic generalized epilepsy. These trials are difficult, as there are fewer patients who are treatment resistant, and seizures tend to be less frequent than in partial onset seizure syndromes. Typically, these studies will enroll patients with one or more generalized tonic clonic convulsions per month. Other seizure types that occur in idiopathic generalized epilepsy (absence, myoclonus) are allowed and are counted, but are not included in the primary outcome, which is usually % reduction in generalized tonic clonic convulsions. As in the other trials, a 2–3 month baseline will be followed by randomization to adjunctive test drug or placebo. The treatment period is usually 6 months in duration.

By convention, indications are usually granted by regulatory authorities for the primary seizure type that is studied, with an indication of the syndrome where appropriate. Therefore, a successful study as described above would lead to an indication for 'generalized tonic clonic convulsions associated with idiopathic generalized epilepsy'.

Additional study designs

Trials to assess effectiveness of antiepileptic drugs as monotherapy are complex, primarily because placebo is ethically almost impossible to employ in a patient with active epilepsy. To address this concern, a trial design was introduced which was known as the 'pseudo-placebo withdrawal to monotherapy study in treatment resistant partial onset seizures' [37]. In this study design, patients are randomized to treatment with an experimental drug or placebo, after which baseline therapy is withdrawn over 2–8 weeks. A true placebo is not utilized as the comparison to reduce the likelihood of status epilepticus or secondary generalization. The comparison arm can consist of a minimally effective dose of either the same investigational drug or of any other therapy presumed to be less effective than the test drug. A starting dose of valproic acid (15 mg/kg) has been employed in a number of trials for this purpose. Outcome is assessed in terms of 'failures' and 'completers.' Failure is determined on the basis of escape criteria, such as doubling of seizure frequency, occurrence of generalized tonic-clonic seizures or increase in seizure severity. If more patients receiving the experimental drug at a therapeutic dose in monotherapy can complete the trial, without fulfilling escape criteria, than patients receiving the less effective comparator in monotherapy, the treatment is considered effective. Over time, concern arose about randomizing patients to a less effective therapy, and most recently, a historical control has been compiled, which uses a meta-analysis of the escape rate from the pseudo-placebo arms of all of the relevant trials, to create a 'virtual placebo arm', against which active drugs can be measured [42]. The FDA has agreed to accept trials which use the historical control at the comparator arm for approval of drugs as monotherapy [43]. In contrast, the European regulatory authorities have not accepted this design, and prefer active control non-inferiority trials in newly diagnosed patients (described above).

The time to event design has been mentioned above. This design can be used to study subjects with more rare outcomes of interest, and is being explored as a regulatory endpoint. This design has been used to study seizure clusters, by measuring time to seizure cessation [22]. It could also be used to study a severe seizure type such as primary generalized tonic clonic seizures [44]. Cross over trials are rarely used in epilepsy. The disadvantages of a crossover trial include a much longer duration, risk of patients dropping early, and, more importantly, a potential unblinding of the trial (see Chapter 10). This is of most concern in a trial which compares placebo to active treatment. Patients may be able to discern a difference in side effects when switching from placebo to drug, or vice versa. There may be carryover effects (that is, long-lasting effects) of treatment, which would impact on the initial portion of the second treatment phase [44]. For these reasons, the Food and Drug Administration as well as European Medicines Agency do not favor such trials.

Clinical testing of antiepileptic drugs often considers children separately because of the age-related changes in both brain and overall physiological and biochemical status that occur during childhood along with the age dependency of certain seizure types and epileptic syndromes. Most studies on antiepileptic drugs have considered children to be less than 12 years, and have included those aged 12 years and over in trials designed primarily for adults. However, a recent statement by the European Medicines Agency suggested that focal epilepsy in children is similar enough to its adult counterpart, that 'the results of efficacy trials performed in adults could to some extent be extrapolated to children provided the dose is established … [46].'

There are a number of severe epilepsy syndromes that occur in infants and young children, such as West syndrome, severe myoclonic epilepsy in infants, and myoclonic astatic epilepsy which deserve separate trials.

Safety issues

Common side effects of antiepileptic drugs tend to be CNS related (dizziness, drowsiness, diplopia, concentration difficulties) and tend to increase with dose. Behavioral disturbances (irritability, depression, psychosis) are also seen. It may be difficult to determine the true extent of these dose-related adverse events, because most of these trials are add-on. Pharmacodynamic interactions with baseline antiepileptic drugs will tend to amplify apparent toxicity from the new drug. In one study, toxicity developed in 90% of patients who were converted from monotherapy to polytherapy with standard agents [47]. Idiosyncratic side effects, such as hypersensitivity syndromes, pancreatitis, hepatic failure and renal calculi, occur with one or several marketed antiepileptic drugs, and may occur months to years after initiation of the drug. Thus, if they occur over the course of a trial with a new intervention, it may be difficult to determine if they are related to the drug of interest, or the background medication. Patients who are receiving marketed antiepileptic drugs associated with more frequent serious adverse events, such as felbamate (aplastic anemia up to 1 in 3000) and vigabatrin (irreversible visual field defects 30%) are often excluded from participation in trials.

A placebo control is extremely helpful in assessing whether some adverse events are truly related to the intervention being tested, rather than related to the underlying epilepsy. Certain adverse events, such as sudden death, depression, and psychosis, are more common in patients with epilepsy than in the population at large.

One safety issue that is currently challenging those conducting clinical trials is the recent FDA determination that all antiepileptic drugs may cause suicidal thoughts and behaviors [48]. It is likely that screening for suicidal thoughts will be required during future clinical trials. Studies are currently underway to find the best screening tool to identify this effect.

Sudden unexplained death in epilepsy patients is a concern for clinical trials. The rate of sudden unexplained death in epilepsy patients in clinical trials has been estimated at 0.3/100 patient years. In the past, there have been some concerns that certain drugs increase the rates of sudden unexplained death in epilepsy patients, and this may be difficult to confirm or refute in studies without a control group, such as long-term extension studies after randomized trials. However, several analyses have indicated that the rate is consistent with the expected rate for patients with frequent uncontrolled seizures [49].

Implementation issues

One of the persistent difficulties in antiepileptic drug development is the selection of the appropriate dose of the drug. There are cost pressures to move a drug quickly through development, but as with all new therapies, it is prudent to proceed only when there is a reasonable assessment of optimal dosing. A selection of a dose that is too low will result in a study that does not meet its endpoints for efficacy. A dose that is too high will suffer from a high drop-out rate. Dose selection is complicated by the fact that there may be a great deal of interindividual variability in drug metabolism, leading to over dosing in some cases and under dosing in others. This is particularly true, as a proportion of patients may be receiving one of the antiepileptic drugs that is hepatic enzyme inducing, which will lead to relatively lower serum concentrations in that subset of patients. Often, dose will not be adjusted to account for these pharmacokinetic interactions. One possible solution was used in a trial of topiramate, in which the drug was titrated to a fixed serum concentration rather than a fixed dose [50]. However concentration controlled trials are complex and difficult to perform.

Another issue is that the placebo response rate for clinical trials in epilepsy may be increasing. The rate of responders to placebo in epilepsy trials has been variable over time [51]. The factors that contribute include more reliable antiepileptic drug intake [52], regression to the mean (described above), and potential reduction of patient stress when enrolled in a trial and obsessively supervised. There has also been an increase in failure of clinical trials to separate active drug arms from placebo. Two recent large development programs led to failed trials (carisbamate, brivaracetam) [53]. Studies performed in the 1990s were often done at a few very experienced centers that were resource intensive, leading to solid outcome data. More recently, individual centers have been unable to enroll the same number of subjects, probably due to the rising number of previously approved therapies. A patient is unlikely to try a new chemical entity when an already approved one may be available. The result is that less experienced investigators with less intensively screened subjects enroll in studies. These factors tend to lead to errors such as counting events that are not seizures or to enrolling subjects with the wrong syndrome, thus narrowing the difference between placebo and treatment arms. Currently there are efforts to improve the quality of outcomes by assessing each investigator's seizure descriptions. Another proposed solution is to widen the possible patient pool by using new trial designs such as the time to n-th seizure design to reduce patient burden, and hopefully increase enrollment.

Challenges and controversies

It is always difficult to determine what risks are appropriate for patients to be subjected to. Most patients enter trials with investigational drugs because they have failed many standard drugs, and continue to have seizures that impair their quality of life. They may also be influenced by the promise of free medical care or free drug. However, with so many available marketed drugs, patients may be approached to enter clinical trials before they have failed a number of marketed drugs. This issue also arises in trials to obtain a monotherapy approval, which in Europe are typically done in patients with newly diagnosed epilepsy. It may be hard for an investigator to decide how much information should be available about a drug, before it is reasonable to start newly diagnosed patients on it, when they have so many other options.

Another common concern in epilepsy studies, is that many patients may have some or considerable cognitive disturbance. Many studies require patients to be capable of signing their own consent. However, it is not common to perform any specific testing to determine whether the patient is truly capable of understanding what is being asked of them.

Trial duration is an issue in epilepsy trials. Ideally, a clinical trial should last for as long as possible, to assess whether a new therapy will be successful over the long term. Unfortunately, epilepsy trials are performed in patients with severe, treatment resistant epilepsy and frequent seizures. It is not benign to maintain these patients on the same therapy for a prolonged period of time without intervening, as is the case in the placebo arm of randomized trials. Moreover, patients are reluctant to be randomized knowing that they will receive no active treatment for an 8–12 week baseline ended 3-months treatment phase. Efforts are underway to consider new trial designs, such as time to n-th seizure, which would allow patients who were doing poorly to exit sooner and yet provide adequate trial duration to assess treatment effect.

As noted above, monotherapy trial design remains extremely controversial. In the US at the present time the accepted trial design is historical control conversion to monotherapy in treatment resistant partial onset seizures. In Europe, the accepted trial design is monotherapy active control non-inferiority study in newly diagnosed patients. Discussions with regulatory agencies continue, to try and harmonize monotherapy trial designs [54].

Many have questioned the generalizability of epilepsy trials that are performed for registration of new drugs. The majority of these trials enroll patients with very frequent treatment resistant seizures, who may not be representative of the bulk of the patients will ultimately receive the treatment.

References

1. Kandel ER, Schwartz JH, Jessell TM. *Principles of Neural Science*. 3rd edition. New York: Elsevier. 1991.

2. Porter RJ. Antiepileptic drugs: future development. *Epilepsy Res* Suppl 1993; **10**: 69–77.

3. Herman ST. Epilepsy after brain insult: targeting epileptogenesis. *Neurology* 2002; **59**(Suppl 5): S21–6.

4. Kwan P, Brodie MJ. Refractory epilepsy: mechanisms and solutions. *Expert Rev Neurother* 2006; **6**: 397–406.

5. White HS, Smith MD, Wilcox KS. Mechanisms of action of antiepileptic drugs. *Int Rev Neurobiol* 2007; **81**: 85–110.

6. Jung MJ, Lippert B, Metcalf BW, *et al.* gamma-Vinyl GABA (4-amino-hex-5-enoic acid), a new selective irreversible inhibitor of GABA-T: effects on brain GABA metabolism in mice. *J Neurochem* 1977; **29**: 797–802.

7. Lynch BA, Lambeng N, Nocka K, *et al.* The synaptic vesicle protein SV2A is the binding site for the antiepileptic drug levetiracetam. *Proc Natl Acad Sci USA* 2004; **101**: 9861–6.

8. Perucca E, Gram L, Avanzini G, *et al.* Antiepileptic drugs as a cause of worsening seizures. *Epilepsia* 1998; **39**: 5–17.

9. White HS, Wolf HH, Woodhead JH, *et al.* The National Institutes of Health Anticonvulsant Drug Development Program: screening for efficacy. *Adv Neurol* 1998; **76**: 29–39.

10. Barton ME, Klein BD, Wolf HH, *et al.* Pharmacological characterization of the 6 Hz psychomotor seizure model of partial epilepsy. *Epilepsy Res* 2001; **47**: 217–27.

11. Loscher W and Leppik IE. Critical re-evaluation of previous preclinical strategies for the discovery and the development of new antiepileptic drugs. *Epilepsy Res* 2002; **50**: 17–20.

12. van Luijtelaar EL and Coenen AM. Two types of electrocortical paroxysms in an inbred strain of rats. *Neurosci Lett* 1986; **70**: 393–7.

13. Marescaux C, Vergnes M, and Depaulis A. Genetic absence epilepsy in rats from Strasbourg – a review. *J Neural Transm* 1992; **35**(Suppl 1): 37–69.

14. Mager DE, Woo S, and Jusko WJ. Scaling pharmacodynamics from in vitro and preclinical animal studies to humans. *Drug Metab Pharmacokinet* 2009; **24**: 16–24.

15. Berg AT, Berkovic SF, Brodie MJ, *et al.* Revised terminology and concepts for organization of seizures and epilepsies: report of the ILAE Commission on Classification and Terminology, 2005–2009. *Epilepsia* 2010; **51**: 676–85.

16. Seino M. Classification criteria of epileptic seizures and syndromes. *Epilepsy Res* 2006; **70** (Suppl 1): S27–33.

17. Kwan P and Brodie MJ. Early identification of refractory epilepsy. *N Engl J Med* 2000; **342**: 314–9.

18. Kwan P, Arzimanoglou A, Berg AT, *et al.* Definition of drug resistant epilepsy: consensus proposal by the ad hoc Task Force of the ILAE Commission on Therapeutic Strategies. *Epilepsia* 2009; **51**: 1069–77.

19. Bergey GK. Evidence-based treatment of idiopathic generalized epilepsies with new antiepileptic drugs. *Epilepsia* 2005; **46** (Suppl 9): 161–8.

20. Arzimanoglou A, French J, Blume WT, *et al.* Lennox-Gastaut syndrome: a consensus approach on diagnosis, assessment, management, and trial methodology. *Lancet Neurol* 2009; **8**: 82–93.

21. Ramael S, Daoust A, Otoul C, *et al.* Levetiracetam intravenous infusion: a randomized, placebo-controlled safety and pharmacokinetic study. *Epilepsia* 2006; **47**: 1128–35.

22. Dreifuss FE, Rosman NP, Cloyd JC, *et al.* A comparison of rectal diazepam gel and placebo for acute repetitive seizures. *N Engl J Med* 1998; **338**: 1869–75.

23. Marciani MG, Gigli GL, Stefanini F, *et al.* Effect of carbamazepine on EEG background activity and on interictal epileptiform abnormalities in focal epilepsy. *Int J Neurosci* 1993; **70**: 107–16.

24. Milligan N, Dhillon S, Oxley J, *et al.* Absorption of diazepam from the rectum and its effect on interictal spikes in the EEG. *Epilepsia* 1982; **23**: 323–31.

25. Efficacy of felbamate in childhood epileptic encephalopathy (Lennox-Gastaut syndrome). The Felbamate Study Group in Lennox-Gastaut Syndrome. *N Engl J Med* 1993; **328**: 29–33.

26. Glauser TA, Cnaan A, Shinnar S, *et al.* Ethosuximide, valproic acid, and lamotrigine in childhood absence epilepsy. *N Engl J Med* 2010; **362**: 790–9.

27. Cramer JA. Seizure measurement in clinical trials. *J Epilepsy* 1998; **11**: 256–60.

28. Cramer JA, Perrine K, Devinsky O, *et al.* Development and cross-cultural translations of a 31-item quality of life in epilepsy inventory. *Epilepsia* 1998; **39**: 81–8.

29. Leone MA, Beghi E, Righini C, *et al.* Epilepsy and quality of life in adults: a review of instruments. *Epilepsy Res* 2005; **66**: 23–44.

30. Fisher R, Salanova V, Witt T, *et al.* Electrical stimulation of the anterior nucleus of thalamus for treatment of refractory epilepsy. *Epilepsia* 2010; **51**: 899–908.

31. Cramer JA, Mintzer S, Wheless J, *et al.* Adverse effects of antiepileptic drugs: a brief overview of important issues. *Expert Rev Neurother* 2010; **10**: 885–91.

32. Ben-Menachem E, Sander JW, Privitera M, *et al.* Measuring outcomes of treatment with antiepileptic drugs in clinical trials. *Epilepsy Behav* 2010; **18**: 24–30.

33. Gazzola DM, Balcer LJ, and French JA. Seizure-free outcome in randomized add-on trials of the new antiepileptic drugs. *Epilepsia* 2007; **48**: 1303–7.

34. Pledger GW and Sahlroot JT. Alternative analyses for antiepileptic drug trials. *Epilepsy Res* 1993; **10** (Suppl): 167–74.

35. Brodie MJ, Richens A, and Yuen AW. Double-blind comparison of lamotrigine and carbamazepine in newly diagnosed epilepsy. UK Lamotrigine/Carbamazepine Monotherapy Trial Group. *Lancet* 1995; **345**: 476–9.

36. Kasteleijn-Nolst Trenite DG, Marescaux C, *et al.* Photosensitive epilepsy: a model to study the effects of antiepileptic drugs. Evaluation of the piracetam analogue, levetiracetam. *Epilepsy Res* 1996; **25**: 225–30.

37. Devinsky O, Faught RE, Wilder BJ, *et al*. Efficacy of felbamate monotherapy in patients undergoing presurgical evaluation of partial seizures. *Epilepsy Res* 1995; **20**: 241–6.

38. Ketter TA, Malow BA, Flamini R, *et al*. Anticonvulsant withdrawal-emergent psychopathology. *Neurology* 1994; **44**: 55–61.

39. Wilensky AJ. Protocol design. *Epilepsy Res* 1993; **10** (Suppl): 107–13.

40. Glauser T, Kluger G, Sachdeo R, *et al*. Rufinamide for generalized seizures associated with Lennox-Gastaut syndrome. *Neurology* 2008; **70**: 1950–8.

41. The US Gabapentin Study Group. The long-term safety and efficacy of gabapentin (Neurontin) as add-on therapy in drug-resistant partial epilepsy. *Epilepsy Res* 1994; **18**: 67–73.

42. French JA, Wang S, Warnock B, *et al*. Historical control monotherapy design in the treatment of epilepsy. *Epilepsia* 2010; **51**: 1936–43.

43. Perucca E. When clinical trials make history: Demonstrating efficacy of new antiepileptic drugs as monotherapy. *Epilepsia* 2010; **51**: 1933–5.

44. Biton V, Sackellares JC, Vuong A, *et al*. Double-blind, placebo-controlled study of lamotrigine in primary generalized tonic-clonic seizures. *Neurology* 2005; **65**: 1737–43.

45. Richens A. Proof of efficacy trials: cross-over versus parallel-group. *Epilepsy Res* 2001; **45**: 43–7; discussion 9–51.

46. Guideline on clinical investigation of medicinal products in the treatment of epileptic disorders. EMEA. 2010. http://www.ema.europa.eu/pdfs/human/ewp/056698enrev2.pdf.

47. Schmidt D. Two antiepileptic drugs for intractable epilepsy with complex-partial seizures. *J Neurol Neurosurg Psychiatry* 1982; **45**: 1119–24.

48. French JA. Obstacles encountered in designing antiepileptic drug trials. *Epilepsy Res* 1993; **10** (Suppl): 81–9.

49. Walczak T. Do antiepileptic drugs play a role in sudden unexpected death in epilepsy? *Drug Saf* 2003; **26**: 673–83.

50. Christensen J, Andreasen F, Poulsen JH, *et al*. Randomized, concentration-controlled trial of topiramate in refractory focal epilepsy. *Neurology* 2003; **61**: 1210–8.

51. Guekht AB, Korczyn AD, Bondareva IB, and Gusev EI. Placebo responses in randomized trials of antiepileptic drugs. *Epilepsy Behav* 2010; **17**: 64–9.

52. Cramer J, Vachon L, Desforges C, *et al*. Dose frequency and dose interval compliance with multiple antiepileptic medications during a controlled clinical trial. *Epilepsia* 1995; **36**: 1111–7.

53. Sperling MR, Greenspan A, Cramer JA, *et al*. Carisbamate as adjunctive treatment of partial onset seizures in adults in two randomized, placebo-controlled trials. *Epilepsia* 2010; **51**: 333–43.

54. French JA and Schachter S. A workshop on antiepileptic drug monotherapy indications. *Epilepsia* 2002; **43** (Suppl 10): 3–27.

Chapter

26

Insomnia

Michael E. Yurcheshen, Changyong Feng, and J. Todd Arnedt

Overview

Chronic insomnia affects up to 10% of American adults and exacts a major personal and societal burden. Chronic insomnia has been linked to reduced quality of life, increased risk for psychiatric and substance use disorders, and exacerbates comorbid health conditions [1–3]. The total costs of insomnia to the health care system are highly significant, with one recent study estimating that average direct and indirect costs for younger adults with untreated insomnia were more than $1200 greater than for adults without insomnia [4].

Amongst the neurological conditions outlined in this textbook, insomnia shares its dual objective and subjective nature with other conditions. Current therapy has both a biological and behavioral basis. For the purposes of this chapter, circadian rhythm disorders, which involve a mismatch between the biological timing system and preferred sleep and wake cycles, are considered pathophysiologically separate from insomnia, and will not be discussed.

Biological basis for intervention

Insomnia is a sleep disorder characterized by complaints of difficulty initiating sleep, maintaining sleep, waking too early, or sleep that is chronically experienced as non-restorative or poor in quality. These complaints occur despite adequate opportunity and circumstances for sleep, and individuals attribute some form of daytime impairment (e.g., fatigue, neurocognitive deficits, mood disturbance) to the sleep problems [5].

Primary insomnia

Primary insomnia can be considered a condition of hyperarousal, and is defined as an insomnia disorder that is not directly caused by another medical, sleep, or mental disorder, or by the direct physiological effects of a substance [5]. The current prevailing psychological construct about primary insomnia is the Spielman '3P' model [6]. This model suggests that an individual has 'predisposing' factors that may increase individual susceptibility to insomnia. Identified inherent characteristics that are considered predisposing factors include a familial history of light or disrupted sleep and psychological characteristics such as a tendency to worry excessively and over concern with personal well-being. 'Precipitating' factors are triggering events that initiate a bout of insomnia. Some examples of precipitating conditions include physical stressors (i.e., acute illness, pain), psychiatric stressors (clinical depression, mania), or social stressors (either positive or negative). Once insomnia has been initiated, 'perpetuating' factors, counterproductive associations and habits, can maintain it over time, even after the original precipitating event has disappeared or has been managed. The perpetuating factors that have received most attention include behavioral strategies to compensate for poor sleep (i.e., napping), efforts to deal with the consequences of insomnia (i.e., excessive caffeine intake), pre-sleep cognitive arousal, and negative sleep-related beliefs and attitudes (i.e., worry about inability to sleep and daytime consequences as a result of sleep loss, unrealistic sleep expectations).

Comorbid insomnia

Comorbid insomnia is more common than primary insomnia. Although there is some debate about the directionality of the relationship, comorbid insomnia is thought to be caused primarily by a concurrent medical, sleep, or psychiatric disorder, or to be the direct result of another substance. Until recently, most clinical trials have focused on primary insomnia; however,

Table 26.1 Neurotransmitters involved in sleep and wakefulness

Transmitter	Wakefulness	NREM sleep	REM sleep	Examples of sleep related agonists/upregulators	Examples of sleep related antagonists
Acetylcholine	x		x		Tricyclic antidepressants
Monoamines	x			Amphetamines	
Histamine	x				Diphenhydramine
Glutamine	x				
Adenosine					
Serotonin		x			
GABA		x		Benzodiazepines, Benzodiazepine receptor agonists	
Hypocretin (orexin A)	x		x		Under development

recruitment of appropriate subjects with this disorder is often difficult, given its relative rarity compared to comorbid insomnia. The frequency of comorbid insomnia is now becoming a recognized phenomenon in clinical trials planning. Some recent comparative efficacy trials have examined responses to pharmacologic interventions in cohorts with primary vs. comorbid insomnia [7].

Brief mention should be made of some of the more established neural pathways responsible for initiating and maintaining sleep and wakefulness, as they are putative therapeutic targets. Wakefulness, non-REM sleep, and REM sleep are separate but functionally interconnected states, and are modulated by different neurotransmitter systems. Glutaminergic, cholinergic, and monoaminergic pathways ascending from the brainstem serve critical roles in maintenance of wakefulness [8]. By contrast, non-REM sleep regulation relies largely on GABAergic pathways, ascending from a portion of the reticular activating system and descending from the anterior hypothalamus [9]. To date, most of the developed neuropharmacologic agents for insomnia have focused on these pathways, specifically in the form of GABAergic manipulation. Additional neurotransmitter systems contribute to non-REM sleep. For instance, serotonergic pathways are based largely in the midbrain, and like many of the pathways responsible for wakefulness, have ascending cortical and septal projections. Substantial complexity was introduced into the known basic sleep-wake mechanisms in the late 1990s with the discovery of hypocretin (orexin A). These centers primarily localize to the posterior hypothalamus,

but have widespread connections, and play a role in REM sleep regulation [10–12]. This neurotransmitter, however, is involved in more than REM-sleep, and has an impact on wakefulness as well. Similarly, acetylcholine, a neurotransmitter also involved in wakefulness, also contributes to REM sleep regulation. Coordination between these various states is complicated, and the details of these patterns are emerging.

Some studies of insomnia suggest that disruption of these mechanisms will result in sleep-wake dysregulation. For instance, in animal models, lesions of the ventrolateral preoptic nucleus in the hypothalamus result in a substantial decrease in NREM and REM sleep [13, 14]. For most individuals with insomnia, however, such distinct lesions are not present. There are several convergent areas of research using different techniques that lend support to hyperarousal in insomnia. It is unclear how the psychological and biological state of hyperarousal relates to the 3P model, and how it causes dysregulation of these neural pathways.

With this as background, interventions for insomnia have been non-pharmacologic, pharmacologic, or both [15]. Drawing a distinction between psychological and pharmacologic interventions may prove arbitrary, as both types of interventions may ultimately result in biological change.

Non-pharmacologic interventions

Cognitive behavioral therapy for insomnia (CBT-I) has become the gold standard therapy for primary insomnia and has demonstrated efficacy for comorbid insomnia [16]. This multimodal intervention incorporates therapeutic interventions targeting behavioral factors (maladaptive sleep habits, irregular sleep scheduling) and cognitive factors (worry, beliefs, apprehension about sleep) that are believed to perpetuate insomnia over time. Other examples of individual non-pharmacologic interventions for insomnia include, but are not limited to, stimulus control, relaxation therapy, paradoxical intention, and biofeedback [16]. Early studies evaluated the efficacy of individual behavioral therapies and CBT-I via in-person individual treatment format, but more recent trials have expanded to effectiveness studies with treatment modalities ranging from group therapy to telephone consultations to internet-delivered CBT-I [17].

Pharmacologic interventions

Pharmacologic agents with hypnotic properties via several different mechanisms have been evaluated in clinical trials. In the past 10–20 years, many of these trials have studied novel drugs targeted to some of the neurological pathways outlined above.

Regarding the aforementioned neural networks responsible for wakefulness, REM sleep, and non-REM sleep, pharmacologic agents generally act either as sleep 'agonists', or wakefulness 'antagonists'. Table 26.1 summarizes some of the known neurotransmitter systems involved with sleep, and examples of neurotherapeutic agents that act at these targets (benzodiazepine receptor agonists, benzodiazepines, hypocretin antagonists, antihistamines, anticholinergics).

The ideal hypnotic would be a safe, effective agent that preserved sleep macro and micro architecture. It would also be free of side effects (dependency, rebound insomnia, residual daytime sleepiness, medication interactions, etc.) while working rapidly and on a known therapeutic target [18].

Goals of intervention

In general, there are two major goals when treating insomnia:
1) Treat for resolution of/improvement in sleep disruption
2) Treat to improve the associated neurocognitive and medical consequences of insomnia

Compared to hypnotics, CBT-I seems to have a more sustained effect, and perhaps an additional benefit of disease modification [19].

Conditions associated with/exacerbated by insomnia include depression, as well as a host of other neurophysiological complaints including altered concentration, energy levels, attention and vigilance, and motivation [20, 21]. Motor vehicle accidents have also been linked to sleepiness, which can be associated with insomnia [22]. Emerging evidence links some insomnia with hypertension [23, 24]. The studies that have linked insomnia to these conditions have been small, and have some methodological limitations, thereby hindering their use as primary outcome measures.

Study populations

As outlined, insomnia can be primary or comorbid. Most early insomnia trials generally focused on subjects with primary insomnia, however, some calls for clinical trials in comorbid insomnia have been sounded [25].

Furthermore, insomnia is, in many ways, a disorder studied in the developed world. Clinical trials for insomnia are generally conducted in populations that have an awareness of the functional impact of sleep loss, as well as the luxury to consider this disorder as a significant concern.

Special populations

It is estimated that up to 90% of insomnia is comorbid, and psychiatric disease and pain are likely the inciting factors in the majority of these cases [26]. Consequently, there is a significant need for exploratory and confirmatory clinical trials for such conditions. The converse is also true, and the impact of insomnia on these inciting conditions is becoming increasingly recognized. This represents an opportunity to conduct clinical trials that evaluate outcomes on the underlying condition, as the concurrent insomnia is addressed. There is some argument to include more detailed criteria for sleep disturbance as part of the operational definition of many of these conditions, especially in psychiatric disease. Sleep disturbances are varied, though, and finding sufficient uniformity in a potential study population can be a barrier to design and recruitment. These types of studies are far smaller and rarer than would be expected when considering the prevalence of comorbid insomnia in these populations [27].

Insomnia is more common amongst women, and, as a result, many clinical trials have a preponderance of female subjects [28]. Perhaps one of the best studied insomnia subpopulations is menopausal women. These trials can be challenging, in part because there are several contributing factors to the insomnia [29]. Furthermore, although these subjects could certainly be included in standard insomnia trials, there has been substantial interest in alternative agents that are generally not considered hypnotics/soporifics in other populations [30, 31]. Specifically, hormone replacement therapy has been studied as a targeted treatment for menopausal insomnia, often with contradictory results [32–34].

Another condition that warrants mention is paradoxical insomnia (also known as sleep state misperception). This condition is characterized by objectively normal sleep duration, continuity, and architecture in an individual with complaints of gross sleep disturbances [5]. Although misjudgment of sleep time is a feature of most forms of insomnia, patients with paradoxical insomnia have minimal daytime impairments with a *grossly* disproportionate perception of sleep time compared to objective measurements. This is a challenging patient population to treat, and no clinical trials to date have evaluated the efficacy of pharmacologic or non-pharmacologic therapeutics on this condition.

Properties of measurement tools

Clinical measures

A variety of objective and subjective measures have a role in clinical insomnia trials. Practical considerations of these measures are introduced here, but their application in clinical trials is detailed below ('Clinical trial designs and analytical methods used in development').

Subjective measures

Sleep diary

In both pharmacologic and non-pharmacologic clinical trials of insomnia, sleep diaries are often the primary outcome measure of treatment efficacy. One advantage of daily sleep diaries is the ability to evaluate sleep over days to weeks, providing a more complete picture than polysomnography or other short-term measures. The information is typically averaged over the assessment period, with calculation of key sleep parameters: sleep onset latency (time to fall asleep for the first time), number of awakenings during the night, wakefulness after sleep onset, total sleep time, sleep efficiency (total sleep time/time in bed × 100), and sleep quality. Investigators often select primary and secondary sleep diary outcomes based on the patient selection criteria

(e.g., sleep onset vs. maintenance insomnia) or putative mechanisms of the treatment under evaluation. Sleep diaries can be used as stand-alone tools, or as an adjunct to objective measures such as actigraphy.

Questionnaires

Several questionnaires are utilized in clinical trials. These include the Insomnia Severity Index (ISI), which measures the characteristics and severity of the condition, and the Pittsburgh Sleep Quality Index (PSQI), which is a measure of general sleep disruption [35–37]. The Women's Health Initiative Insomnia Rating Scale (WHIIRS) is used in appropriate populations [38, 39]. Depending on the protocol, measures of daytime sleepiness, such as the Epworth Sleepiness Scale (ESS) or Stanford Sleepiness Scale (SSS), can be appropriate [40, 41].

Collateral clinical and neurocognitive measures

Other subjective measurements are available to measure the *impact* of insomnia or sleep deprivation on performance. The range of these measures is wide, and will vary depending on the individual protocol and what it seeks to measure. These tests often include psychomotor vigilance tasks. These occasionally also take the form of objective measurements. For instance, the 'steer clear' test, a driving simulator that measures surrogates of driving performance, has been used in clinical trials in insomnia and sleep deprivation [42].

Objective measures

Polysomnography

There are several objective tests that are relevant in insomnia trials. Of these, polysomnography (PSG) remains the gold standard. It remains the only reliable method by which sleep stages can be detected, and is the most accurate measure of sleep continuity variables (sleep latency, sleep efficiency, wake after sleep onset, number of arousals) that are often important in these trials. More invasive measures can be taken during PSG monitoring (for instance, blood pressure readings or long-line blood draws). This said, PSG has significant limitations as a research tool. In-lab studies with type 1 devices (as opposed to type 2, 3, or 4 devices that are considered ambulatory) are sometimes prohibitively expensive to use in research protocols [43]. In addition, polysomnography is subject to certain systemic artifacts, including 'first night effect' where sleep architecture can be disrupted simply by virtue of being observed in a foreign environment with surface instrumentation.

Table 26.2 Methods of evaluating sleep and insomnia in clinical trials

Method	Examples	Advantages	Disadvantages
Questionnaire	ISI, PSQI, ESS, SSS[a]	Many validated. Simple to complete. Can have validated cut-offs to differentiate normal from pathology.	Each questionnaire has limitations of what it is able to measure. Can suffer from floor effects.
Sleep diaries		Simple to complete. Prospective. Longitudinal data.	Requires significant subject effort. Adherence can drop over time.
Actigraphy		Can provide longitudinal, objective data about sleep.	More involved than questionnaires. Some cost involved. Not as reliable as PSG to determine sleep and wakefulness. Does not always correlate with PSG data in insomnia subjects.
Portable polysomnography monitoring		Less expensive than in-lab polysomnography. Can provide longitudinal data about sleep.	Many devices cannot determine sleep staging.
In-lab monitored polysomnography		Best method for determining sleep staging.	Expensive. Does not provide longitudinal data about sleep. Subject to 'first night' effect

[a] See text for abbreviations.

A run-in night is often utilized in protocols, especially for large, phase 3 trials. During this night, data are usually recorded, but are rarely used as a baseline for analysis. Lastly, polysomnography provides no longitudinal data about sleep. It does create a detailed 'snapshot' of an individual night's sleep, but this is insufficient to judge sleep objectively over weeks or months.

Actigraphy

Actigraphy, another objective measurement tool for sleep, utilizes movement (or more correctly, the lack thereof) as a surrogate for sleep. This wristwatch size and shaped unit is worn by the subject, sometimes for weeks at a time. The information is then downloaded for recording and analysis. Although actigraphy data is useful to measure sleep over a sustained period of time, and to confirm objectively what is recorded in subjective sleep journals, it does not permit measurement of sleep stages and is less accurate in measuring sleep parametrics (sleep latency, etc.) than polysomnography.

Biomarkers and their relationship to biological targets

Polysomnography and actigraphy are physiologically more precise in detecting and quantifying sleep latency and sleep disruption than clinical interview, sleep diaries, or questionnaire data, and could be considered neurophysiological extensions of clinical measurements that allow improved sensitivity in identifying sleep characteristics. There are spectral analysis data that suggest faster EEG frequencies are present in sleeping individuals with primary insomnia [44–46]. This finding lends some support to a theory of hyperarousal contributing to insomnia; however, not all studies have yielded similar results [47].

Observational studies have identified biomarkers in related sleep disturbances, (i.e., melatonin levels and Period (Per) gene secretegogues in circadian rhythm disturbances); however, there are no analogous serum markers identified to date in primary or comorbid insomnia.

Some observational studies have evaluated biomarkers for the *sequelae* of insomnia. For instance, inflammatory markers have been explored in forced sleep deprivation [48]. It remains to be seen whether Spielman's 3P model of insomnia will eventually lend itself to the identification of biomarker surrogates.

Clinical trial designs and analytical methods used in development

The studies highlighted below are examples of some recent clinical trials that evaluated non-pharmacologic,

pharmacologic, or dual therapies for insomnia. They utilize a host of study designs, including the gold standard: randomized controlled double-blind clinical trials. Some of the trials are considered to be seminal in the field. Others were selected as examples of trials that had some methodological or biostatistical limitations in order to highlight challenges or advances in the implementation of such studies.

Examples of clinical trials

Non-pharmacologic based trials

Espie *et al.* conducted a randomized, controlled clinical trial to study the effectiveness of CBT delivered by primary care nurses [49]. The study aimed to evaluate effectiveness of CBT over weeks to months. Patients with chronic insomnia were randomized with equal probability to two treatments: CBT or self-monitoring control (SMC). The SMC patients entered the treatment replication phase, receiving an identical treatment to the CBT group after 6 weeks. The authors concluded that CBT was an effective intervention as evidenced by both its initial superiority over SMC, and by the replication of a similar outcome with deferred treatment.

This is a half crossover study. Since each individual serves as his/her own control, the influence of covariates other than the treatment assignment is reduced. Also, crossover designs are usually statistically efficient, and require fewer subjects than do non-crossover designs. This is closely related to the first point, as the crossover design generally reduces the variation of the pre- and post-treatment difference. This efficiency is an advantage in insomnia trials, where both variability within the condition and recruitment difficulties can be barriers to conducting the trial.

Despite these advantages, both the order of administration of treatment, and carry-over effects between treatments, can confound the estimates of the treatment effect. For these reasons, crossover designs are not ideal for large-scale insomnia trials until carryover effect can be minimized or disproven. See Chapter 10 for a further discussion of crossover designs.

Other studies have evaluated efficacy of different types of psychological interventions for insomnia. In a comparative efficacy trial, Lichstein *et al.* studied the treatment effect of three psychological treatments (relaxation, sleep compression, and placebo therapy) on older adults with insomnia [50]. Seventy-four participants were randomized to three treatment groups with equal probabilities. Sleep diary data demonstrated

efficacy of all methods, although this finding was not demonstrated with PSG.

Although the use of objective PSG data in this trial lends objective data, this trial has a number of shortcomings that are common in the study of psychological interventions. For instance, like the Espie trial, it is difficult to blind subjects for psychological treatment. The trial also uses some statistical methods that are limiting, although concerns are not necessarily specific to insomnia trials.

A handful of clinical trials have been designed to evaluate non-pharmacologic interventions on comorbid insomnia. Currie *et al.* studied the effect of CBT on participants with insomnia secondary to chronic pain [51]. Fifty-one subjects finished the study. Using self-report measures and actigraphy, a CBT group showed significant improvement at 7 weeks and again at 3 months, as compared to a wait list control group.

The imputation of missing data in this trial was performed using an intention to treat principle; one that introduces significant uncertainty into the final comparisons and therefore conclusions. Since this publication, increasing emphasis has been placed on subject retention in clinical trials. Furthermore, other statistical methods have been developed for imputation of missing data [52]. The use of a repeated measure analysis of variance to study outcomes is no longer considered ideal in longitudinal studies. For future studies that study insomnia longitudinally, other methods such as the linear mixed-effect model and generalized estimation equation (GEE) methods could be considered [53, 54].

Pharmacologic-based clinical trials

Roth *et al.* studied the treatment effect of eszopiclone (ESZ) over 1 year. After 6 months of double-blind, randomized, placebo-controlled treatment with eszopiclone, the study was extended for an additional 6 months in an open-label phase [55]. In effect, there are two groups (placebo-ESZ) and (ESZ-ESZ) in this report. The analyses indicated that significant improvement in sleep and daytime function was evident in those switched from double-blind placebo to 6 months of open-label eszopiclone therapy. In addition, improvements were noted and sustained in the ESZ-ESZ group as well. This trial uses a different design in order to gather long-term data, although half of the trial was open label. There are significant limitations to using an open-label design, but this trial highlights the difficulty in designing ethically appropriate studies that will maximize subject retention while still gathering long-term data about insomnia.

Krystal *et al.* conducted a randomized, double-blind, placebo-controlled parallel-group multi-center study that aimed to evaluate long-term efficacy and safety of zolpidem on patients with chronic primary insomnia [56]. Patients were randomized at a rate of 2:1 to two groups: treatment (669) and placebo (349). The subjective sleep measures, including sleep onset latency (SOL), total sleep time (TST), number of awakenings (NAW), wake after sleep onset (WASO), quality of sleep (QOS), and next day functioning were assessed daily through the Patient Morning Questionnaire (PMQ) while the patients global impression (PGI) and Clinical Global Impression-Improvement scale (CGI-I) were assessed every 4 weeks. The total study lasted 6 months. The study demonstrated that the zolpidem extended-release treatment was statistically superior to the placebo at each time point of assessment for PGI, CGI-I, TST, WASO, QOS, SOL and NAW. The treatment provided sustained and significant improvements in sleep onset and maintenance, and improved next-day concentration and morning sleepiness. The design of the study is the clearest among all clinical trials discussed here. The advantage of a longitudinal design is to study both the time trend of outcome variables, and the effect of covariates (for example, treatment indicator) on those outcome variables in the same model. In the data analysis, the authors compared the outcome variables of two groups at each assessment time point. Although intuitive, this type of analysis should only be used for a very preliminary analysis. Given the relatively large sample size, semiparametric methods for longitudinal studies (such as GEE, linear mixed model, or generalized linear mixed model) can be used to analyze the data efficiently [53, 54, 57].

Dual therapy and comparative efficacy trials

Recently, there has been interest in using pharmacologic and non-pharmacologic treatment in combination to treat insomnia. Hypnotics can produce rapid symptomatic relief, but the results are often not sustained. Conversely, CBT-I is generally intensive, but often results in sustained improvement. A dual approach represents an uncommon opportunity in neurology.

Morin *et al.* conducted a randomized controlled trial of subjects with persistent insomnia designed to: 1) evaluate the short and long-term effects of CBT-I, singly and combined with zolpidem and 2) compare

the efficacy of maintenance strategies in optimizing long-term outcomes [15]. Initially, the subjects were randomized to either CBT-I or dual therapy. After 6 weeks, the CBT cohort was randomly split in two. One half was selected to no treatment, and the remaining half continued with CBT. Likewise, the dual therapy group was split in two, with one half randomly transferred to CBT-I treatment only. The extended treatment was stopped after 6 months, but the cohorts were studied for an additional 6 months in follow-up. In the short term, both CBT-I and dual therapy showed efficacy; long-term benefits were maintained for the dual therapy turned CBT-I group. Although the randomization procedure and data analysis were complicated, this study explores a much needed treatment strategy, one with previous little data to support it. Furthermore, it represents an evaluation with active treatment comparisons, a rarity in insomnia trials.

Lastly, in a comparative efficacy trial, aimed to evaluate active treatments using *objective* measures, Sivertsen, *et al.* examined short- and long-term clinical efficacy of CBT and pharmacologic treatment in older adults experiencing chronic primary insomnia [19]. This was a randomized, double-blinded, placebo-controlled trial, with subjects randomized to three groups: CBT, sleep medication, and placebo medication. The treatment period was for 6 weeks, with 6 months follow-up for the two active treatment groups. With polysomnography, they found that CBT was more effective than medication over both the short and long term in certain sleep parameters (efficiency, slow-wave sleep, and total wake time). The study was subject to a host of limitations (small sample size, no blinding for CBT group, last value carried forward for missing data), but does address comparative efficacy using objective methods.

General consideration of design and data analysis

Parallel / crossover design

For crossover insomnia trials, it is difficult to determine exactly how long a washout period is required for psychological interventions, such as CBT-I. For instance, in the Espie trial, the placebo group switched over to the CBT-I treatment after 6 weeks [49]. There are also some issues in estimating the treatment effect of CBT-I, specifically due to the delayed start of CBT-I in some subjects. For instance, the CBT-I evaluated vs.

placebo in the first 6 weeks, may be fundamentally different from the CBT-I that is delayed for 6 weeks.

Sample size

Sample size is one of the most important considerations in clinical trials. Some studies have a sample size too small (for example, in the Sivertsen trial) to make a meaningful statistical inference. As an example, some of the above studies highlighted above set power at 80% while others at 90% [19].

Length of follow-up

Clinical trials for insomnia have examined both the short- and long-term effect of treatment. Several studies of hypnotics have examined the efficacy and safety (i.e., the risk of dependency) of these agents for periods up to 6 months in duration [55]. Some non-pharmacologic intervention trials have examined treatment periods longer than this. Future studies that use a commonly accepted standard for short- and long-term treatment periods will help to standardize treatments and facilitate comparative efficacy.

Blindness and placebo effect

In clinical trials with medication as the treatment modality, blinding is simple to perform and maintain, for both the patients and researchers. For CBT-I, blinding is somewhat more difficult. Most trials to date have used wait list controls or minimal intervention comparisons, but some trials have used behavioral placebos successfully.

Primary objective/primary outcome (end point)

Ideally each clinical trial should have only one primary objective, and one primary outcome. Since insomnia is a complicated problem, most clinical trials have several primary objectives and primary outcomes.

Standards for efficacy and special safety issues

Significant progress has been made in developing and testing pharmacologic and non-pharmacologic treatments for insomnia; however, variability remains across clinical trials in the assessment of efficacy and safety [58]. Early studies focused nearly exclusively on changes in sleep parameters with treatment, but the importance of including collateral clinical measures and relevant assessments of daytime functioning has become increasingly recognized.

Subjective

Diary data

Efficacy of insomnia interventions is commonly determined by comparing diary means and/or proportions between a treatment and control group before and after treatment using appropriate standard tests of statistical significance. Magnitude of treatment effects are often expressed in terms of effect size using the d-statistic [59]. Results from several meta-analyses of insomnia treatment studies indicate that pharmacologic and non-pharmacologic insomnia therapies produce medium to large effect sizes on key subjective sleep parameters [60, 61].

Indicators of clinical significance go beyond the inferential statistical analysis and enable investigators to predict whether treatment-related changes are likely to produce meaningful improvements in subjects' daily lives. Although no consensus exists on how to define clinically meaningful improvements, some possible approaches include comparing sleep improvements to normative comparisons (e.g., mean sleep latency ≤30 minutes), using collateral information from significant others and clinicians, and documenting the proportion of responders and remitters to insomnia based on an accepted criterion.

Collateral clinical and neurocognitive measures

A thorough assessment of insomnia treatment efficacy includes administration of collateral clinical measures. In many trials, related conditions include depression (Beck Depression Inventory), anxiety (State-Trait Anxiety Inventory), fatigue (Multidimensional Fatigue Inventory), and quality of life (SF-36).

Although no standards exist for establishing efficacy, CBT-I trials have included clinician- and significant-other ratings of insomnia symptoms and severity, reasoning that an efficacious treatment should evidence changes in sleep and functioning that are noticeable to others [62]. The Clinical Global Impressions Scale, in particular the Improvement subscale, is commonly used in pharmacologic insomnia studies as a secondary measure of treatment efficacy.

Patients with insomnia frequently complain about deficits in cognition, most notably in the domains of attention, concentration, and memory, yet few clinical trials of insomnia have incorporated these measures as outcomes. Because neurocognitive deficits can be mild and selective, the role of neurocognitive tests in insomnia clinical trials has been restricted to quantifying residual daytime impairment following nighttime hypnotic administration [63].

Objective

Polysomnography

Polysomnography is considered the gold standard for measurement of sleep in hypnotic trials and is also used as a measure of treatment efficacy in behavioral insomnia trials. Because insomnia has a large subjective component, PSG is essentially never the sole measure of efficacy in clinical trials. It is often used to exclude subjects with other sleep disorders, and is increasingly used as a pre-post measure of treatment efficacy. Key sleep continuity parameters, such as total sleep time and sleep efficiency (total sleep time/planned sleep time × 100) are generally measured. This approach may substantially increase Type I error rates (depending on sample size), therefore, defining primary and secondary PSG endpoints based on expected mechanisms of treatment is a preferred approach.

Actigraphy

The use of actigraphy as a measure of efficacy is appealing because it seems to balance the benefits of daily sleep diaries (continuous recording over days to weeks in the home environment) with those of overnight PSG (objective measure of sleep). Actigraphy is generally most useful as a secondary and complementary measure of treatment efficacy and in situations when PSG is not practical.

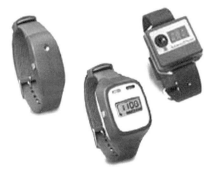

AW-2, AW-Spectrum, AW-Score

Figure 26.1. Examples of actigraphy units. They are intended to be worn on the non-dominant wrist. Many units come with event markers and/or with light sensors. The actigraphs can store several weeks' worth of wake-sleep information. These data can be downloaded, stored, and analyzed using a PC. Images courtesy of Philips Respironics, Murrysville, PA.

Efficacy in comorbid populations

In comorbid insomnia trials, determination of treatment efficacy is based on changes in both sleep *and* the accompanying condition. For example, Fava and colleagues found that remission rates to depression were higher in subjects who received 8 weeks of combined fluoxetine and eszopiclone, compared to those who received fluoxetine plus placebo [64]. In this study, the primary endpoint of efficacy was change in psychiatric symptomatology rather than sleep. Primary efficacy outcomes have also been measured in terms of markers for dependency and pain [65, 66].

Safety measures

In pharmaceutical insomnia trials, as with other pharmacologic treatment studies, it is standard to include laboratory studies, vital signs, electrocardiograms, and self-report scales. These measures are included to document side effects, and adverse events while studying the experimental and placebo agents, whether related or unrelated to the study treatment. Residual daytime sedation and its consequences on daytime functioning is a unique focus of safety evaluations in insomnia clinical trials. In clinical trials involving hypnotic dependent individuals, the Clinical Institute Withdrawal Assessment (CIWA) – Benzodiazepines assesses the type and severity of symptoms that may be related to discontinuation of the medication.

Implementation issues

Recruitment

Insomnia is extremely prevalent in the general population, with as many as one in three individuals complaining of persistent insomnia in a given year [67]. Nevertheless, recruitment issues and challenges are common in insomnia clinical trials. Community advertisement can result in samples of primarily non-treatment seeking participants. These individuals are characteristically different from treatment-seeking individuals in primary care or specialty settings, which may impact on the generalizability of findings [68]. The use of prescription or non-prescription sleep agents, or other CNS active medications are also frequent exclusions, and the common use of these drugs is a significant barrier to recruitment. As a result, selection bias may be an issue in many trials, since only volunteers who: 1) can tolerate a withdrawal from their hypnotics, 2) desire to discontinue these agents, or 3) are not currently on sleep agents are likely to volunteer. As a result, this bias can potentially compromise the external validity of the study. Few clinical trials in insomnia are multi-site studies, resulting in suboptimal samples in terms of geographic and racial/ethnic diversity. Moreover, while insomnia disproportionately affects older rather than young adults, most randomized trials to date have been carried out with middle-aged samples, with notable exceptions [61].

Sample selection

One challenge unique to insomnia clinical trials is the lack of standards for the insomnia diagnosis. Criteria differ across three widely used nosologies, the *Diagnostic and Statistical Manual of Mental Disorders, Fourth Edition – Text Revision (DSM-IV-TR)*, the *International Classification of Diseases (ICD-9-CM and ICD-10)* and the *International Classification of Sleep Disorders Second Edition (ICSD-2)*, with investigators using all three for sample selection. Recent efforts have been made to address the heterogeneity in insomnia definitions across trials by deriving a consensus definition for insomnia research [69]. In addition, frequency, severity, and duration are important dimensions to insomnia, but there has been little agreement about what or how cutoffs should be used for study inclusion [70].

Duration of treatment

A methodological challenge relevant to both pharmacologic and non-pharmacologic insomnia trials is determining the duration of treatment. The duration of therapy in a particular study is likely the result of a variety of factors, including the specific research questions, known properties of the treatment under investigation, and practical and methodological considerations. Despite evidence that a significant proportion of individuals with chronic insomnia use hypnotic agents for longer than indicated, very few pharmaceutical trials have evaluated nightly or non-nightly use of these agents beyond 1 month, with median treatment duration of just 1 week [71]. More recent medication trials have been enhanced methodologically by the inclusion of placebo lead-ins to evaluate placebo response and lead-outs to evaluate the sustainability of treatment effects after acute therapy [72]. Issues about treatment duration have also been evident in non-pharmacologic insomnia trials [16].

Appropriate control group

Nearly all pharmacologic insomnia trials to date have compared active treatments to pill placebos, yet a more appropriate question involves the relative risks and benefits of pharmacologic therapies with similar or different mechanisms of action. One of the most commonly used control conditions in non-pharmacologic trials is a wait-list condition. As discussed in other chapters in this book, this introduces both ethical considerations and concerns that post-treatment differences cannot be ascribed to the specific treatment provided vs. non-specific factors associated with participating in a research trial. More recent clinical trials have used behavioral placebos against which to compare active CBT-I treatments, allowing for more specific interpretation of observed treatment-related differences [73, 74]. Given the recruitment challenges inherent in insomnia trials, crossover or single-case designs may be reasonable alternatives to randomized controlled parallel trials in certain circumstances, with the caveats noted above ('Properties of measurement tools') that washout periods should be reasonably known.

Frequency of assessments

Repeated assessments in randomized clinical trials are crucial for determining efficacy of therapies, but the frequency of these assessments is a topic of significant debate. While the frequency of assessments in a given trial is guided by a number of considerations, insomnia trials should include, at a minimum, baseline assessments to characterize symptom status at study entry, post-treatment assessments to measure treatment efficacy, and some follow-up assessment to ascertain durability of gains following acute discontinuation of treatment. In addition, assessing outcomes during the course of therapy allows for the determination of treatment response trajectories and process-outcome relationships [75].

Subject retention

A primary challenge to any clinical trial is subject retention. More than one-third of active treatment participants and one-half of placebo participants discontinued their respective treatments in the longest controlled trials of a pharmacologic insomnia therapy (6 months) [63, 76]. In general, attrition rates in large-scale randomized behavioral insomnia trials are lower than rates in medication trials. However, attrition rates increase significantly for behavioral trials that are not in-person, such as internet-based insomnia treatment trials [77].

Future directions

Clinical trials examining insomnia are in their early stages, and there is significant controversy regarding optimal treatment approaches and duration, and the measurement of efficacy outcomes.

For instance, trials using two active drugs or therapies (i.e. study drug vs. active control) are rare, however, comparative effectiveness trials are critical for identifying differentiating factors among subjects that are related to treatment response/non-response. Ideally, these trials would involve drugs or therapies posited to target different mechanisms of disease. Better access to funding outside of industry-sponsored sources could help with this challenge. The few trials evaluating pharmacologic vs. non-pharmacologic interventions have been encouraging, and could serve as a model for this type of trial.

To date, most clinical trials have focused on treatments for primary insomnia. Both comorbid insomnia, and special patient populations (such as menopausal insomnia or insomnia in the elderly or in children) deserve unique attention. Given subject variability, it is not clear that the results from previous hypnotic trials can be generalized to these groups that have some fundamental differences when compared to a general primary insomnia population.

In general, hypnotic trials have evaluated efficacy over short-term periods, weeks to months. Given the chronicity of the condition, trials evaluating long-term use of hypnotics are important and should be prioritized. Trials that examine long-term adherence to therapies, and sustainability of treatment gains, are needed. Perhaps more importantly, the safety profile of these pharmacologic agents, in terms of dependence and other effects, needs to be evaluated, as many patients remain on these drugs for years.

Insomnia is a complicated process, and afflicted individuals are different from one another in a variety of ways. To date, consistent genetic, physiological, and psychological profiles of insomnia have not been identified. Moreover, the characteristics of responders vs. non-responders in clinical trials are understudied. By identifying phenotypes of insomnia, treatment can potentially be more targeted in the future.

Safety outcomes have heretofore generally been excluded in non-pharmacologic treatment trials. It has been assumed that CBT, biofeedback, relaxation therapy, and other techniques have few treatment risks, but the evidence behind this assumption in an insomnia population is lacking. Studies evaluating the safety profile of these types of treatments are needed.

Lastly, cost analysis in insomnia treatment has been largely excluded from clinical trials. A few population-based studies have examined the direct and indirect costs of untreated insomnia [4]. Studies designed to measure economic productivity, offset by costs of the therapy, are lacking. Outcomes should also be examined in terms of utilization of health care resources and treatment satisfaction.

These gaps in knowledge should serve as a basis for future clinical trials in this rapidly expanding field.

References

1. Breslau N, Roth T, Rosenthal L, *et al*. Sleep disturbance and psychiatric disorders: a longitudinal epidemiological study of young adults. *Biol Psychiatry* 1996; **39**: 411–8.

2. Katz DA and McHorney CA. The relationship between insomnia and health-related quality of life in patients with chronic illness. *J Fam Pract* 2002; **51**: 229–35.

3. Taylor DJ, Mallory LJ, Lichstein KL, *et al*. Comorbidity of chronic insomnia with medical problems. *Sleep* 2007; **30**: 213–8.

4. Ozminkowski RJ, Wang S, Walsh JK. The direct and indirect costs of untreated insomnia in adults in the United States. *Sleep* 2007; **30**: 263–73.

5. American Academy of Sleep Medicine. International classification of sleep disorders, 2nd edition.: Diagnostic and coding manual. Westchester, Illinois, American Academy of Sleep Medicine. 2005.

6. Spielman AJ, Glovinsky P. The varied nature of insomnia. In: Hauri PJ, ed. *Case Studies in Insomnia*. New York, Plenum Press. 1991; 1–15.

7. Edinger JD, Olsen MK, Stechuchak KM, *et al*. Cognitive behavioral therapy for patients with primary insomnia or insomnia associated predominantly with mixed psychiatric disorders: A randomized clinical trial. *Sleep* 2009; **32**: 499–510.

8. Jones BE. Toward an understanding of the basic mechanisms of the sleep-waking cycle. *Behavior Brain Sci* 1978; **1**: 495.

9. Jones BE. The organization of central cholinergic systems and their functional importance in sleep-waking states. *Prog Brain Res* 1993; **98**: 61–71.

10. De Lecea L, Kilduff TS, Peyron C, *et al*. The hypocretins: hypothalamus-specific peptides with neuroexcitatory activity. *Proc Natl Acad Sci* 1998; **95**: 322–7.

11. Gautvik KM, de Lecea L, Gautvik VT, *et al*. Overview of the most prevalent hypothalamus-specific mRNAs,

as identified by directional tag PCR subtraction. *PNAS* 1996; **93**: 8733–8.

12. Sakurai T, Amemiya A, Ishii M, *et al.* Orexins and orexin receptors: a family of hypothalamic neuropeptides and G protein-coupled receptors that regulate feeding behavior. *Cell* 1998; **92**: 573–85.

13. Saper CB, Chou TC, and Scammell TE. The sleep switch: hypothalamic control of sleep and wakefulness. *Trends Neurosci* 2001; **24**: 763–71.

14. Saper CB, Scammell TE, and Lu J. Hypothalamic regulation of sleep and circadian rhythms. *Nature* 2005; **437**: 1257–63.

15. Morin CM, Vallieres A, Guay B, *et al.* Cognitive behavioral therapy, singly and combined with medication, for persistent insomnia: A randomized controlled trial. *JAMA* 2009; **301**: 2005–15.

16. Morin CM, Bootzin RR, Buysse DJ, *et al.* Psychological and behavioral treatment of insomnia: Update of the recent evidence (1998–2004). *Sleep* 2006; **29**: 1398–414.

17. Ritterband LM, Thorndike FP, Gonder-Frederick LA, *et al.* Efficacy of an internet-based behavioral intervention for adults with insomnia. *Arch Gen Psychiatry* 2009; **66**: 692–8.

18. Mendelson WB, Roth T, Cassella J, *et al.* The treatment of chronic insomnia: drug indications, chronic use and abuse liability. Summary of a 2001 New Clinical Drug Evaluation Unit Meeting Symposium. *Sleep Med Rev* 2004; **8**: 7–17.

19. Sivertsen B, Omvik S, Pallesen S, *et al.* Cognitive behavioral therapy vs zopiclone for treatment of chronic primary insomnia in older adults: A randomized controlled trial. *JAMA* 2006; **295**: 2851–8.

20. Tsuno N, Besset A, and Ritchie K. Sleep and depression. *J Clin Psychiatry* 2005; **66**: 1254–9.

21. Roth T and Ancoli-Israel S. Daytime consequences and correlates of insomnia in the United States: Results of the 1991 National Sleep Foundation Survey. II. *Sleep* 1999; **22**: S354–S8.

22. Powell NB, Schechtman KB, Riley RW, *et al.* Sleep driver near-misses may predict accident risks. *Sleep* 2007; **30**: 331–42.

23. Vgontzas AN, Liao D, Bixler EO, *et al.* Insomnia with objective short sleep duration is associated with a high risk of hypertension. *Sleep* 2009; **32**: 491–7.

24. Lanfranchi PA, Pennestri M-H, Fradette L, *et al.* Nighttime blood pressure in normotensive subjects with chronic insomnia: Implications for cardiovascular risk. *Sleep* 2009; **32**: 760–6.

25. Stepanski E and Rybarczyk B. Emerging research on the treatment and etiology of secondary or comorbid insomnia. *Sleep Med Rev* 2006; **10**: 7–18.

26. Lichstein K, Gellis LA, Stone K, *et al.* Primary and secondary insomnia. In: Pandi-Perumal SR, Monti JM, ed. *Clinical Pharmacology of Sleep*. Berlin: Birkhauser Basel; 2006.

27. Zucker TL, Samuelson KW, Muench F, *et al.* The effects of respiratory sinus arrhythmia biofeedback on heart rate variability and posttraumatic stress disorder symptoms: a pilot study. *Appl Psychophysiol Biofeedback* 2009; **34**: 135–43.

28. Liljenberg B, Almqvist M, Hetta J, *et al.* The prevalence of insomnia: the importance of operationally defined criteria. *Ann Clin Res* 1988; **17**: 1–7.

29. Moline M, Broch L, Zak R. Sleep in women across the life cycle from adulthood through menopause. *Med Clin N Am* 2004; **88**: 705–36.

30. Dorsey CM, Lee KA, and Scharf MB. Effect of zolpidem on sleep in women with perimenopausal and postmenopausal insomnia: a 4-week randomized, multicenter, double-blind, placebo-controlled study. *Clin Therap* 2004; **26**: 1578–86.

31. Joffe H, Petrillo L, Viguera A, *et al.* Eszopiclone improves insomnia and depressive and anxious symptoms in perimenopausal and postmenopausal women with hot flashes: a randomized, double-blinded, placebo-controlled crossover trial. *Am J Obstet Gynecol* 2010; **202**: 171.e1–.e11.

32. Best NR, Rees MP, Barlow DH, *et al.* Effect of estradiol implant on noradrenergic function and mood in menopausal subjects. *Psychoneuroendocrinology* 1992; **17**: 87–93.

33. Schiff I, Regestein Q, Tulchinsky D, *et al.* Effects of estrogens on sleep and psychological state of hypogonadal women. *JAMA* 1979; **242**: 2405–7.

34. Pickett CK, Regensteiner JG, Woodward WD, *et al.* Progestin and estrogen reduce sleep disordered breathing in postmenopausal women. *J Appl Physiol* 1989; **66**: 1656–61.

35. Buysse DJ, Reynolds III CF, Monk TH, *et al.* The Pittsburgh Sleep Quality Index: A new instrument for psychiatric practice and research. *Psychiatry Research* 1989; **28**: 193–213.

36. Morin CM. *Insomnia: Psychological assessment and management.* Barlow DH, ed. New York, The Guilford Press, 1993.

37. Bastien CH, Vallières A, and Morin CM. Validation of the Insomnia Severity Index as an outcome measure for insomnia research. *Sleep Med* 2001; **2**: 297–307.

38. Levine DW, Bowen DJ, Kaplan RM, *et al.* Factor structure and measurement invariance of the women's health initiative insomnia rating scale. *Psychol Asses* 2003; **15**: 123–36.

39. Levine DW, Kripke DF, Kaplan RM, *et al.* Reliability and validity of the Women's Health Initiative Insomnia Rating Scale. *Psychol Assess* 2003; **15**: 137–48.

40. Johns MW. A new method for measuring daytime sleepiness: The Epworth Sleepiness Scale. *Sleep* 1991; **14**: 540–5.

41. Hoddes E, Dement W, and Zarcone V. The development and use of the Stanford Sleepiness Scale (SSS). *Psychophysiol* 1972; **9**: 150.

42. Findley LJ, Fabrizio MJ, Knight H, *et al*. Driving simulator performance in patients with sleep apnea. *Am Rev Respir Dis* 1989; **140**: 529–30.

43. Standards of Practice Committee of the American Sleep Disorders Association. Practice parameters for the use of portable recording in the assessment of obstructive sleep apnea. *Sleep* 1994; **17**: 372–7.

44. Freeman R. EEG power in sleep onset insomnia. *Electroencephal Clin Neurophysiol* 1986; **63**: 408–13.

45. Merica H, Blois R, and Gaillard JM. Spectral characteristics of sleep EEG in chronic insomnia. *Eur J Neurosci* 1998; **10**: 1826–34.

46. Krystal AD, Edinger JD, Wohlgermuth WK, and Marsh GR. NREM Sleep EEG frequency spectral correlates of sleep complaints in primary insomnia subtypes. *Sleep* 2002; **25**: 630–40.

47. Bastien CH, LeBlanc M, Carrier J, *et al*. Sleep EEG power spectra, insomnia, and chronic use of benzodiazepines. *Sleep* 2003; **26**: 313–7.

48. Irwin MR, Wang M, Ribeiro D, *et al*. Sleep loss activates cellular inflammatory signaling. *Biol Psychiatry* 2008; **64**: 538–40.

49. Espie CA, Inglis SJ, Tessier S, *et al*. The clinical effectiveness of cognitive behaviour therapy for chronic insomnia: implementation and evaluation of a sleep clinic in general medical practice. *Behav Res Ther* 2001; **39**: 45–60.

50. Lichstein KL, Riedel BW, Wilson NM, *et al*. Relaxation and sleep compression for late-life insomnia: a placebo- controlled trial. *J Consult Clin Psychol* 2001; **69**: 227–39.

51. Currie SR, Wilson KG, Pontefract AJ, *et al*. Cognitive-behavioral treatment of insomnia secondary to chronic pain. *J Consult Clin Psychol* 2000; **68**: 407–16.

52. Little RJA and Rubin DB. *Statistical Analysis with Missing Data*, 2nd edition. Hoboken, NJ, John Wiley & Sons, 2002.

53. Laird NM and Ware JH. Random-effects models for longitudinal data. *Biometrics* 1982; **38**: 963–74.

54. Liang KY and Zeger SL. Longitudinal data analysis using generalized linear model. *Biometrika* 1986; **49**: 623–30.

55. Roth T, Walsh JK, Krystal A, *et al*. An evaluation of the efficacy and safety of eszopiclone over 12 months in patients with chronic primary insomnia. *Sleep Med* 2005; **6**: 487–95.

56. Krystal AD, Erman M, Zammit GK, *et al*. Long-term efficacy and safety of zolpidem extended-release 12.5 mg, administered 3 to 7 nights per week for 24 weeks, in patients with chronic primary insomnia: A 6-month, randomized, double-blind, placebo-controlled, parallel-group, multicenter study. *Sleep* 2008; **31**: 79–90.

57. McCulloch CE, Searle SR, Neuhaus JM. *Generalized, Linear, and Mixed Models*, 2nd edition. New York, John Wiley & Sons. 2008.

58. Buysse DJ, Ancoli-Israel S, Edinger JD, *et al*. Recommendations for a standard research assessment of insomnia. *Sleep* 2006; **29**: 1155–73.

59. Cohen J. *Statistical Power for the Behavioral Sciences*. 2nd edition. New York, Academic Press. 1988.

60. Morin CM, Culbert JP, and Schwartz SM. Nonpharmacological interventions for insomnia: a meta-analysis of treatment efficacy. *Am J Psychiatry* 1994; **151**: 1172–80.

61. Irwin MR, Cole JC, and Nicassio PM. Comparative meta-analysis of behavioral interventions for insomnia and their efficacy in middle-aged adults and in older adults 55+ years of age. *Health Psychol* 2006; **25**: 3–14.

62. Morin CM, Colecchi C, Stone J, *et al*. Behavioral and pharmacological therapies for late-life insomnia: a randomized controlled trial. *JAMA* 1999; **281**: 991–9.

63. Krystal AD, Walsh JK, Laska E, *et al*. Sustained efficacy of eszopiclone over 6 months of nightly treatment: Results of a randomized, double-blind, placebo-controlled study in adults with chronic insomnia. *Sleep* 2003; **26**: 793–9.

64. Fava M, McCall WV, Krystal A, *et al*. Eszopiclone co-administered with fluoxetine in patients with insomnia coexisting with major depressive disorder. *Biol Psychiatry* 2006; **59**: 1052–60.

65. Edinger JD, Wohlgemuth WK, Krystal AD, *et al*. Behavioral insomnia therapy for fibromyalgia patients: A randomized clinical trial. *Arch Intern Med* 2005; **165**: 2527–35.

66. Morin CM, Bastien C, Guay B, *et al*. Randomized clinical trial of supervised tapering and cognitive behavior therapy to facilitate benzodiazepine discontinuation in older adults with chronic insomnia. *Am J Psychiatry* 2004; **161**: 332–42.

67. Ohayon MM. Epidemiology of insomnia: what we know and what we still need to learn. *Sleep Med Rev* 2002; **6**: 97–111.

68. Davidson JR, Aime A, Ivers H, *et al*. Characteristics of individuals with insomnia who seek treatment in a clinical setting versus those who volunteer for a randomized controlled trial. *Behav Sleep Med* 2009; 7: 37–52.

69. Edinger JD, Bonnet MH, Bootzin RR, *et al.* Derivation of research diagnostic criteria for insomnia: Report of an American Academy of Sleep Medicine Work Group. *Sleep* 2004; **27**: 1567–96.

70. Lichstein KL, Durrence HH, Taylor DJ, *et al.* Quantitative criteria for insomnia. *Behav Res Ther* 2003; **41**: 427.

71. Nowell PD, Mazumdar S, Buysse DJ, *et al.* Benzodiazepines and zolpidem for chronic insomnia: a meta-analysis of treatment efficacy. *JAMA* 1997; **278**: 2170–7.

72. McCall WV, D'Agostino R, and Dunn A. A meta-analysis of sleep changes associated with placebo in hypnotic clinical trials. *Sleep Med* 2003; **4**: 57–62.

73. Edinger JD, Wohlgemuth WK, Radtke RA, *et al.* Cognitive behavioral therapy for treatment of chronic primary insomnia: a randomized controlled trial. *JAMA* 2001; **285**: 1856–64.

74. Manber R, Edinger JD, Gress JL, *et al.* Cognitive behavioral therapy for insomnia enhances depression outcome in patients with comorbid major depressive disorder and insomnia. *Sleep* 2008; **31**: 489–95.

75. Morin CM. Measuring outcomes in randomized clinical trials of insomnia treatments. *Sleep Med Rev* 2003; **7**: 263–79.

76. Walsh JK, Krystal AD, Amato DA, *et al.* Nightly treatment of primary insomnia with eszopiclone for six months: Effect on sleep, quality of life, and work limitations. *Sleep* 2007; **30**: 959–68.

77. Ström L, Pettersson R, and Andersson G. Internet-based treatment for insomnia: A controlled evaluation. *J Consult Clin Psych* 2004; **72**: 113–20.

Chapter

27

Clinical trial planning: An academic and industry perspective

Cornelia L. Kamp and Jean-Michel Germain

Clinical trial planning overview

Implementing large scale clinical trials is a logistical challenge for both academic investigators and companies. The purpose of this chapter is to describe the planning process for a clinical trial. Successful clinical trials rely on scientific, clinical, and operational excellence. It requires not only the optimal protocol or study design, but also the appropriate experience and expertise in project planning and management. Much of the battle is won or lost in the planning stages when risks can be assessed and mitigated in advance. Table 27.1 provides an overview of key clinical trial activities that need to be planned ahead and managed throughout the trial. In this chapter, we use the example of large, global studies, but the basic principles in planning a trial are the same regardless of trial size.

Project planning

Project and trial management

The study or project team's primary responsibility is to deliver clinical trials that meet the clinical study plan objectives. A clear definition of roles and responsibility among the team members and effective processes are necessary to successfully manage the multiple steps associated with study planning, initiation, implementation, publication, and ultimate closeout. Here, we will primarily focus on reviewing key roles of the sponsor or coordinating center (e.g., academic coordinating center, contract/clinical research organization (CRO) or sponsor) and the site team.

Study team members

Running multi-center clinical trials requires a matrix team approach across multiple organizations/institutions and numerous individuals within each entity. A sample clinical trial team is included in Figure 27.1. These may vary across different settings and the figure is merely an illustration of the typical study team components including:

- Steering Committee (SC): primary responsibility is for the scientific and clinical conduct of the study, typically used in investigator-initiated studies conducted in academic medical centers
- Sponsor: typically the company or investigator with overall responsibility for the trial
- Operational Team: with the Project Manager as the team leader
- Enrolling Site Team
- Data Safety Monitoring Board (DSMB), or Safety Monitoring Board (SMC)
- Independent Medical Monitor: individual charged with reviewing day to day safety of randomized subjects and answering site questions about inclusion/exclusion criteria
- Vendor Teams which include central laboratory, primary and secondary drug packaging/labeling/distribution, central ECG, electronic diaries, electronic patient reported outcomes (ePROs), etc.
- Endpoint Adjudication Committee (EAC)
- Others as may be required by unique trial designs.

A large phase 3, global trial may have hundreds of study team members, each contributing a unique component to the success of the trial, while smaller proof-of-concept or single site studies will have a more manageable team size of ~10–20 individuals.

Most study management models in the pharmaceutical industry rely on a *study* or *project manager* (PM). This role may vary from one company to another but responsibilities remain very similar. The PM is primarily accountable for the execution of the study, leading the study team, and coordinating the various

Clinical Trials in Neurology, ed. Bernard Ravina, Jeffrey Cummings, Michael P. McDermott, and R. Michael Poole. Published by Cambridge University Press. © Cambridge University Press 2012.

Table 27.1 Clinical trial overview

	Study planning	Study start-up	Study maintenance	Study analysis/ reporting
Planning	Study Planning/Tracking/Communication			
Projects/studies	Synopsis/Protocol/Amendment			
	ICF/ICF Amendment			
	Advertising			
	Hold/Early Termination			
Project/study documents	Investigators Brochure/Annual Update			
Service providers	CRO & Vendors Selection			
	CRO & Vendors Agreements			
		Budgets & Payments		
Investigational product(s)	Manufacturing/Packaging/Labeling/Stability Program/Management of Expiry Dates/Distribution			
		Accountability/Reconciliation		
Specimens	Specimen Planning	Specimen Collection and Tracking		Specimen Analysis
Regulatory affairs	IND/CTA/CTX/CTN/IMPD			
	Safety Reporting			
Investigational sites	Sites Identification/ Selection	Sites Qualification		
		Confidentiality Agreements / Clinical Study Agreements		
		Financial Disclosure		
		Study Training		
		Enrolment Planning & Tracking		
			Enrolment	
	Development of Monitoring Plan	Monitoring		
Data management	CRF Development			
	Database set-up			
		Data Collection/Editing/Review/Data Monitoring Committee		Data Reporting
	Statistical Analysis Plan/Study Programming/Interim Analysis			Data Analysis
	Randomization Code			Code Release
Documents management	Study Documents Translation/Trial Master Files Maintenance			
QA	Audits & Inspections/Inspection Readiness			
Project communication	Study Registration/Publication/Scientific Communication/Meetings			
Compliance	Compliance Management/Training			

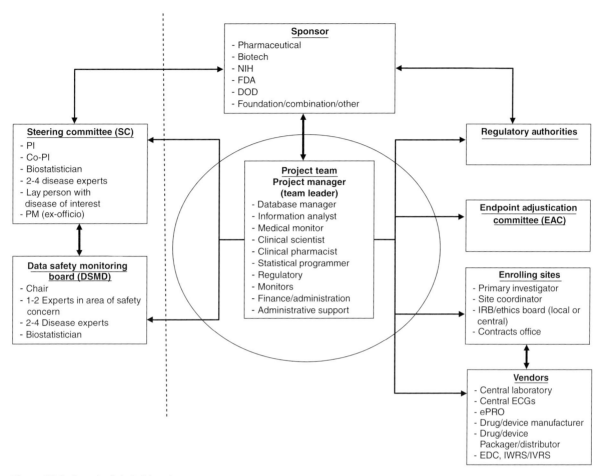

Figure 27.1. Sample clinical trial study team.

functional areas (i.e., biostatistics, regulatory, data management, monitoring groups, vendors etc.) as well as external partners, committees (SC, DSMB, EAC) and providers of services such as central laboratory, ECG provider, or drug/device manufacturer, to achieve study objectives and milestones. Other responsibilities include risk analysis and management, adherence to the approved budget, as well as the optimization of operational efficiency. In essence the PM is tasked with ensuring the study is completed on-time, with high quality and within budget.

The *site manager* (SM) or *clinical research associate* (CRA) is generally the main point of contact for investigational sites. The SM's primary responsibility is executing the monitoring plan, and ensuring sites comply with Good Clinical Practice (GCP) and International Conference on Harmonisation (ICH), Code of Federal Regulations (21 CFR Part 11) and other regional or local regulatory requirements, as applicable. The CRA is responsible for site initiation, collection of regulatory documents, and monitoring as well as for overseeing the study progress and delivering operational and protocol training to site personnel.

Site organization relies on multiple specialties and area of expertise, but the primary site team roles are those of the *principal investigator* (PI) and *site coordinator*. Since the complexity of studies has significantly increased over the last several years, sponsors have been looking for efficient, well-qualified, and well-trained investigative teams, which have technical, organizational, and administrative skills [1, 2]. The PI is responsible for the overall conduct of the study at his/her site. This includes overseeing the study progress, patient selection and safety, as well as compliance with the federal, state, and local regulatory requirements. The investigator may delegate his/her responsibilities to other qualified members of the team via the use of a delegation of authority log, but ultimately remains the sole person responsible for the overall conduct of the study and site [3].

The site coordinator is typically responsible for coordinating clinical activities at the site level, managing standard operating procedures (SOPs), site personnel training records, contacts with CRAs or companies subcontracted by the sponsor such as central laboratories, interactive voice/web response system, or data management. This position relies on excellent organization and communication skills and is generally held by a study nurse with established experience in clinical trials.

Communication strategy

Efficient communication across the entire study team, is a requisite for successful execution of clinical trials (Figure 27.1). Site personnel will have to communicate and collaborate with various internal and external partners. These partners may be at diverse locations around the world and language and cultural barriers may present a challenge for communications.

Because the management of clinical trials relies on activities from individuals sitting in various functional domains, departments, or institutions, the sponsor or CRO project team must ensure that the clinical study plan is aligned with site, vendor, and functional area objectives and that all study teams' members understand the overall strategy and objectives. This is especially true when conducting multi-center, worldwide clinical trials, where the operational team must ensure that all study steps are implemented consistently across sites and regions. Therefore, regular meetings with key team members, whether these are teleconferences, web-based, and in-person meetings are required to ensure a common understanding of study priorities, challenges, timelines, and budget.

From a project management perspective, clinical trials sponsors value a single point of accountability with the CRO/vendors, with frequent and regular updates to ensure the appropriate oversight of the execution plan.

Service providers

CRO selection and management

The use of CROs (either academic or for-profit) has significantly increased over the last decade. Whether the sponsor is a large biopharmaceutical company or a small one, the reasons for outsourcing activities are often the same: lack of resources or lack of in-house expertise, and large projects involving many sites in multiple regions of the world [4].

When selecting a CRO, most sponsors prioritize the CRO's experience in the target therapeutic area or indication, its worldwide experience, or its expertise in a specific region. Other important selection criteria generally include the proposal for the implementation and the execution of the project (resources allocation, sites, and countries), budget, as well as the working relationship between the sponsor and the CRO as both parties will need to develop a close collaboration.

The choice of a CRO should stem results from a thorough evaluation process performed in collaboration with staff with relevant expertise (e.g., site monitoring). The assessment of the CRO should include the evaluation of written SOPs.

In general, when selecting a CRO or any other vendors, it is critical to put together a Request for Proposal (RFP) document that clearly defines the services being requested. The more specific the RFP is, including anticipated key timeline milestones such as first patient enrolled, enrollment duration, last patient enrolled, number of sites, or number of countries, the more realistic and comprehensive the CRO/vendor proposal will be and the more accurate the budget will be. The industry standard is to submit an RFP to a minimum of two or three CROs/vendors for the requested service. The process of requesting RFPs and evaluating returned proposals often helps identify gaps, inconsistencies, or deficiencies in the protocol.

The contract agreement and the scope of work (SOW) which formalizes and delineates the proposal for services should clearly include detailed obligations to be assumed by the CRO, vendors etc. as well as detailed descriptions of all activities with associated costs and timelines. Also, to preclude any conflict of interest the agreement should clearly state the responsibilities for each party. As an example, Table 27.2 provides a non-exhaustive list of activities and associated responsibilities. More complex studies may include SOWs with even greater clarity of roles including codes like P = primary creation, R = Review, A = approval, O = oversight, etc. as many tasks involve input from multiple groups within the sponsor, CRO, or other vendors. The greater the clarity to the defined roles and responsibilities in the planning phase of the study the greater the likelihood for tasks being completed on-time.

Table 27.2 Planning and implementation scope of work

Task/description	Investigator	Medical team	Project team	Data management/ biostastistics	Clinical pharmacy	CRO
		Sponsor				
A. Protocol development						
Develop, refine protocol		X				
Develop informed consent form (study template)		X				
Develop informed consent form (site specific)	X					X
Develop sites & monitor training material		X	X			
B. Study preparation						
Identify regulatory requirements for protocol submission to IRB/IEC & local regulatory bodies						X
Develop/review procedures for reporting serious adverse events to sponsor, IRB, IEC, local regulatory bodies		X	X			X
Package, label, study medication					X	
Develop database and CRF				X		
C. Sites selection and qualification						
Develop criteria for sites selection		X	X			
Identify medically appropriate study sites						X
Conduct sites qualification visits						X
Develop clinical study agreement with sites	X					X
Obtain & file site documentation (CVs, financial disclosure forms, 1572 FDA forms) & regulatory documents						X
D. Study start-up						
Submit protocol and protocol-related documents to IRB/IEC and local regulatory bodies	X					X
Follow-up on submission/ approval status	X					X

Table 27.2 (*cont.*)

Task/description	Investigator	Medical team	Project team	Data management/ biostastistics	Clinical pharmacy	CRO
		Sponsor				
Conduct site initiation visits						X
Distribute CRF to sites				X		X
E. Study maintenance						
Oversee subject recruitment and enrollment			X			X
Safety reporting to IRB/IEC and local regulatory bodies	X					X
Ship study medication to sites as required					X	X
Run consistency & edit checks, derivations, batch validations				X		
Follow-up on queries resolution						X
Monitor sites according to monitoring plan						X
F. Study closure						
Ensure resolution of all issues at site level	X					X
Conduct study medication reconciliation					X	X
Perform site closeout visit						X
Inform IRB/IEC and local authority of trial end	X					X

In an attempt to gain efficiency and to avoid repeating the same process for each study, most biopharmaceutical companies have now developed Master Services Agreements (MSAs) with preferred CRO and other vendors or are now entering strategic partnerships and alliances with CROs and other vendors.

Data Management vendor selection/management

Sponsors often contract for data management services. Activities generally range from database and Case Report Form (CRF) design to database lock, including clinical data collection, validation and editing, coding, transfer, and, occasionally, analysis and reporting. As with any other clinical trial related activities, data management is governed by GCP and ICH. Therefore, as part of the vendor selection process the

sponsor must ensure that the vendor complies with the existing regulations [5] through adequate SOP documentation, for all steps. Critical steps include but are not limited to:

- **CRF data entry**: Whether the protocol uses paper CRF or electronic-CRF (e-CRF) the investigator remains responsible for the accuracy, completeness, legibility, and timeliness of the data reported in the CRF.
- **Data entry**: For paper CRF, double-data entry with third party verification is considered standard practice. In case additional clinical data from external vendor(s) (e.g., central laboratory) is expected, the format of the data to be received, as well as the frequency of transfer, is to be agreed to and documented in the Data Management

and Data Validation Plan (DMP) prepared with the data vendor and approved by the sponsor. The clinical data that require derivation such as calculated scores must be identified together with the raw data it is derived from. The DMP is a living document that is updated throughout the study as modifications to the data management criteria are agreed to with the sponsor.

- **Editing and validation**: The clinical trial sponsor and the data vendor must agree on standard validations to be performed on an ongoing basis, with appropriate documentation in the DMP. All alterations to the database (addition, deletion, and update) must have a complete and searchable audit trail, and can only be performed by authorized, qualified, and trained personnel. For protocols using e-CRF, clinical data can only be entered by site personnel.

- **Management of queries**: To address inconsistencies and potential data entry errors from site personnel, queries, or clarifications on data collected in the CRF are sent by data management personnel directly to the investigational sites. The DMP defines upfront all data that will be queried. This can include for example range checks for an assessment where each question can only be answered 1–4 as an acceptable response or logic checks across CRFs such as querying the subject demography indicated as male on the CRF while a 'yes' response for pregnancy is provided on the laboratory CRF.

- **Coding and dictionary**: The coding of adverse events and medications is required to ensure a standardized reporting. For the coding of adverse events, MedDRA (Medical Dictionary for Regulatory Affairs) is the standard in use from phase 1 to phase 4 clinical [6]. The European Directive 2001/20/EC [7] requires that adverse reaction terms be coded according to MedDRA when reporting suspected unexpected serious adverse events (SUSARs) [8]

- **Data quality check**: As per ICH E6 GCP [9] quality checks on pre-determined samples must be conducted to ensure that validated processes have been used for the transformation of the data.

- **Safety Data Management**: Serious adverse event (SAE) data entered in the clinical database is to be reconciled vs. the safety database used for the collection of serious adverse events.

- **Database lock**: The lock of the database occurs after all clinical data including data from external vendors (e.g., central laboratories, ePROs, Interactive Web/Voice Response System (IWRS/IVRS)) have been received, edited, and after all discrepancies have been resolved. At the time of database lock, all permissions to add, delete, or modify clinical data are revoked. For studies that require a per-protocol interim analysis, the lock of the database can occur while the study still includes active subjects

Laboratory and ECG vendor selection/management

Central laboratories

The use of central laboratories for routine testing (blood chemistry, hematology, and urine analysis) and other biological specimens is now very common in clinical trials. It developed in the late 1980s from the need for clinical trial sponsors to collect and report data in a more consistent way. In the mid and late 1990s, with the extension of clinical trials in emerging markets (Latin America, Eastern Europe) and more recently in Asia/Pacific and India, the use of central laboratories continued to develop so that it is now well established for the monitoring of safety parameters, and also for the collection of biochemical or biological efficacy data (if applicable).

When outsourcing biological samples testing to a central laboratory, clinical trial sponsors are looking for:

- consistent methodology for both the collection and the testing of biological specimens
- consistent reporting (i.e. consistent normal ranges across sites)
- consistent SOPs
- high quality data
- global services
- efficient shipping, tracking and reporting systems
- contingency plans
- high quality services to sites
- responsiveness.

Unless the central laboratory considered has already been selected as a preferred provider of services by the sponsor, the assessment process should include a review of SOPs and ideally a visit of the facility and ancillary sites, if possible.

315

The contract agreement and scope of work should clearly identify the parameters which are tested together with the methodology and associated costs, as well as detailed information on timelines associated with the shipment, receipt, analysis, and reporting of data. A primary point of contact and accountability for reporting to the sponsors, as well as a primary point of contact for both site personnel and site monitors should also be identified.

ECG vendors

Cardiac safety issues identified post New Drug Application (NDA) (21 CRF part 314) approval, starting in the late 1990s are some of the reasons that several drugs have been pulled from the market such as Sertindole (atypical antipsychotic) and Terfenadine (antihistaminic) or required significant labeling changes [10]. As a result of these findings, clinical ECG evaluation of novel agents is now required by the regulators. The recommendation was made to clinical trial sponsors to conduct and analyze clinical studies to assess the potential of a drug to delay cardiac repolarization [11]. The effect on cardiac repolarization, also known as 'Thorough QT/QTc Trial' is evaluated in healthy volunteers unless the drug cannot be studied in that population due to unacceptable tolerability, such as cytotoxic agents. With additional data collected in phase 3, 12-lead ECG monitoring is a widely used safety measure to identify drug-induced cardiac adverse effects.

Clinical trial sponsors increasingly rely on ECG vendors that provide standardized ECG collection and reading that limit variations and inconsistencies that are frequently observed between investigational sites. The selection process for ECG vendors are not too different from those used when selecting a CRO and should focus on the following specific relevant criteria:

- management of ECG equipment (shipping process, supplies management)
- query process
- transmission timing and process from the site to the ECG vendor
- turnover time between ECG acquisition, central reading and data transfer back to the site and to the sponsor
- training program for site personnel and CRAs, and
- customer service.

Other vendors

Similar to central ECG readers and central laboratories, the use of vendors providing central imaging solutions (MRI, β-CIT, PET, DEXA, etc.) has recently developed specially in the fields of neurology and oncology. As medical imaging is more and more accepted as a surrogate marker of disease progression, there has been increased needs for more standardization in the acquisition and the review of images. In the context of global clinical trials, the study team must ensure that when contracting this activity to an external partner, enough resources and adequate customer service is provided to sites with a 365/24/7 help desk. This is of critical importance as the vendor is likely to have responsibilities for qualifying and training sites for image acquisition and for developing and providing sites with image acquisition protocol.

Similar precautions would apply to other technologies such as electronic Patient Reported Outcomes (e PRO) which have been progressively replacing paper-based diaries when collecting data directly from subjects. As the cost associated with such technology is substantial, the study team and vendor must ensure that the technology and the proposed devices are really suitable for use in the study (e.g., multiple country trials, special populations: pediatric, elderly subjects). The most important question that needs to be addressed is whether the subjects can actually use the technology as required. It may be necessary to test the technology in a few patients before using it in a clinical trial.

Other solutions such as IWRS/IVRS are discussed below ('IWRS/IVRS and IRT used to manage clinical supply inventories').

Clinical trial budgets

The cost of conducting clinical trials continues to increase. A median phase 3 study of 800 subjects, 50 sites and 2 years from First Subject First Visit (FSFV) to Last Subject Last Visit (LSLV) can cost upwards of $25 million or $36 000/day [12]. The cost of bringing one compound to market over a 12 year period in 2000 dollars was ~$802 million [13]. In short, conducting clinical trials is an expensive undertaking and appropriately budgeting for a clinical trial, whether a single center proof-of-concept study or a large, multi-center, multi-year global phase 3 trial, it is of utmost importance to avoid budget shortfalls, which are common.

Budgeting for clinical trials is an art form given the number and varied types of services required. Given the maturity of the CRO, and associated vendor industry (e.g. central lab, interactive response system (IRT), electronic data capture (eDC) ECG providers, ePRO, etc.), most clinical trial services providers have a good understanding of the cost of doing business. What typically creates havoc in most clinical trial budgets are all the unexpected challenges such as the need to add visits, efficacy or safety measures, slow enrollment, and problems with drug availability.

The most important step to creating a realistic budget is to develop a detailed scope of work document clearly delineating all aspects of conducting the trial and the responsible groups (see Table 27.1). The greater the granularity the more precise the budget can become. Established pharmaceutical, biotech companies, and CROs have historical data that can be applied to the creation of each new budget and also rely on experienced operational functional group leaders to review budgets and provide input on the number and type of labor unit required for each activity. The budgeting process is a team effort that requires the review and input of all operational stakeholders. This includes obtaining a minimum of two or three proposals for each type of service that will be outsourced and providing the vendors with the most current protocol and realistic timeline for key milestones (see below 'Timelines').

When budgeting for a global trial the budget should also factor in anticipated fluctuations in currency exchange rates. Most vendors stipulate pricing in the currency of the parent company so that the sponsor must consider the impact of currency fluctuations. Multi-year studies also need to take into account inflation and increases in labor rates associated with annual merit increases that occur at most companies.

Components of a clinical trial budget

Most industry budgets are created on a unit activity basis (e.g. (# monitoring visits/site) × (# of sites) × (cost per routine monitoring visit) = total routine monitoring budget). Investigator-initiated studies conducted within academic institutions and funded by NIH, FDA, DOD are often based on a percent effort basis (e.g. Project manager 50% effort in Year 01–02; 35% effort Year 03). Regardless of which method is used, the key is attempting to estimate the total effort required based on a final protocol and schedule of activity. The key components of a typical clinical trial are broken down into the main categories below. A non-inclusive budget driver template can be found in Appendix 27.A. As most of the general trial costs are covered in the

template by key category, not all are discussed within the section below, only a few are highlighted.

Investigational medicinal product supply

There are many components to investigational medicinal product (IMP) costs, including a full understanding of the supply chain: procurement of the active pharmaceutical ingredient (API), excipients, components (bottles, caps, labels, etc.), manufacturing, analytical testing, dissolution testing, stability program, packaging, labeling, distribution, custom costs, and accountability/returns/destruction. Obtaining detailed information on the various costs from the appropriate suppliers early and accounting for inflation and applicable overage (see below 'Quantities of IMP to order') will insure adequate funds are budgeted for this critical component. If the IMP is still in early development phases, additional funds need to be allocated to formulation development and testing. Additionally, studies that include a comparator(s) will require comparable effort for its procurement and often come at considerable cost and matching placebo may not be readily available if a drug is not in clinical development.

Investigator-initiated studies often try to obtain IMP directly from the manufacturer at no-cost. As part of initial grant submissions, investigators may obtain a letter of support from the manufacturer indicating that the manufacturer will provide the IMP. However, as most grant funding takes anywhere from 1 to 3 years to obtain, depending on the review cycle, company priorities, leadership changes, mergers and acquisitions, and the general economy often interfere with these letters of support being upheld. These letters of support are not legally binding. Therefore, investigators often end up scrambling to find funds to cover this critical piece of the study.

Operational team effort

Whether budgeting the time and effort for tasks as percent effort or based on unit activity, the unit activity efforts for the responsibility of each functional area need to be identified in order for the appropriate unit cost and number of units or percent effort to be calculated correctly. Clinical trial budgets typically include costs for project management, data management, medical writing, biostatistics, regulatory, clinical supplies support, meeting planning, investigator training, and administrative activities; the list goes on, depending on the complexity and size of the study. In the budget template provided in Appendix 27.A, costs are broken down by unit of activity within the various functional areas.

Committees and consultants

Budgeting for the various committees and consultants required for the conduct of a study, whether a DSMB, adjudication committee, scientific advisory committee, or specific consultants requires determining the membership, frequency of meetings, and compensation per meeting. The budget should include the contingency for impromptu meetings by the DSMB if safety issues emerge.

Data management and interactive response system

Budgets for electronic data capture systems and paper CRFs do have certain shared features, including the actual database build, hardware/software and maintenance fees, and creation of the Data Management Plan (DMP). For studies involving paper CRFs, the cost for the reproduction of each CRF binder, typically created as 3 part no carbon required (NCR) and the cost for the shipping of completed CRFs and data queries need to be factored in. Likewise budgeting for an IRT solution, includes the hardware/software and maintenance fees, along with transaction fees and 365/24/7 help desk support. Costs for IRT systems vary broadly by the provider, so obtaining multiple bids will help determine the scope of the solution required.

Monitoring

The monitoring budget is determined based on the monitoring plan, which describes the planned number and type of visits per site. Generally this will include a pre-study visit [for those sites not previously used by a company or not used over a set period of time (e.g. 2 years], one site initiation visit, routine monitoring visits, and one closeout visit (see Chapter 28). The duration for visit type includes time and effort for visit preparation, travel to/from the site, on-site monitoring time, and time for report writing and follow-up. Many companies have metrics on average time for each type of activity and budget accordingly. For example pre-study visits are allocated at 14 hours, initiation visits at 17 hours, and routine and closeout visits at 24 hours for all associated activities.

The other key component for the monitoring budget is the travel which typically includes: airfare, car rental, hotel, meals, and incidentals. In an effort to reduce the travel budget many companies have moved towards a regional-based monitoring strategy to reduce travel time and airfare, ideally with monitors living within driving distance of most of the sites they monitor.

Vendors

Depending on the protocol requirements the services of one or more vendors may be required. In most studies, central laboratory services are required for routine safety laboratories. Laboratory fees typically include cost per safety assays (clinical chemistry, hematology, urinalysis and pregnancy tests). Other specialty assays may be required. For pharmacokinetic (PK) studies, budgeting for the PK assays is also required and may require a different vendor. In addition to the actual assay, laboratory budgets also need to factor in kits for blood and urine specimen collection and shipment to the laboratory, associated courier fees, and storage fees as some samples could be kept for a period of time which exceeds study duration. If frozen specimens are transported, additional costs for dry ice, special shipping packs must also be included.

Other vendors that may be required include central ECG costs, electronic diaries, holter monitoring services etc.

Site costs

In most cases, site payments are the single largest budget item (~ 50–70%). The site budget typically includes the following components: a per-subject fee (PFS), IRB/EC fees, one time non-reimbursable start-up fee, and other per-occurrence costs.

Per subject fee

The per subject fee (PSF) is based on the protocol schedule of activities and the assessments conducted at each visit. Appendix 27.A provides a template for how the budget would typically be determined. Many companies have access to costing databases that help with determining reimbursement rates for typical procedure types that are often regionally based. In most cases, companies will determine a range for the PSF recognizing that costs in larger metropolitan areas will generally be greater than costs in small cities and that costs vary from country to country. The PSF should factor in the anticipated screen failure rate, such that these additional costs, typically some percentage of the cost of the screening and baseline visit are also added to the total budget.

As part of the PSF calculation, costs that are standard of care (SOC) costs, typically covered by insurance, need to be flagged. If companies are reimbursing the SOC costs as part of the PSF then sites need to ensure that processes are in place to prevent billing these costs to insurance. Many companies put very stringent language into their agreements with sites to prevent sites from 'double-dipping'. For many NIH funded studies SOC costs are determined up front and the costs for these are not budgeted as part of the PSF so that sites would bill insurance.

It is critical to get input from local and regional staff regarding the proposed PSF as in some cases the PSF may be significantly more than what is typically received for a comparable study.

IRB/EC fees

The study budget needs to factor in the average cost per IRB/EC initial review and approval of the protocol, ICF, investigator brochure, and ideally any advertising materials. Additionally, the budget needs to factor in annual IRB/EC renewals for the total duration of the study and some assumption regarding the anticipated number of amendments. On average this may be one or two amendments per year. Also, the budget should factor in some percentage of investigator turn-over that also requires IRB/EC review and approval.

One-time non-reimbursable start-up fee

Start-up costs, regardless of actual enrollment, are often requested by experienced sites to cover the labor effort associated with getting a site up and running. It includes reimbursement for time and effort spent preparing the IRB/EC submission, time spent reading the protocol, training site staff and source document creation, time spent by the investigator and coordinator at an investigator training meeting and an on-site initiation visit, getting systems and processes in-place for conducting study visits, etc. The start-up fee may vary based on the complexity of the protocol and added resources, equipment, materials, etc. that may need to be obtained.

General office/clinic costs

The budget should also include costs for copying, faxing, phone usage, courier, long-term storage, materials (paper, gloves, folders, etc.), specialty equipment, or space.

Other per-occurrence costs

Other per-occurrence site costs for consideration include time and effort for serious adverse effect processing, amendments, pharmacy set-up fees, local advertising (e.g. newspaper, radio, etc. advertising creation time, plus actual advertising costs) and others that may be study specific.

Budget management

The person who manages the budget during the trial must have first hand knowledge of whether or not the study is running according to plan or if unexpected costs are being incurred due to study delays or new protocol requirements. This person is often the PM. It is critical that the person responsible for the budget communicates early and often regarding anticipated shortfalls so that sponsors can make plans to raise additional funds or for investigators to go back to the funding source or an alternate funding source to obtain additional funding. Like many construction projects, clinical trials typically cost more than originally budgeted and sponsors and investigators should plan accordingly.

Timelines

As the person responsible for ensuring the study is completed with high quality, within the budget and on time, the PM (this may be the PI for investigator-initiated trials conducted at academic institutions) needs to go through a thorough and detailed preparation phase, planning all possible activities, tasks, or actions that need to be accomplished during the life of the project. The project team and the PM generally rely on using a standard template developed from previous experiences and which identifies the different steps together with the duration of each step. Most project teams or PMs use a countdown approach where the main goal is identified as the final task and all activities that need to take place to achieve that goal are defined. Since conducting clinical trials includes hundreds of tasks, it is not uncommon to breakdown the timelines by study phase (e.g. 'study planning and set-up'; 'study execution', 'study reporting') with the main objective for each phase identified as a final task (e.g. '80% of sites initiated', 'last subject last visit', 'final clinical study report signed-off'). This document is then used routinely to measure the progress of the study by tracking the completion of each step, for reporting purposes, and also to identify potential deviations from the original plan and put in place the appropriate corrective actions or contingency plans.

Elements of realistic timelines

The proper planning of clinical trial activities requires that each process and associated tasks be understood as some activities can be run in parallel while other activities must be sequential. Most project teams develop project timelines based on historical data and recent experience. However, in order to improve the accuracy of the planning, it is critical for the PM to obtain the appropriate input from key players from the team (internal or external) such as data management, clinical pharmacy, site monitoring or regulatory affairs staff, investigative sites, and other functional areas, and to obtain endorsement on the timeline from the project team and from the management. As the study proceeds, it is important that the planning document be updated with actual dates in real time and shared regularly with individuals from the study team that are accountable for deliverables, especially if there are major shifts in achieving key milestones. For instance, if enrollment goes significantly quicker than originally planned then downstream milestones, like database lock would be shifted forward. The data management group and biostatistical group need to be informed of this early on to ensure resources are made available earlier than originally planned.

Discussion of critical timelines milestones

Study planning and set-up phase

The main goal of the planning and set-up phase is generally the initiation of all sites or at least of a certain number of sites. To ensure accurate planning one needs to identify all of the steps leading to site activation. For global clinical trials, the regulatory step is probably one of the most challenging as spelled out in 'Regulatory requirements' (see below). In preparation for the initiation of sites, others items that need to be planned ahead and tracked down during the set-up phase include:

- protocol and protocol-related documents (informed consent form (ICF), CRF, investigator's brochure, regulatory documents, monitoring plan).
- IMP (manufacturing, labeling, packaging)
- contracts with vendors and investigator sites
- other clinical supplies and material (laboratory kits for blood testing, ECG machines, investigator's manuals, electronic diaries, etc.)
- site training strategy and materials
- monitoring documents (e.g., monitoring plan)
- data management activities: database set-up and validation, statistical analysis plan (SAP), clinical data review and validation plan, etc. (see Figure 27.1).

Study start-up phase

The end of the study planning phase is generally defined by the first subject enrolled or the First Subject First Visit (FSFV). In the biopharmaceutical industry, this key milestone is one of the most scrutinized by upper management as it really signals the beginning of the study. The FSFV is often associated with key financial pay-outs, which is critical information for stockholders and potential investors in publically traded companies and often coincides with a major press release. Assuming that all previous steps and previous key milestones have been achieved and that sites have everything they need to get started, the FSFV milestone depends upon the site's ability to recruit subjects. A comprehensive site feasibility study (see Chapter 28) conducted during the planning phase can help the project team in validating the planning strategy as well as identifying unforeseen risks and developing contingency plans.

Study execution

The Last Subject Last Visit (LSLV) milestone signals the end of the trial. Every PM has faced situations where enrollment is running behind schedule, with missed targets and milestones. The key for timely completion of a clinical trial relies on a protocol that is feasible and on sites that can recruit enough patients within the project time frame. Site feasibility assessment must be conducted early during the planning phase to identify those sites that have access to the applicable patient population, and that have the experience and infrastructure necessary to conduct the study.

Database lock and database freeze

Terminology for "locking/freezing" of the database varies from company to company. What is important is the general process for securing the database to further changes following treatment unblinding. The database lock is a procedure used to prevent data from being modified or altered when multiple users have access to the database. Generally it takes place after all data from investigative sites and any external vendors are received, checked for completeness, reviewed, edited, and all queries and issues have been resolved. The clinical data can either be locked at site, patient, or study level depending on the completeness status of the database. The locked database is then used by the biostatistician and the clinical programmer to ensure that their final programs are suitable and allow the proper analysis, per the Statistical Analysis Plan (SAP), of the data. Treatment codes are then assigned to each subject, per the original randomization, before the database is frozen. As this stage no additional changes can be made to the database. Should any update need to be made to a frozen database, this can only be made by users that have privileged access to the database.

In order to meet CFR 21 part 11 and other regulatory requirements, the database must include an audit trail for recording and tracking all activities from individuals responsible for the development and maintenance of the clinical database.

Reporting

The final timeline activities associated with true completion of a clinical trial include the reporting requirements as spelled out in Chapter 28.

Investigational products: drug or device

The success of any clinical trial depends on the availability of adequate quantities of the investigational product (IP): drug or device (herein 'clinical supplies or IP'). Clinical supplies are frequently a bottleneck especially in investigator-initiated studies. Inadequate time is spent in the planning phases understanding the complexity of the clinical supply chain, which includes the availability of the API, excipients, and components (bottles, caps, kit boxes, pill counters, dosing syringes, etc.), understanding the manufacturing timeline and complexity, availability of an appropriate stability program, understanding possible delays at customs, and the time required for primary and secondary packaging, labeling, and distribution. Unfortunately, clinical supplies are not straightforward commodities readily available in the marketplace. As such, a dedicated person needs to be identified in the planning phase of a trial, through LPLV, whose primary responsibility is to ensure appropriate quantities of clinical supplies are available when and where they are needed in a continuous, uninterrupted fashion.

Most pharmaceutical and biotech companies have clinical supply departments whose sole responsibility is to focus on all aspects of the IP used in a clinical trial. Investigator-initiated studies do not typically have this luxury and in many cases academic investigators are not properly trained in all aspects of IP manufacture, procurement, testing, and all other regulatory aspects of manufacturing IP, etc. An in-depth review of supply chain management in the drug industry can be found in [14].

Clinical supplies used in clinical trials must be manufactured according to current Good Manufacturing Practices (cGMPs). The 'c' stands for 'current,' reminding manufacturers that they must employ technologies and systems which are up-to-date in order to comply with the regulations that are set forth in the Federal Food, Drug, and Cosmetic Act (Chapter IV for food, and Chapter V, Subchapters A, B, C, D, and E for drugs and devices). Good Manufacturing Practice regulations in the US are defined in 21 CFR parts 210 and 211, and Guideline on the Preparation of Investigational New Drug Products, March 1991 [15], and in the European Union are defined in the Clinical Trials Directive 2001/20/EC [16]. According to cGMPs manufacturers, processors, and packagers of drugs, medical devices, some food, and blood products are required to take proactive steps to ensure that their products are safe, pure, and effective. The regulations require a quality approach to manufacturing, enabling companies to minimize or eliminate instances of contamination, mix-ups, and other errors. Failure of firms to comply with cGMP regulations can result in serious consequences including recall, seizure, fines, and jail time. Issues including record-keeping, personnel qualifications, sanitation, cleanliness, equipment verification, process validation, and complaint handling are addressed by cGMP regulations. Most cGMP requirements are very general and open-ended, allowing each manufacturer to decide individually how to best implement the necessary controls. This provides much flexibility, but also requires the manufacturer to interpret the requirements in a manner best suited for their individual business. When selecting vendors in the clinical supply chain it is critical that each vendor adheres to cGMPs.

There are key terms used throughout the supply chain that defined in 21 CFR part 210.3:

- **API (active pharmaceutical ingredient):** Any component that is intended to furnish pharmacologic activity or other direct effect in the diagnosis, cure, mitigation, treatment, or prevention of disease, or to affect the structure or any function of the body of man or other animals. The term includes those components that may undergo chemical change in the manufacture of the drug product and be present in the drug product in a modified form intended to furnish the specified activity or effect.
- **Drug substance:** Active pharmaceutical ingredient (API) or 'raw drug substance'
- **Drug product:** A finished dosage form, for example, tablet, capsule, solution, which contains an active drug ingredient generally, but not necessarily, in association with inactive ingredients. The term also includes a finished dosage form that does not contain an active ingredient but is intended to be used as a placebo [17].

Device classification

The FDA has established classifications for approximately 1700 different generic types of devices and grouped them into 16 medical specialties referred to as panels. Each of these generic types of devices is assigned to one of three regulatory classes (class I through class III) based on the level of control necessary to assure the safety and effectiveness of the device (see Chapter 19). Determining what class a device is categorized in and the regulatory requirements can be found on the FDA device website [18] and within the regulations 21 CFR parts 862–892.

Stability testing of drug substance and drug product

The purpose of stability testing is to provide evidence on how the quality of a drug substance or drug product varies with time under the influence of a variety of environmental factors such as temperature, humidity, and light, and to establish a re-test period for the drug substance or a shelf life for the drug product and recommended storage conditions. As part of the cGMP regulations, the FDA has adopted the standards of the ICH [19] which requires that drug products bear an expiration date determined by appropriate stability testing (21 CFR 211.137 and 211.166). The stability of drug products is required to be evaluated over time in the same container-closure system in which the drug product is marketed or being provided to subjects participating in the clinical trial. In some cases, accelerated stability studies can be used to support tentative expiration dates in the event that full shelf-life studies are not available. When a firm changes the packaging or formulation of a drug product, stability testing must be repeated.

The description of the stability program includes the list of tests to be performed, analytical procedures, acceptance criteria, test time points, storage conditions, and duration of the study. Standard stability programs for solid dosage forms are delineated in the FDA guidance document [20]. The stability program should be conducted for as long as the IMP will be used in the field and a minimum of 1-month accelerated stability data should be available before any materials are used in the field.

- **Expiration dates (marketed product):** The expiration date on marketed product is based on the data obtained from the stability program collected from three individual production size batches in its original closed container. The date does not mean that drug was unstable after a longer period; it means only that real-time data or extrapolation from accelerated degradation studies indicate that the drug will remain stable through that date.
- **Retest dates (investigational product):** The date assigned by the manufacturer after which the drug substances need to be examined (retested) to ensure that they remain within suitable specifications for use in the manufacture of a drug product.

For many investigator-initiated studies, planning and budgeting for stability programs is often overlooked. This is an important aspect of the clinical drug supply expiry dating, which in turn affects all study timelines, and should remain at the forefront of the investigator's responsibilities to fulfill this requirement.

Methods for blinding the IP

Varying methods are available for creating a placebo-to-match (PTM). This includes manufacturing identically matching tablets, capsules, powder, IVs, oral solutions, devices, etc. Attempting to create a PTM for marketed tablets/capsules is often complicated by branding either engraved or printed on a tablet/capsule, which cannot be readily duplicated on the PTM. One of the most common forms of blinding oral dosage forms is over-encapsulation of tablets or capsules, thus allowing for an identically matched final capsule in all physical attributes: size, color, shape, imprints, taste, smell, solubility, etc.

- **Over-encapsulation:** Over-encapsulation of marketed product, changes the formulation of the original dosage form. The effectiveness of tablets/capsules relies on the drug dissolving in the gastrointestinal tract. Over-encapsulated marketed product should be tested to ensure comparable dissolution to the original formulation. This can sometimes be difficult to achieve especially with controlled release (CR) or extended release (ER) type products [21].

Any time double-blind materials are created for use in a clinical trial, testing should be conducted to ensure that patients, investigators, site coordinators, and other members of the project team are unable to distinguish active product from placebo. Engaging the help of the biostatistician to develop formal testing methodology (e.g., total number of matched pairs to test and SAP) can ensure the integrity of the blind from a product standpoint prior to study launch.

In those cases where it is not possible to make a PTM or where it is not cost effective, other blinding methods may be used. For example, for an in-patient early proof-of-concept study, an unblinded pharmacist may administer the IP to a blind-folded subject. Any unblinded staff should have no other role in the study and should not discuss the study with any other project team members.

Clinical supply labeling and packaging

The labeling requirement for IP is determined by the regulations of the countries in which the study will be conducted. In general, label text for IP includes, but is not limited to the following: study protocol identification, investigational caution statement, storage conditions of the product, administration directions, expiry or re-test date of the material, name and address of the sponsor, manufacturer, and /or distributor. If conducted in multiple regions, appropriate certified translations are required. Determining upfront if all clinical supplies will have the same labels (e.g., booklet labels allow for multiple languages such that the same clinical supplies can be used for all regions) or if clinical supplies will be region-specific will aid in determining the quantities needed. Consulting with the applicable region regulations during the planning phase will ensure materials are appropriately labeled and avoid the necessity for rework of the supplies. Knowing the container system sizes upfront helps determine appropriate label size and thus total label content that can be included without running into space constraints. Most vendors that deal with packaging and labeling are well versed in the labeling regulations.

Subject use considerations

Formulation of IMP affects subject compliance. There are several key items to take into consideration when thinking about optimizing subject compliance. Large tablets/capsules may be difficult for older subjects with neurological conditions to swallow. Mixing IMP with food/liquid may cause weight gain if daily dosing requirements are frequent. Volume of IMP distributed may make transporting IMP home from the clinic difficult. Likewise, the packaging and labeling may also affect compliance. Use of child-resistant caps or blister packets may make it too difficult for subjects to open the container or worse yet, once opened, not be able to close again. Small label text or poorly differentiated labels may cause confusion if there is more than one container that must be opened per each dose. All of these factors need to be considered early on in the planning phase to ensure that the packaging configuration does not negatively impact compliance, thereby skewing study results.

Quantities of IMP to order

The following general formula can be used to determine an initial estimate of the amount of investigational drug that will be needed for a given treatment arm. Although protocols generally specify time interval between patient's visits, most protocols also allow for some flexibility (window) to allow a subject to come earlier or later. This visit window should be taken into consideration for estimating the quantity of investigational drug required for the trial and one should assume that all subjects would come later than by required by the protocol (e.g. the visit may provide for a month 3 visit with a ± 7 day window. A subject could therefore be seen at 3 months (day 91) plus 1 week (day 98) and still be within the protocol requirements. Day 98 would be considered the plus 7 day side of the visit window).

Total amount of study drug for arm #1 = [(Dosage strength × doses/day) × (# dosing days/subject + plus side of each visit window) × (total number of subjects in treatment arm] × overage (e.g. 1.30 for 30% overage).

It is best to calculate quantities based on the final packaging configuration as in the example provided; final unit dose count may not always coincide with the count contained in the final kit configuration per subject.

Overage accounts for manufacturing waste, loss, damage, extra supplies at the sites that may never be used, and allows for the ability to bring additional sites on-board quickly in the event of slow enrollment. Overage estimates vary based on many factors and may be in the range 15–30%. Overage can be decreased via use of an IRT (see below). Similar calculations can be computed for determining the number of devices required in a device study; however given high costs of many devices, overage requirements are typically much lower.

Forecasting IMP needs

While knowing the total quantity of investigational product required for the duration of the study is a relatively straight forward calculation, what is less obvious is determining how much IMP is required at the start of the study and when to manufacture subsequent batches. This becomes especially tricky and important for larger long-term trials. Factors that influence a forecasting algorithm include: site activation rates; enrollment rates; premature withdrawals; the re-test or expiry date; lead time required to order and receive API, excipients and components; lead time and cost associated with the manufacture of multiple batches; possible challenges in matching active product with an identical matching placebo on multiple manufacturing runs (e.g., color variation between batches can significantly affect whether materials are truly identical, thus impacting the study blind); storage constraints of bulk product at the vendor packaging site; and transportation and customs (for international shipments) time and costs for multiple shipments. Plans must be put in place early in the study to forecast appropriate quantities of IMP to avoid two major pitfalls: 1) producing too much IMP at the start of the study that expires before it can be used (e.g. delayed study start, lower than expected enrollment); and 2) not manufacturing enough IMP such that there is an IMP shortage (e.g. enrollment quicker than anticipated). Forecasting reports should be reviewed and adjusted regularly during the course of the study taking into account actual enrollment rates, enrollment projections, and actual premature withdrawals and permanent drug suspensions, to determine timing of subsequent manufacturing/packaging runs.

IWRS/IVRS and IRT used to manage clinical supply inventories

An integrated solution for the optimization and the management of the drug supply chain in clinical trials is provided by IWRS/IVRS or most recently Interactive Response Technology (IRT). It enables seamless 365/24/7 management of randomization, drug/device supply, patient diary data, laboratory samples, treatment disclosure information, temperature excursions of drug product, and drug returns and reconciliation, all through a web-based platform that can be accessed anytime via the Internet or the telephone. There are many vendors that now offer this service compliant with 21 CFR part 11 (regulations covering computerized systems used in clinical investigations) [4]. Many companies are now utilizing some form of IRT to: help manage complex packaging configurations and titration schedules, to proactively manage global expiry and label updates, to dissociate the enrollment ID # from the drug kit thus allowing the IP to be non-subject specific, and to provide real-time visibility into accountability documentation, including inventory updates and a complete view of the entire supply chain throughout the process and across all sites. The IRT systems maintain site and depot inventory reports that give immediate access to real-time shipment information and dynamic updates

to drug status and readily allow for changes to site supply strategies at a site or regional level. There are multiple advantages to using these systems including savings in overall amount of drug required, just in time delivery to the sites when needed, accurate study progress, and enrollment information, and ease in the overall management of the drug inventory. However, as clinical trials are more complex (e.g., multiple cohorts, stratified randomization, adaptive design, etc.) the team and the vendors must plan for enough time for the design, development, and validation of the tools. Also, the clinical team should bear in mind that any future change in the design of the study (e.g. randomization, treatment arms) could have a significant impact on the study timelines and budget as the system could go through extensive changes requiring additional work and re-validation.

For large and long-term (more than a 12-month study duration) phase 3 neurological studies where there is routine resupply (e.g. every 3, 4, or 6 months), possible stability issues, and significant drug costs, the use of an IRT is something that should be considered initially in the planning phases of the trial.

Transportation and storage considerations

The IP is transported within the clinical supply chain regularly between manufacturing facilities, to the primary and secondary packagers, to the central depot for distribution to the sites, and including the return of used/unused IP. The chain of custody for a shipment may be quite complex. Factoring in all of the possible temperature fluctuations throughout the chain of custody is critical for ensuring the integrity of the product once received by the sites. Should temperature excursions be identified by site personnel they should be promptly reported to the sponsor so that the impact on IP stability can be assessed before it is dispensed to subjects.

Supplies that are temperature sensitive may require special temperature-controlled and monitored shipping in order to ensure constant temperature throughout the chain of custody. This is often accomplished via the development of special packaging that has been validated (shipping studies have been conducted from central depot to sites in countries furthest from the depot to ensure package maintains the appropriate temperature for the duration of the shipping period and may also include testing of the IP following brief temperature excursions to ensure the IP is still useable). Temperature monitoring devices are often included in shipments to monitor and record the temperature throughout the transport of the IP.

If shipping internationally, it is critical to establish a communication link between shipper, consignee, custom broker, importer of record, and transport provider [22]. It is important that import approval is obtained *before* shipping to avoid delays and ensure that the transport provider has a clear understanding of transportation requirements (e.g., temperature-controlled trucks). Most of the large couriers have been working with industry for years to help address some of these issues and can often provide significant advice in managing the logistics for international transportation of temperature-sensitive IP prior to shipping. Those involved with the actual shipping process should also be knowledgeable and trained on the International Air Transport Association (IATA) regulations, which include guidelines for packaging and labeling diagnostic specimens, and use of hazardous materials like dry ice used for cold chain supplies [23].

Additionally, when exporting clinical materials, regulatory compliance with government agencies in both the originator and destination countries must be ensured prior to shipping.

Factoring in lead time to transport material from one location to another is an important factor in ultimately determining lead time for ordering supplies and ensuring IP arrives where it is required (i.e., at the sites) when there are patients ready to be enrolled. The impact of transportation costs on the overall study budget should not be forgotten, keeping in mind that these costs are significantly affected by fluctuations in fuel prices.

Most sites have limited room temperature secured storage capabilities, and as non-cGMP compliant facilities, they do not always have appropriate temperature/humidity monitoring capabilities. These storage constraints should be factored in when considering how much IP should be shipped as part of a site's initial set of supplies and any restock supplies. The storage requirements typically become more problematic for frozen or refrigerated IP.

As part of the items to be checked during on-site monitoring visits, the sponsor monitor or CRA will ensure the adequate delivery, storage conditions, and proper administration of IP. Proof of documentation to verify that sites have properly stored the IP may be requested throughout the study duration (i.e., if returning to distributor or site to site transfers, etc.).

Accountability, reconciliation and destruction

Regulatory agencies mandate that all IP manufactured for use in clinical trials have cradle-to-grave tracking for accountability, reconciliation, and destruction [24]. Terms are defined as follows:

- **Accountability**: The amount of IP dispensed to a subject vs. the amount returned by the subject, which takes into account missed doses, lack of compliance, lost IP, and any study drug suspensions. This is typically documented at the subject level on a 'drug accountability log' using the smallest dosage level (e.g. tablet, capsule, ml, mg etc.) and monitored routinely by the CRA during on-site monitoring visits.

- **Reconciliation**: This is the amount of IP manufactured, amount released to the packager, shipped to the clinical sites, dispensed to the subjects, returned from the subjects, and destroyed. The amount of IP remaining at each site at a closeout in addition to what was dispensed to the subjects should be equivalent to the amount received during the course of the trial. The following key variables are typically tracked through the life cycle of the manufacture of the IP to its final destruction: Batch/lot #, kit #, site #, subject #, date dispensed, date returned, amount returned, destruction date, and quantity.

- **Destruction**: The process of destroying all remaining IP at the conclusion of a study after all reconciliation has been completed, using the appropriate documented method for destruction (e.g., incineration, landfill etc.).

Numerous regulations, both cGMP and GCPs address accountability, reconciliation, and destruction including 21 CFR parts 312, 210, 211 and ICH guidelines. The life cycle of IP is complex transitioning from a manufacturing environment that must adhere to cGMPs to a clinical environment bound by GCPs.

For complete and accurate drug accountability, reconciliation, and destruction it is essential that all companies involved in the supply chain, including any monitoring groups, and the participating clinical sites have SOPs in place to address these critical aspects of the IP. Planning for these essential elements at the start of the study will ensure that they are tracked by all stakeholders in the supply chain.

The use of IRT can greatly facilitate complete and accurate drug accountability and reconciliation as well as documentation of destruction, especially if deployed at the start of the study with key supply chain stakeholders having clear visibility and input into the system [25].

When conducting clinical trials in the European Union, IMPs may only be used after being released by a trained or certified Qualified Person (QP) [25]. Products that are imported from countries outside the EU are subject to a release by a QP. The release will be at the QP's discretion, but will be based on a quality assessment of the manufacturing site and review of batch records. The depth of assessment will be dependant upon the recognized standards of GMP in that country.

Data management

Similar to any other phase of the project, clinical data management activities must be identified and planned ahead during the planning phase of the study. The project team with representatives from key functional areas (data management, programming, biostatistics, medical/clinical) should get together to set the direction and execute the database build and data analysis requirements. The critical items required for database lock include:

- the build and test of the study database, automatic edit checks, and derivations
- database structure and variable naming conventions should follow the Clinical Data Interchange Standards Consortium (CDISC) conventions. CDISC is a global, open, multidisciplinary, non-profit organization that has established standards to support the acquisition, exchange, submission and archive of clinical research data and metadata. CDISC standards are vendor-neutral, platform-independent and freely available via the CDISC website at www.cdisc.org.
- the definition of electronically collected data vs. eCRF or paper CRF collected data such as laboratory data or ePRO data
- the definition of data transfer requirements
- the identification and set-up of blinding requirements
- the confirmation and validation of automated data flags including automated flags for prior concomitant treatments, or the automated flags for treatment emergent adverse events as opposed to adverse events
- the definition of the data cleaning, review and validation processes, including standard validations
- the definition of data presentation (e.g. clinical data listings)
- the confirmation of successful transfer of test data from the different vendors.

Even if all clinical data management activities are planned ahead, the project team still relies on the investigative sites and services providers such as ECG vendor or central laboratory to enter clinical data into the CRF/eCRF or transfer the data to the sponsor on a regular basis. It is therefore critical to ensure that well-trained and qualified personnel either at the sponsor or on site is dedicated to this activity and is either following-up with sites or vendors, or is directly responding to clinical data management queries, in a timely manner. Again, adequate resources at sites, availability of dedicated personnel as well as the experience of the site in clinical trials are critical aspects that need to be evaluated when selecting potential sites and investigators to ensure the successful execution of a clinical trial.

Coding of clinical data

Case Report Forms are used to collect various subjects' information such as medical diagnosis, medical history, adverse events, and concomitant treatments. Although instructions for completion of CRFs are aimed to harmonize the CRF data entry process, the nature of clinical trials involving investigative sites from different practices or background, and different cultures, lead to a lot of variation in the data entered in the CRF fields. In an effort to standardize and harmonize the reporting of information across sites and countries, the coding of clinical data is a critical step when building-up the integrated clinical database.

The medical coding system is therefore a harmonization system relying on the use of medical dictionaries which provide matching terms for terms entered in the CRF. Various dictionaries exist and can be used as references. The most commonly used include the WHO Drug Dictionary Enhanced (WHO DDE) for coding of concomitant medications [30], and for the coding adverse events, COSTART (Coding Symbols for a Thesaurus of Adverse Reaction Terminology), and MedDRA (Medical Dictionary for Regulatory Activities) are frequently used. [26].

The main objective of MedDRA, which was developed as an ICH initiative, is to standardize the communication between the industry and the regulators through all phase of the drug development cycle including investigational and marketed drugs. The Maintenance and Support Services Organization reviews and maintains MedDRA on a regular basis, so that the data management group must always ensure the most current version is used.

Biostatistics and programming

The statistical analysis plan

The SAP is a document that provides a detailed description of the statistical analysis described in the protocol including, detailed procedures, methodology, and statistical techniques for running the statistical analysis. The objectives of the SAP are multiple. It documents the rationale for the choice of the statistical model applied to the statistical analysis and provides evidence that the analysis is performed in a pre-specified manner. Ultimately, it should contain enough information for the analysis to be repeated by the reviewing authorities.

Guidance documents giving directions to sponsors for the design, conduct, and analysis of clinical trials have been released by regulatory authorities, in the various regions, and should be used as a reference when planning the statistical analysis [27].

Drafting the SAP typically begins shortly after the protocol synopsis is finalized. It is generally prepared by the biostatistician and reviewed by key study team members: clinical pharmacokineticist (e.g., for phase 1 studies), statistical programmer, DSMB, medical team members, steering committee members, health outcome group (if applicable), or regulatory affairs representatives.

The information required in the SAP includes information on:

- study design
- study objectives
- sample size and statistical power
- randomization and blinding techniques
- interim analysis requirements
- primary and secondary endpoints and comparison of interest
- assessments methods for endpoints
- other endpoints and ancillary data
- treatment groups for analysis
- handling of missing data
- statistical software used
- references.

The SAP must also contain a description of the populations studied and analyzed (e.g., 'all randomized', 'intent-to-treat', 'per-protocol' populations). Although the primary analysis is typically run on 'all randomized subjects' population, there may be circumstances that lead to excluding individual subjects from the full analysis. The criteria used to define the different populations of patients must be justified and documented in

the relevant section of the SAP. The SAP must be consistent with the statistical section of the protocol, and must be revised according to any subsequent protocol amendment, if applicable. In order to permit the development and the validation of the required analysis programs, the SAP must be completed as early as possible, preferably before enrollment begins and in any case before the study is unblinded (for blinded studies).

Regulatory requirements

The PM needs to have a clear understanding of the different regulatory requirements (e.g., required documents, translation), process (local ethics committee, versus central ethics committee, national drug agency), and timelines associated with submitting and obtaining local regulatory clearance for the study. Standard delays and turn around time for obtaining IRB/IEC and regulatory approval may range from a couple of weeks to a couple of months. In Europe, the European Medicines Agency (EMEA) established guidelines and guidance documents requesting that applications for clinical trials authorization from the competent authorities and ethics committee be reviewed within 60 days of a valid application [28]. In the US, the FDA must respond to a new investigational new drug application within 30 days [29]. For global trials the PM must seek advice from internal regulatory or CRO staff or from local site monitors or affiliates to make sure about country specific submission processes and requirements.

Importantly, it should not be assumed that the submission of the protocol and its approval will happen at the same time for all sites. Local differences must be considered when planning study start-up activities and setting up start-up objectives and realistic timelines.

Conclusion

Properly planning and appropriately resourcing for the conduct of a clinical development program or a single clinical trial is an important upfront investment that takes time, input from key stakeholders, and needs to be taken seriously. In most cases active planning can easily take 6–9 months. Just like a construction company would not begin to build a multi-billion dollar hotel, without the fully approved architect's blueprints and all applicable zoning and building approvals, a clinical trial should not be started without first having a fully fleshed out and realistic plan that includes: a realistic study timeline; budget; applicable resources and well defined project team and other required

Appendix 27.A Template clinical trial overall budget

A non-inclusive template of typical clinical trial costs

Task title	Resource title	Rate per hour	Number of units	Total hours	Total USD ($)	Comments/assumptions
Protocol development tasks						
Full protocol development						
Protocol amendments						Assume minimum of 1/year
Protocol review						
Start-up tasks						
Country specific regulatory submissions (e.g. IND, CTA, etc)						
Country and site feasibility						Based on # countries/sites required
Identify and recruit sites						
Pre-study site qualification visits						
Develop, assemble and distribute operations manual						
Develop, assemble and distribute site regulatory binder						
Develop, translate and distribute ICF						
Site budget and contract development/negotiation						
Central file set-up						
Investigator meeting planning and preparation						
Investigator training material						
Investigator meeting travel and attendance						
Project kick-off/training meetings						Depending on # of vendors there may need to be one with the CRO and then each of the vendors. For academic centers these kick-off meetings may be between departments or units and vendors.
IRB/EC initial submissions						Average IRB costs in the US for initial submissions is ~ $2500
Regulatory document collection (site specific)						

Ideally obtain 2–3 bids for each type of vendor required (central lab, ECG, electronic diaries, IVRW etc.)

RFP develop, distribution and analysis for all vendors

Vendor selection, budget/contract negotiations

Clinical supplies (drug or device)

Project management

Cost of drug or device

Materials (exipients, components, etc.)

Label printing charges plus translation

Primary manufacturing

Secondary packaging/labeling

Receipt

Storage

Distribution

Analytical/dissolution/stability fees

Courier shipping charges

Custom fees

Returns/destruction

Central laboratory costs

Central ECG costs

Any other vendor costs (paper CRF binders, IRT, ePRO, holter monitoring etc.)

Site monitoring tasks

Develop and maintain site monitoring plan

Site initiation visits

Routine monitoring visits

Site closeout visits

Site management tasks

Draft and maintain site management plan

Administer grant payments to sites

Maintain central files (trial master file (TMF))

Task title	Resource title	Rate per hour	Number of units	Total hours	Total USD ($)	Comments/assumptions
Newsletter development distribution						Based on frequency expected (e.g. monthly, quarterly, etc.)
Annual IRB renewals (review time)						Time for PM to review each site's annual IRB renewal
Project management tasks						
Tracking of enrollment and key milestones						
Provide and document training for all operational project team members						
Routine internal and external team meetings/teleconferences and creation of minutes						
Review trip reports						
Overall project management during study start-up, implementation and close-out						
Vendor management and external committee management and payments						
External committees and consultants						
Data Safety Monitoring Board						# of members × number of meetings × payment/member
Steering Committee						# of members × number of meetings × payment/member
Endpoint Adjudication Committee						# of members × number of meetings × payment/member
Consultants						
Data management tasks						
Draft and maintain data management plan						
Case report form (CRF) d+B44evelopment+B64						
CRF design, review and approval						
CRF printing and distribution (paper studies)						
Develop, assemble and distribute CRF completion instructions						
Electronic data capture (EDC) (including electronic diaries and other eRPO devices						
Develop design specifications						

Site assessment, provisioning and training

Design and validate EDC system

Deploy system and support end-users

License fees (if applicable)

EDC help desk support

Database development

Design, test and implement database

Annotate CRFs

Set-up and maintain medical coding dictionaries (e.g., AEs, concomitant medications, medical history, etc.)

Documentation of database design and edit checks (range checks and cross form logic checks)

Double data entry costs (paper studies)

Tracking, storing and logging CRFs (paper studies)

Data entry

If a paper study data entry costs are driven by the actual process, including any double data entry fees etc.

Data review

The data management system will define all the steps in the review process

Database coding

Using the appropriate data dictionary code AEs, Concomitant medications, medical history etc. and resolve and discrepancies

Review and approval of applicable coding reports

Electronic data transfers

Design file format transfer specifications

Design, test and validate data transfer files

Provide electronic data transfer files

Depending on the # of external vendors and frequency of file transfer, cost per file transfer (varies by vendor) determine total budget. If combined data from all sources need to go elsewhere, also factor in those costs

Task title	Resource title	Rate per hour	Number of units	Total hours	Total USD ($)	Comments/assumptions
Database finalization						
Identify and perform all database finalization activities						
Perform subject acceptability criteria and flag subjects						Identify those patients that do not meet protocol inclusion/exclusion criteria or had other protocol violations to determine which patients can be included in the various analyses (e.g. per protocol, intention-to-treat, completors etc.)
Authorization and sign-off on database lock						
Site closeout tasks						
Provide sites with corrections report (paper studies only)						
Provide sites with pdf of all data or CD and obtain investigator sign-off (EDC only)						
ECC site closeout and decommissioning						
QC of data management activities vs. clinical study report (CSR)						
Biostatistics tasks						
Development and finalization of statistical analysis plan (SAP)						
Development of SAP tables, listing and figures (shells)						
Derived data programming						
Programming tables, figures, listings and graphs						
Validation/QC of tables, figures, listings and graphs						
Interim analysis production and QC (if applicable)						
Final statistical analysis and QC						
Site budget						
Site IRB costs						
IRB/EC initial submissions						Average IRB costs in the US for initial submissions is ~ $2,500

Item	Notes
IRB/EC amendment fees	
IRB/EC annual review/renewal fees	On average assume ~ 1/year
Per subject fee (PSF)	
Cost per subject based on PSF (see Fig. 27A.1)	PSF is based on the final protocol schedule of activities (SOA). Any changes to the SOA typically result in a modification to the PSF and amendments to the site subcontracts
Other site costs	
Local advertising (creation and placement) (e.g. newspaper, radio, newsletters, flyers etc.)	
Site labor cost per amendment (independent of IRB/EC costs)	Two types of amendments: 1) administrative that do not require reconsenting of subjects, but require personnel effort on the submission, 2) those that require modification to the ICF and thus reconsenting of subjects
One time non-reimbursible site start-up fee	Funds required for the upfront effort put forth by site personnel before any subjects can be enrolled, including time for IRB submission activities, subcontracts, training of personnel etc.
Per occurrence SAE processing	
Pharmacy set-up fee	
Specialty equipment that may require purchase	
Site archiving costs (sorting, boxing and documenting items for archive)	
General office supplies that may be independent of PSF, including things like dry ice for shipments	

Task title	Resource title	Rate per hour	Number of units	Total hours	Total USD ($)	Comments/assumptions
Courier fees						
Institutional indirect rates						For academic institutions the indirect rate for pharmaceutically, foundation and NIH sponsored studies vary and can range anywhere from 0% to 75%

Reporting/publication tasks

Task title	Resource title	Rate per hour	Number of units	Total hours	Total USD ($)	Comments/assumptions
Publication plan and publication creation						
Publication reprint costs						
Regulatory submissions (IND, CTA etc); include required annual submission and final end of study submission						
Regulatory submissions (IND safety letters, SUSARs)						
Development and implementaiton plan for informing sites, subjects of study results						
Submission of required financial reports to SEC and comparable authorities and competent authorities in other countries						

Overall study archive tasks

Task title	Resource title	Rate per hour	Number of units	Total hours	Total USD ($)	Comments/assumptions
Sorting, boxing and documenting materials to be archived						
Central files management & long-term off-site storage/ retrieval costs						
Total Clinical Trial Budget ESTIMATE					$ –	

General comments

1. For each item, determine resource that will perform the task and the associated hourly rate, which should include applicable Facilities and Administration (F&A) rates.

2. Once final budget has been created, consider applying a 'fudge factor' to the total budget, anywhere from 10 to 20% depending on preceived level of unknown

3. Attempt to get a minimum of 2–3 bids from each vendor type required. The bidding process typically identifies protocol inconsistencies, deficiencies and significant valuable input can be gained from the expertise from the various vendors.

4. If conducting study in multiple countries or if vendors are located in other countries, factor in anticipated fluctuations in currency exchanges rates that are likely to occur during the course of multi-year studies. Hedge against significant negative changes.B24

Sample Per Subject Fee Budget Template (Based on final protocol Schedule of Activities)													
ASSESSMENTS	Unit cost	Screening	Baseline	Visit 1 Day 1	T1	Visit 2	Visit 3	T2	Visit 4	Visit 5	Premature withdrawal visit/end of study	Total per subject fee	Unsched visit
Timeframes				Titration					Maintenance				
Study day	SC	0	1	2	7	8	9	14	50	80		
Written informed consent												-	
Update screening projections form													
Inclusion/exclusion review												-	
Medical history / demographics												-	
Physical/neuro examinations												-	
Brief physical/neuro examinations												-	
ECG 12-lead												-	
Vital signs / weight												-	
Total functional capacity (TFC)												-	
MMSE												-	
Concomitant medication review												-	
Enrollment log												-	
Safety laboratory procedures												-	
Pharmacokinetics												-	
Hospital stay for pharmacokinetics												-	
UPDRS												-	
Dispense study drug												-	
Dosage log												-	
Drug accountability / compliance												-	
Adverse events log												-	
Adverse events follow up												-	
Coordinator time and effort												-	
Worksheet prep / data entry												-	
Investigator time and effort												-	
Total direct costs	-	-	-	-	-	-	-	-	-	-	-		-
F&A at XX% (include institutional rate)	-	-	-	-	-	-	-	-	-	-	-		-
Total per subject fee	-	-	-	-	-	-	-	-	-	-	-		-

Notes: Detemine % of screen failures that will be reimbursed and at what rate (e.g., full screening visit and portion of baseline visit); Determine reimbursement rate for premature withdrawals

Figure 27A.1. Sample Per Subject Fee Budget Template (Based on final protocol Schedule of Activities).

committees (e.g., Steering Committee, DSMB); assessment of protocol feasibility; appropriate sites selection, qualification and site training; a realistic recruitment strategy; well defined CRFs; a fully validated database with appropriate edit and logic checks; a fully developed DMP and SAP and applicable regulatory approvals. A well-laid-out plan will ensure a smooth execution of the trial which is discussed in detail as part of the implementation phase in Chapter 28.

References

1. Getz K, Wenger J, Campo R, *et al*. Assessing the impact of protocol design change on clinical trial performance. *Am J Ther* 2008; **15**: 450–5.

2. Getz K, Campo, R, Kaitin K. Variability in protocol design complexity by phase and therapeutic area. *Drug Inform J* 2011; **45**: 413–20.

3. FDA Guidance. Investigator responsibilities–protecting the rights, safety and welfare of study subjects. http://www.fda.gov/downloads/Drugs/GuidanceComplianceRegulatoryInformation/Guidances/UCM187772.pdf

4. Getz K. Ominous clouds over outsourcing. Applied Clinical Trials. 2010. http://appliedclinicaltrialsonline.findpharma.com/appliedclinicaltrials/CRO%2FSponsor/Ominous-Clouds-OverOutsourcing/ArticleStandard/Article/detail/686210?contextCategoryId=37194. (Accessed August 8, 2011.)

5. 21 CRF Part 11. Electronic Records; Electronic Signatures – Scope of Application. http://www.fda.gov/RegulatoryInformation/Guidances/ucm125067.htm. (Accessed August 8, 2011.)

6. MedDRA MSSO Medical Dictionary for Regulatory Activities, Maintenance, and Support Services. http://www.meddramsso.com. (Accessed August 8, 2011.)

7. Directive 2001/20/EC of the European Parliament and of the Council of 4 April 2001 on the approximation of the laws, regulations and administrative provisions of the Member States relating to the implementation of good clinical practice in the conduct of clinical trials on medicinal products for human use. http://www.eortc.be/Services/Doc/clinical-EU-directive-04-April-01.pdf. (Accessed August 8, 2011.)

8. EudraVigilence. Information for sponsors of non-commercial clinical trials. Reporting Rules of SUSARs to EudraVigilance for commercial and non-commercial sponsors of clinical trials conducted in the EEA. http://eudravigilance.ema.europa.eu/human/index03.asp. (Accessed August 8, 2011.)

9. European Medicines Agency. ICH Topic E6 (R1). Guideline for Good Clinical Practice. http://www.ema.europa.eu/docs/en_GB/document_library/Scientific_guideline/2009/09/WC500002874.pdf. (Accessed August 8, 2011.)

10. 21 CFR 314. Applications for FDA Approval to Market a New Drug. http://www.accessdata.fda.gov/scripts/cdrh/cfdocs/cfcfr/CFRSearch.cfm?CFRPart=314. (Accessed August 8, 2011.)

11. ICH E14. Clinical Evaluation of QT/QTc Interval Prolongation and Proarrhythmic Potential for Non-Antiarrhythmic Drugs. 2005. http://www.fda.gov/downloads/RegulatoryInformation/Guidances/ucm129357.pdf. (Accessed August 8, 2011.)

12. Li G. Site Activation, The Key to more Efficient Clinical Trials. Avanstar Communications Inc. 2008.

13. DiMasi JA, Hansen RW and Grabowski HG. The price of innovation; new estimates of drug development costs. *J Health Econ* 2003; **22**: 151–85.

14. Rees, H. Supply Chain Management in the Drug Industry: Delivering Patient Value for Pharmaceuticals and Biologics. 2011.

15. FDA Guideline on the preparation of Investigational New Drug Products. 1991. http://www.fda.gov/downloads/Drugs/GuidanceComplianceRegulatoryInformation/Guidances/ucm070315.pdf. (Accessed August 8, 2011.)

16. Commission Directive 2003/94/EC of 8 October 2003. Laying down the principles and guidelines of good manufacturing practice in respect to medicinal products for human use and investigational medicinal products for human use. 2003. http://ec.europa.eu/health/files/eudralex/vol-1/dir_2003_94/dir_2003_94_en.pdf. (Accessed August 8, 2011.)

17. ICH Harmonized Tripartite Guideline Comparability of biotechnological/biological products subject to changes in their manufacturing process. http://www.ich.org/fileadmin/Public_Web_Site/ICH_Products/Guidelines/Quality/Q5E/Step4/Q5E_Guideline.pdf. (Accessed August 8, 2011.)

18. FDA Guideline. Device Classification. 2009. http://www.fda.gov/MedicalDevices/DeviceRegulationandGuidance/Overview/ClassifyYourDevice/default.htm. (Accessed August 9, 2011.)

19. The International Conference on Harmonisation of Technical Requirements for Registration of Pharmaceuticals for Human Use (ICH). http://www.ich.org/. (Accessed August 8, 2011.)

20. FDA Guidance for Industry. Q1A (R2) Stability Testing of New Drug Substances and Products. 2003. http://www.fda.gov/downloads/RegulatoryInformation/Guidances/ucm128204.pdf. (Accessed August 8, 2011)

21. What is Tablet Dissolution Testing? 2011. http://www.tabletdissolution.com/education/dissolution/index.php. (Accessed August 8, 2011.)

22. Lis F, Gourley D, Wilson D, and Page M. Global Supply Chain Management. Applied Clinical Trials. 2009. http://appliedclinicaltrialsonline.findpharma.com/appliedclinicaltrials/article/articleDetail.jsp?id=602049&pageID=1&sk=&date=. (Accessed August 8, 2011.)

23. International Air Transport Association. http://www.iata.org/index.htm. (Accessed August 8, 2011.)

24. Dowlman N, Kwak M, Wood R, *et al*. Managing the Drug Supply Chain with eProcesses. *Appl Clin Trials* 2006; **15**: 40–5.

25. European QP Association. Qualified Persons in Europe. http://www.qp-association.eu/qualified_person_qp_regulation.html, (Accessed August 8, 2011.)

26. Medical Dictionary for Regulatory Activities. Maintenance and Support Services Organization (MedDRA MSSO). http://www.meddramsso.com/. (Accessed August 8, 2011.)

27. European Medicines Agency. Science Medicines Health. Clinical efficacy and Safety Guidelines Introduction. http://www.ema.europa.eu/htms/human/humanguidelines/efficacy.htm. (Accessed August 8, 2011.)

28. ICH Topic E6 (R1). Guideline for Good Clinical Practice. http://www.ema.europa.eu/docs/en_GB/document_library/Scientific_guideline/2009/09/WC500002874.pdf. (Accessed August 8, 2011.)

29. FDA Code of Federal Regulations. 21 CFR Part 312.40. http://www.accessdata.fda.gov/scripts/cdrh/cfdocs/cfcfr/CFRSearch.cfm?fr=312.40. (Accessed August 8, 2011.)

30. WHO Drug Dictionary Enhanced (WHO DDE). http://www.umc-products.com/DynPage.aspx (Accessed November 20, 2011).

28

Clinical trial implementation, analysis, and reporting: An academic and industry perspective

Cornelia L. Kamp and Jean-Michel Germain

Clinical trial implementation overview

The successful implementation of any clinical trial depends on careful planning as described in Chapter 27. With a realistic timeline, budget and a detailed scope of work for all study activities the actual execution of the trial should be relatively straightforward. The focus during the implementation phase is on monitoring the study progress which includes: overall subject recruitment and retention activities, timeliness of Case Report Form (CRF) entry, observation of any site, safety laboratory or data trends that may need to be addressed, and ensuring adequate IP is available as needed. Additionally, the project manager (PM) will be managing the project against the overall budget, pre-defined timeline, and scope of work, and communicating proactively and frequently to all key stakeholders about any changes that have downstream ramifications.

Successful project teams are *flexible* in managing the trial, planning for major milestones, and addressing day-to-day operational issues as they arise. The more time spent properly planning the execution of the trial, the fewer headaches endured during the study implementation.

This chapter will review the key implementation steps and outline key aspects to be considered and monitored, as well as key requirements to comply with throughout the execution phase, from sites selection to reporting of results.

Protocol feasibility

Whether it is performed internally or outsourced to a clinical research organization (CRO), the protocol feasibility should rely on criteria developed and agreed by relevant representatives from the project

team (medical, project management). The team should agree on the minimum qualifications required for each principal investigator (PI) and/or sites to participate in the study. These criteria should assess the site experience and the qualifications of the site as well as the chance for achieving the recruitment/retention target. The feasibility study is usually conducted through a survey to potential sites and includes selection criteria such as:

- site setting (hospital vs. private practice)
- catchment area (large hospital, large city, regional center)
- patient referral system (physician network)
- site experience in the same disease area with indications on previous performance (number of subjects enrolled, recruitment period associated and retention rates)
- site experience in similar study design (e.g., placebo-controlled trial)
- information on recruitment potential (number of new patients seen every month)
- anticipated recruitment rate and recruitment strategy
- advertisement possibility
- comments on eligibility criteria
- confidence in obtaining regulatory and Institutional Review Board (IRB)/ Independent Ethics Committee (IEC) approval ('were trials with similar design recently approved?')
- frequency of IRB/IEC meetings
- information on the anticipated delay between protocol submission to IRB/IEC and/or local regulatory body approval and site activation
- site technology and infrastructure is consistent with the protocol requirements (MRI equipment,

Clinical Trials in Neurology, ed. Bernard Ravina, Jeffrey Cummings, Michael P. McDermott, and R. Michael Poole. Published by Cambridge University Press. © Cambridge University Press 2012.

central pharmacy or adequate space for proper storage of study medication, availability of refrigerator or freezer, etc.)

- site experience in collaborating with external vendors (interactive response system (IRT), central laboratories) or using specific technology such as electronic Case Report Forms (eCRFs), or electronic patient diaries
- site personnel training on FDA, International Conference on Harmonisation (ICH), Good Clinical Practice (GCP) and other applicable regulatory requirements based on region
- site previous exposure to inspections (FDA, European Medicines Agency (EMEA), Drug Enforcement Agency (DEA) for controlled substances, or local drug agency)
- availability of dedicated staff (sub-investigator, study coordinator)
- evaluation of concurrent studies (ongoing or planned) that could compete with the proposed trial
- principal investigator's interest in participating in the study.
- availability of site standard operating procedures (SOPs)

Sites selection, qualification and training

Site selection

Beside a 'well-designed' protocol, the site selection process is probably one of the most challenging and critical steps of the project, as the performance of sites both in terms of subject recruitment, retention and quality of the data submitted can impact the outcome of a trial.

Good Clinical Practices require sponsors to select investigators that are qualified by education, training and experience to assume responsibility for the proper conduct of clinical trials [1]. Investigators must also meet all qualifications specified by the applicable regulatory requirements and provide evidence of their qualifications (through an up-to-date curriculum vitae or other relevant document) upon request by the sponsor, IRB, IEC, and regulatory authorities

In Europe, the current regulation requires that documentation and information on the qualification and training of the principal investigator in GCPs be sent to the ethics committee for review and approval. The ethics committee must also approve the quality

of the investigative sites including the availability of adequate resources and personnel. Therefore, the purpose of the site selection process is to identify sites that have the appropriate experience and expertise with the disease or the indication studied, access to the right population of patients, adequate organizational capabilities and familiarity with clinical trials requirements and regulations.

Site qualification

For sites that have previous experience with the clinical trial sponsor, a review of the site's previous performance may also provide valuable information on the recruitment rate, drop-out rate, quality of the data (query rate, protocol violations, and audit findings), site collaboration and responsiveness (submission of CRF data, response to queries).

In order to ensure that meaningful data is obtained from the feasibility study, it should be conducted with a mature version of the protocol synopsis with no anticipated major changes. A change in any of the eligibility criteria could have a significant impact on the patient population and the site's ability to recruit.

The identification of potential investigators can be based on a variety of sources including literature, publications, network, and input for local staff, including Site Monitor (SM) or Clinical Research Associate (CRA), local affiliates or marketing. As a first step in establishing potential future collaboration with sites and PIs, most clinical trial sponsors generally rely on locally trained and experienced internal or outsourced resources for the administration of the feasibility survey. Ultimately, the qualification of the sites to participate in the study is based on the review of the site selection documents including both surveys and on site visit monitoring reports (see 'Sites Monitoring') by the appropriate project team members. For regulatory inspection purposes, the clinical trial sponsor should be able to document the selection and qualification process for all sites, and the compliance with its own requirements, so that the filing of the relevant documentation in the Trial Master Files (see 'Monitoring of Quality') is appropriately completed.

In order to ensure that sites are meeting their objectives and sponsor's recruitment expectations, the performance of the sites must be monitored closely after sites are activated, meaning that sites have started to actively enroll subjects into the trial. Also, the quality of the clinical data submitted by the sites should be assessed throughout the sites' participation with different tools including the review of CRA monitoring visit reports, clinical data, trending, and site audits (see also 'Monitoring of Quality')

Site training

Site personnel must be adequately trained to ensure smooth execution of a clinical trial. In Europe, the EU Directive requires that information documenting the qualification of the PI, the training of the PI in GCP as well as his/her experience in investigational research be reviewed by the Ethics Committees [2]. In the US, FDA also requires similar documentation [3]. For global multicentre trials, the general approach adopted by sponsors has been to complete all training during global and/or local investigator's meetings. Although the investigator's meeting is an important training vehicle, it is sometimes organized several months before a site can get started. Therefore, sponsor representatives must plan for enough time during the site initiation visit to go again through important messages from the investigator's meeting and study procedures. All training should be documented so that it can be provided in case of regulatory inspection. Throughout the execution of the trial the CRA will play a key role in monitoring site adherence to the trial procedures and requirements and in identifying any needs for training (new personnel on site) and retraining in case of non-adherence. Training requirements are obviously not limited to site personnel but also include any team members at the sponsor, CRO, or vendors.

Site monitoring

In accordance with GCP, including the ICH Guidelines for GCPs, sponsors must ensure that the following key aspects are respected [4, 5]:

- The rights and well-being of human subjects are protected.
- The reported trial data are accurate, complete and verifiable from source documents.
- The conduct of the trial is in compliance with the currently approved protocol/amendment(s), GCP, and with the applicable regulatory requirements.

Site monitoring, therefore, requires on-site visits conducted by well-trained study personnel (SM, or CRA). On-site visits are usually performed according to pre-agreed criteria defined in a global monitoring plan (MP) which generally includes information such as the frequency of site monitoring visit, the items and

data to be verified and compared with source documents including all [a information in original records and certified copies of original records of clinical findings, observations, or other activities in a clinical trial necessary for the reconstruction and evaluation of the trial. Source data are contained in source documents (original records or certified copies)]. [ICH E6]. Additionally the MP typically requires a complete tour of the facilities where any aspect of the study will be conducted, for example ancillary sites such as an imaging unit or clinical pharmacy. The MP also spells out the process for escalating issues and the resolution process. The MP is a critical document for the standardization of monitoring aspects especially when site monitoring activities are outsourced to an external vendor, or when a study is conducted in various geographic locations. The extent and the nature of site monitoring visit depend on the objectives and purpose of the visit.

Site initiation visit

Prior to enrolling any subjects in a study the PI as well as site personnel must be trained in GCP as well as on protocol specific requirements and study procedures, and have to understand their role and responsibilities in the conduct of the study. Although training could already have been dispensed as part of the investigator's meeting, the SM or CRA will plan for a specific site initiation visit to ensure that the investigator and site staff understand the protocol and GCP. During this visit the SM or CRA will also check the completeness and the accuracy of all study documentation will make sure that all regulatory and IRB/IEC approvals have been received and will confirm the qualification of the site for participating in the study.

Regular site monitoring visit

After the first patient is enrolled, the site will receive regular site monitoring visits as described in the GMP. During these visits, the monitor will ensure that the trial is conducted and that the data are recorded and reported in compliance with the protocol requirements, the sponsor SOPs, the international regulation and local regulation as applicable. The monitor will generally focus on ensuring the proper documentation of subject's informed consent (ICF), the compliance with the requirement for reporting safety information, managing and storing clinical supplies including investigational medicinal product (IMP). The monitor will also verify that current study documentation is maintained on site, including study records, such as updated list of study personnel, training records, list of all subjects enrolled, communication with IRB/IEC and delegation of authority log.

Every on-site visit has to be documented on site and in the sponsor central repository. The monitor has responsibility for preparing a monitoring visit report describing the data which were verified, the findings as well as the corrective actions taken. The monitor has responsibility for following-up on all findings until resolution by the site or the sponsor.

Routine study closure

The routine closure of most clinical trials includes the following:

- All sites should have a final site closeout monitoring visit prior to database lock to ensure all data queries have been addressed, and to ensure that the data in the database agrees with the source documentation.
- During the final site closeout monitoring visit, the CRA should perform a full account of all used and unused investigational product (IP) including drug and devices and prepare IP for final return to the sponsor or destruction of any used/unused IP at each participating center following institutional policy. Final reconciliation of all IP by the study sponsor or designee is also required. The CRA will also ensure appropriate closure of all monitoring issues identified during the course of the study.
- Return or destruction of any other clinical supplies such as ECG machines, personal digital assistants if used for patient reported outcomes, or paper CRF binders.
- Notification of each site's IRB/IEC that the site is no longer actively enrolling subjects and that the database has been locked. Some IRBs/IECs require that the study remain open until the primary manuscript has been published.
- All site files must be prepared for archive and long-term storage. If an electronic data capture system was used, each site must be provided with a final complete CD of their data [6].
- FDA Code of Federal Regulations (CFR 21 312.56) contains record retention requirements for IRB records.
- FDA CFR 21 312.57 contains record retention requirements for financial disclosures.
- CFR 21 312.62 contains record retention requirements for drug disposition and case histories.

- Following the lock of the database, all user permissions to modify the clinical trial database, are disabled, so that no further changes to the data can be made.
- All vendors should be notified about study completion to ensure final study tasks and invoicing are completed in a timely matter and to avoid unnecessary expenditures by vendors. The members of the project team and the vendors would be responsible for ensuring all documentation for the study was appropriately filed and ultimately archived according to the regulations and applicable internal SOPs.
- Final reporting requirements as delineated in 'Clinical trial reporting'.

All entities involved in the conduct of clinical trials should have SOPs in place for the orderly closeout of a clinical trial. Dinnett *et al.* provide lessons learned on study closeout experience from the large multi-center study of Prospective Study of Pravastatin in the Elderly at Risk [7].

Recruitment and retention plan

Recruitment

Much has been previously written in the literature about the importance of recruitment and retention of subjects for the timely completion and success of any clinical trial [8]. The key is ultimately to have a well-defined recruitment and retention plan available at the start of the study with a realistic enrollment timeline with robust contingencies plans that are implemented as soon as enrollment falls behind. While much research has been done identifying barriers to recruitment, slow enrollment continues to plague most clinical trials, including those in neurological disorders. Regardless of the funding source, most studies are being completed behind schedule by at least 1 or more months. Recent data suggests that as many as 80% of studies finish enrollment at least 1 month behind schedule [9]. There are few, if any, reports of studies completing enrollment ahead of schedule. Recruitment starts with site selection (see above 'Sites selection and qualification and training'). Identifying sites with an appropriate patient pool, with a qualified and experienced investigator/study coordinator team is of utmost importance in ensuring successful recruitment.

Pharmaceutical companies and CROs have spent significant effort during the past decade or more looking at methods to enhance recruitment, including more sophisticated advertising, targeted databases and interactive websites, educational brochures for subjects [10], better training of staff recruiting subjects, increasing the per subject fee, etc. One trend that has been noted by researchers at Tufts Center for the Study of Drug Development is the fact that protocols have become more complex over the past decade [11, 12, 13]. More frequent visits and more assessments per visit often add lots of 'nice to have' but not 'need to have' data, collectively driving up the costs of clinical research and hampering effective recruitment efforts as subject and site burden increases.

In many cases the calculation used to determine the enrollment duration is unrealistic. This includes attempting to squeeze a study timeline into a grant timeline or an overall drug development plan. In many cases, project teams determine the enrollment duration by taking the total sample size, divided by the anticipated enrollment rate (e.g. number of subjects enrolled/month), and divided by the total number of sites. For example a phase 3 Parkinson's disease (PD) study of 600 subjects with an enrollment rate of 1 subject/site/month at 40 centers, the enrollment duration, using this simplistic formula will be calculated to be 15 months (600 ÷ 1subject/site/month ÷ 40 sites = 15 months). The calculation assumes that all sites will be activated (ready to start enrolling subjects, meaning all regulatory documents are in-house, IRB/IEC approval has been obtained, clinical trial agreements are in-place and clinical supplies are available at the site (investigational agent, laboratory kits, etc.) at the exact same time. Unfortunately, this is typically not the case, especially for global trials that involve sites in countries that have different timing for the submission and the review of protocol and regulatory documents.

Published data suggest average site activation of 100 days [14]. In addition to factoring on site activation time, additional time must be factored in for the delay from site activation to first enrollment, which from unpublished data has averaged an additional 83 days. Clearly more robust formulas should be developed when calculating the enrollment duration taking into account these very real staggered site activation profiles, plus factoring in reduced enrollment during holiday months (e.g., late November and December and summer vacation months) thereby developing a realistic enrollment timeline from the start.

Recruitment plans need to be specific to the disease and disease stage being recruited. What works for one group of patients does not necessarily transfer to another population. Gathering data about prior enrollment rates for other randomized controlled trials can help in determining realistic enrollment rates and number of sites to include. For example published data for newly diagnosed PD subjects suggest an enrollment rate of 0.83 subjects/site/month [15], regardless of the funding source or clinical trial infrastructure.

Recruitment of women and minorities

From 1977 to 1993, the FDA forbade early-stage testing of most medication on women of child-bearing potential for fear of causing birth-defects. It was not until 1993 with the NIH revitalization act that NIH established guidelines for the inclusion of women and minorities in clinical trials [16, 17, 18]. In 1997, the Food and Drug Modernization Act recommended inclusion and documentation of race and ethnicity and analysis thereof. While significant strides have been made in the past 15 years to include more women and minorities, there is still a significant shortage of women and minority participation in clinical trials [19, 20, 21, 22, 23, 24]. In fact, clinical trial participation rates by race for new drug applications (NDAs) submitted between 1995 and 1999 showed a distribution of 88% white, 8% black, 1% Hispanic, and 3% Asian [25]. There is still much to be done to get minority participation rates to coincide with the actual distribution of race and ethnicity distribution of the US population.

Materials used for successful enrollment of minorities should be culturally appropriate and translated in the applicable languages. Having investigator, coordinator or other study staff of the same race/ethnicity often helps to remove cultural barriers and build trust, allowing for greater enrollment of the targeted group.

While NIH grant submission forms require a clear breakdown of anticipated enrollment by race, ethnicity, and gender few NIH studies achieve the targeted enrollment distribution. Likewise, while regulatory authorities would like to see a diverse patient population as part of the data used for an NDA or CTA, there are no regulatory requirements that insist on certain targets. Most NDA/CTA submissions also fall short of the target distribution of the racial/ethnic and gender distributions based on population census in the given region [25].

Retention

Retention starts with recruitment. Identifying the right subjects that meet all protocol inclusion and exclusion studies, who fully understand the purpose of their participation for the *entire duration* of the study and who are committed to follow the study visits and assessments as required. Experienced investigators/ coordinators can often determine up front which subjects are most likely to remain in the study for the full duration and will make a decision not to enroll those subjects who although may meet inclusion/exclusion criteria are not apt to remain committed for the long haul. During the site selection process it is important to gather information on site retention rates in prior studies to avoid including those sites who may be high enrollers, but who fail to follow the vast majority of subjects to study completion. Poor subject retention can have a significant negative impact on the outcome of a trial. The chance of showing efficacy can be compromised by a high premature withdrawal rate and/or a high lost to follow-up rate.

Experienced investigator/coordinator teams understand the importance of building and maintaining a strong relationship throughout the duration of the study. This includes open communication during in-person visits, regular follow-up by phone, and a true attempt to understand what the subject and their spouse/caregiver/significant other and family are going through as part of participation. Efforts to eliminate barriers to attend routine visits can help ensure continued participation. This could include; the reimbursement for costs associated with travel; pre-paid phone card; childcare; food; parking; home visits; week night and weekend clinic hours; offering a car service for pick-up/drop-off; and efforts to minimize the entire duration of study visits by keeping assessments involving other departments such as MRI, or assessments by a neuropsychologist, on time so as to avoid large gaps between assessments.

In some studies payment to subjects for time and effort may be allowed. The compensation cannot be coercive in nature, must be prorated based on visits completed, and should be done in compliance with local regulatory requirements (as the regulation may vary from one country to another). In most cases it should be reviewed and approved by the IRB/IEC and the amount and timing of the compensation is generally disclosed in the ICF.

Understanding the intensity of assessments at each protocol visit and the unique situation of each subject in the study can help an investigator/coordinator team in determining specific barriers to ongoing retention to that subject that could be eliminated often with minimal additional effort by the study team.

The literature is rich with articles on various tools used to ensure subject retention, especially in long-term studies where in-person study visits may be infrequent; every 6 months to 1 year (e.g. birthday and anniversary cards, hand written thank you notes following visits or for special efforts, gift cards for protocol milestones, newsletters reporting ongoing status of the study, etc.) [26, 27]. Budgeting for these types of retention initiatives prior to study start is critical for their success.

The industry as a whole has been paying specific attention to recruitment and retention issues in all clinical trials. There are numerous vendors available that specialize in recruitment/retention initiatives and there are a plethora of training courses available specifically addressing this particular challenge in conducting clinical trials [28].

Retention rates in many neurological disorders are relatively high, with premature withdrawal rates about 10–20% [29, 30]. The sample size calculations must include contingencies for the anticipated premature withdrawal rate to ensure that enough subjects complete the full study for the analysis to be meaningful.

Quality management

Inspections to confirm GCP at investigator sites have been occurring for many years. Originally driven by the FDA, the environment has been changing over the last decade as not only the FDA, but also other regulatory agencies from either Europe, Japan, and other countries are now routinely conducting GCP site inspections. It is therefore critical for sites to get prepared for such audits.

Preparing for inspection

Local regulatory agencies can perform GCP inspections as part of a national surveillance program of clinical trials, coordinated by the EMEA or the FDA before marketing authorization. As opposed to the FDA, the EMEA does not employ any full time inspector, but appoints an inspection team by gathering inspectors from two or three different European countries. For inspections related to marketing authorization, the focus of the site inspection will be primarily on the integrity and validity of the data, on the ethical standards, adherence to the protocol, training and qualifications of the study personnel as well as on specific issues that could be identified during the review process of the application dossier/NDA. These inspections can be announced but are frequently unannounced.

The specific items that may be checked during a GCP inspection [31] include but are not limited to:

- **Legal and administrative aspects**: communication with the IRB/IEC and local regulatory bodies, to ensure that IEC/IRB and local regulatory approvals were obtained for the protocol and its amendment(s) and ICF before the study start. Additionally, that all subjects enrolled in the study signed the ICF prior to any study assessments being completed and any ICF amendments prior to conducing new protocol requirements dictated by the protocol amendment(s).
- **Organizational aspects**: documentation of delegation of responsibility by the PI, staff qualification, CVs, responsibilities, experience, availability of PI and site personnel, training program and training records, SOPs, contract between the sponsor and the investigator as it relates to delegation of responsibility but not the budget component.
- **Facility and equipment**: proper use, adequacy and validation of procedures and equipment (including documentation of routine calibration) used for the conduct of the trial.
- **Management of biological samples**: conditions of collection, storage and shipment, shipping documentation.
- **Organization of the documentation**: general documentation available, signed, dated and filed on site, trial subject's documents available including source documents, ICF documents, CRFs.
- **Monitoring and audit**: review of signed and dated ICF, ICF approval documentation by IRB/IEC, and documentation of the consent process.
- **Trial subject data**: study conducted according to the approved protocol, source data verification, corrections of CRF data according to ICH/GCP.
- **Characteristics of subjects included:** accuracy of eligibility criteria as compared to source data, documentation of protocol violations.
- **Efficacy and safety assessments**: consistency between CRFs and source documents.
- **Concomitant therapies**: managed according to protocol requirements and recorded in the source documents and in the CRF.
- **Management of IP**: review of shipping records, drug or device labels, IP accountability

documents, destruction (if applicable), treatment compliance, storage conditions, randomization procedures (IRT), and unblinding.

The most common findings from FDA or EMEA GCP inspections of investigator sites are related to the management of IMP, trial management and study oversight, essential documents, delegation of tasks and functions, as well as qualification and training of investigators and site personnel [32].

Monitoring of quality

Sponsors are required to have an internal quality assurance system which includes quality control and auditing [33]. Generally independent from the research and development team, the audit or quality assurance groups routinely perform audits of investigator sites, vendors, clinical trial processes and systems, trial master files, but also conduct pre-inspection activities.

In biopharmaceutical companies audit activities are usually planned before the protocol starts. The auditors and the project team generally agree on an audit plan which includes a minimum number of sites to be audited. This plan can be revised during the execution of the study based on the performance of the sites both in terms of recruitment and quality. However, as clinical trials may involve dozens or even sometimes hundreds of sites, only a small proportion are ultimately selected for an audit. It is therefore critical that all sites and institutions running clinical trials get prepared and develop quality management tools to maximize compliance and quality in the execution of clinical trials.

Sites, institutions, and project teams from the sponsor can address and limit most deficiencies found on audits by developing simple tools such as checklists, or ongoing quality checks based on the identification of trends.

Document checklist: The following items are examples of critical site level documents that can be tracked for filing in the sponsor or institution central repository or Trial Master File:

- updated and signed CVs of investigators, sub-investigators and other key site personnel involved in subject assessments
- investigator's meeting documentation and materials
- statement of investigator (FDA form 1572)
- certification of disclosure of financial interest
- request for shipment of clinical supplies

- confirmation of receipt of clinical supplies
- completed drug dispensing and inventory records
- IRB/IEC approved ICF
- IRB/IEC approved protocol and amendment(s)
- IRB/IEC composition/organization
- IRB annual report
- delegation of site responsibilities and signatures record
- sponsor approved protocol signed and dated by the PI
- acknowledge receipt of Investigator's Brochure and Safety Reports
- site monitoring trip reports
- site monitoring sign-in-log
- site monitoring correspondences (including documentation on closure of outstanding monitoring issues)
- site monitoring visit follow-up letters.
- subject master list.

Analysis of trends: the systematic and regular review of specific items can also help the sponsor to monitor the overall quality of the study, and to address potential gaps. For example, the regular review and analysis of monitoring issues reported in site monitoring reports can be very useful to identify recurrent site issues and determine the needs for additional training for sites or CRAs, or the needs for vendors to improve their performance. Reports on subject screening, enrollment, retention, timeliness of data entered into the database, number of queries and time to resolution of queries can provide overall site performance information. Reports looking at overall safety lab trends and overall adverse events that are reviewed regularly by medical staff can provide early safety signals in a blinded fashion.

Compliance and quality management by both sites and sponsors requires constant attention from all team members from conception to final regulatory reporting. The progress of a trial must be assessed by performance metrics but also by developing and generalizing quality assessment measures, as high quality data and compliance with the current regulations and current processes could make the regulatory approval process smoother and could therefore lead to the drug being available on the market sooner.

Database management and lock

When planning for a clinical trial the team must agree early enough on the technology to be used as this will shape the timeline for the project. The use of advanced electronic data capture (eDC) technology has drastically changed the clinical data management area, by expediting the retrieval and clean-up of data and therefore saving time and money on the data management process. Where it could take up to several months with paper CRF studies between the Last Patient Last Visit (LPLV) and the freeze of the database, it now takes a couple of days or a couple of weeks with eDC technology.

Whether the clinical trial uses paper CRF or eDC system, the investigational sites, the project manager and data management staff play a key role in ensuring the database is completed on time. Most sponsors require that clinical data be entered in the CRF within 2 days of the subject's visit. Site monitors make sure that site personnel are adequately trained in methods to enter clinical data in CRF fields. It is also expected that data management staff edit and clean-up the data on an ongoing basis to address missing data or data discrepancies. The project manager and data management group are responsible for closely monitoring the status of the database both for timeliness and quality of data. The project manager usually holds regular meetings with clinical data management representatives (especially when approaching database finalization or interim analysis) to address potential issues as they arise.

Routine study closure and early termination

The early termination of a study must be done in an orderly manner and plans should be put in place at the start of the study outlining the procedure that would be followed in the event of an early termination of a study [34, 35]. This will avoid potentially missing notification to key players and avoid the chaos often associated with the early termination of studies.

The steps followed to complete a routine close out of a study are delineated in 'Routine study closure' (see above) and are the same things that need to be completed in the event of early termination. In the event that a study is terminated early regardless of the reason (safety, futility, etc.), each actively participating subject must be notified that the study has been stopped prematurely, including the reason why the study has been stopped. Each subject should be given instructions for stopping the use of the IP, plans for return of the IP, and scheduling of a final visit for each study subject.

Depending on the local regulation and the reason for early termination, expedited reporting to IRB/IEC and/or local Board of Health may be required.

Following the notification of the participating study subjects, all of the other study team members, including the various vendors must be informed of the early termination of the study along with instructions for the orderly conclusion of their service and contract issues associated with the early termination.

Clinical trial reporting

Reporting the results of clinical trials is not just the publication of a peer-reviewed manuscript. There are several important parts, each serving different purposes as defined further below. The order in which reporting occurs is important. Delineating a comprehensive reporting plan, at the start of the study, encompassing all six elements described below, is essential to ensuring the timeliness, completeness and transparency of reporting trial results, regardless of the study outcome.

US Securities and Exchange Commission (SEC) and equivalent reporting requirements

According to Section 13 or 15 (d) of the Securities Exchange Act of 1934, publically traded companies must report *material corporate events* on a more current basis, beyond the required standard quarterly and annual reports [36]. Material corporate events are those events that may affect a company's stock price. Examples of material corporate events include the results (positive or negative) of a completed clinical trial, stopping a study for safety concerns or futility, for safety reasons, lack of enrollment, etc. Information is submitted to the SEC using Form 8-K within 4 days of a material corporate event [37, 38]. Regulation FD provides that when an issuer discloses material non-public information to certain individuals or entities – generally, securities market professionals, such as stock analysts, or holders of the issuer's securities who may well trade on the basis of the information – the issuer must make public disclosure of that information. In this way, the new rule aims to promote full and fair disclosure [39].

Securities and Exchange Commission reporting requirements supersede the requirements of disclosing study results, or the halting of an ongoing clinical trial, to the research participants, site investigators,

and coordinators. Most publically traded companies will file Form 8-K and in addition issue a press release. Immediately upon meeting the SEC disclosure requirements, critical players in the clinical trials process, the participants, and the site investigators and coordinators, should be informed.

Notification of study results to research participants and site investigators and coordinators

While research participants are essential to the conduct of any clinical trial study, they are often the last group to be made aware of study results. Following any SEC and non-US comparable financial reporting requirements, the subjects, caregivers, and the sites that participated should be the next group that are formally made aware of study results, including any therapeutic and/or public health recommendations. In one clinical trial in Huntington's disease, the investigators used a three-part communication plan to disseminate the study results: 1) a media release from the principal investigators posted on the Huntington' disease website and emailed to the Huntington's community; 2) a telephone call from the site investigator or coordinator at each site to the participants providing the results and next steps; and 3) a joint teleconference for the investigators, sponsors, research participants, and caregivers to listen to the results and ask questions [40]. Other means for disseminating study results include having each site send a letter to each of their research participants with the results included in lay language plus the name and phone number of a contact person to call with questions, along with the participant's actual treatment assignment information and copies of the published abstract(s) and/or manuscript(s).

IRB/IEC Notification

Pursuant to 21 CFR parts 312.64 (d) (Investigator reports), 312.66 (Assurance of IRB review) and 56.109 (2) (f) (IRB review of research) Investigators must inform the IRB of any changes to an ongoing study which includes notifying the IRB when a study has been completed. This alleviates the IRB from its obligation of continuing review of a research protocol that has been completed. Most institutional and for-profit IRB's have clear procedures for what must be submitted to an IRB at the conclusion of a study and what the IRB defines as a completed study.

In Europe, according to article 10 (c.) of the Directive 2001/20/EC, the sponsor of a clinical trial must notify the competent authority of member state(s) concerned that the clinical trial has ended. This end of clinical trial notification must be submitted within 90 days of the end of the clinical trial as defined in the protocol. Should the trial be prematurely terminated, the notification must be submitted expeditiously (within 15 days). The sponsor is also required to file an end of clinical trial notification when the sponsor decides not to commence or not to resume (after a hold) a clinical trial. In such a case, it is not required to follow the expedited reporting process.

Regulatory submissions

While many aspects of the reporting requirements are similar, there are some differences across countries and regions. With the emergence of the International Conference on Harmonisation of Technical Requirements for Registration of Pharmaceuticals for Human Use (ICH) starting in April 1990, significant effort has been made to bring together the regulatory authorities of Europe, Japan, and the US, and experts from the pharmaceutical industry in the three regions to discuss scientific and technical aspects of product registration and streamline the regulatory submission process in these regions, including the submission of Clinical Study Reports (CSR) at the conclusion of a study [41, 42]. While significant progress has been made with harmonizing the process within these three regions there are still distinct differences even within these three regions let alone in the rest of the world. A few of the differences are addressed below. Before embarking into new regions it is critical that regulatory experts from the given region are included early in the process to ensure all post-study reporting requirements are completed.

US Food and Drug Administration

21 CFR part 312.33 (Annual Reports) requires annual investigational new drug (IND) updates within 60 days of the anniversary that the IND application went into effect. This annual report includes detailed reporting of the outcome of completed studies, via the submission of a CSR as delineated in 21 CFR part 312.33 (3) and ICH E3 (Structure and Content of Clinical Study Reports) [42].

European Medicines Agency

Similar to the reporting requirements in the US, the EMEA also requires the submission of a CSR, but the EMEA regulations require the CSR be submitted to the competent authority of each member state within 1 year of the end of clinical trial notification

Health Canada

Similar to the US reporting IND requirements, the Therapeutic Products Directorate (TPD) of the Health Products and Food Branch (HPFB) within Health Canada requires the submission of a clinical trial application (CTA) before conducting research in Health Canada (C.05.006). A CTA is specific to a given protocol vs. a development program for a compound for a given indication (e.g. an IND in the US). Unlike the US, an annual report does not need to be submitted to the CTA, but an updated Investigators Brochure must be submitted annually. Additionally, Health Canada must be notified within 15 days of the completion of a clinical trial (C.05.007) or the premature termination of the trial (C.05.015.(1)) [43]. These notifications are submitted via a cover letter and any supporting documentation.

Other countries

All countries have specific regulations relating to conducting clinical trials and their ultimate reporting. Understanding those requirements prior to study launch is critical to keeping a study on track. There are numerous companies that specialize in offering regulatory support of clinical research that can often help navigate the process thereby avoiding missteps for first time studies in countries where the investigator/sponsor does not have prior regulatory experience.

The regulatory reporting requirements for gaining regulatory approval to market new drugs, via the submission of the electronic Clinical Technical Document (eCTD) in the various countries and regions is beyond the scope of this book. Readers seeking more information on this topic should review 21 CRF part 314 (Applications for FDA to Market a New Drug), ICH regulations [44], and other applicable regulations in the country of interest.

Peer-reviewed publications

Failure to publish an adequate account of a well designed clinical trial is often regarded as a form of scientific misconduct [45]. Reporting is essential to evidence-based medicine. Reporting has many venues, but peer-reviewed original contributions in journals remain the highest form of data dissemination. Publication of clinical trial results should follow the reporting requirements as outlined in **Con**solidated **S**tandard of **R**eporting **T**rials (**CONSORT**) [46]. CONSORT has become the standard for reporting clinical trials including a 22 item checklist and a diagram for documenting the flow of participants through the four stages of a clinical trial: enrollment, intervention allocation, follow-up, and analysis. Most major journals require CONSORT standards be followed. Knowing the requirements of CONSORT will ensure that critical data about the study cohort is complete, accurate, balanced, devoid of bias, and is published according to the pre-specified outcome. Ultimately, including the data elements from CONSORT allows the readers to assess the validity of the results and allows for greater ease of comparison between clinical trials. Even with CONSORT in-place reporting of RTC is not always complete [47].

Transparency in publication has become of utmost importance, not only in presenting all of the data collected in an accurate and comprehensive manner but also the transparency of authorship contributions. Full disclosure of authorship contribution, including those of sponsors or any medical writers that have been hired has become necessary to avoid the practice of ghostwriting that emerged in the mid 2000s [48].

To keep trial documents compliant and transparent, the following publication planning guidelines can be used from organizations like International Society for Medical Publication Professionals (www.ismpp.org), American Medical Writers Association (www.amwa.org), and Pharmaceutical Research and Manufacturers of America www.phrma.org/publications.

In 2004, the International Committee of Medical Journal Editors (ICMJE) published their clinical trials registration policy requiring the prospective registration (prior to first patient enrolled) of all interventional studies in order for ICMJE journals to even consider publishing the results of a study. The ICMJE accepts registration in several registries including the US registry (www.clinicaltrials.gov), AUS/NZ registry, ISRCTN, Japan Registry, Netherlands registry, and any of the primary registries that participate in the WHO International Clinical Trial Portal. The policy applies to any trial that started recruitment on or after July 1, 2005 (see May 2005 editorial and Frequently Asked Questions for details of the current ICMJE policy including the definition of applicable trials, acceptable registries, timing of registration, and required data items)[49, 50].

Publication bias exists in favor of significant, 'positive' results and larger, multi-center, NIH-sponsored trials. There are many sources of this bias including the decision by investigators or journal editors not to publish negative or seemingly uninteresting results. Conflicts of interest exist at both the sponsor level and the investigator level when it comes to publications [51]. Additionally, the publication rate of abstracts and summaries exceeds full reports, creating media sampling bias. More stringent conflict-of-interest disclosures by ICMJE, related to financial relationships between sponsors and authors, will likely evolve in the coming years.

Government registry: Basic results reporting requirements

Currently there are about two dozen international clinical trial registries available. The majority of these registries are voluntary registries while a few, like the one in the US (www.clinicaltrials.gov) are mandatory. Many registries are set up to adhere to the World Health Organization (WHO) registry requirements for content, quality and validity, accessibility, unique identification, technical capacity, and administration. WHO Primary Registries meet the requirements of the ICMJE (http://www.who.int/ictrp/network/primary/en/index.html).

The clinical trials registry in the US was prompted by policy makers via the FDA modernization act of 1997 (FDAMA 1997) to increase clinical trial transparency through the public disclosure of key information about clinical trials. Under the Food and Drug Administration Amendments Act 2007 (FDAAA): US Public Law 110–85, Title VIII requires study sponsors or investigator to not only register their trials prior to the first subject being enrolled, but additionally, study summary results must be reported/posted within one year after the actual or estimated completion date, whichever is earlier (http://prsinfo.clinicaltrials.gov) on the www.clinicaltrials.gov registry. Completion date is defined in the legislation as the date that the last patient in a trial is evaluated for the primary outcome. This leaves very little time for investigators and sponsors to get a peer-reviewed manuscript in the public domain before needing to post the summary results on www.clinicaltrials.gov. The ICMJE does not consider results data posted in the tabular format required by ClinicalTrials.gov to be prior publication [49]. As the regulations regarding clinical trial registration and result posting continues to evolve, reviewing the current regulations at the time of starting a clinical trial will help ensure appropriate clinical trial reporting via the registry(ies) at the conclusion of the study [52].

Conclusion

A therapeutically focused team with clinical experts (investigator sites and sponsor clinical team) as well as a proficient and efficient project management team is key to the successful conclusion of a clinical study. Enhanced communication between well-trained key players, well-defined processes and procedures, and appropriate oversight by the sponsor throughout the project life, are also prerequisites.

One should not forget that an objective without a plan is just a wish, so that the team should get involved very early in thorough planning, flexible enough to allow adaptation to emerging situations.

References

1. ICH Topic E6 (R1). Guideline for Good Clinical Practice. 2009. http://www.ema.europa.eu/docs/en_GB/document_library/Scientific_guideline/2009/09/WC500002874.pdf. (Accessed August 9, 2011.)

2. EudraLex – Volume 10 Clinical Trials Guidelines. Detailed guidance on the application format and documentation to be submitted in an application for an Ethics Committee opinion on the clinical trial on medicinal products for human use. http://ec.europa.eu/health/files/eudralex/vol10/12_ec_guideline_20060216_en.pdf (Accessed August 8, 2011.)

3. FDA Guidance Document. Investigator Responsbilities – Protecting the Rights, Welfare and Safety of Study Subjects. 2009. http://www.fda.gov/downloads/Drugs/GuidanceComplianceRegulatoryInformation/Guidances/UCM073122.pdf. (Accessed August 8, 2011.)

4. FDA Guidance: Guideline for the monitoring of Clinical Investigations. Docket Number 82D-0322. 1988.

5. ICH E5 – Good Clinical Practice: Consolidated Guideline. 1996. http://www.fda.gov/downloads/Drugs/GuidanceComplianceRegulatoryInformation/Guidances/UCM073122.pdf. (Accessed August 8, 2011.)

6. CDISC, Electronic Source Data Interchange (eSDI) Group. Leveraging the CDISC Standards to Facilitate the use of Electronic Source Data Within Clinical Trials, Version 1. 2006. http://www.cdisc.org/esdi-document. (Accessed August 8, 2011.)

7. Dinnett EM, Mungal M, Kent JA, et al. Closing out a large clinical trial: lessons from the Prospective Study of Pravastatin in the Elderly at Risk (PROSPER). Clin Trials 2004; 1: 545–52.

8. Kamp C and Shinaman A. Participant recruitment and retention in clinical trials. In: Dunn C and Chadwick G (eds). Protecting Study Volunteers in Research: A Manual for Investigative Sites. Boston, MA, CenterWatch. 2002.

9. The Center for Information & Study on Clinical Research Participants (CISCRP). Clinical Trial Facts and Figures for Health Professionals. http://www.ciscrp.org/professional/facts.htm. (Accessed August 8, 2011.)

10. Clinical Research Educational Material. http://www.ciscrp.org/professional/store/index.html. (Accessed August 8, 2010.)

11. Getz K, Wenger J, Campo R, et al. Assessing the impact of protocol design changes on clinical trial performance. Am J Ther 2008; 15: 450–7.

12. Getz K. First things first: patient recruitment. Scrip 2008; 3371: III–IV.

13. Getz K, Campo R, and Kaitin K. Variability in protocol design complexity by phase and therapeutic area. Drug Inf J 2011; 45: 413–20.

14. Li G. Site Activation: The Key to More Efficient Clinical Trials. Pharmaceutical Executive. 2008. http://license.icopyright.net/user/viewFreeUse.act?fuid=NjU3OTMwMA%3D%3D. (Accessed August 8, 2011.)

15. Kamp C Shinaman A, Kieburtz K, et al. Do clinical trial infrastructures impact enrollment rates and baseline demographics in early Parkinson's disease (PD) studies? Mov Dis 2004; 19(Suppl 9): S198.

16. Fortune T, Wright E, Juzang I, et al. Recruitment, enrollment and retention of young black men for HIV prevention research: experiences from The 411 for Safe Text Project. Contemp Clin Trials 2009; 31:151–6.

17. NIH Revitalization Act of 1993. U.S. Congress Public Law 103–43. (National Institute of Health Revitalization Amendment. Washington, DC. 1993. http://grants.nih.gov/grants/funding/women_min/guidelines_amended_10_2001.htm. (Accessed August 8, 2011.)

18. Food and Drug Administration. Guideline for the Study and Evaluation of Gender Differences in the Clinical Evaluation of Drugs, Notice. Fed Reg 1993; 58: 39405–16.

19. Meinert CL, Gilpin AK, Unalp A, et al. Gender representation in trials. Control Clin Trials 2000; 21: 462–75.

20. Vidaver RM, Lafleu B, Tong C, et al. Women subjects in NIH-funded clinical research literature: lack of progress in both representation and analysis by sex. J Womens Health Gend Based Med 2000; 9: 495–504.

21. Merkatz RB and Junod SW. Historical background of changes in FDA policy on the study and evaluation of drugs in women. *Acad Med* 1994; **69**: 703–7.

22. McCarthy CR. Historical background of clinical trials involving women and minorities. *Acad Med* 1994; **69**: 695–8.

23. Wermeling DP and Selwitz AS. Current issues surrounding women and minorities in drug trials. *Ann Pharmacother* 1993; **27**; 904–11.

24. Killien M, Bigby JA, Champion V, *et al*. Involving minority and underrepresented women in clinical trials: The National Centers of Excellence in Women's Health. *J Womens Health Gend Based Med* 2000; **9**: 1061–70.

25. Evelyn B, Toigo T, Banks D, *et al*. Participation of racial/ethnic groups in clinical trials and race-related labeling: a review of new molecular entities approved 1995–1999. *J Natl Med Assoc* 2000; **93**(**12 Suppl**):18S–24S.

26. Levkoff S and Sanchez H. Lessons learned about minority recruitment and retention from the Centers on Minority Aging and Health Promotion. *Gerontologist* 2003; **43**: 18–26.

27. Stahl SM and Vasquez LJ. Approaches to improving recruitment and retention of minority elders participating in research: examples from selected research groups including the National Institute on Aging's Resource Centers for minority Aging Research. *Aging Health* 2004; **16**(Suppl 5): 9S–17S.

28. Drug Information Association (DIA) Training Courses. http://www.diahome.org/DIAHome/Search/UrlListEO.aspx#Training%20Course. (Accessed August 8, 2011.)

29. Galpern W. The NINDS NET-PD Investigators. A pilot clinical trial of creatine and minocycline in early Parkinson Disease: 19-month result. *Clin Neuropharmacol* 2008; **31**: 141–50.

30. Holloway R. Parkinson Study Group. Pramipexole vs. levodopa as initial treatment for Parkinson disease: A 4-year randomized controlled trial. *Arch Neurol* 2004; **61**: 1044–53.

31. Procedure for Preparing GCP Inspection Requested by the EMEA. 2007. http://www.ema.europa.eu/docs/en_GB/document_library/Regulatory_and_procedural_guideline/2009/10/WC500004455.pdf. (Accessed August 8, 2011.)

32. European Medicines Agency Annual Report of Good Clinical Practices Inspectors Working Group. 2009. http://www.ema.europa.eu/docs/en_GB/document_library/Annual_report/2010/04/WC500089199.pdf. (Accessed August 8, 2011.)

33. ICH Topic E6 (R1). Guideline for Good Clinical Practice. http://www.ema.europa.eu/docs/en_GB/document_library/Scientific_guideline/2009/09/WC500002874.pdf. (Accessed August 8, 2011.)

34. Shepherd R, Macer JL, and Grady D. Planning for closeout – from Day One. *Contemp Clin Trials* 2008; **29**: 136–9.

35. The Center for Information & Study on Clinical Research Participants (CISCRP). Unanticipated Closing of a Clinical Trial. http://www.ciscrp.org/downloads/articles/CISCRP_Article_UnanticipatedClosingofTrial.pdf (Accessed August 8, 2011.)

36. US Securities and Exchange Act of 1934. http://www.sec.gov/about/laws/sea34.pdf. (Accessed August 8, 2011.)

37. US Securities and Exchange Commission. Form 8K. http://www.sec.gov/answers/form8k.htm (Accessed August 8, 2011.)

38. US Securities and Exchange Commission. Fair Disclosure Regulation, FD. http://www.sec.gov/answers/regfd.htm. (Accessed August 8, 2011.)

39. US Securities and Exchange Commission. Final Rule: Selective Disclosure and Insider Trading. http://www.sec.gov/rules/final/33-7881.htm. (Accessed August 8, 2011.)

40. Dorsey ER, Beck C, Adams M, *et al*. Communicating clinical trial results to research participants. *Arch Neurol* 2008; **65**: 1590–5.

41. ICH-E3. Structure and Content on Clinical Study Reports. http://www.ich.org/products/guidelines/efficacy/efficacy-single/article/structure-and-content-of-clinical-study-reports.html. (Accessed August 8, 2011.)

42. FDA Guidance. Structure and Content of Clinical Study Report. http://www.fda.gov/downloads/RegulatoryInformation/Guidances/UCM129456.pdf. (Accessed August 8, 2011.)

43. Health Canada. Guidance for Clinical Trial Sponsors. Clinical Trial Application. 2001. http://www.hc-sc.gc.ca/dhp-mps/alt_formats/hpfb-dgpsa/pdf/prodpharma/ctdcta-ctddec-eng.pdf. (Accessed August 8, 2011.)

44. ICH M4: The Common Technical Document. http://www.ich.org/products/ctd.html. (Accessed August 8, 2011.)

45. Chalmers I. Underreporting research is scientific misconduct. *JAMA* 1990; **263**: 1405–8.

46. *JAMA* 1996; **276**: 637–9. Updated *Ann Intern Med* 2001; **134**; 663–94; www.consortstatement.org.

47. Toerien M, Brookes ST, Metcalfe C, *et al*. A review of reporting of participant recruitment and retention in RCTs in six major journals. *Trials* 2009; **10**: 52.

48. PLoS Medicine Editors. Ghostwriting: the dirty little secret of medical publishing that just got bigger. *PLoS Med* 2009; **6**: e1000156.

49. International Committee of Medical Journal Editors. Frequently Asked Questions About Clinical Trial Registration. http://www.icmje.org/faq_clinical.html. (Accessesd August 8, 2011.)

50. Collier R. Prevalence of ghostwriting spurs calls for transparency. *CMAJ* 2009; **181**: E161–2.

51. Dunn C and Chadwick G (ed). *Protecting Study Volunteers in Research: A Manual for Investigative Sites.* Boston, MA, Thompson CenterWatch. 2002.

52. ClinicalTrials.Gov. Protocol Registration System. http://prsinfo.clinicaltrials.gov/. (Accessed August 8, 2011.)

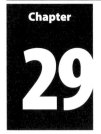

Chapter

29

Academic-industry collaborations and compliance issues

D. Troy Morgan

Introduction

The demand for clinical research has increased dramatically in recent years. Total spending on medical research in the US has doubled over the past decade to nearly $95 billion dollars a year [1]. While this dramatic expansion has created a vast array of opportunities for clinical researchers, there has also been an unprecedented rise in regulatory and compliance obligations for sponsors and investigators alike. The public and law makers have become extremely skeptical of industry sponsored research due to concerns of potential bias and inducement. Over the last 25 years, drug and device makers have displaced the federal government as the primary source of research financing and this industry support has become vital to many university research programs [2]. However, industry relationships with physicians and academic medical institutions are under intense scrutiny and will become even more challenging in the future.

> We cannot live in a nation where drug companies are less than candid, hide information and attempt to mislead the public. When they manipulate or withhold data to hide or minimize findings about safety and/or efficacy they put patient safety at risk, US Senator Charles Grassley [3]

Although recent enforcement actions and headlines have given rise to some areas of concern, the future of breakthrough therapies depends on the successful collaboration of industry and clinical researchers. This chapter is intended to serve as an introduction to the compliance landscape associated with conducting clinical research in today's challenging environment.

Clinical trial fair market value and enforcement trends

Clinical trials have become the center stage of recent enforcement activity and government inquiry. Regulators such as the Department of Justice (DOJ) have clearly signaled that their focus is on industry-physician financial relationships. In response to recent allegations that researchers were failing to disclose payments from pharmaceutical companies, such as a world renowned Harvard psychiatrist who failed to disclose $1.6 million dollars in consulting fees [3], a US Senate committee lead by Senator Charles Grassley launched several investigations into the nature of financial arrangements between industry and researchers. The focus of these investigations was to determine if the payments made to the physicians were in anyway considered excessive (e.g., above fair market value) or inappropriate.

The Centers for Medicare & Medicaid Services (CMS) defines 'fair market value' as the compensation that would be included in a service agreement as the result of bona fide bargaining between well-informed parties to the agreement who are not otherwise in a position to generate business for the other party [4]. Because regulators provide little guidance on how fair market value compensation should be determined, sponsors and investigators must rely on their own methodologies. A range of methods to set compensation for clinical research has emerged, including: 1) an institution's own past practice; 2) compensation surveys; 3) the use of independent third parties to conduct fair market value assessments; 4) benchmarks such as the Medicare reimbursement rate for a given procedure; and 5) a combination of these methods or other methods altogether [5].

Clinical Trials in Neurology, ed. Bernard Ravina, Jeffrey Cummings, Michael P. McDermott, and R. Michael Poole. Published by Cambridge University Press. © Cambridge University Press 2012.

Every payment set forth in a clinical trial budget agreement should represent the fair market value for the services rendered and must not be determined in any manner that takes into account the volume or value of any referrals or business otherwise generated between the investigator and the sponsor.

- Payments should be based on the actual work performed; and need a transparent method of taking into account the core activities or elements necessary for each type of clinical study the company conducts;
- Payments should not be based on opportunity cost, to determine a fee amount; even if it seems reasonable it may not be acceptable since it is not based on the actual services performed;
- Hourly rates should be determined based on objective criteria such as training, specialty, research experience, type of work being performed, and other factors, including a basis for increasing or decreasing base rates.

It is important for sponsors and investigators to document every transaction in order to ensure the integrity of the research and to avoid even the appearance of inducement. The approach for determining fair market value fees for clinical trials described above meets the type of requirements that should be done to ensure that this integrity is met, the process is transparent; it is based on the actual activities performed by consultants conducting a company's clinical research, and establishes hourly rates based on objective factors. Sponsors and investigators should use these strategies as a risk mitigation effort to ensure that their transactions are defendable against regulatory scrutiny and government inquiry.

Emerging disclosure and transparency requirements

US physician payments Sunshine Act (Sunshine Act)

The US Physician Payments Sunshine Act (Sunshine Act) was signed into law on March 23, 2010 as part of the Patient Protection and Affordable Care Act. The Sunshine Act requires manufacturers of drug, device, biologics, and medical supplies covered under Medicare, Medicaid to report payments on an annual basis to the department of Health and Human Services (HHS). Manufacturers must begin recording all

transfers of value on January 1, 2012. The information must be reported to HHS by March 31, 2013 and continue on an annual basis. In turn, HHS will post this information on a searchable public database, which is scheduled to be available on September 30, 2013. The database will contain the name, business address, specialty, and National Provider Identifier of the covered recipient. Manufacturers will also report the amount and date of payment, form of payment, cash or cash equivalent, in-kind items or services, stock, stock options, or ownership, interest or dividend, and the nature of the payment. If the payment is related to marketing, education, or research specific to a covered drug, device, biologic, or medical supply, the name of the product must also be reported [6].

The Sunshine Act is part of a growing body of 'aggregate spend' global legislations whose intentions are to collectively address the following: 1) Increased transparency with regard to payments made to health care providers by industry; 2) Statutory reporting from pharmaceutical manufacturers for said payments; and, 3) Monitoring and regulating spend per physician.

Aggregate spend is the total, cumulative amount spent by companies on individual health care professionals and organizations through consulting fees, grants, honoraria, travel and other consideration. The health care reform law requires health care providers like physicians, physician groups, and teaching hospitals to disclose payments and transfers of value, whether cash or in-kind. All of these instances must be aggregated into an electronic form, along with the physicians' National Provider Identifier (NPI) and submitted to the federal government annually.

The Sunshine Act is one of the more demanding disclosure regulations for the industry because any transfer of value, with some minor exceptions for amounts under $10, needs to be reported annually and will be made available to the public. This level of reporting and transparency is unprecedented and will not only require a tremendous amount of work, but will also be visible to the media, competitors, regulatory agencies, and others. Compensation such as investigator meeting fees, meals and accommodations, business courtesies, and other things of value such as leased equipment must be included [7]. In addition to this new federal law, individual states have also adopted their own tracking and reporting requirements. The federal government included a clause in the Sunshine Act to indicate that federal laws preempt individual state laws to the extent that they require the reporting of the same information. Unfortunately, current state laws require the reporting of different items to a broader audience and therefore escape federal preemption. Additionally, several countries outside of the US are in the process of introducing similar transparency laws [7].

The FDA – Disclosure of financial interests and arrangements of clinical investigators

On February 2, 1998, the FDA published a final rule requiring anyone who submits a marketing application of any drug, biological product, or device to submit certain information concerning the compensation to, and financial interests of, any clinical investigator conducting clinical studies covered by the rule. The financial disclosure regulations were intended to ensure that financial interests and arrangements of clinical investigators that could affect the reliability of data submitted to the FDA are identified and disclosed by the applicant.

To protect research integrity, NIH require researchers to report to universities earnings of $10 000 or more per year, for instance, in consulting money from makers of drugs also studied by the researchers in federally financed trials. Universities manage financial conflicts by requiring that the money be disclosed to research subjects, among other measures.

The FDA is also expanding its audit scope to include review of the financial disclosures before, during and after the clinical trial, and is randomly selecting clinical investigators to review the financial transactions between sponsors and investigators to ensure that there is no conflict of interest. In the past this type of documentation was viewed as a minor part of the process. However, with the increasing pressure from the transparency trends it has gone from a minor part to a significant part of the audit process. If this is disclosed and there is a conflict of interest, such as payments reaching the threshold, the investigator may be disqualified from participating in the clinical trial. Investigators should consider managing their relationships with industry sponsors to ensure that they do not exceed these minimum thresholds.

As much as investigators would like to work with the sponsor outside of the clinical trial environment for consulting and other advisory capacities, such as speaker engagements, an investigator will need to take proactive steps to monitor that these engagements do not preclude them or disqualify them from participating in future clinical studies with the sponsor during

any given period of time. The government is requesting that the investigator report any and all significant payments of other sorts (SPOOS), substantial payments or other support provided to an investigator that could create a sense of obligation to the sponsor. (e.g. honoraria, consulting fees, grant support for laboratory activities and equipment or actual equipment for the laboratory/clinic).

The financial disclosure requirement applies to any clinical study submitted in a marketing application that the applicant or the FDA relies on to establish that the product is effective, and any study in which a single investigator makes a significant contribution to the demonstration of safety. The final rule requires applicants to certify the absence of certain financial interests of clinical investigators or to disclose those financial interests. If the applicant does not include certification and/or disclosure, or does not certify that it was not possible to obtain the information, the agency may refuse to file the application [8].

Under the applicable regulations of (21 CFR) an applicant is required to submit to FDA a list of clinical investigators who conducted covered clinical studies and certify and/or disclose certain financial arrangements as follows:

1. Certification that no financial arrangements with an investigator have been made where study outcome could affect compensation; that the investigator has no proprietary interest in the tested product; that the investigator does not have a significant equity interest in the sponsor of the covered study; and that the investigator has not received significant payments of other sorts; and/or

2. Disclosure of specified financial arrangements and any steps taken to minimize the potential for bias [9].

Disclosable Financial Arrangements:

A. Compensation made to the investigator in which the value of compensation could be affected by study outcome. This requirement applies to all covered studies, whether ongoing or completed as of February 2, 1999.

B. A proprietary interest in the tested product, including, but not limited to, a patent, trademark, copyright or licensing agreement. This requirement applies to all covered studies, whether ongoing or completed as of February 2, 1999.

C. Any equity interest in the sponsor of a covered study, i.e., any ownership interest, stock options, or other financial interest whose value cannot be readily determined through reference to public prices. This requirement applies to all covered studies, whether ongoing or completed;

D. Any equity interest in a publicly held company that exceeds $50 000 in value. These must be disclosed only for covered clinical studies that are ongoing on or after February 2, 1999. The requirement applies to interests held during the time the clinical investigator is carrying out the study and for 1 year following completion of the study; and

E. Significant payments of other sorts, which are payments that have a cumulative monetary value of $25 000 or more made by the sponsor of a covered study to the investigator or the investigators' institution to support activities of the investigator exclusive of the costs of conducting the clinical study or other clinical studies (e.g., a grant to fund ongoing research, compensation in the form of equipment or retainers for ongoing consultation or honoraria) during the time the clinical investigator is carrying out the study and for 1 year following completion of the study. This requirement applies to payments made on or after February 2, 1999 [10].

If the FDA determines that the financial interests of any clinical investigator raise a serious question about the integrity of the data, the FDA will take any action it deems necessary to ensure the reliability of the data including: Initiating agency audits of the data derived from the clinical investigator in question; Requesting that the applicant submit further analyses of data, e.g., to evaluate the effect of the clinical investigator's data on the overall study outcome; Requesting that the applicant conduct additional independent studies to confirm the results of the questioned study; and Refusing to treat the covered clinical study as providing data that can be the basis for an agency action.

There are significant penalties for non-compliance. If a sponsor or investigator unknowingly fails to report a single instance, there will be a $1000 to $10 000 fine that is limited to $100 000 annually. However, if the parties knowingly fail to report a transfer of value, there will be a $10 000 to $100 000 fine that is limited to $1 000 000 annually and an investigation will be opened by the federal government.

In complying with these rules, sponsors and applicants are urged to use reasonable diligence and judgment to collect this information. If sponsors/applicants find it impossible to obtain the financial information

in question, applicants are urged to explain why this information was not obtainable and document attempts made in an effort to collect the information. Additionally, the disclosure forms must also be signed and dated by a responsible corporate official or representative of the applicant (e.g., the chief financial officer) and the investigators involved in the study.

Industry guidance

PhRMA Code on interactions with health care professionals and conduct of clinical trials

The Pharmaceutical Research and Manufacturers of America (PhRMA) is a trade group that represents research-based pharmaceutical and biotechnology companies. It has created a voluntary code, commonly known as the PhRMA Code, which sets standards for the health care industry's interactions with health care professionals. The purpose of the Code is to ensure that interactions are focused on supporting medical education, informing health care professionals about products, and providing medical or scientific information. The PhRMA Code sets standards for many different aspects of the health care industry, such as consultant arrangements, speaker programs, and industry support of independent medical education, business courtesies, gifts, and training of company representatives [9].

In 2009, PhRMA updated its model Principles on Conduct of Clinical Trials and Communication of Clinical Trial Results to help assure that clinical research conducted by America's pharmaceutical research and biotechnology companies continues to be carefully conducted and that meaningful medical research results are communicated to health care professionals and patients. Some of the key changes in the revised Principles are increased transparency about clinical trials for patients and health care professionals, enhanced standards for medical research authorship, and improved disclosure to better manage potential conflicts of interest in medical research.

The following voluntary principles have been adopted by PhRMA to clarify its members' relationships with other individuals and entities involved in the clinical research process and to set forth recommended standards of practice for the industry.

The key issues addressed are:

- Protecting Research Participants – Clinical research should be conducted in a manner that recognizes the importance of protecting the safety of and respecting research participants. Our interactions with research participants, as well as with clinical investigators and the other persons and entities involved in clinical research, recognize this fundamental principle and reinforce the precautions established to protect research participants.

- Conduct of Clinical Trials – Clinical research should be conducted with the highest quality, including trials and observational studies, to test scientific hypotheses rigorously and gather bona fide scientific data in accordance with applicable laws and regulations, as well as locally recognized good clinical practice. When conducting multinational, multi-site trials, in both the industrialized and developing world, ensure that standards based on the Guideline for Good Clinical Practice of the ICH are followed. In addition, clinical trial protocols are reviewed by independent Institutional Review Boards and Ethics Committees as well as national clinical trials health authorities.

- Ensuring Objectivity in Research – Clinical research will respect the independence of the individuals and entities involved in the clinical research process, so that they can exercise their judgment for the purpose of protecting research participants and to ensure an objective and balanced interpretation of trial results.

- Providing Information About Clinical Trials – Sponsors and investigators are committed to the transparency of clinical trials. They recognize that there are important public health benefits associated with making appropriate clinical trial information widely available to health care practitioners, patients, and others. Such disclosure must maintain protections for individual privacy, intellectual property, and contract rights, as well as conform to legislation and current national practices in patent law. Availability of information about clinical trials and their results in a timely manner is often critical to communicate important new information to the medical profession, patients and the public. Additionally, sponsors are responsible for receipt verification of data from all research sites for the studies we conduct; we ensure the accuracy and integrity of the entire study database, which is owned by the sponsor.

In sponsoring and conducting clinical research, PhRMA places great importance on respecting and protecting the safety of research participants. Principles for the conduct of clinical research are set forth in internationally recognized documents, such as the Declaration of Helsinki and the Guideline for Good Clinical Practice of the International Conference on Harmonisation. The principles of these and similar reference standards are translated into legal requirements through laws and regulations enforced by national authorities, such as the FDA.

PhRMA has a longstanding commitment of supporting its members through the development of model standards of conduct for the health care industry. The PhRMA code of conduct and model standards for clinical research are the foundation of the majority of ethics and compliance programs today and should be a reference guide for any organization or practitioner involved in clinical research.

Fraud and abuse regulations that govern research and development activity

The Federal Anti-Kickback Statute

One of the most influential laws governing the health care industry in the US is the Federal Anti-Kickback Statute, 42 U.S.C. § 1320a-7b(b). This statute prohibits individuals or entities from knowingly and willfully offering, paying, soliciting or receiving remuneration to induce referrals of items or services covered by Medicare, Medicaid, or any other federally funded program. Remuneration means anything of value given, directly or indirectly, overtly or covertly, in cash or in kind, to a health care provider and includes, but is not limited to cash, free goods, free services, and payments for items, services, or data at above fair market value.

The Anti-Kickback Statute is an intent-based statute and may be violated if *any one purpose* of the transaction or practice is to induce referrals or the purchasing, leasing, or ordering of any item or service, or the recommending of or arranging for such activities, even if there are other legitimate purposes for the transaction or practice.

The *any one purpose* doctrine is a critical analysis that must be applied to any engagement between health care providers and industry. This can be a complicated analysis due to the fact that even though an engagement meets all of the threshold criteria of a reasonable and necessary transaction, if the contributing factor of the amount of compensation or element of the engagement has the appearance to induce, it could create a risk to both parties as potential violation. The subjective nature of this doctrine requires parties involved in clinical research to determine what level of risk they are willing to assume for the amount of compensation involved for the contracted services. Additionally, the subjective nature of the negotiation of services by industry and investigators and the any one purpose doctrine creates a paradigm of risk that must be carefully analyzed to ensure the appropriate level of justification and documentation will defend the transaction.

In evaluating whether any particular business transaction or practice violates the Anti-Kickback Statute, the government may consider whether the transaction or practice has the potential to: increase costs to a Federal Health Care Program, beneficiaries, or enrollees; increase the risk of over-utilization or inappropriate utilization; raise patient safety or quality-of-care concerns; or interfere with appropriate clinical decision-making.

While the anti-kickback law is broad, the Office of Inspector General (OIG) at the US Department of Health and Human Services issued 'safe harbor' rules in 1991, identifying specific types of activities not subject to enforcement actions under the anti-kickback statute as long as various conditions are satisfied [10].

The safe harbor rules cover such activities as investments in publicly traded companies, joint ventures, rentals of space or equipment, personal services agreements, sales of practice, discounts, and other arrangements. The safe harbor of particular relevance to clinical research is the 'personal services safe harbor.'

This personal services safe harbor allows for common business practices, such as consulting arrangements, subject to certain valid business need and fair market value requirements. The arrangement must be in writing and be signed, specify the services to be rendered, specify the length and time of the engagement, last for at least 1 year, provide the aggregate compensation and be consistent with fair market value, not include services to 'promote' a business arrangement, not exceed the reasonable and necessary business purposes of the arrangement. Generally, as long as the service falls within the boundaries of these safe harbors, an anti-kickback law violation has not occurred. Conduct that falls outside a safe harbor does not mean an individual or entity automatically has violated the law. However, compliance with the safe harbor requirements will protect a transaction from anti-kickback scrutiny by the OIG and the Justice Department.

A violation of the Anti-Kickback Statute is a criminal offense, which constitutes a felony punishable by a fine of not more than $25 000 per offense and/or imprisonment for up to 5 years. A conviction also will lead to mandatory exclusion from participation in Federal Health Care Programs and may also lead to civil monetary penalties of up to $50 000 for each violation, plus damages of three times the amount of the remuneration.

The following are recommendations that can be taken to reduce the risk of anti-kickback violations in clinical research: 1) Both the sponsor and the investigator must ensure that only reasonable compensation is paid and received for valid business purposes; 2) All payments for services must be consistent and objective based on the complexity and amount of time for the services, but also must be justifiable for the background and qualifications of the provider; 3) All compensation must only be paid for reasonable necessary services and procedures; 4) There must be an objective and defendable scientific purpose for the research with a well defined protocol; 5) Ensure that the study is objective, unbiased, necessary, and that the payments do not reflect the physician's ability to generate business; 6) Establish clear methodology to determine a reasonable study size [11].

The False Claims Act

The False Claims Act (31 U.S.C. §§ 3729–3733) is a US law that imposes liability on persons and companies who defraud governmental programs. The law includes a whistleblower provision that allows people who are not affiliated with the government to file actions on behalf of the government. Persons filing under the Act stand to receive a substantial portion, 15–25%, of any recovered damages. The government has recovered nearly $22 billion under the False Claims Act between 1987 and 2008 and has received significant media attention in recent years.

There have been many developments and recent enforcement actions with matters involving clinical research where the False Claims Act and Anti-Kickback statute have the focus of the investigation. A common theme with recent enforcement actions are duplicative fees whereby an investigator has already been paid for a service and is additionally being reimbursed by the federal government for the same procedure, or unnecessary procedures that are not required for standard of care or the clinical research in question. Investigators should be aware that due to the recent increase in whistleblower claims that anyone including their internal staff, associated pharmacists and third parties, as well as CROs and patients, could be a potential whistleblower, if they have evidence of what could be construed as a false claim or potential kickback.

The Act establishes liability when any person or entity improperly receives from or avoids payment to the Federal government. The Act prohibits: knowingly presenting, or causing to be presented a false claim for payment or approval; knowingly making, using, or causing to be made or used, a false record or statement material to a false or fraudulent claim; conspiring to commit any violation of the False Claims Act; knowingly making, using, or causing to be made or used a false record to avoid, or decrease an obligation to pay or transmit property to the government [11].

The most commonly used of these provisions are the first and second, prohibiting the presentation of false claims to the government and making false records to get a false claim paid. By far the most frequent cases involve situations in which a defendant, usually a corporation but on occasion a health care practitioner, overcharges the federal government for goods or services. Other typical cases entail failure to test a product as required by the rigorous government specifications or selling defective products.

There have also been a series of cases whereby the government has prosecuted organizations and individuals for false claim billing as they relate to the clinical trial setting. More specifically, submitting false service records or samples in order to show better-than-actual performance, double billing – charging more than once for the same procedure or service, up-coding employee work – billing at doctor rates for work that was actually conducted by a nurse or resident intern and billing for research that was never conducted; falsifying research data.

Pharmaceutical manufacturers can only promote approved uses of their approved products. Manufacturers are strictly prohibited from promoting investigational products or unapproved uses of approved products. Promotion of an investigational product or an unapproved use of an approved product is not allowed under the law. Only a product or the particular use of a product that has been approved by the FDA is deemed to be safe and effective can be promoted.

The False Claims Act not only imposes liability on those who submit the false claims, but has also been used against those who are determined to cause the submission of the claims. Enforcement can take the form of government action or a private party bringing a civil action in the name of the government.

The following are recommendations that can be taken to reduce the risk of False Claims Act violations in clinical research: 1) Avoid any appearance of Anti Kick back Statute violations; 2) Prohibit billing for free services; 3) Do not encourage billing for free services; 4) Include a 'no billing for free services' provision in agreements; 5) Do not double bill for study services; 6) Prohibit practices that encourage double billing; 7) Include a 'no double billing' provision in agreements [12].

The Foreign Corruption Practices Act

Another significant law that governs research and development activities is the The Foreign Corrupt Practices Act, 15 U.S.C. §§ 78dd-1, (FCPA). The FCPA prohibits corrupt payments to foreign officials for the purpose of obtaining or keeping business. Specifically, the anti-bribery provisions of the FCPA prohibit the willful use of any means of interstate commerce corruptly in furtherance of any offer, payment, promise to pay, or authorization of the payment of money or anything of value to any person, while knowing that all or a portion of such money or thing of value will be offered, given or promised, directly or indirectly, to a foreign official to influence them in their official capacity, induce the foreign official to do or omit to do an act in violation of their lawful duty, or to secure any improper advantage in order to assist in obtaining or retaining business for or with, or directing business to, any person. The FCPA is interpreted broadly and the definition of a government official includes health care practitioners who are employed by state and federal health care institutions [13].

The anti-bribery provisions of the FCPA apply to all US persons and certain foreign issuers of securities. With the enactment of certain amendments, the anti-bribery provisions of the FCPA were expanded to include foreign firms and persons who cause, directly or through agents and third parties, an act in furtherance of such a corrupt payment to take place within the territory of the US.

Under the Act, the person making or authorizing the payment must have a corrupt intent, and the payment must be intended to induce the recipient to misuse his official position to direct business wrongfully to the payer or to any other person. Additionally, the FCPA does not require that a corrupt act succeed in its purpose. The offer or promise of a corrupt payment can constitute a violation of the statute.

The FCPA prohibits any corrupt payment intended to influence any act or decision of a foreign official in his or her official capacity, to induce the official to do or omit to do any act in violation of his or her lawful duty, to obtain any improper advantage, or to induce a foreign official to use his or her influence improperly to affect or influence any act or decision.

The Act applies to payments to any public official, regardless of rank or position. The FCPA focuses on the purpose of the payment instead of the particular duties of the official receiving the payment, offer, or promise of payment, and there are exceptions to the anti-bribery provision for facilitating payments for routine governmental action [12].

The FCPA prohibits corrupt payments through intermediaries. Therefore, it is unlawful to make a payment to a third party, while knowing that all or a portion of the payment will go directly or indirectly to a foreign official. The term 'knowing' includes conscious disregard and deliberate ignorance. The elements of an offense are essentially the same as described above, except that in this case the 'recipient' is the intermediary who is making the payment to the requisite 'foreign official.'

The FCPA also requires companies in the US to meet its accounting provisions [14]. These accounting provisions, which were designed to operate in tandem with the anti-bribery provisions of the FCPA, require corporations covered by the provisions to: 1) make and keep books and records that accurately and fairly reflect the transactions of the corporation and 2) devise and maintain an adequate system of internal accounting controls.

The following criminal penalties may be imposed for violations of the FCPA's anti-bribery provisions: corporations and other business entities are subject to a fine of up to $2 000 000; officers, directors, stockholders, employees, and agents are subject to a fine of up to $100 000 and imprisonment for up to 5 years. Moreover, under the Alternative Fines Act, the actual fine may be up to twice the benefit that the defendant sought to obtain by making the corrupt payment. Finally, fines imposed on individuals pursuant to the FCPA are deemed to be punitive and may not be paid by their employer or principal.

The UK Anti-Bribery Act

The UK Bribery Act 2010 (c.23), effective July 1, 2011, is an Act of the Parliament of the United Kingdom that covers the criminal law relating to bribery. The Bribery Act applies to UK citizens, residents and companies established under UK law. In addition, non-UK companies can be held liable for a failure to prevent bribery if they do business in the UK.

The Act has been described as 'the toughest anti-corruption legislation in the world,' raising the bar above the standard set by the US Foreign Corrupt Practices Act (FCPA). It is more stringent than other anti-corruption laws because it covers not only bribes or inducement to government officials, but it also covers bribes to non-government officials, including UK health care practitioners. The Act also broadens the jurisdictional reach of the UK anti-bribery laws to cover bribery worldwide by individuals who are UK nationals or are ordinarily resident in the UK, and organizations that conduct some portion of their business in the UK. The Act specifically prohibits the issue of facilitation payments, which was not a focus of the FCPA [13].

The UK Act represents a new tool for regulators and prosecutors, whose earlier efforts at criminal enforcement of anti-bribery laws against companies were constrained by limitations in attributing criminal misconduct to organizations. The Act redefines the substantive criminal elements of bribery, including a new general offense that covers domestic and foreign bribery, and a separate, stand-alone foreign bribery offense that introduces standards similar in scope to the US Foreign Corrupt Practices Act. It also repeals the pre-existing criminal anti-bribery laws in the UK and creates a new bribery offense imposing liability on organizations whose employees or representatives engage in bribery in the UK or abroad.

There are four general offenses to the UK Bribery Act.

1) Offering, promising or giving a bribe – active bribery.
2) Requesting, agreeing to receive or accepting a bribe – passive bribery.
3) Bribery of a foreign public official.
4) Failure by a commercial organization to prevent a bribe being paid to obtain or retain business or a business advantage [15].

The UK Bribery Act introduces an offense of corporate failure to prevent bribery. In addition, a company or corporate entity is culpable for bribes given to a third party with the intention of obtaining or retaining business for the organization or obtaining or retaining an advantage useful to the conduct of the business by their employees and associated persons, even if they had no knowledge of those actions. There is also personal liability for senior company officers that turn a blind eye to board-level bribery.

A company can invoke in its defense that it had adequate procedures designed to prevent persons associated from undertaking misconduct. However, a company must prove that it had 'adequate procedures' in place during the time of the offense.

The following procedures must be in place for an organization to be considered in compliance with the UK Act [16]:

- Proportionate Procedures – An organization must show proportionate risk mitigation procedures based on the risk and complexity of their business.
- Top Level Commitment – The organization must be able to demonstrate top level commitment to mitigating bribery risk. Examples include internal and external communications from senior leadership tailored to establish an anti-bribery culture.
- Risk Assessment – Periodic, risk based, and documented anti-bribery risk assessments demonstrating corrective actions and continual risk mitigation.
- Due Diligence – Proportionate and risk based with respect to third parties
- Communication and Training – Communication and training (internal and external) regarding bribery prevention policies
- Monitoring & Review – Monitoring procedures designed to prevent bribery and make improvements where necessary

The penalties for committing a crime under the Act are imprisonment for up to 10 years with unlimited fines and the potential for the confiscation of property, as well as the disqualification of directors. The Act has a near-universal jurisdiction, allowing for the prosecution of an individual or company with links to the UK, regardless of where the crime occurred. Additionally, a company or an individual is automatically and perpetually debarred from competing for public contracts where it is convicted of a corruption offense under the UK Act.

The UK Act poses a multi-dimensional risk to investigators, academic medical institutions and sponsors alike. Everyone involved in clinical research activities with a nexus in the UK should be vigilant to ensure that payments made and consideration received involving clinical research be reasonable and necessary, appropriately documented and is not considered an inducement or kickback pursuant to the requirements of the Act [17].

Conclusion

Clinical research is our investment in the future of public health. Every effort we make today defines the treatment therapies and potential cures of tomorrow. Many different entities and individuals contribute to the safe and appropriate conduct of clinical research, including not only sponsoring companies but also regulatory agencies; investigative site staff and medical professionals who serve as clinical investigators; hospitals and other institutions where research is conducted; and Institutional Review Boards and Ethics Committees.

While most organizations and practitioners have no intention of violating compliance requirements in this area, little guidance is available, which makes adherence to compliance difficult. At a minimum, sponsors and investigators must be able to show that research-related payments and activities are reasonable, necessary and in no way create an unethical outcome and ensure public trust.

References

1. The Associated Press. $95 Billion a Year Spent on Medical Research. 2005. http://www.msnbc.msn.com/id/9407342/ns/health-health_care/t/billion-year-spent-medical-research/ (Accessed August 9, 2011.)

2. Congress of the United States: Congressional Budget Office. Research and Development in the Pharmaceutical Industry. 2006. http://www.cbo.gov/ftpdocs/76xx/doc7615/10–02-DrugR-D.pdf (Accessed August 9, 2011.)

3. Harris G, Carey B. Researchers Fail to Reveal Full Drug Pay. 2008. http://www.nytimes.com/2008/06/08/us/08conflict.html (Accessed August 9, 2011.)

4. Federal Register. Final Rule, Stark II, Phase II Regulations. 2004.

5. The Center for Health & Pharmaceutical Law & Policy. Conflicts of Interest in Clinical Trial Recruitment & Enrollment: A Call for Increased Oversight. 2009. http://law.shu.edu/programscenters/healthtechIP/upload/health_center_whitepaper_nov2009.pdf (Accessed August 9, 2011.)

6. Sullivan T. Physician Payment Sunshine Provision: Patient Protection Affordable Care Act Passed the House. 2010. http://www.policymed.com/2010/03/physician-payment-sunshine-provisions-patient-protection-affordable-care-act.html (Accessed August 9, 2011.)

7. 111th Congress. S.301 Physician Payments Sunshine Act of 2009. http://thomas.loc.gov/cgi-bin/query/z?c111:S.301.IS: (Accessed August 9, 2011.)

8. FDA Guidance. 21CFR 54.4 [b].

9. FDA: US Food and Drug Administration. Financial Disclosure by Clinical Investigators. 2001. http://www.fda.gov/RegulatoryInformation/Guidances/ucm126832.htm (Accessed August 9, 2011.)

10. PhrMA. Principles on Conduct of Clinical Trials and Communication of Clinical Trial Results. http://www.phrma.org/about/principles-guidelines/clinical-trials (Accessed August 9, 2011.)

11. Federal Register. Proposed Rules: 42 CFR Part 1001. 2002. http://oig.hhs.gov/fraud/docs/safeharborregulations/MedicareSELECTNPRMFederalRegister.pdf (Accessed August 9, 2011.)

12. Steiner. Clinical Research Law and Compliance Handbook. Jones and Bartlett Publishers, 2005, 182.

13. Wikipedia. False Claims Act. 2011. http://en.wikipedia.org/wiki/False_Claims_Act. (Accessed August 9, 2011.)

14. The False Claims Act: A Primer. http://www.justice.gov/civil/docs_forms/C-FRAUDS_FCA_Primer.pdf (Accessed August 9, 2011.)

15. The United States Department of Justice. Foreign Corrupt Practices Act. http://www.justice.gov/criminal/fraud/fcpa/. (Accessed August 9, 2011.)

16. Atkins M. Introduction to the UK Bribery Act. 2011. http://www.financierworldwide.com/article.php?id=8188. (Accessed August 9, 2011.)

17. Foreign and Commonwealth Office. The UK Bribery Act. 2011. http://www.fco.gov.uk/en/global-issues/conflict-minerals/legally-binding-process/uk-bribery-act. (Accessed August 9, 2011.)

Index

Abciximab in Emergency Stroke Treatment Trial–II (AbESTT-II), 246
abuse liability, 13
actigraphy, 299, 303
active arm comparator designs, 265
active controls, 13, 143, 201–202
active-control trials, 135
acute ischemic stroke, 242
Acute Stroke Therapy by Inhibition of Neutrophils (ASTIN) study, 247
acute stroke treatment, 243
  recruitment, 252
acute stroke trials
  consent, 251
  early and middle development studies, 247
  endpoint measures, 245
  recruitment, 252
  subject recruitment, 251
  surrogate consent, 251
ADAGIO trial, 116–117, 122
adaptive design, 91, 93, 97, 98, 247
  assessment, 92
  definition, 91
  neurological trials, 96
  sample size re-estimation design, 95
  sample size re-estimation methods, 95
adaptive design type, 92, 98
Adaptive Designs Working Group (ADWG), 91
adaptive dose-finding study, 97
adaptive randomization, 94, 251
adaptive seamless design, 95–97
adaptive trials, 13
ADAS-Cog, 101
  scale, 230
  score, 32, 230
adverse drug event
  manufacturer responsibility, 161
  physician reporting survey, 162
adverse drug event factors, 160–161
adverse drug event reporting, 163, 164
  statins, 162
Adverse Event Reporting System (AERS), 163
aggregate spend, 353

Albumin in Acute Stroke (ALIAS) trial, 247
ALS, 273
  biomarker, 278
  disease models, 273
  futility design studies, 279
  lead-in design, 279
  motor neuron death, 273
  mouse model, 273–274
  phenotypic heterogeneity, 275
  selection designs, 279
  symptomatic management, 274
  symptomatic treatment, 282
  therapies, 273
ALS clinical trials, 273, 275, 279
  dosage, 280
  dropout rate, 281
  drug interactions, 280
  eligibility criteria, 275, 281
  enrollment, 281
  missing data, 278
  random effects model, 278
  sample size, 280
ALS trial outcome measure, 275
ALS trials
  statistical techniques, 278
ALS trials outcome measure
  longitudinal outcomes, 278
  MUNE, 276
  muscle strength, 276
  survival, 276
  vital capacity, 276
ALSFRS-R, 276, 278
ALSSQOL, 278
alternate dosing formulations, 15
alternative hypothesis, 60
alternative hypothesis of superiority, 137
Alzheimer's disease, 11, 14, 19, 25, 29, 113, 132, 203, 204, 227
  behavioral outcomes, 233
  biological signatures, 228
  characteristics, 229
  diagnosis, 229
  diagnostic criteria, 238
  disease-modifying therapies, 238
  molecular changes, 228
  pathology, 227–228
  prevention, 236

progression, 233
  treatment, 229
Alzheimer's disease Assessment Scale, 103
Alzheimer's disease Cooperative Study-Activities of Daily Living (ADCS-ADL), 232
Alzheimer's disease modification
  randomized withdrawal design, 236
  staggered start design, 236
  trial duration, 238
Alzheimer's disease trials, 227, 230, 233, 239
  drug safety, 235
  efficacy, 236
  enrollment issues, 237
  minority recruitment, 237
  phase I clinical trials, 234–235
  phase II clinical trials, 235
  phase IIa trials, 235
  phase IIb trials, 235
  phase III trials, 235
  placebo group decline, 237–238
  safety measures, 237
  study partner, 237
amyloid imaging, 75
Amyotrophic lateral sclerosis (ALS). See ALS
animal CNS disease models, 21
animal model, 21–22
antegrade reperfusion, 243
antiepilepsy drugs (AEDs), 202
antiepileptic drug development, 291
antiepileptic drug safety, 291
antiepileptic drugs, 284
  mechanism, 285
antiepileptic drugs trials
  children, 291
Anti-Kickback Statute, 356
  violation, 357
Antiplatelet Trialist Collaboration (APTC) endpoint, 170
any one purpose doctrine, 356
aplastic anemia, 164
Appel rating scale, 278
Arrhythmia Suppression Trial (CAST), 130
as treated analysis, 66
aspirin, 6

asymptomatic intracranial hemorrhage (ICH), 244
ataluren, 25
atrial fibrillation, 6
Avonex Combination Trial, 265
Aβ imaging, 25
Aβ plaques, 227

Barthel Index, 245
baseline severity, 249
baselines, 108
basic exposure requirements, 14
Belmont Report, 174, 183
BENEFIT Trial, 265
Best Pharmaceuticals for Children Act (BPCA), 199
beta-amyloid (Aβ1–42), 74
BEYOND Trial, 265
bias, 42
binary outcomes, 107
biochemical biomarkers, 74
bio-creep, 143
bioequivalence, 136
biological therapies, 5
biomarker adaptive designs, 95
biomarkers, 20, 23, 71, 73–74, 127, 243
    pharmacodynamic markers, 20
    type 0 biomarker, 23
    type 1 biomarker, 23
    type 2 biomarker, 24
Biomarkers Definitions Working Group
    conceptual model, 71
blinding, 43, 45, 136
blood brain barrier, 22, 23
blood-CSF barrier, 24
Bonferroni method, 40
botulinum toxin, 5
brain atrophy, 268
brain imaging, 180
    incidental findings, 180
    studies, 11
brain intervention study risk, 176

C-11 labeled donepezil, 11
calcitonin gene-related peptide (CGRP), 97
calcitonin gene-related peptide (CGRP) receptor, 96
cancer futility designs, 220
cancer therapy, 275
Cardiac Arrhythmia Suppression Trial (CAST), 71, 130
carotid endarterectomy, 6
carrier-mediated and receptor-mediated transport, 23
carryover, 104
case series, 163
CDP, 47
celecoxib, 170

censored data, 107
Center for Devices and Radiological Health (CDRH), 206
central laboratories, 315
central laboratory criteria, 315
cerebral beta-amyloid, 11
cerebral infarction, 242
cerebrovascular disease, 1
cGMP regulations, 321
characteristics of instruments, 76
child epilepsy, 291
China, 1
cladribine, 266
Class I medical devices, 207, 209
Class I neurological devices, 208
Class II medical devices, 208
Class III medical devices, 209
clincal trials scope of work (SOW), 312
clinical care, 174
clinical data management, 326
Clinical Dementia Rating Scale (CDR), 232–233
clinical development, 8, 13, 15, 17
    early stage, 9
    late stage, 13–15
    middle stage, 11, 13
clinical drug safety trials, 170
clinical endpoint
    late phase acute stroke study, 246
clinical enrollment duration, 342
clinical equipoise, 175, 176, 178
Clinical Global Impression, 29
clinical guidance documents, 16
Clinical Interview Based Impression of Change (CIBIC), 232
clinical investigators, 182
clinical post-marketing safety assessment, 161
clinical research
    competent only policy, 192, 193
clinical research associate (CRA), 311
clinical research consent, 188
clinical research organizations (CROs), 312
Clinical Study Reports (CSR), 347
clinical supplies, 321
clinical supply chain, 321
clinical supply labeling, 323
clinical trial budget, 316, 317
    budget management, 319
    committees, 318
    components, 317
    currency fluctuations, 317
    data management costs, 318
    IRB/EC costs, 319
    monitoring budget, 318
    vendors, 318
clinical trial design
    entry and exclusion criteria, 30
    timeline, 30

clinical trial team, 309
    communication, 312
clinical trials, 1, 2, 5, 9, 29
    candidates, 177
    caregiver participation, 182
    censoring, 36
    central laboratories, 315
    cognitively impaired subjects, 192
    committees, 148
    critical public engagement, 183
    data management services, 314
    data review, 147
    design, 15, 28
    design protocol, 28
    drug safety hypothesis, 169
    eligibility criteria, 182
    endpoint, 244
    enforcement, 352
    implementation, 338
    interpretation of results, 201
    intervention risks, 177
    investigational agent access, 182
    management, 312
    participation, 189
    patient exclusion, 182
    payment, 353
    planning, 319, 327
    planning process, 309
    prospective registration, 176
    publication bias, 348
    quality assurance system, 344
    recruitment, 341
    registries, 348
    regulatory requirements, 327
    reporting, 346
    reporting and transparency, 353
    results dissemination, 346
    results publication, 347
    retention, 342–343
    safety, 9
    set-up phase, 320
    site audits, 344
    site monitoring, 339–340
    site qualification, 339
    site selection process, 39
    site training, 340
    subject payment, 343
    timelines, 319
    vendors, 316
clinically isolated syndrome (CIS), 259
cluster headaches, 101
CNS drug delivery, 23
CNS targets, 21
CNS trial challenges, 173
CNS trials
    aggressive interventions, 177
    ethical research, 183
    risks, 183
    trial enrollment, 177

Code of Federal Regulations, 73
cognitive behavioral therapy for
      insomnia (CBT-I), 296
collateral perfusion, 243
Combination Drug Selection Trial, 85
comorbid insomnia, 295
comparative effectiveness studies, 6
comparative selection trial, 88
complete two-period design, 118
    participant allocation, 120
    statistical model, 118–119
compliance and quality management,
      345
concomitant medications, 10
conditional power, 154–155
confidence interval, 33, 63
confirmatory trials, 93, 98
    adaptations, 94
confounding, 179
Consolidated Standard of
      Reporting Trials (CONSORT).
      See CONSORT
continual reassessment method, 92
    stopping criteria, 93
continuous outcomes, 106
control group, 30–31, 42
controlled clinical trial, 42
Coronary Drug Project (CDP), 47
correlative and marker studies, 180
CRFs, 326
CRM. See continual reassessment
      method
    modified approaches, 93
crossover design, 101, 110
    2-treatment 2-period design, 101
    AB:BA design, 103, 107
    matched crossover design, 109
    parallel design, 103
crossover insomnia trials, 301
crossover trials, 101
    applications, 101
    baselines, 109
    logistical challenges, 111
    sample size, 101
    sequence effects, 104
    two-stage approach, 108
    with carryover, 105
    without carryover, 105
CSF measurement, 24

Data and Safety Monitoring Board
      (DSMB), 94
data monitoring committee, 148, 149
data monitoring committee
      objectivity, 150
data vendor regulation compliance,
      314
database freeze, 320
database lock, 320, 326

DATATOP study, 114
DATATOP trial, 115, 121
decision-making capacity, 190–191
Declaration of Helsinki, 174–176, 181,
      183
deep brain stimulation (DBS), 218
deep brain stimulation devices, 210
demonstration of effectiveness, 197
Deprenyl and Tocopherol Antioxidative
      Therapy of Parkinsonism
      (DATATOP) trial, 114
device classifications, 322
Disability Assessment for Dementia
      (DAD) scale, 232
disease modification, 113
    modifying effect, 203
    modifying effect study, 203
disease prevention effect study, 204
disease prevention study
    surrogate marker, 204
disease progression treatment, 203
disease-modifying effect, 124
DMC, 159
DMC Charter, 149
donepezil, 101, 107
dopamine agonist, 218
dopaminergic medication, 218, 219,
      222–223
    sleep attacks, 222
dose-response relationship, 11
dose-response study, 96
drop out, 66
drug approval, 197
drug safety, 160
    active surveillance systems, 164, 165
    case definitions, 167
    clinical efficacy trials, 169
    clinical trials, 168
    clinical trials constraints, 168
    drug definition, 167
    observational epidemiological
          study, 165
    post-market clinical trials, 168
    profile trials, 205
    relative risk, 165
    study approach, 171
drug safety issue identification, 161
drug safety profile, 160
drug safety program, 160
drug stability testing, 322
drugs, lack of increase, 3
drugs, cost, 1
DSMB, 96, 98
Duchenne muscular dystrophy
      (DMD), 25
dyskinesias, 218
dystrophin, 25

early exploratory (phase I) trials, 92
early phase studies

candidates, 177
early stage clinical trials, 69
early trial termination, 154, 345
Early vs. Late L-dopa in Parkinson
      Disease (ELLDOPA) trial, 115
ECG vendor criteria, 316
ECG vendors, 316
EDSS, 262, 268
EDSS scale, 262
effect size, 250
efficacy, 11, 150, 154
    in vivo model, 9
    proof-of-efficacy-trials, 12
    therapeutic efficacy, 11
efficacy and safety endpoints, 11
efficacy trials, 168
electronic data capture (eDC)
      technology, 345
eligibility, 48
eligibility criteria, 249
endovascular mechanical treatments,
      248
endpoint, 76, 136
    model, 70
endpoint selection, 12
enrichment design, 132
enrichment design trial
      methods, 127
enrichment design trials, 127
    advantages, 128, 130, 133
    carryover effects, 132
    complete enriched enrollment, 128
    generalizability, 131
    Kopec mathematical
          model, 129
    limitations, 130
    partial enriched enrollment, 128
    planning considerations, 131
    recruitment efficiency, 131
    responder definition method, 129
    sample size, 129
    sensitivity, 129
    strengths, 129
    subject response, 128
epilepsy, 284
    photoparoxysmal response, 288
epilepsy clinical designs
    monotherapy trial design, 292
epilepsy clinical trials
    adverse event frequency, 287
    assessment of efficacy, 286
    definitive proof of efficacy studies,
          289
    dose-finding study, 289
    drug efficacy, 288
    electroencephalogram (EEG), 287
    exit criteria, 288
    failed trials, 292
    outcome measures, 287–288
    placebo response rate, 292

populations, 285
presurgical inpatient study, 289
quality of life scales, 287
seizure clusters, 287
seizure freedom, 288
sudden unexplained death, 291
trial duration, 292
epilepsy drug delivery, 286
epilepsy drug efficacy studies, 289
epilepsy drug models, 285
epilepsy open label extension
study, 290
epilepsy regulatory studies, 289
epilepsy syndromes, 284
epilepsy treatment resistance, 284
Epworth Sleepiness Scale, 222
equal carryover, 105
equivalence, 135–137, See non-
inferiority
equivalence trials, 135, See non-
inferiority trials
eszopiclone (ESZ), 300
ethical criteria, 187
ethical study design, 175
ethics research
justice, 181
EU clinical trials, 326
European Medicines Agency, 16
evaluable subjects analysis, 65
Expanded Disability Status Scale
(EDSS), 21
experimental autoimmune
encephalomyelitis (EAE), 257
experimental autoimmune
encephalomyelitis (EAE) model
limitations, 258
exploratory outcomes, 29

fair market value compensation, 352
false claim billing, 358
False Claims Act, 357–358
violations, 358
family-wise error rate, 150–151
FCPA, 359
FDA, 3
FDA Adverse Event Reporting System,
162
FDA MedWatch program, 161
Federal Anti-Kickback Statute.
See Anti-Kickback Statute
Federal Drug Agency, 5
Federal Food, Drug, and Cosmetic Act
Medical Device Amendments of
1976, 206–207
Federal Regulations 21 Code, 200
felbamate, 164
financial disclosure regulations, 354
financial disclosure requirement, 354
fingolimod, 266
First Subject First Visit (FSFV), 320

flexible design methods, 152
focal dystonia, 5
Food and Drug Administration
Modernization Act (FDAMA),
197
Food, Drug, and Cosmetic Act (the
Act), 197
Foreign Corrupt Practices Act.
See FCPA
fully sequential designs, 155
funding mechanisms, 98
funding research (US), 3
futility analysis, 81, 154
futility assessment, 97
futility design, 78, 80–81, 248
criterion of superiority, 79
neuroprotective agents, 78
sample size, 82
single-arm design, 79, 84
two-arm design, 79
futility design hypotheses, 79
futility outcome, 81
sensitivity, 80
specificity, 80
type I error, 80
type II error, 80
futility design pitfalls, 83
historical control data, 84
sample size, 83

G93A SOD1, 273
gadolinium-enhancing
lesions, 257
Gaucher's disease, 5
GCP inspections, 343–344
General Practitioner Research
Database, 167
generalized onset seizures, 286
genomics studies, 75
Glasgow Outcome Scale, 59
global outcome measures, 232
global statistics, 246
GMP, 340
Good Clinical Practice
(GCP), 159
Good Manufacturing Practice (GMP).
See GMP
group sequential adaptive
randomization design, 97
group sequential methods, 151
development, 154

hazard function, 37
hazard ratio, 38
Health Canada, 347
health-related quality-of-life
(HR-QOL) scales, 263
hemorrhagic transformation, 244
HESDE, 142
historical controls, 201, 248

historical evidence of sensitivity
to drug effects (HESDE).
See HESDE
human drug development, 21
human drug exposures, 22
human medical research, 174
policies, codes and regulations, 174
regulations, 175
welfare of volunteers, 174
human pharmacokinetics, 10
human pharmacology, 10
human research ethics, 173, 175
human research risk, 173
human volunteer studies, 15
Humanitarian Device Exemption
(HDE), 210–211
Humanitarian Use Device (HUD), 210
Huntington's disease, 346
hypotheses, 31
'one sided' alternative hypothesis, 31
null hypothesis, 31
two sided alternative hypothesis, 31
hypothesis of non-inferiority, 144
hypothesis tests, 150

ICH Guideline E3, 141
IDE application, 211
IDE exempt studies, 212
IDE study, 211
IHAST, 53–54
imaging biomarkers, 75
imiglucerase (Cerezyme), 5
IMP formulation, 323
IMP quantities, 323
IMP quantity forecasting, 323
income of countries, 1
infarction, 243
informed consent, 187, 188, 194
capacity assessment, 190
decision-making capacity, 190
emergency exceptions, 253
probability statements, 189
subject understanding, 189
therapeutic motivation, 194
informed consent forms, 188
insomnia, 295
associated conditions, 297
biomarkers, 299
diagnosis criteria, 304
diary data, 302
intervention goals, 297
neural pathways, 296
perpetuating factors, 295
pharmacologic agents, 297
precipitating factors, 295
sleep diaries, 298
treatment efficacy, 302
insomnia clinical trials, 297, 299
blinding, 302
CBT trials, 300

comparative effectiveness trials, 305
comparative efficacy trial, 301
controls, 304
dual approach, 301
duration of treatment, 304
efficacy, 303
efficacy and safety, 302
frequency of assessments, 304
hypnotic trials, 305
improvement indicators, 302
menopausal women, 297
neurocognitive tests, 302
psychological interventions, 300
questionnaires, 298
recruitment, 303
retention, 304
safety outcomes, 305
sample size, 302
institutional review board (IRB), 188
intention to treat (ITT), 46–47
intent-to-treat (ITT)
    principle, 136
    strategy, 141
Interactive Response Technology (IRT). *See* IRT
interferon β, 259–260
interim analysis, 49, 151, 157, 250
    sample size, 158
internal pilot designs, 95
International Committee on Harmonisation Guidelines, 14
International Conference on Harmonization (ICH), 163
intra-class correlation, 103
Intraoperative Hypothermia for Aneurysm Surgery Trial (IHAST) 53
intra-parenchymal delivery, 23
investigational device exemptions (IDE), 211
investigational medicinal products (IMP), 317
Investigational Product (IP). *See* clinical supplies
investigational research plan, 211
IP
    accountability, reconciliation and destruction, 325
    cradle-to-grave tracking, 325
    storage, 325
    transportation, 325
IRB notifications, 346
IRT, 324
ischemia, 242
ischemia trials, 243
    superiority, 250
ITT strategy, 144
IV rt-PA pilot study, 247

Kaplan-Meier curve, 37

large simple trial, 170
    ibuprofen safety, 170–171
last observation carried forward (LOCF), 48, 67
Last Subject Last Visit (LSLV), 320
late exploratory (phase II) trials, 93
Latin square design, 110
L-DOPA, 23
Lennox-Gastaut Syndrome, 286, 290
levetiracetam, 285
Levin-Robbins-Leu (LRL) sequential selection procedures, 86–87
levodopa, 217–218, 222
    melanomas, 222
life expectancy, 1
likelihood-based approach, 111
linomide, 266
lipophilic compounds, 23
log-rank test, 38
Long-term disability trials, 221
LRL. *See* Levin-Robbins-Leu (LRL) sequential selection procedures

Mainland-Gart's approach, 107
manual muscle testing (MMT), 276
marginal approach, 107
masking, 249, *See* blinding
material corporate events, 346
maximum tolerated dose (MTD), 92
Mechanical Embolus Removal in Cerebral Ischemia (MERCI) trials, 248
MedDRA dictionary, 326
medical coding system, 326
medical devices, 206
    legally marketed device, 209
    premarket approval, 210
    regulatory framework, 207
    substantial equivalence, 209
Medical Devices Advisory Committee, 213
Medical Devices Dispute Resolution Panel, 213
medical devices premarket notification, 209
metabolomic approaches, 75
microdialysis, 24
middle phase studies, 250
mild cognitive impairment (MCI), 190, 228
minorities enrollment material, 342
missing at random (MAR), 66
missing completely at random (MCAR), 66
missing data, 66
missing data mechanism, 111
    missing at random (MAR), 111

missing completely at random (MCAR), 111
    not missing at random (NMAR), 111
missing not at random (MNAR), 66
mitoxantrone, 266
mixed carryover effect,, 109
mixed effects model, 107
mixed model repeated measures, 123
MMT, 276
model-based development, 11
modified Rankin scale, 245–246
monotonic spending function, 153
mortality, 137
MRI, 76
MRI measure
    brain atrophy, 263, 264
MS Functional Composite (MSFC), 262
MS trials
    adaptive designs, 269
MTD. *See* maximum tolerated dose
multi-center trial, 252
multiple ascending dose studies, 10
multiple dose studies, 10
multiple hypothesis testing, 144
multiple imputation, 67, 123
multiple sclerosis (MS), 5, 76, 178, 257
    adverse events, 265
    anti-inflammatory therapy, 258
    disease free, 268
    disease-modifying therapy, 258
    drug development, 258
    early treatment, 260
    gray matter pathology, 258
    hypotheses, 258
    multiple trials, 266
    relapse and treatment, 267
    severity drift, 266
    subtypes, 259
    symptom-based therapies, 258
    MRI measures, 264
    MRI studies, 263
multiple sclerosis trials
    enrollment, 260
    entrance criteria, 260
    informative enrollment, 260, 262
    MRI outcome measures, 268
    recruitment, 266
multiplicity, 151, 158

N of 1 trials, 110
natalalizumab, 5, 265
National Commission for the Protection of Human Subjects of Biomedical and Behavioral Research, 174
National Institutes of Health, 17
National Multiple Sclerosis Society policies, 178

NDLM, 96
NET-PD futility studies, 81, 84
  additive two-arm design, 82
  control group, 81
  placebo parameter, 82
  single-arm study, 81
  two-arm design, 82
NET-PD network, 78
neuritic plaques, 227
neurofibrillary tangles, 227–228
neuroimaging, 11
neuroinflammation, 258
neurointerventional devices, 206
neurological device market, 206
Neurological Devices Advisory Panel,
    213
neurological worsening, 244
neuropathic pain, 19
neuroprotection, 242, 268
Neuropsychiatric Inventory
    (NPI), 233
Neuropsychological Test Battery
    (NTB), 231
neuropsychological testing, 263
Neuro-QOL projects, 69
neurostimulation de
  vices, 206
neurotherapeutics, challenges, 5
neurotrophic factor development, 20
New Drug Applications (NDA), 16
NIH Anticonvulsant Screening
    Program, 285
NIH Biomarkers Definitions Working
    Group, 71
NIH Toolbox, 69
NINDS rt-PA acute stroke study, 248
NINDS rt-PA trial, 246
no-adverse effect level (NOAEL), 10
non-inferiority, 142, 250
non-inferiority margin, 122, 138, 169
non-inferiority trials, 169–170
  assay sensitivity, 142–143
  choice of margin, 141–142
  patient noncompliance, 141
  sample size, 140
non-invasive imaging techniques, 24
non-significant risk device
  studies, 211
non-validated CNS interventions, 183
no-pharmacologic effect dose
    (NOPED), 10
normal distribution, 55
novel therapeutic, 19
nuisance parameters, 94, 103–105
null hypothesis, 46, 60
Numeric Pain Rating Scale, 12
Nuremberg Code, 174, 176

observational epidemiological studies,
    170

retrospective cohort study, 166
observational epidemiological study,
    165
  case control studies, 167
  cohort study, 165
  cohort study design, 166
  cohort study restrictions, 166
  confounding, 165
  prospective cohort studies, 166
  restrospective cohort design, 166
observational epidemiologic study
    designs
  case-control studies, 165
  cohort studies, 165
observational epidemiologic study
  case-control study, 168
  nested case-control, 167
ocular coherence tomography (OCT),
    264
open label dose escalation studies, 247
Open Report, 148
open-label dose-escalation studies,
    247
open-label safety extension studies, 15
ordinal outcome scales
  dichotomous treatment, 246
ordinal outcomes scales
  trichotomous treatment, 246
orphan diseases, 200
orphan drug approval, 200
orphan drug effectiveness, 200
orphan drugs, 5
outcome measures, 69, 76
outcome-adaptive dose-finding
    design, 97

paradoxical insomnia, 298
parallel group designs, 114
Parkinson's disease, 1, 19, 101, 107,
    113–114, 163, 179, 215
  causes, 215
  comparative effectiveness trials, 222
  confirmatory (phase III) clinical
    trials, 220
  disability, 219
  early trials, 217
  impulse control disorders, 222
  long term disability trials, 221–222
  medication, 168
  motor complications, 218, 219
  motor features, 215
  neuropathology, 215
  non-motor features, 216
  off time, 218
  phase II clinical trials, 220
  pilot trials, 221
  suicide, 222
Parkinson's disease modification, 221
  clinical trial, 221
  patient population, 223

statistical analysis, 221
Parkinson's disease progression,
    219–220, 223
  clinical trials, 220
  monitoring devices, 219
  survival endpoint, 219
Parkinson's disease trials, 216, 218
  disease progression modification,
    219
  missing data, 223
  outcome measures, 219
partial onset seizures, 286
passive spontaneous reporting system,
    162
patient follow-up, 137
patient non-compliance, 141
patient population, 14
patient reported outcome (PRO), 12,
    69
patient selection, 11, 249
Pediatric Research Equity Act (PREA),
    199
pediatric studies, 199–200
pediatric study safety data, 199
pediatric written requests (PWRs), 200
pediatric written responses, 200
penumbral salvage, 243
per subject fee (PSF), 318
per-protocol analysis, 141, 144
pervasive developmental disorder, 101
PET imaging studies, 75
pharmaceutical promotion, 358
Pharmaceutical Research and
    Manufacturers of America
    (PhRMA). See PhRMA
pharmacodynamic marker, 25
pharmacodynamic modeling, 11
pharmacodynamic studies, 264
pharmacokinetic modelling, 11
pharmacologic agents, 113
pharmacologic properties, 9
phase I trial, 177
phase 1 trial design objectives, 177
phase 1 trial risks, 177
phase I clinical trials, 74, 264
  approaches, 92
phase II clinical trials, 74, 264
phase III clinical trials, 264
PhRMA adaptive dose ranging studies
    working group, 93
PhRMA Code, 355
PhRMA principles, 355
Physicians Withdrawal Checklist, 12
Pittsburgh Imaging agent B (PIB), 11
placebo control trial ethics, 178
placebo controls, 178
  principles of justice, 181
placebo group, 202
placebo response
  rates, 12

placebo responses, 179
placebo-to-match (PTM). *See* PTM
polysomnography (PSG), 298–299, 303
population, 53, 54
population distribution, 54–56
population parameters, 54
population standard deviation, 57
positron emission tomography (PET), 11, 75
post-market drug safety, 160–161
pre-approval drug safety assessment, 160
PRECISION trial, 170
preclinical experiments, 176
    researcher responsibility, 177
pre-IDE process, 212
pre-IDE submission, 213
premarket approval (PMA), 214
primary insomnia, 295
primary outcome, 29
primary progressive multiple sclerosis (PPMS), 257, 260
principal investigator (PI), 311
principle of responsiveness, 181
PROACT I, 243
progressive multifocal leukoencephalopathy (PML), 265
project manager (PM), 309
proteomics, 75
protocol feasibility, 338
PROUD trial, 116, 118
pseudo-placebo withdrawal study, 290
PTM, 322
public Advisory Committee meetings, 16
Public Health Service Act, 197
putative disease related pathways, 21
p-value, 65

QALS trial, 85
quality control monitoring, 46
Quality of Life-AD (QOL-AD), 234

radio-labeled receptor ligands, 24
random effects models, 107
random error, 42, 44, 45, 50
randomization, 65, 136
randomization allocation ratio, 249
randomized clinical trial, 31, 135
randomized controlled stroke trials, 247
randomized controlled therapeutic trials, 147
randomized controlled trial, 136, 178
randomized start trials, 128, 204
randomized withdrawal trials, 204
    outcome measure, 202
rapid endpoint, 85
recanalization, 242, 243

recruitment and retention plan, 341
recruitment and retention plans, 342
regression models, 67
regulatory reporting requirements, 347
relative risk. *See* hazard ratio
remyelination strategies, 258
Request for Proposal (RFP), 312
research ethics, 174
    fair research design, 181
    justice, 181
    principles, 175
research participants, 3
Resource Utilization in Dementia (RUD) scale, 233
response adaptive design, 109
response-adaptive randomization, 94
reverse multiplicity problem, 144
reverse placebo effect, 131
rhabdomyolysis, 166
riluzole, 280
routine trial closure, 341, 345
RRMS trials
    placebo-controlled trials, 265
    relapse number, 262
rt-PA treatment, 251

safe harbor rules, 357
safety and tolerability issues, 12, 15
safety and tolerability profile, 14
safety endpoints, 69
safety of research participants, 356
safety or tolerability issues, 11
safety pharmacology studies, 9
safety studies, 155
sample mean, 52
sample size, 33, 94, 250
sample size adjustment, 251
sample size re-estimation, 15
statistical analysis plan, 327
schizophrenia, 19
secondary outcomes, 29
secondary progressive MS (SPMS), 257
Securities Exchange Act of 1934, 346
seizure diary, 286–287
seizure prophylaxis, 6
seizures, 284
selection design, 78
selection of endpoints, 76
selection procedures, 84–86
    indifference zone approach, 85
    sequential selection procedures, 85
sensitivity analyses, 48
sequential monitoring, 94
serious adverse events (SAEs), 161, 244
serotoninergic effects, 11
serotonin-norepinephrine reuptake inhibitors, 11

severe impairment battery (SIB), 232
sham control studies, 223
sham surgical approach, 43, 218
sham surgical controls, 179, 223
    conditions of use, 179, 180
    ethical critique, 179
    intervention studies, 179
shift analysis, 246, 247
sICH, 250
significance level, 62, 151
significant risk device, 211
simple carryover, 110
simple random sample, 54
single ascending dose studies, 9
single dose studies, 10
single imputation, 67
single photon emission computerized tomography (SPECT), 75
single treatment arm studies, 248
site coordinator, 312
site manager (SM), 311
Site Monitoring Visit (SMV), 340
sliding dichotomy analysis, 246
SMV, 341
societal benefit, 3
solanezumab, 25
spending functions, 153
SPORTIF III trial, 138, 141–142
standard deviation, 53
standard of care (SOC) costs, 318
state biomarker, 73
statistical software, 155, 157
    EAST, 157
    ldBounds package, 155
    R-project, 155
    SAS, 156
statistics, 52–53
step-forward randomization, 252, 252
stopping boundaries, 152, 155, 157
    Haybittle-Peto method, 152
    O'Brien and Fleming method, 152–154
    Pocock method, 152, 154
stratification factors, 48
stroke prevention, 6
stroke prevention trials, 253
Stroke Prevention using Oral Thrombin Inhibitor in Atrial Fibrillation (SPORTIF) III trial. *See* Sportif III trial
Stroke Therapy Academic Industry Roundtable (STAIR) recommendations, 242
Stroke–Acute Ischemic NXY Treatment II (SAINT II) trial, 246
stroke-specific outcome measures, 245
structural imaging, 76
Student's *t*-distribution, 55

study forms, 46
substantial evidence of effectiveness, 197
   clinical trials, 200–201
   single trial elements, 198
   single trials, 198
sufficient washout periods, 107
Sunshine Act, 353
superiority, 250
superiority to placebo, 142
superiority trial, 137
   patient noncompliance, 140
   sample size, 140
surrogate consent, 191
surrogate endpoint, 71
surrogate markers, 198, 203
   clinical outcomes, 198, 199
   studies, 198
surrogate outcome measures, 71
symptomatic and disease-modifying effects, 113
symptomatic intracranial hemorrhage (sICH), 244

T2 hyperintense lesions, 263
Tacrine Consortium study, 132
tau, 227
TEMPO trial, 116
test of significance, 32
therapeutic development, 19
therapeutic development programs, 71
therapeutic misconception (TM), 193

time to event trial, 290
tissue plasminogen activator, 97
TNK trial, 251
TOAST (III) trial, 147, 150
   data monitoring committee, 149
tolerability profile, 10
tolerable dose range, 10
trait biomarker, 73
treatment approval, 203
treatment by period interaction, 104
trial monitoring, 159
trial termination, 159
Tufts quantitative neuromuscular examination (TQNE), 276
two-arm non-inferiority trial
   sample size, 140
two-period design, 114, 221
   ADAGIO trial, 120
   additional treatment, 121
   delayed start design, 116, 118
   eligibility criteria, 120
   evaluation, 121
   limitations, 124–125
   missing data, 123
   multiple statistical testing, 122
   period duration, 120
   primary analyses, 121–123
   PROUD, 120
   sample size, 124
   withdrawal design, 115, 116
two-stage adaptive dose-ranging design, 96

type I error, 61, 150, 151
type II error, 61

UK Bribery Act, 359
unblinding, 132
unequal carryover, 106
unexpected adverse drug events, 161
Unified Parkinson's Disease Rating Scale (UPDRS), 216, 219
United States drug safety system, 161
unvalidated surrogate markers, 198
US Physician Payments Sunshine Act (Sunshine Act), 353

variability, 53
variance, 53
virtual biotechnology firms, 5

warfarin, 6
washout periods, 132
Wilcoxon-rank sum test, 106
women and minority participation, 342

ximelagatran, 138, 141

zolpidem, 301

α spending function, 153, 154